ORGANIC SPECTROSCOPY

(NMR, IR, Mass and UV)

ORGANIC SPECTROSCOPY
(NMR, IR, Mass and UV)

Dr. S.K. Dewan
MSc (Gold Medalist) PhD (Edinburgh)
Professor of Organic Chemistry
Deptt. of Chemistry, M.D. University, Rohtak (Haryana), India
Ex-Postdoctoral Research Fellow, University of Wales, UK
Ex-Research Scientist, Ranbaxy Research Labs, Delhi
Ex-Pool Officer, National Chemistry Laboratory, Pune

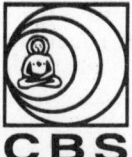

CBS

CBS Publishers & Distributors Pvt. Ltd.

New Delhi • Bengaluru • Chennai • Kochi • Kolkata • Mumbai
Hyderabad • Uttarakhand • Nagpur • Patna • Pune • Jharkhand

ISBN: 978-81-239-1906-5

First Edition: 2010
Reprint: 2012, 2017, 2019, 2020

Published by **Satish Kumar Jain** and produced by **Varun Jain** for
CBS Publishers & Distributors Pvt. Ltd.,
4819/XI Prahlad Street, 24 Ansari Road, Daryaganj, New Delhi - 110002
delhi@cbspd.com, cbspubs@airtelmail.in • www.cbspd.com
Ph.: 23289259, 23266861, 23266867 • Fax: 011-23243014

Corporate Office: 204 FIE, Industrial Area, Patparganj, Delhi - 110 092
Ph: 49344934 • Fax: 011-49344935
E-mail: publishing@cbspd.com • publicity@cbspd.com

Branches:
• *Bengaluru:* 2975, 17th Cross, K.R. Road, Bansankari 2nd Stage,
  Bengaluru - 70 • Ph: +91-80-26771678/79 • Fax: +91-80-26771680
  E-mail: cbsbng@gmail.com, bangalore@cbspd.com
• *Chennai:* No. 7, Subbaraya Street, Shenoy Nagar, Chennai - 600030
  Ph: +91-44-26681266, 26680620 • Fax: +91-44-42032115
  E-mail: chennai@cbspd.com
• *Kochi:* Ashana House, 39/1904, A.M. Thomas Road, Valanjambalam,
  Ernakulum, Kochi • Ph: +91-484-4059061-65
  Fax: +91-484-4059065 • E-mail: cochin@cbspd.com
• *Kolkata:* 6-B, Ground Floor, Rameshwar Shaw Road, Kolkata - 700014
  Ph: +91-33-22891126/7/8 • E-mail: kolkata@cbspd.com
• *Mumbai:* 83-C, Dr. E. Moses Road, Worli, Mumbai - 400018
  Ph: +91-9833017933, 022-24902340/41 • E-mail: mumbai@cbspd.com

Representatives:
• Hyderabad: 0-9885175004   • Nagpur: 0-9021734563
• Patna: 0-9334159340   • Pune: 0-9623451994
• Jharkhand: 0-9811541605   • Uttarakhand: 0-9716462459

Printed at:
J.S. Offset Printers, Delhi (India)

To
STUDENTS AND TEACHERS
of
**Chemical Sciences, Biochemistry,
Biophysics, Biotechnology**
and
Pharmaceutical Sciences

Once you have carefully chosen a goal to contribute to the society, go for it wholeheartedly. Don't be afraid, no mountain is too big to climb even if you climb at your own pace. Along the path though, there may be sorrows and pain, but there also lies a great happiness. Anytime, you learn and create something new, for others to learn and enjoy, you have progressed well. That will bring you accomplishment, inner peace and self growth as you have attempted to make other's life easy and happy. You feel contented as you have contributed your mite to the global society to which you owe too much to repay. Always envision today as a gift... tomorrow as another and add a meaningful page to the diary of each new day, making the society happy and wise. A person's life is too short whereas a society's life is long, man is mortal but society is immortal as generations after generations keep coming.

S.K. Dewan

Preface

The book in your hands is a consequence of repeated requests made to me over the years by many upper level undergraduate, graduate and post-graduate students and postdocs doing organic chemistry, inorganic chemistry, pharmacy (pharmaceutical sciences, B. Pharma and M. Pharma.), bio-chemistry, bio-technology and bio-physics as well as some teachers. In fact, some of these students had tears in their eyes while making the request so that I was left with no option but to say yes to their demand. I am grateful to Almighty for having bestowed upon me the quality to help those who so require. I ardently believe that one must also make attempts to contribute towards upliftment of the global society without whose shelter one could not survive. In fact, I feel that it is the moral duty of a person to share one's knowledge and skills with the society otherwise these meet their end with the demise of the person, a stark reality of life – everyone who gets birth has got to leave this world for ever, one day or the other, I believe that, advancement in science should aim at aiding the global society in all possible ways, particularly from the point of view of health (consider, for example, the development of NMR into MRI). This book has been written with that aim in mind. Science progresses bit by bit, it is not one man's job. Years of sincere thinking and hardwork carried out by a large number of persons over so many years gives birth to new scientific ideas, fosters and promotes these. I am hopeful this book will succeed in that direction. I feel satisfied in that through this mission I have tried my maximum to excite, inspire and challenge the readers about the topics discussed and science, in general. Of particular concern are the thought-provoking questions in the Intext Exercise boxes within each Chapter that I have framed myself. The topics have been introduced, explained and then expanded, a step at a time to the advanced level in a didactic approach.

As the best way to learn thoroughly any subject is to solve the relevant problems, the text has hundreds covering a vaste range from simple to difficult ones. At the same time, I have tried not to extend their number of a level that would prove counter-productive, keeping in view the stark reality that excess of everything is bad. The idea is to attract, rather than distract or repel the readers. Suggestions are always welcome. Kindly take time out to write to me at the following address:

sharwankumardewan@yahoo.com and sharwandewan@rediff.com.

Sharwan K. Dewan
Rohtak

Acknowledgements

I am sincerely indebted to all those who I have met in my life, here in India and in the U.K., (where I stayed put for over half-a-decade) for however short a duration as I believe, I have always learnt positively from their attitude which in my view is necessary for doing positive task like writing of a textbook such as this, now in your hands. I am particularly indebted to my teachers who taught me at any levels for nursery up to the Ph.D. level. I am grateful to stalwarts of science who publish and thus serite science and society — American Chemical Society, Royal Society of Chemistry, Angew Chem. Int. Ed., Engl., Wiley, Elsevier, Aldrich, Sadtler, Varian, JEOL, Spectral Database for Organic Compounds, S.D.B.S. etc. Perhaps Chemical Sciences would not have progressed so rapidly to the extent we find them today if these stalwarts were not to come to its aid.

Several persons have helped me in bringing out this edition of the book and I am highly thankful to each one of them individually. I am also thankful to Mr. Satish Kumar Jain and Mr. Vinod Kumar Jain of CBS Publishers & Distributors Pvt. Ltd., Delhi, for its publication in a short time.

Suggestions and comments for its improvement are welcome.

Sharwan K. Dewan

Contents

Basis of ID-NMR Spectroscopy

1.1. MAGNETIC PROPERTIES OF ATOMIC NUCLEI AND OLD CONCEPT OF NMR

The atomic nuclei like protons having non-zero radii act as microscopic magnets because they are charged and spinning. Therefore, they are associated with a magnetic moment, μ of their own as shown in Fig. 1.1.

Atomic nuclei (which act as microscopic magnets) when placed in an externally applied magnetic field, B_0, experience a couple or torque and are forced to align themselves with B_0 just as a compass needle does in the earth's magnetic field as shown in Fig. 1.2. However, it should be noted that the magnetic moment of a spinning nucleus does not orient itself with the direction of the applied field B_0, *however strong the field*, unlike a non-spinning bar magnet. Further, the nucleus can be considered just analogous to a top i.e. it behaves as a spinning top. As a top (or a gyroscope) starts precessing (wobling) under the earth's gravitational field, in a similar manner, the spinning nuclei start precessing around the applied magnetic field B_0 rather than rotating as they possess angular momentum (Fig. 1.2). The frequency with which the nuclei

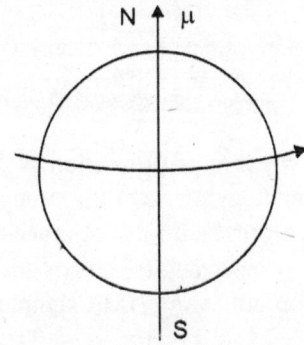

Fig. 1.1. The spinning nucleus behaving as a tiny magnet.

precess is called Larmor frequency ν_0, which is related to gyromagnetic ratio γ and B_0 as shown in equation 1.1 whereby, γ represents the ratio of the nuclear magnetic moment, μ to the nuclear angular momentum ($\gamma = \mu/L$).

$$\nu_0 = \gamma \frac{B_0}{2\pi} \qquad ....(eq.\ 1.1)$$

Thus, for a proton having $\gamma = 2.675 \times 10^8 \ T^{-1} \ rad \ s^{-1}$ placed in a magnetic field of 2.35 T, the Larmor precession frequency ν_0 will be :

$$v_0 = \frac{2.675 \times 10^8 \times 2.35 \times 7}{2 \times 22}$$

$$= 1.000 \times 10^8 \text{ Hz} = 100 \text{ MHz}$$

Hence, the precession rate of protons about B_0 along z axis is about 100 MHz (plus or minus a few hundred Hz). In fact, this is the origin of the term 100 MHz spectrometer for a spectrometer built with a 2.35 T magnetic field strength i.e. the strength of the NMR instrument.

The Larmor Precession Frequency v_0, will be different for different nuclei even at the same field strength B_0. This is because they differ in their nuclear strength, the y. Thus, for ^{13}C nucleus γ = 1/4th of that of

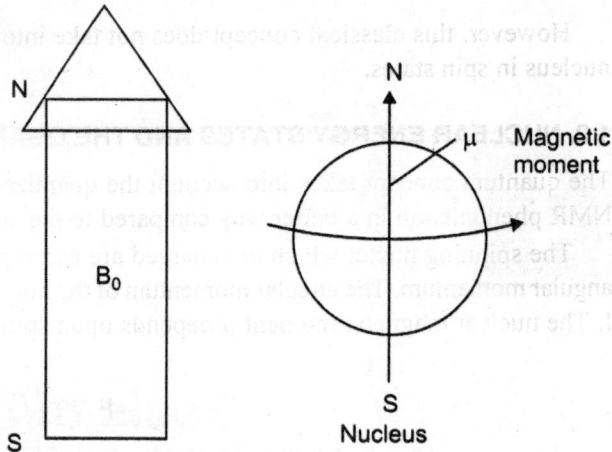

Fig. 1.2. This figure shows a nucleus being aligned with the applied field.

proton. Therefore, γ for ^{13}C at 2.35 T will be 1/4th of that of proton i.e. 100 MHz ÷ 4 = 25 MHz.

γ for deuterium (D or ^2H) is 1//7th of total of ^1H, and y for nitrogen −15 (^{15}N) is 1/10th of that of ^1H· Accordingly, they will require proportionate frequencies.

Obviously, greater the strength of applied field B_0, greater the Larmor precession frequency or the rate of the precession.

The rate of precession has been found to be millions of rotations per second and lies in the radio frequency range of tens or hundreds of megahertz (MHz). It is given by :

$$\omega_0 = 2 \text{ M } v_0 = y.B_0$$

so, the rate of precession is dependent upon the strength of the applied field, B_0 as well as on the magnetogyroratio or the strength of the nuclear magnet y. As different nuclei have different values of y, therefore, their rates of precession about a constant magnetic field Bo will be different.

When a radiofrequency equal to the Larmor precession frequency V_0 is applied, the nucleus resonates and produces an NMR signal (Fig. 1.3).

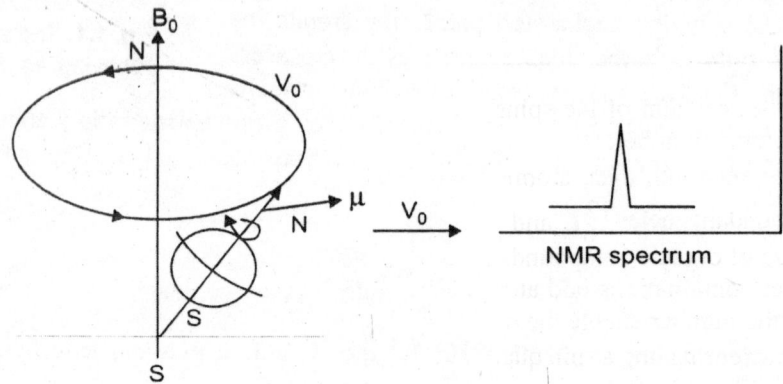

Fig. 1.3. The precessing nucleus under the influence of external applied field, B_0.

However, this classical concept does not take into account the quantum concept of behaviour of a nucleus in spin states.

1.2 NUCLEAR ENERGY STATES AND THE QUANTUM CONCEPT OF NMR

The quantum concept takes into account the quantized spin states of the nuclei and thus explains the NMR phenomenon in a better way compared to the earlier described classical model.

The spinning nuclei which are charged are associated with a magnetic moment, μ and a quantized angular momentum. The angular momentum of the nuclei is determined by nuclear spin quantum number, I. The nuclear magnetic moment μ depends upon spin number I as shown in the following equation:

$$\mu = \gamma \cdot I \cdot \frac{h}{2\pi}$$

where γ is called the magnetogyro ratio. It is an inherent property of the nucleus. μ is expressed in Ampere metre^2, (B_0 is expressed in Tesla in S.I. units such that 1 Tesla = 10^4 Gauss), h is the Planck's constant.

The spin quantum number I is constant for a nucleus and can have values such as 0, $\frac{1}{2}$, $\frac{3}{2}$, $\frac{5}{2}$, 3, $\frac{7}{2}$ etc. i.e. integrats or half-integrals, in general as shown in Table 1.1 and Table 1.2.

Table 1.1. Some elements with spin quantum number

Spin quantum numbers	Elements
0	^{12}C, ^{16}O, ^{32}S, ^{34}S
$\frac{1}{2}$	^{1}H, ^{13}C, ^{15}N, ^{19}F, ^{28}Si, ^{31}P, ^{77}Se, ^{103}Rh, ^{195}Pt
1	D, ^{14}N
$\frac{3}{2}$	^{11}B, ^{33}S, ^{35}Cl, ^{37}Cl, ^{79}Br, ^{81}Br
$\frac{5}{2}$	^{17}O, ^{27}Al, ^{127}I
3	^{10}B

The spin I is the resultant of the spins of the protons and neutrons. It can be obtained from the atomic mass and atomic number:

In general, elements with even atomic number and even atomic mass have zero spin. Example include the most abundant nuclei $^{12}_{6}C$ and $^{18}_{8}O$ (this is a good news indeed as this leads to simplification of the NMR spectra of organic compounds otherwise the spectra could be very complicated as we will see later). All other combinations-odd atomic mass and odd or even atomic number and even atomic mass and odd atomic number enable the nuclei to possess a spin other than zero.

Now, when a nucleus having a spin quantum number I, other than zero is placed in an external field, Bo, then it can assume $2I + I$ spin states. Thus an element with a I equal to $\frac{1}{2}$, can assume $\left(2 \times \frac{1}{2} + I \right)$

Table. 1.2. Magnetic properties of some important nuclei

Isotope	Natural abundance (%)	Spin (I)	$\gamma \times 10^{-7}$ (rad $T^{-1}s^{-1}$)
^1H	99.98	1/2	26.7519
^2D	0.016	1	4.106
^{10}B	18.83	3	2.875
^{11}B	81.17	3/2	8.583
^{12}C	98.89	0	–
^{13}C	1.11	1/2	6.726
^{14}N	99.63	1	1.933
^{15}N	0.037	1/2	– 2.711
^{16}O	99.76	0	–
^{17}O	0.037	5/2	– 3.627
^{19}F	100	1/2	25.167
^{27}Al	100	5/2	6.971
^{28}Si	92.28	0	–
^{29}Si	4.67	1/2	– 5.314
^{31}P	100	1/2	10.829
^{32}S	95.06	0	–
^{33}S	0.74	3/2	2.052
^{77}Se	7.58	1/2	5.101
^{195}Pt	33.7	1/2	5.752

two spin states. Thus, hydrogen can adopt two spin states $+\frac{1}{2}$ and $-\frac{1}{2}$ as shown in Fig. 1.4. $+\frac{1}{2}$ spin state is aligned with Bo at an angle of 45° from the $+z$ axis (Fig. 1.5) while the $-\frac{1}{2}$ spin state is aligned at an angle of 45° with respect to Bo, the applied magnetic field (Fig. 1.6) from the $-z$ axis.

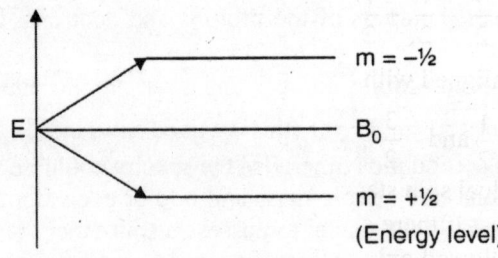

Fig. 1.4. Two spin states (energy levels) of a nucleus with $I = \frac{1}{2}$ in an applied magnetic field, Bo (such as D, ^{14}N).

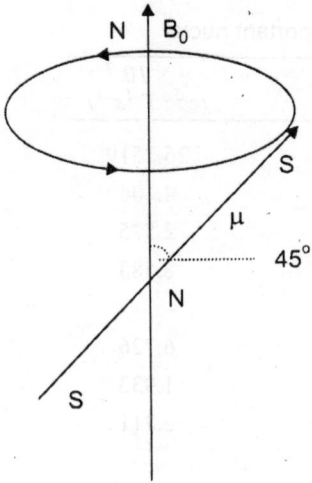

Fig. 1.5. α-spin state aligned at 54.7° w.r. to B_0 from the z axis.

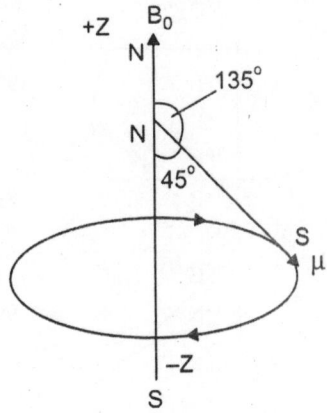

Fig. 1.6. β-spin state aligned at 135° w.r. to Bo.

Intext Exercises

1. What are the orientations of spin in deuterium?
   Hint : See Fig. 1.7.
2. What are the orientations of B-11?
   Hint : See Fig. 1.9.

Elements with I equal to 1 (such as D, ^{14}N) can have (2 × 1 + I) three spin states as shown in Fig. 1.6, i.e. −1, 0 and +1 which are respectively aligned w.r. to B_0 at 45°, 90° and 135° as shown in Fig. 1.7.

For an element with $I = \dfrac{3}{2}$ (such as ^{11}B, ^{35}Cl,

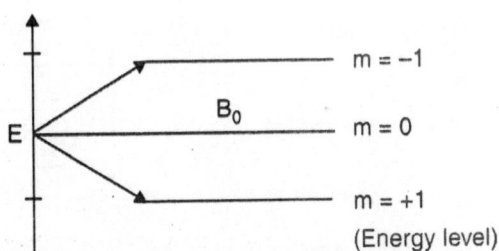

Fig. 1.7. Thres spin states (energy levels) of a nucleus with $I = I$ in an applied magnetic field, B_0. Examples D, 11B, 37Cl, 79Br, 81Br.

^{37}Cl, ^{79}Br, ^{81}Br etc.) four spin states (2 × 3 + I) are possible (see Fig. 1.9) i.e. $-\dfrac{3}{2}, -\dfrac{1}{2}, +\dfrac{1}{2}, +\dfrac{3}{2}$. Two spin states $+\dfrac{1}{2}$ and $+\dfrac{3}{2}$ are aligned with the applied field, while the other two, $-\dfrac{1}{2}$ and $-\dfrac{3}{2}$ are opposed to the applied field.

In conclusion, the individual spin states follow the order +1, (I − 1)....(−1 +1), −I. It should be noted that **selection rules** tell us that if there are more than two spin-states (orientations) as per the formula (2I + I), the transitions are allowed only between the adjacent spin states as the energy difference, ΔE between any two states is constant. So the selection rule for transitions permit that m_I can only change by one unit. In other words, $\Delta m_I = \pm 1$.

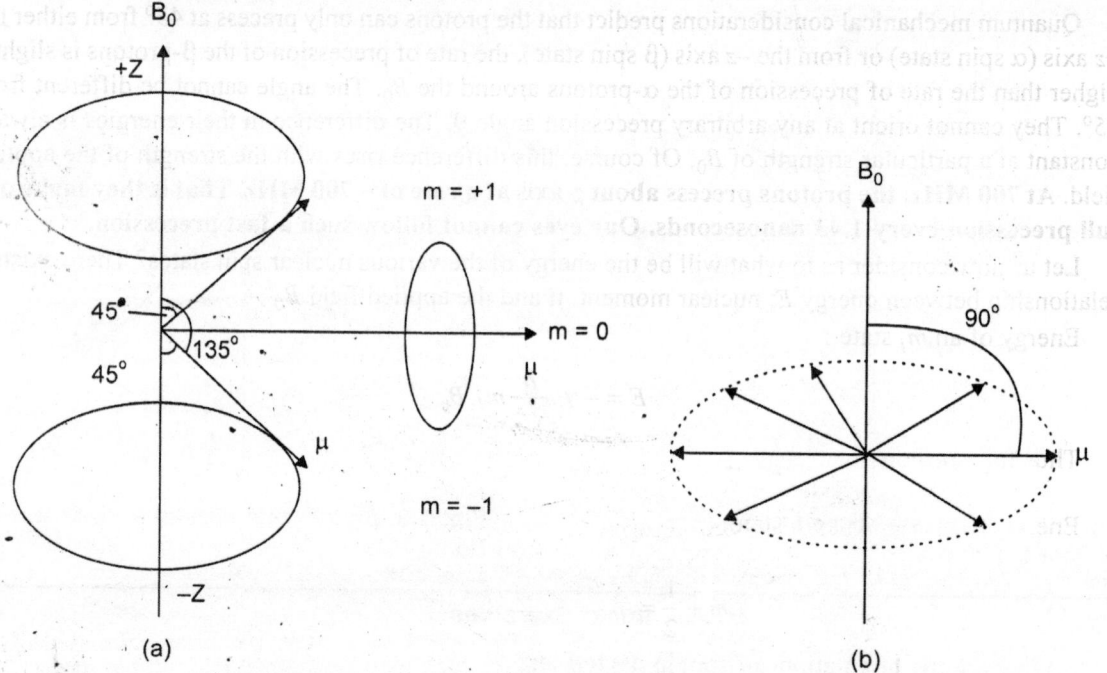

Fig. 1.8. (a) The three spin states of a nucleus with $I = 1$, (b) the spin state with $m = 0$.

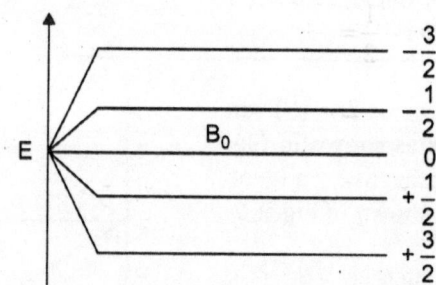

Fig. 1.9. One spin state of a nucleus with $I = \dfrac{3}{2}$ in an applied magnetic field B_0.

1.3 ENERGY OF SPIN STATES

For the sake of convenience, we shall study the case of proton (or the hydrogen). As a proton (or the hydrogen). As a proton has $I = \dfrac{1}{2}$, it can adopt two spin states $+\dfrac{1}{2}$ and $-\dfrac{1}{2}$ in presence of the applied magnetic field B_0 as shown in Fig. 1.3. That means that in one spin state $\left(m = +\dfrac{1}{2} \right)$ (called a) is aligned at an angle of 45º from the +z axis with the applied B_0 (Fig. 1.10) and in another spin state, $m = -\dfrac{1}{2}$ (called 13) it is aligned against to the applied field (Fig. 1.10) at an angle of 45º from the −z axis (Fig. 1.10c).

Quantum mechanical considerations predict that the protons can only precess at 45° from either the +z axis (α spin state) or from the −z axis (β spin state), the rate of precession of the β-protons is slightly higher than the rate of precession of the α-protons around the B_0. The angle cannot be different from 45°. They cannot orient at any arbitrary precession angle θ. The difference in their energies is always constant at a particular strength of B_0. Of course, this difference rises with the strength of the applied field. **At 700 MHz, the protons precess about z-axis at a rate of ~ 700 MHz. That is they make one full precession every 1.43 nanoseconds. Our eyes cannot follow such a fast precession.**

Let us now consider as to what will be the energy of the various nuclear spin states? There exists a relationship between energy E, nuclear moment, μ and the applied field B_0 :

Energy of an m_I state :

$$E = -\gamma \cdot \frac{h}{2\pi} m_I B_0$$

Thus for a proton :

Energy of $m + \frac{1}{2}$ (α-spin state) :

$$Em + \frac{1}{2} = -\gamma \cdot \frac{h}{2\pi} \frac{1}{2} \cdot B_0 \left(m_I = +\frac{1}{2} \right)$$

Energy of $m - \frac{1}{2}$ (β-spin state) :

$$Em - \frac{1}{2} = -\gamma \cdot \frac{h}{2\pi} - \frac{1}{2} \cdot B_0 \left(m_I = -\frac{1}{2} \right)$$

$$= +\gamma \cdot \frac{h}{2\pi} - \frac{1}{2} \cdot B_0$$

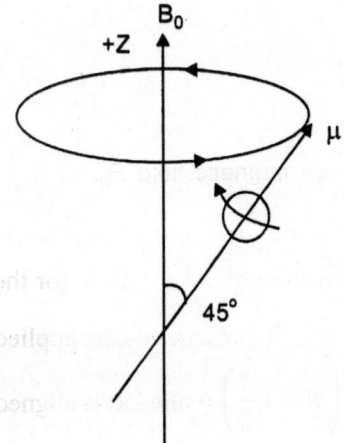

Fig. 1.10a. The $+\frac{1}{2}$I spin of proton.

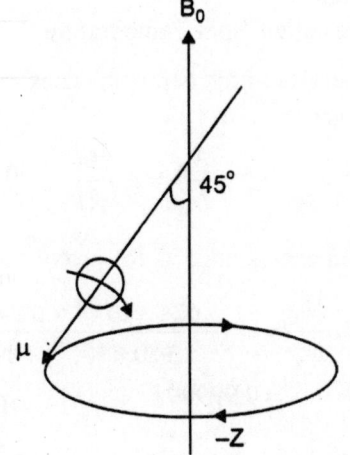

Fig. 1.10b. The $-\frac{1}{2}$I spin of proton.

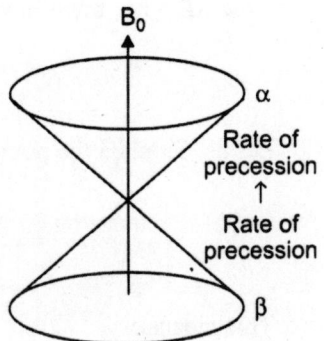

Fig. 1.10c. The α and β spin states of protons.

So, it is clear that the energy of the β $\left(m - \dfrac{1}{2}\right)$ spin state is higher than that of the α $\left(m + \dfrac{1}{2}\right)$ spin state.

Now $\Delta E = E_2 - E_1$:

$$= \frac{\gamma.h}{2\pi} \frac{1}{2} B_0 - \left(-\gamma \frac{h}{2\pi} \cdot \frac{1}{2} B_0\right)$$

$$= \frac{\gamma h}{2\pi} \frac{1}{2} B_0 + \gamma \frac{h}{2\pi} \frac{1}{2} B_0$$

$$= 2 \frac{\gamma h}{2\pi} \cdot \frac{1}{2} B_0$$

Energy

$$\Delta E = \gamma \cdot \frac{h}{2\pi} B_0$$

1.4 BOLTZMAN POPULATION EXCESS

From the above discussion, it seems logical to assume that some (slightly more than) fifty percent of the protons will be in the α-spin state, while the other slightly less than fifty percent population will be in the β-spin state. In fact, by using Boltzman distribution equation, it turns out that there is a slight excess of the protons in the α-energy level, the lower spin state. If N_B and N_A are the populations of nuclei in the β- and α-spin states respectively, then the ratio is given by the following equation :

$$\frac{N_\beta}{N_\alpha} = e^{-\frac{\Delta E}{kT}}$$

where k is the Boltzman constant (1.380×10^{-23} Jk^{-1} per molecule)
h = Planck's constant (6.624×10^{-34} J sec)
T = Absolute temperature called 'Spin Temperature'

ΔE is the difference in the energies of the two spin states.

Now $\Delta E = h\nu$, therefore, we get :

$$\frac{N_\beta}{N_\alpha} = e^{-\frac{h\nu}{kT}}$$

Let us calculate the population excess at 25°C for protons at 60 MHz.

$$\frac{N_\beta}{N_\alpha} = e^{-\frac{6.624 \times 10^{-34} \times 60 \times 10^6}{1.380 \times 10^{-23} \times 298}}$$

$$= 0.99999I$$

This means :

$$\frac{N_\beta}{N_\alpha} = \frac{1000000}{1000009}$$

Hence, if one million protons are present in the higher energy β-spin state, then there are 1 million +9 protons in the lower energy α-spin state. Let us have a feel of this excess from the sample size point of view. An NMR sample contains about 20 molecules. Of these protons the α spin state contains an excess of about 10^{11} spins relative to β spin state at 700 MHz (16.45 T) at 25°C.

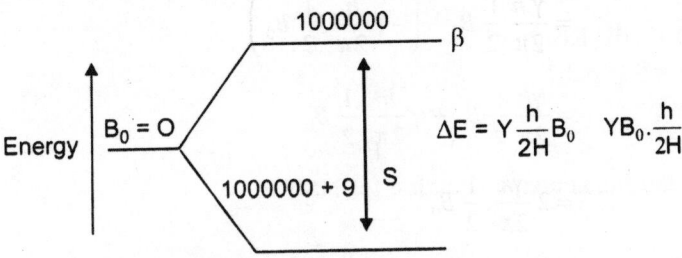

Fig. 1.11. Nuclear Zeeman splitting energy, ΔE.

The reason for almost equal populations of the nuclei in both the spin states is that the energy difference between the two energy levels α and β is very small (this is not so in case of u.v. or i.r. spectroscopy). ΔE, the Nuclear Zeeman Splitting Energy is the difference in energy between these two spin states (Fig. 10.12) is given as under :

$$\Delta E = h\nu_0 = \nu_0 \text{ is called Larmor frequency}$$

Now $$\nu_0 = y \cdot \frac{B_0}{2\pi} \qquad ...(A)$$

where Y is the magnetogyro constant and B_0 the applied field strength.

$$\therefore \Delta E = h \cdot y \cdot \frac{B_0}{2\pi}$$

Thus, for protons with $y = 2.675 \times 10^8$ T^{-1} rad sec^{-1} at 298 K (25°C) and at $B_0 = 7.05\ T$.

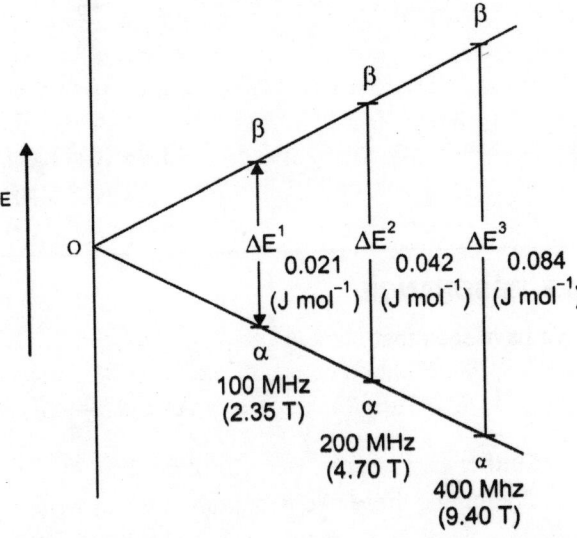

Fig. 1.12. Increasing ΔE with increasing magnetic field strength.

$$\Delta E = 6.624 \times 10^{34} \times 2.675 \frac{10^8 \times 7.05 \times 7}{2 \times 22}$$

$$= 0.0315 \text{ J/mol}$$

As can be seen, this energy difference is very small. It needs to be noted that ΔE is proportional to the strength of the magnetic field B_0. So, if B_0 is lesser than 7.05 T, ΔE would be still small as shown in Fig. 1.13. If it has higher value than this, ΔE would rise proportionately. However, this population does not reach more than 0.001%.

Intext Exercise

3. Calculate the nuclear Zeeman splitting energy for the spin states of proton at 25°C for B_0, 7.05 T, $Y_H = 2.67 \times 10^8$ T^{-1} rad sec^{-1}. $h = 6.624 \times 10^{34}$ joules sec.

4. What will be the energy needed for observing NMR signal for hydrogen at a field strength of 4.7 T?

   Given: $h = 9.5 \times 10^{14}$ Kcal/mol,

   $\qquad y = 2.7 \times 10^8$ rad T^{-1} s^{-1}

   Ans. We know :

   $$E = h\nu$$

   We also know the fundamental equation for NMR :

   $$\nu = y \cdot \frac{B_0}{2\pi}$$

   Putting the value of g into equation for E, we get :

   $$E = h \cdot y \cdot \frac{B_0}{2\pi}$$

   $$= 9.5 \times 10^{-14} \times 2.7 \times 10^8 \times \frac{4.7 \times 7}{2 \times 22}$$

   $$= 1.9 \times 10^{-5} \text{ Kcal mol}^{-1}$$

   $$= 1.9 \times 10^{-5} \times 10^3 \text{ cal mol}^{-1}$$

   $$= 1.019 \text{ cal mol}^{-1}$$

1.5 RESONANCE

We have seen that :

$$\Delta E = \gamma \cdot \frac{h}{2\pi} B_0$$

Further $\qquad\qquad\qquad \Delta E = h\nu$

Combining these two equations, we can write :

$$h\nu = \gamma \cdot \frac{h}{2\pi} B_0$$

or,

$$\nu = \gamma \cdot \frac{h}{2\pi} B_0$$

The frequency of radiomagnetic radiation ν, required is actually equal to Larmor precession frequency ν_0 of the nucleus in the α-spin state. In other words, we can say that when a nucleus having magnetogyro ratio γ is placed in a magnetic field, B_0, it will resonate or give a resonance signal at a frequency ν if supplied to it. In fact, this is the equation in our hands which can help us predict the frequency that will be equal to the Larmor frequency required for resonance of any nucleus having magnetogyroratio γ at any particular value of applied magnetic field B_0.

Geometry of the NMR Experiment

If we apply an alternating magnetic field B_A with radiofrequency V^1 to the nucleus precessing in the applied field B_0, then it can provide the required ΔE if it rotates in the plane of the precession with a frequency V^1 equal to Larmor frequency V_0 of the nucleus as shown in Fig. 1.13. Technically speaking, an alternating field B_1 is applied that is perpendicular to B_0 and a radiofrequency V^1 equal to the Larmor frequency V_0 is provided and a resonance signal is obtained as the proton flips from α spin to the β-spin state.

What is done technically is that we gradually vary the radiofrequency, keeping the magnetic field B_0, constant. When this radiofrequency

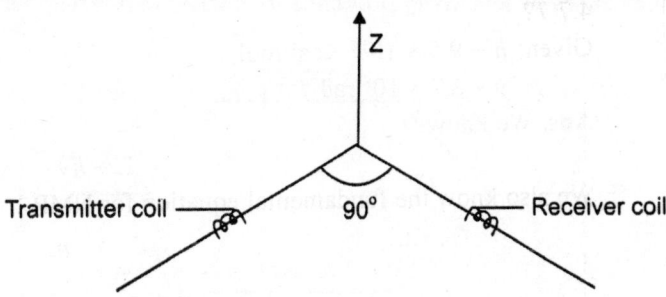

Fig. 1.13. Geometry of the resonance phenomenon.

becomes equal to that of the Larmor precession frequency v_0, the nucleus gives a resonance signal in the NMR spectrum as it flips from the lower energy α spin state to the higher energy β spin state.

When a radiofrequency of 60 MHz is applied to the protons $\left(I = \dfrac{1}{2} \right)$ at a fixed magnetic field strength of 1.41 Tesla (14,092 gauss), protons flip from the lower energy α-spin state to the higher energy β-spin state after absorption of energy equal to ΔE ($h\nu$). Of course, if B_0 is increased, then the frequency of the electromagnetic radiation required to bring protons into resonance, will also increase. Thus, for example the radio frequency v_0 required for the protons at a magnetic field, B_0 of 7.05 T will be equal to 300 MHz.

$$v_0 = \frac{\gamma \cdot B_0}{2\pi}$$

$$= \frac{2.675 \times 10^8 \times 7.05 \times 7}{2 \times 22}$$

$$v_0 = 2.675 \times 10^8 \text{ rad T}^{-1} \text{ s}^{-1}$$

$$= 300.1 \text{ MHz}$$

Thus, when the protons are placed in an NMR spectrometer operating at a fixed field of 7.05 T, they will resonate at a radiofrequency of 300 MHz, rather than at 60 MHz. Such a spectrum is called **frequency sweep spectrum**.

It should be noted that, it is more convenient to keep the radiofrequency constant and vary the magnetic field, till a resonance signal is obtained. That is to say if the protons are subjected to a fixed radiofrequency of 60 MHz, then they give a resonance signal when a field strength equal to 1.41 T is applied (and if the radiofrequency is fixed at 300 MHz, then the field strength of 7.05 T is required). Such a spectrum is called **field sweep spectrum**.

1.6 SENSITIVITY PROBLEMS IN NMR

Theoretically speaking, it seems easy to obtain an NMR signal but in practice, it is very difficult to do that. This is in striking contrast to the situation in i.r. and u.v. spectroscopy where it is relatively easy to obtain a good spectrum as sensitivity problems are hardly encountered. The question arises as what are the causes of sensitivity problems in NMR and how can we do away with them.

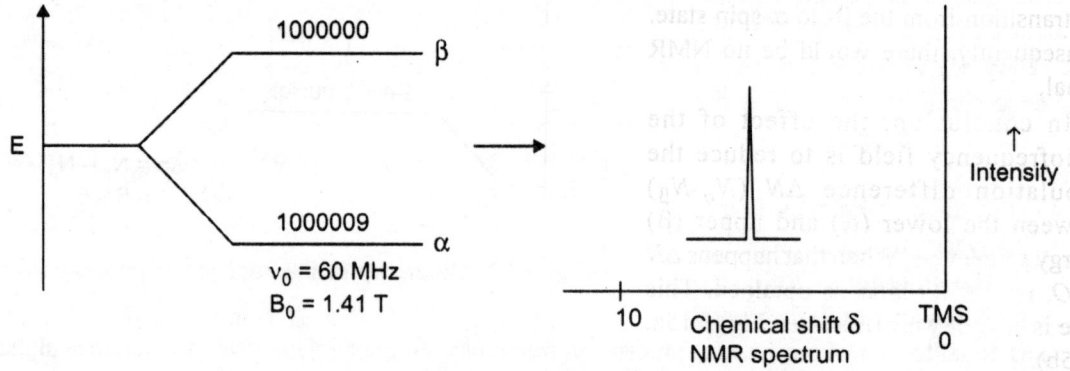

Fig. 1.14. Mechanism of production of NMR spectrum.

1.6.1 Absorption, Induced Emission and Saturation

We have learnt that when a nucleus from α-spin state absorbs a photon ($h\nu$) where ν the radiofrequency is exactly equal to the Larmor frequency ν_0, it goes into the β-spin state. Although the probability of spontaneous emissions from β- to the α-spin state does exist, it is negligible. On the other hand the possibility of **induced emission** is just as probable as the radiation induced excitation (or we can say that the coefficient of absorption and induced emission are equal in NMR spectroscopy). In other words, it means that as a nucleus flips from α- to β-spin state, at the same time a nucleus from the β-spin state jumps down to the α-spin state by absorption of energy ($h\nu$, $\nu = \nu_0$). This phenomenon is also called **stimulated emission.** (Remember it is the net excess of downward transitions which forms the basis for the action of lasers!) Both these transitions (α to β and β to α) occur constantly.

The rate of the "absorption" process is proportional to the population of the nuclei present in the given sample in the α-spin state. Similarly, the rate of the "induced emission" process is proportional to the population of the nuclei present in the given sample in the β-spin state.

Fortunately, there are slightly more nuclei in the lower energy α-spin state compared to the higher energy β-spin state as per Boltzman distribution law. The net effect should be that energy be absorbed by the excess nuclei present in the α-spin state. However, during the process of absorption of energy more nuclei will go from the lower energy α-spin state to the upper energy β-state as compared to the reverse emission process. Therefore, this overall process gives rise to a signal in the NMR spectrum. However, the signal will be very weak and only momentary in nature, particularly in view of the fact that there will be a tendency for the small excess of nuclei present in the α-state to get diminished eventually. In other words, the two spin-states are likely to become equally populated i.e. $N_\beta = N_\alpha$ in due course. This would happen when the rate of the induced emission process becomes equal to the rate of the absorption process. So, a net initial absorption of energy occurs until N_β becomes equal to N_α.

Under the conditions when $N_\beta = N_\alpha$, there would be no net transfer of energy from the radiofrequency applied. This is because the obtainable signal due to transition from α to β, spin state is exactly cancelled due to the obtainable signal from the transition from the β- to α-spin state. Consequently, there would be no NMR signal.

In conclusion, the effect of the radiofrequency field is to reduce the population difference ΔN $(N_\alpha - N_\beta)$ between the lower (α) and upper (β) energy spin levels. When that happens $\Delta N \to O$, no NMR signal is obtained. This state is called **saturation** (see Fig. 1.15a, 1.15b).

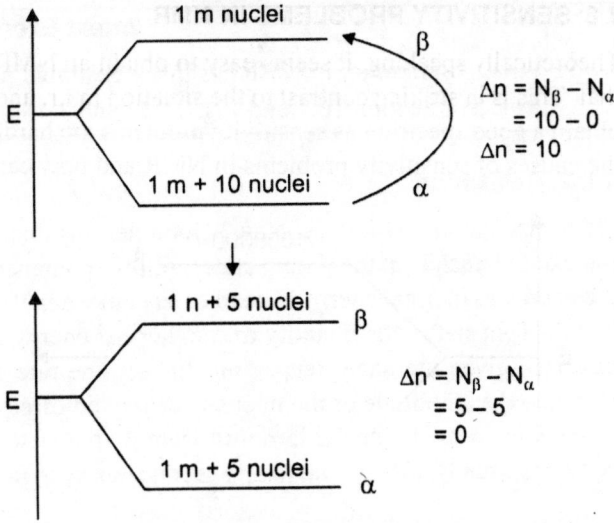

Fig. 1.15a. The saturation state in NMR : No signal!

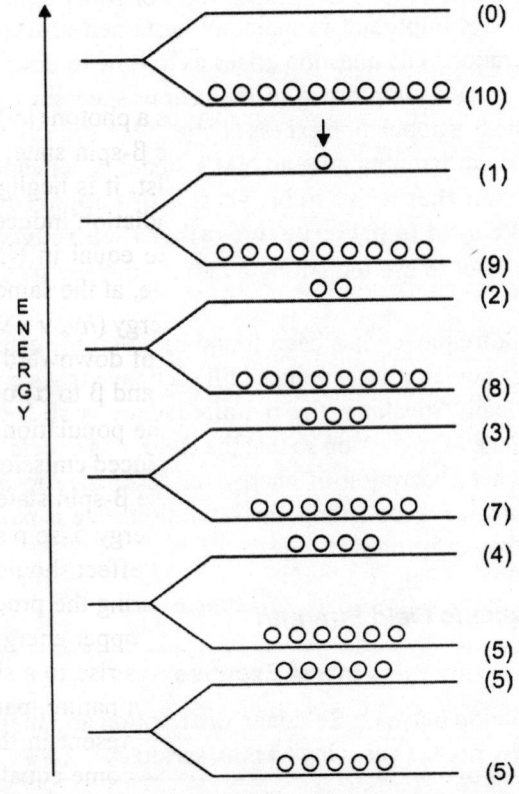

Fig. 1.15b. Gradual attainment of saturation phenomenon as N_α decreases from 10 to 5 and as N_β increases from 0 to 5 so that $N_\beta = N_\alpha$. No signal is obtained at this stage.

1.6.2 Relaxation

Here, also nature favours us. How? Good news is that, it is observed that there is a mechanism which the excited nuclei (in the β-spin state) follow spontaneously to return to the α-spin state. They release the energy as thermal energy instead of as photons in the form of molecular motion as they return (from β- to α-spin state), the quantity of the thermal energy is released so less as photons. This mechanism has been given the name relaxation In fact, the rate of the saturation phenomenon depends on two factors – the amplitude or the intensity of the radiofrequency used and on the rate of relaxation i.e. the time required by the nuclei to return from β-spin state to α-spin state (the relaxation time). This time period is usually a long time taking seconds or even minutes for some nuclei.

1.6.3 Maintaining Population Excess

1.6.3.1 *Weak Radiofrequency and Relaxation time*

Thus, it is crystal clear that it is important to maintain sustained absorption of the radio-frequency energy in order to avoid saturation. The question arises as to how to do that? That can be done only if the nuclei from the excited β-state jump down to the α-spin state such that there always remains a constant Boltzman population i.e. a population excess of one in 10^6 spins is maintained. This is absolutely essential. It must be remembered that obtaining an NMR signal is dependant on the Boltzman excess. **However, small or insignificant that seems to be, yet it is this apparently insignificant figure that is so significant in NMR! We need to preserve this rather than reduce it during the experiment.**

Evidently, it seems logical not to use too strong a radiofrequency so that the Boltzman population excess is maintained.

Indeed, using a weak radiofrequency has been found to be highly effective. So, what is generally done is that the radiofrequency power input is reduced till such time that a constant resonance absorption response is obtained. Technically speaking, the radiofrequency is so set that the rate of absorption becomes exactly equal to the rate of relaxation so that the Boltzman excess of one spin in 10^6 is actually maintained and that there is net absorption of energy for resonance to occur. If the radiofrequency employed to bring about resonance is too strong, the saturation state is reached very quickly. Hence, a weak radiofrequency source has to be used.

1.6.3.2 *Enhancing the Magnetic Field Strength*

The Boltzman distribution should be dependent upon the applied field strength, B_0. This is because, we have earlier argued that the excess of nuclei in the lower of α-spin state was very slight because of very slight difference in the energies of the α- and β-spin states. So, if a way can be found to increase the difference, ΔE between these two spin states, it is likely that there will be a relatively higher population excess in the lower energy α-spin state. One easy way to accomplish that task will be to increase the strength of the applied field B_0. As the magnetic field strength increases, the rate of precession of the nuclei around this applied field increases so that the difference in the energy of both the α- and the β-spin state, ΔE increases.

As ΔE increases, the population excess i.e. the number of excess nuclei in the α-spin state increases. This is because the thermal energy obtainable from room temperature is no longer sufficient to bring about equal population of the nuclei in both the spin states. That is to say, it is no longer able to excite a large number of nuclei from the α-spin state to the β-spin state. Consequently, there is considerable population excess in higher magnetic field. As the signal intensity is dependent upon the number of excess nuclei contributing to the signal, a good spectrum also called a high resolution spectrum will be the result.

A question arises as to why the NMR spectroscopy is different from i.r. and u.v. spectroscopic methods in which the sensitivity problem is hardly encountered. The reason is that in case of i.r. and u.v. spectroscopy, the Boltzman population excess is large as compared to that in the NMR spectroscopy. In other words, the number of excess molecules in the lower energy ground state is large as compared to higher energy excited state. This is due to the fact that ΔE, the difference in the energy levels is very high at room temperature. Further, the rate of relaxation is very large. Consequently, the undesirable phenomenon of saturation as observed in NMR spectroscopy is not encountered.

The increase in the population excess with field strength can be shown as follows. We have already shown that at 25°C and at 1.41 Tesla (60 MHz), the applied field strength, there are about 1 million nuclei in the β-spin state and 1 million + 9 nuclei in the β-spin state. If we keep the temperature constant i.e. 25°C, but increase the value of B_0 2.35 T (100 MHz) than the number of excess nuclei in the spin state becomes 16. As the B_0 is now doubled to 4.70 T (200 MHz), the population excess also becomes doubled to 32. At 7.05 T (300 MHz), the excess nuclei number 48. At 18.80 T (800 MHz), this excess becomes 128. These results are collected in Table 1.2.

Table 1.2. Relationship between population excess for protons and the field strength, B_0 at 298 K

Field strength (frequency)	Population excess
1.41 (60 MHz)	9
2.35 (100 MHz)	16
4.70 (200 MHz)	32
7.05 (300 MHz)	48
18.80 (800 MHz)	128

This technique is particularly useful for those nuclei which unlike ^1H have very low natural abundance and whose γ are also lower relatively, for example ^{13}C whose natural abundance is 1.1% and whose y is about 1/4 of that of proton. Similarly ^{15}N also falls in this category as its natural abundance is 0.37% and its γ/γ_H is 0.1013. However, it should be noted that the Boltzman excess does not reach more than 0.001%.

1.6.3.3 *Lowering the Spin Temperature*

It is evident from Boltzman distribution equation that the spin temperature T appears in the denominator of the exponent. So, the population excess is inversely proportional to the absolute temperature. Therefore, the Boltzman excess can be increased by lowering down the spin temperature. However, practically speaking, this is not advisable since most of the spectral determination is done at room temperature.

1.6.3.4 *Improving Signal/Noise (S/N) ratio: CATING*

In the NMR spectrum, the signals obtained are very weak if the amount of the sample being observed is very small. The reason is that, certain other signals called Noise are also obtained due to instrument itself. These appear as fluctuations of the baseline in the signal. The S/N ratio may be increased by increasing the concentration of the sample if it is readily available.

Usually, a technique called Computer Averaging of Transients (CAT) is used to increase the S/N ratio. What is done is that the spectrum is scanned many times. The information thus obtained is stored in the computer. The resonance signals are added up while the noise signals go down as they are of random nature. In fact, the S/N ratio is a function of the square root of the scans added up.

$$S/N = f\sqrt{n}$$

where n = number of scans.

This is how, cating provides us a good spectrum despite the very small concentration of the sample solution. If CATing is done for one hundred spectra, then the increase observed in *S/N* ratio is 10:1.

Modern digital computers can accumulate many thousands of scans and therefore, improve the *S/N* ratio to yield a good spectrum worth interpretation.

Cating, however, takes long time to record spectra. For instance, when we are working with a continuous wave spectrometer, the time required to obtain a spectrum is generally 100–500 s. Therefore, the time required to obtain many thousands of spectra will be very long. Thus, if 100 spectra (say) are required for cating for a particular sample, which requires 500 s to obtain one spectrum, the total time required will be 500 × 1000 = 500000 s or 500000/3600 = 1110 min.

Some samples may require even five thousands or even more scans, thus the total time required will still be very long.

Intext Questions

7. What are the causes of sensitivity problems in NMR spectroscopy and how are they overcome? Explain in details.
   Hint : As an answer to this question we have to describe what has been discussed in Section 1.6.

8. How is S/N ratio related to number of scans, n?
   Hint : S/N = $f\sqrt{n}$.

9. How can you maintain population excess during the NMR experiment?
   Hint : Describe Sections 1.6.3.1 to 1.6.3.4 herein.

PROBLEMS

1. Unlike a bar magnet, the magnetic moment of a nucleus does not orient itself with the direction of the applied field, B_0 irrespective of its strength. Why?
   Hint: See Section 1.1.

2. What is gyromagneto ratio, γ? What does it represent?
   Hint: See Section 1.1.

3. What is the equation that relates Larmor precession frequency, ν_0 and γ and B_0?
   Hint: See Section 1.1.

4. Calculate the Larmor precession frequency of a proton with $\gamma = 2.675 \times 10^8\ T^{-1}$ rad s^{-1} placed in a magnetic field of strength 2.35 T and 4.70 MHz.
   Hint: Ans. = 100 MHz and 200 MHz respectively. See Section 1.1.

5. What is the relation between (a) γ_H and γ_D, (b) γ_H and γ_{N-15}, (c) γ_H and γ_C?
   Hint: See Section 1.1.

6. What is the classical concept of NMR?
   Hint: See Section 1.1.

7. Give examples (at least two) of the nuclei with $I = 0, \dfrac{1}{2}, 1$ and $\dfrac{3}{2}$.

8. What is the relation between, μ, γ and I?
   Hint: See Section 1.2.

9. Show the orientations of N–14 or B–11 in an applied magnetic field.
   Hint: See Section 1.2, Fig. 1.7.

10. What is the selection rule in NMR spectroscopy?
    Hint: See Section 1.2.

11. What is the angle of alignment of α-spin state w.r. to applied field, B_0 in nmr spectroscopy of liquid samples?
    Hint: See Section 1.3.

12. At what frequency, do the protons precess at 700 MHz NMR instrument?
    Hint: About 700 MHz (Section 1.3).

13. What is the equation that connects E, γ, and B_0?
    Hint: See Section 1.3.

14. What is Boltzman population excess?
    Hint: See Section 1.4.

15. Calculate Boltzman population excess per protons at 600 MHz at 25°C.
    Hint: Answer = 0.999991, see Section 1.4.

16. What does a Boltzman population excess of 0.99999 mean?
    Hint: See Section 1.4.

17. What is ΔE, the energy difference between the two spin states, α and β at 25°C in a magnetic field of 2.35 T? $\gamma_H = 2.675 \times 10^8\ T^{-1}$ rad sec^{-1}.
    Hint: Ans = 0.0105 J mol^{-1}, see Section 1.4.

18. Explain the terms frequency sweep spectrum and field sweep spectrum.

19. Explain in details the Principle of NMR Spectroscopy.
    Hint: See Section 1.1 to 1.6.
20. What is Boltzman Population Distribution equation?
    Hint: See Section 1.4.
21. What is meant by spin temperature?
    Hint: T in the Boltzman Population Excess equation.
22. Which technique is less sensitive between i.r. (or UV) and NMR spectroscopies and why?
    Hint: See Section 1.6.
23. What is meant by Absorption, Induced Emission and Saturation in NMR?
    Hint: See Section 1.6.1.
24. How can you maintain population excess during an NMR experiment?
    Hint: See Section 1.6.3.
25. Does Boltzman population excess depend upon applied field strength even though B_0 does not picture into the Boltzman distribution equation? Explain.
26. How can S/N ratio be improved by CATing?
    Hint: See Section 1.6.3.
27. On what factors does the amplitude of the NMR signal sensitivity depend?
    Hint: Amplitude of NMR signal = $N\gamma^3 B_0^2 /T$.
    where N is the number of identical spins (nuclei) present in the sample.
    γ is the strength of the nuclear magnet (magnetogyro ratio).
    B_0 is the applied field strength.
    T is the temperature of the spins (nuclei) in Kelvin.
28. Calculate the energy change with the proton nuclear spin of $CHCl_3$ having a shielding constant of 7.25×10^{-6} and a nuclear magnetic moment μ of 1.410620×10^{-26} J T^{-1} at B_0 equal to $1T$. What will be the radiofrequency for the nuclear spin transition?

    Hint: $\Delta E = \dfrac{\mu B_0 (1 - \sigma)}{I}$ where I for $^1H = \dfrac{1}{2}$

    $$= \frac{1.410620 \times 10^{-26} \times 1(7.25 \times 10^{-6})}{2}$$

    $$= 2.82160 \times 10^{-26} \text{ J}$$

    As $\Delta E = h\nu$

    $$\therefore \nu = \frac{\Delta E}{h} = \frac{2.82160 \times 10^{-26}}{6.626196 \times 10^{-34}}$$

    $$= 4.257738 \times 10^7 \text{ Hz}$$

29. What are the sensitivity problems in NMR and how are they overcome?
    Hint: See Section 1.6.

Chemical Shift – Origin and Factors

2.1 INTRODUCTION

All spin-active nuclei resonate at a particular frequency, the resonance frequency or the Larmor frequency in an applied field, which is governed by the equation :

$$\omega = \gamma \cdot B_0 \qquad \qquad ....(\text{Eq. 2.1})$$

where y is the gyromagneto ratio that represents the strength of the magnet and B_0 is the applied magnetic field. Obviously, it is this equation (Eq. 2.1) that makes NMR spectroscopy a useful technique in structure elucidation of compounds in chemistry.

The utility of NMR in chemistry lies in the fact that nuclei with different nuclear strengths i.e. with different y, gyromagneto ratios absorb at different radiofrequencies in a constant magnetic field. And the good news is that we do not get any overlappings as the differences in their resonant frequencies are quite large. Thus, at 2.35 T, while the resonance frequency for proton is 100 MHz, that for carbon is 25 MHz as y for carbon is 1/4th of that of proton.

The major advantage of NMR lies in the fact that the same nucleus when bonded to different nuclei in a molecule does not absorb at one fixed frequency say, at 60 MHz at 1.41 T for proton. This is a good news for us as it enables us to make structural elucidation of the compound as we will see later on.

2.2 DEFINITION

There is always a small variation in the resonant frequencies of different protons in different environments. This small change which is of the order of one part a million is called chemical shift. The concept of chemical shift will become more clear when we consider the strength of spectrometer i.e. its operating frequency. The rate of precession of protons at 800 MHz spectrometer means that the protons precess about B_0 along the Z axis at ~ 800 MHz. Actually the precession rate of the protons is not exactly 800 MHz rather it is very near to 800 MHz i.e. $800 \pm x$ MHz where x is equal to plus or minus a few hundred Hz. **This difference from the operating frequency is called chemical shift. Thus chemical shifts are very small relative to 800 MHz precession rate, only about one millionth of the total rate.**

2.3 THEORY AND MEASUREMENT OF CHEMICAL SHIFTS

The small changes in radiofrequencies are actually due to changes in electronic environment of the nuclei. In other words, the effective field surrounding the nucleus is never identical with the applied magnetic field, B_0. In fact, if we look at NMR as a magnetic phenomenon, which indeed it is, and because electrons also are associated with a magnetic field of their own, we must not neglect this or rather we must imagine some sort of magnetic interaction between the behaviour of nuclei and the electrons in an applied magnetic field. We are not dealing with hydrogens that are bare or present alone in solution. The hydrogens we are dealing with are not isolated but are present in molecules, bonded on to other atoms such as carbon etc. by bonds, which contain electrons.

The small changes in radiofrequencies are actually due to changes in electronic environment of the nuclei. The electrons about the nuclei start circulating around and set up a secondary magnetic field B^1 as shown in Fig. 2.1. This induced field opposes the applied field around the nucleus as per Lenz's law. So, the actual field felt by the nucleus is less than that required for a bare proton, i.e. :

$$B_{eff} = B_0 - B^1$$

Now, this induced field B^1 is proportional to the applied field B_0.

So, we can write $B_{eff} = B_0 - \sigma B_0$:

$$B_{eff} = (1 - \sigma)B_0$$

where σ is the shielding constant in units of parts per million.

Hence, it reduces the nuclear frequency because $\nu_0 = yB_0/2\pi$.

The value of σ is proportional to the electron density of the 1s orbital of the hydrogen. The term σB_0 (B^1) represents the magnitude of the induced secondary field. Under these conditions, higher field is required to cause this proton to give a resonance signal if frequency is kept constant (or a higher frequency is required if the NMR instrument is being operated on a fixed field mode.)

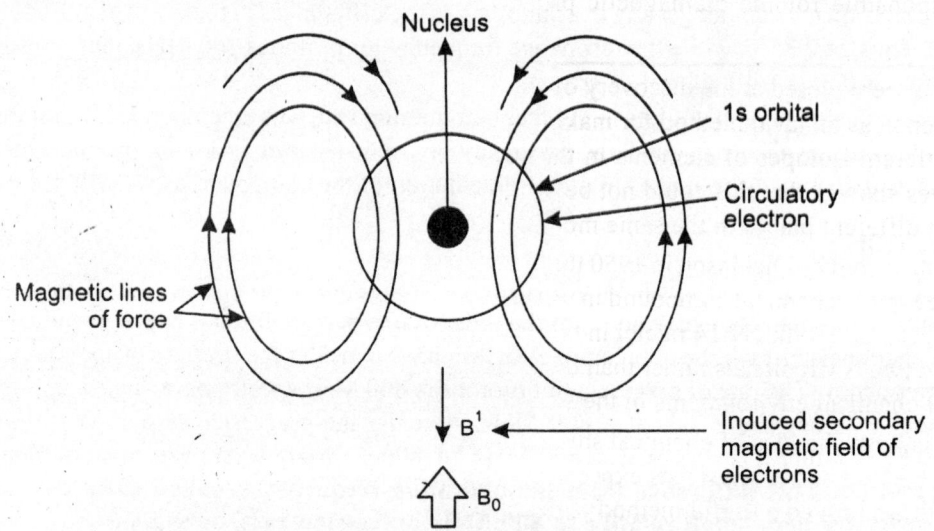

Fig. 2.1a. Shielding by electrons of hydrogen nucleus in an applied magnetic field B_0.

Calculation of σ, the screening constant for a hydrogen atom, a spherical nucleus

Lamb gave a formula with the aid of which the value of σ, the screening constant can be calculated if electron density $\rho(\gamma)$ around the nucleus is known.

$$\sigma = \frac{\mu_0 e^2}{3m_e} \int_0^\infty \gamma e(\gamma) d\gamma$$

γ is the distance from the nucleus and $e(\gamma)$ therefore is a function of this distance γ. μ_0 is the magnetic moment of the electron. m_e is the mass of the electron.

The semi-empirically determined value of σ for protons in a molecule of hydrogen (H_2) has been found to be 26.6×10^{-6}. Thus hydrogen of H_2 is shielded than a bare or an isolated proton.

The nucleus is said to be shielded or screened from B_0, the applied field. Greater the B_0, greater the source of σ. Therefore, the equation :

$$\nu = y \cdot \frac{B_0}{2\pi}$$

Now becomes modified as :

$$\nu = y \cdot B_{eff}$$

or,

$$\nu = y \cdot \frac{B_0}{2\pi} (1 - \sigma)$$

where σ is called the screening constant, a dimensionless quantity. This is also termed diamagnetic screening as it stands responsible for the diamagnetic properties of substances.

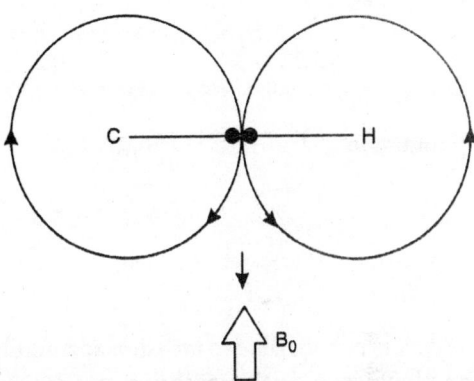

Fig. 2.1b. Shielding by *e* shared pair of electrons around the proton in a C–H bond.

Physicists were plesed at the discovery of the NMR as they thought they would be able to use this phenomenon as an ideal method for making measurements of absolute properties of atomic nuclei – the different isotopes of elements in the periodic table. However, they were dismayed as later researches showed that this could not be done as the precise frequency was different for the same nuclei at different places in the same molecule.

It was discovered by Dickinson in 1950 that the resonance frequency of F-19 ($I = 1/2$) was dependent upon the type of chemical compound in which it was present. Similarly, it was reported in the same year by Proctor Yu that N-14 nuclei in two different chemical environments in NH_4NO_3 solutions exhibited two NMR signals rather than one. Hahn in the same year reported that protons present in different chemical environments in the same compound absorbed at different positions.

So, this is how, the idea of chemical shift came into existence. Although NMR could not serve as an ideal method as per physicists expectations for measuring absolute properties of atomic nuclei, yet NMR has proved a useful method to chemists for making structure elucidation of compounds, which they did not expect at the time the NMR phenomenon was discovered.

Thus, the more shielded proton will appear at lower value of the applied field strength (see Fig. 2.3). That is why, the O–H proton in ethanol appears at the lowest value of the field. This proton will be least shielded because of the high electronegativity of oxygen compared to that of carbon.

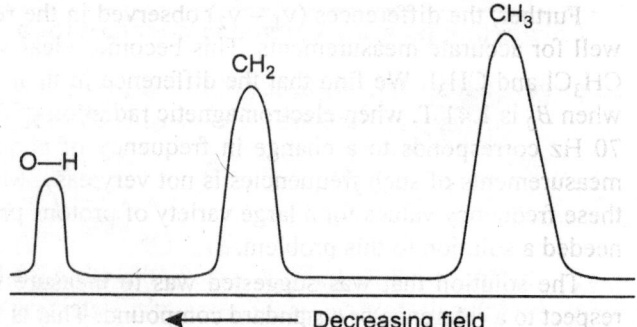

Fig. 2.3. Proton magnetic resonance of ethanol at 60 MHz.

Let us consider two different nuclei having screening constants σ_1 and σ_2, then, their equations of ν versus field strengths will be:

$$\nu_1 = y \cdot \frac{B_0}{2\pi}(1 - \sigma_1) \qquad \text{...(i)}$$

$$\nu_2 = y \cdot \frac{B_0}{2\pi}(1 - \sigma_2) \qquad \text{...(ii)}$$

Subtracting (ii) from (i) will give us :

$$\nu_1 - \nu_2 = y \cdot \frac{B_0}{2\pi}(1 - \sigma_1) - y \cdot \frac{B_0}{2\pi}(1 - \sigma_2)$$

or,

$$\nu_1 - \nu_2 = y \cdot \frac{B_0}{2\pi}(\sigma_2 - \sigma_1) \qquad \text{...(iii)}$$

As, it is not possible to measure accurately the absolute value of applied field, therefore, it is essential not to include B_0 in this equation.

So, let us divide eq. (iii) by eq. (i).

$$\frac{\nu_1 - \nu_2}{\nu_1} = \gamma \cdot \frac{B_0}{2\pi}(\sigma_2 - \sigma_1)$$

$$= \gamma \cdot \frac{B_0}{2\pi}(1 - \sigma_1)$$

or,

$$\frac{\nu_1 - \nu_2}{\nu_1} = \frac{\sigma_2 - \sigma_1}{1 - \sigma_1} \qquad \text{...(iv)}$$

As σ, the screening constant is much less than 1, therefore, the equation (iv) simplifies to :

$$\frac{\nu_1 - \nu_2}{\nu_1} = \sigma_2 - \sigma_1 = \Delta\sigma$$

It is clear, therefore, that the fractional frequency change is equal to the difference in the screening in the environments of two nuclei. This fractional frequency change is called chemical shift, δ :

$$\delta = \frac{\nu_1 - \nu_2}{\nu_1}$$

It should be noted that ν_1 and ν_2 are very large numbers and also differ very slightly from ν_0, the Larmor radiofrequency, which is fixed at a particular value of the applied magnetic field B_0.

Further, the differences $(v_1 - v_2)$ observed in the resonance frequency of protons are too small as well for accurate measurements. This becomes clear when we consider the resonances of protons in CH_3Cl and CH_3I. We find that the difference in their resonance frequencies is a mere seventy Hertz when B_0 is 1.41 T, when electromagnetic radiation of 60 MHz is used. Therefore, such a difference of 70 Hz corresponds to a change in frequency of about one part in ten lakhs (one million). Precise measurements of such frequencies is not very easy. Moreover, it will not be convenient to remember these frequency values for a large variety of protons present in the organic compounds. Therefore, we needed a solution to this problem.

The solution that was suggested was to measure the resonance frequencies of the protons with respect to a reference or a standard compound. That is to say, that the reference chosen should be such that its proton(s) resonate at the extreme right most upfield of the spectrum at highest frequency and the machine be taught to directly measure the differences in Hertz, from this standard, so as to simplify the values. Thus, tetramethyl silane $Si(CH_3)_4$ which was chosen the standard as at that particular point in time as its protons were found to resonate at one extreme of the spectrum compared to any other protons containing compound (i.e. most upfield).

$$\delta = \frac{v_{sample} - v_{reference}}{v_0}.$$

In order to make a chemical shift δ, easy to express, RHS of the equation is multiplied by 10^6. δ is now expressed in ppm. As $v_{sample} - v_{reference}$, the frequency separation is a quantity which is dependant upon the strength of the applied field, therefore, it shall increase with increase in the strength (B_0) of the applied field. But as it is divided by the strength of the applied field, therefore, chemical shift, δ, is independent of the applied field. If it were not so, it could

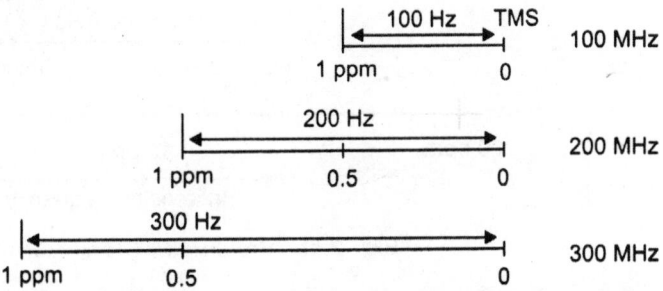

Fig. 2.4a. This figure shows that 100 Hz (1 ppm) at 100 MHz becomes equal to 200 Hz (1 ppm) at 200 MHz and 300 Hz (1 ppm) at 300 MHz. The singlet obtained at 1 ppm on a 100 MHz instrument still appears at 1 ppm on higher strengths i.e. 200 MHz, 300 MHz etc.

have been very confusing because a proton will absorb at different frequencies (in Hz) at different strengths of the spectrometer. Thus, if a proton gave a signal at 60 Hz at 60 MHz, then it would absorb at 100 Hz at 100 MHz and at 200 Hz at 200 MHz spectrometer creating confusion about its identity (as shown in Fig. 2.4a).

Intext Exercises

1. Calculate the radiofrequency at which tetramethyl silane will absorb at an applied field strength 1 T. Given that ΔE is equal to 2.8212×10^{-26} joule and screening constant = 0.

   We know $\Delta E = hn$, where h is Planck's constant = 6.6261×10^{-34} joule sec :

   $$\therefore \quad v = \frac{\Delta E}{h}$$

   $$= \frac{2.8212 \times 10^{-26}}{6.6261 \times 10^{-34}} \, Hz$$

   $$= 4.2576 \times 10^7 \, Hz$$

2. Calculate the chemical shift of $CHCl_3$ proton in NMR, tetramethyl silane being used as a standard. Given $\nu CHCl_3 = 42.577289 \times 10^6$ Hz and $\nu_{TMs} = 42.76981 \times 10^6$ Hz. Note $\nu_0 = \nu_{TMS}$.

$$\delta_{CHCl_3} = \frac{\nu_{CHCl_3} - \nu_{TMS}}{\nu_{TMS}} \times 10^6$$

$$= \frac{42.577289 \times 10^6 - 42.576981 \times 10^6 \times 10^6}{42.57 \times 10^6}$$

$$= 7.23 \text{ ppm.}$$

Thus, the standard TMS appears on the right extreme and is assigned δ as 0.0 ppm. The frequency increases towards left of this standard and the deshielded protons appear on this side; more the deshielding, higher the δ value in ppm. It should be noted that frequency order is opposite to that of the magnetic field B_0. This way, the usual range of protons is up to 20 ppm (Fig. 2.4b), while that for Carbon-13 is about 200 ppm (Fig. 2.4c).

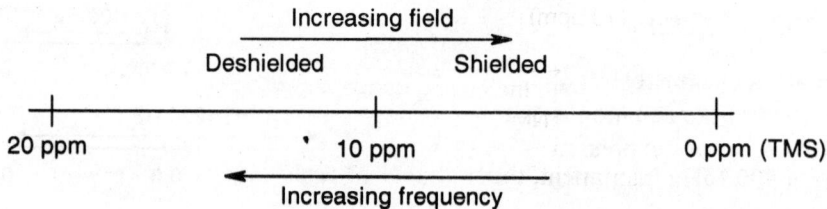

Fig. 2.4b. Proton NMR range of organic compounds.

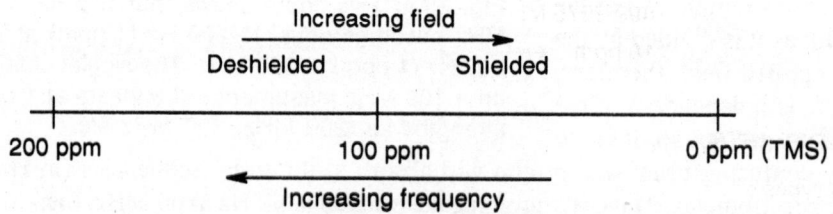

Fig. 2.4c. C-13 NMR range of organic compounds.

It should also be noted that an alternative scale τ (Tau) used earlier was T = 10 − δ, where δ is the chemical shift. Obviously, the reference TMS has the value 10 and accordingly the less shielded protons have smaller and positive values down to zero.

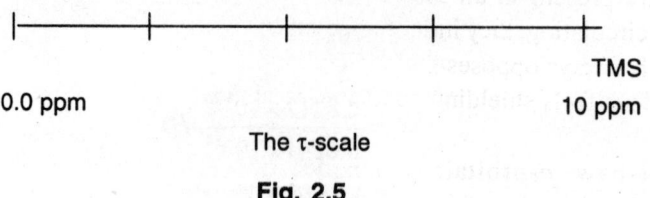

The τ-scale

Fig. 2.5

So, we conclude that the chemical shifts are indeed tiny. In fact, they are expected to be tiny as we are dealing with tiny nuclei or magnets and tiny electrons. Thus, the whole general range of organic protons is only about 10 ppm. If we are working with a 100 MHz NMR machine, the range of these organic protons will be around 99.9995–100.0005 MHz. 0.0005 Hz is equal to 0.0005×10^6 Hz = 5 ppm.

$$500 \text{ Hz} = \frac{500}{100 \times 10^6} \times 10^6 = 5 \text{ ppm}$$

Therefore, frequency of 99.9995 – 100.0005 MHz corresponds to 10 ppm range. It is the graph of these resonant frequencies over a narrow range of frequencies that is centred on the fundamental resonance frequency of a nucleus that is called an NMR spectrum.

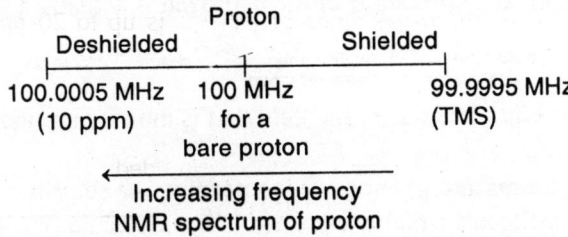

Similarly, on a 500 MHz instrument, the proton NMR spectrum would have the following narrow arrange of frequencies.

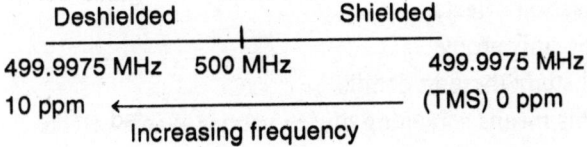

2.4 TYPES OF SHIFTS

Shift is of two types :
1. Diamagnetic shift
2. Paramagnetic shift

2.4.1 Diamagnetic shielding shift

This is a universal type of shielding as it is present in any type of molecule. This shielding arises due to s-electrons which are present in all molecules. When these electrons start circulating, they induce a secondary magnetic field which always opposes the applied field. As a result, the nucleus feels shielding compared to an isolated nucleus.

Protons do not have p-orbitals and hence no p-electrons. That is why, the range of deshielding is small

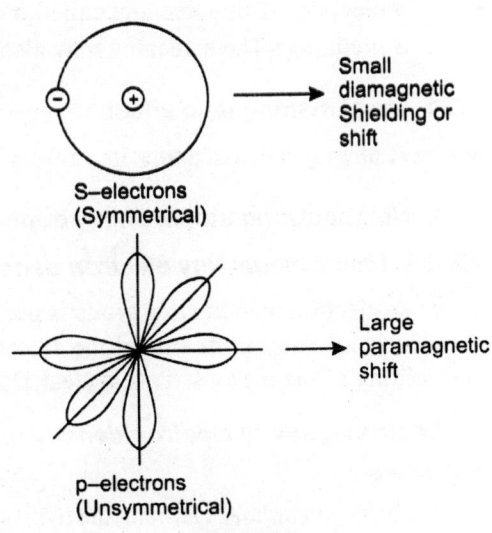

Fig. 2.6.

in protons, 1-10 ppm in general. On the other hand, we find large deshielding in molecules containing p-electrons.

2.4.2 Paramagnetic shift

The paramagnetic shift is caused due to electrons in non-spherical molecules. In such molecules, spherical symmetry is not present. So, p-electrons produce large magnetic fields around the nucleus which reinforce the applied field and thus cause deshielding. This shielding gives rise to paramagnetic shift. This is seen in nuclei such as carbon-13, which unlike hydrogen show very large range of chemical shifts of the order of about 200 ppm.

2.5 PARAMETERS THAT AFFECT CHEMICAL SHIFT

The shielding or the screening constant σ of the hydrogen is actually a sum of following factors :

$$\sigma = \sigma_{\substack{local \\ diamagnetic}} + \sigma_{\substack{neighbouring \\ atoms\ and\ groups}} + \sigma_{electric} + \sigma_{Van\ DW} + \sigma_{medium}$$

1. **σ Local diamagnetic :** It is due to the field that is induced around the nucleus upon application of applied field, B_0.
2. **σ neighbouring atoms and groups :** This screening is a contribution by the neighbouring atoms and groups or substituents which are present in the molecule. The neighbouring atoms or groups or substituents can modify the σ local diamagnetic as following acts :
   (i) Electronegativity effect
   (ii) Resonance effect (+ R or – R)
   (iii) Hybridisation effects
   (iv) Magnetic anisotropy
      We will study these in details.
3. **σ van dw :** This means screening due to vander Waals effects.
4. **σ electric :** This screening called σ electric field is due to electric fields.
5. **σ medium :** The screening may also be caused due to medium effects.

2.5.1 Local diamagnetic effect

We have already discussed this. Its value is 178 ppm for a neutral hydrogen atom as per Lamb's formula.

2.5.2 Neighbouring atoms and groups

2.5.2.1 *Electronegativity electron density effects*

When an electron withdrawing group is present in a molecule (Fig. 20.2), it withdraws and thus reduces the electron density from around the 1s orbital of hydrogen and the value of screening. This leads to deshielding of the protons. This is clear from the following examples.

(i) *Electronegativity electron density effects in neutral molecules*
Examples

(i) *Hydrogen halides* : Among the hydrogen halides, HF, HCl, HBr and HI, the HF is most deshielded whereas the HI proton is least deshielded. The decreasing order of deshielding is:

HF > HCl > HBr > HI

←——— Increasing deshielding

This observation is easy to understand as an effect of the increasing order of electronegativity of the halogen items :

F > Cl > Br > I

4.0 3.2 3.0 2.5 (Electronegativity)

(ii) *Alkyl halides* : The decreasing order of proton chemical shifts of halomethanes are as follows :

$CH_3F > CH_3Cl > CH_3Br > CH_3I$

4.0 2.84 2.45 1.98 (δ ppm)

Again, this reflects the withdrawl of electron density by electronegative halogens. Although in this example, the halogens are not directly attached to the proton as is the case with hydrogen halides,

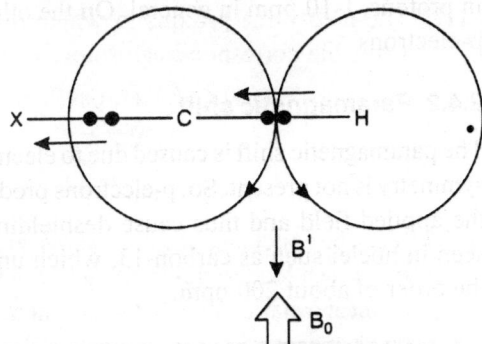

Fig. 2.7. Deshielding of proton due to presence of an electron-withdrawing group. The electron density between C–H bond gets shifted from the centre towards the carbon, which decreases B^1, the induced magnetic field from around hydrogen. So, hydrogen rather gets deshielded.

yet it is clear that electronegative elements can also cause their effect even from a distance along the carbon chain.

(iii) The chemical shifts of protons in compound $(CH_3)_4C$, $(CH_3)_3N$, $(CH_3)_2O$ and CH_3F follow the following decreasing order :

$CH_3F > (CH_3)_2O > (CH_3)_3N > (CH_3)_4C$

4.1 3.2 2.1 0.9 (ppm)

This is in line with the electron-withdrawing ability of the involved electronegative atoms which is :

F > O > N > C

4.0 3.5 3.0 2.5 (ppm)

(iv) The observed chemical shifts of protons in $(CH_3)_4Si$, $(CH_3)_3P$, $(CH_3)_2S$ and $(CH_3)Cl$ is as follows :

CH_3Cl >	$(CH_3)_2S$ >	$(CH_3)_3P$ >	$(CH_3)_4Si$
Methyl	Dimethyl	Trimethyl	Tetramethyl
chloride	sulfate	phosphine	silane (TMS)
–3.0	2.1	0.9	0.00 (ppm)

This again reflects the variation in shift on ground of electronegativity.

(v) While dimethyl ether CH_3OCH_3 protons absorb at S 3.24, the chloromethane protons resonate at 53.0 which in turn are :

CH_3OCH_3 CH_3Cl $CH_3–CH_3$

3.24 3.06 0.26 (ppm)

deshielded compared to protons of ethane, $CH_3–CH_3$.

(vi) The methylene protons to which nitro group in 1-nitropropane is attached appears at δ 4.31, while the corresponding protons of propane absorb at 0.9 ppm.

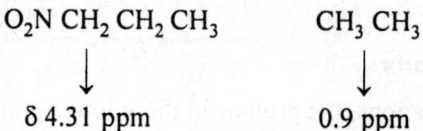

$$O_2N\ CH_2\ CH_2\ CH_3 \qquad CH_3\ CH_3$$

$$\downarrow \qquad\qquad\qquad \downarrow$$

$$\delta\ 4.31\ ppm \qquad\qquad 0.9\ ppm$$

(vii) It can be concluded from the above examples, that the substitution of a proton by an electronegative group can lead to deshielding of the remaining protons in the group. That is there seems to exist a linear relationship between chemical shift and electronegativity. In fact, if more than one electronegative group is present, then deshielding seems to become **additive.**

This is reflected in the following series of chloromethane CH_3Cl, dichloromethane CH_2Cl_2 and chloroform, $CHCl_3$.

	$CHCl_3$	CH_2Cl_2	CH_3Cl
δ ppm	7.3	5.3	3.0

In fact, this becomes more clear from another series :

	$CHBr_3$	CH_2Br_2	CH_3Br
δ ppm	6.8	5.0	2.0

One more example is the iodo-series :

	CHI_3	CH_2I_2	CH_3I
δ ppm	4.9	3.9	2.1

(viii) The slight electronegativity difference between carbon and hydrogen seems to be responsible for the slight differences observed between the chemical shifts of 1°, 2° and 3° hydrogens.

$$
\begin{array}{ccc}
R & R & \\
\diagdown & \diagdown & \\
R\!-\!C\!-\!H & CH_2 & R\ CH_3 \\
\diagup & \diagup & \\
R & R &
\end{array}
$$

δ ppm	1.5	1.3	0.9

We think, it is due to slightly larger electronegativity of carbon compared to hydrogen.

(ix) The deshielding effect of a halogen decreases with distance as expected. This is clear from the following example. In fact, the electronegativity effect almost fades on a proton that is more three carbons far.

	CH_3–Cl	CH_3–CH_2–Cl
δ ppm	3.0	1.5

Thus, the methyl protons in methyl chloride CH_3Cl are deshielded more compared to methyl protons in ethyl chloride.

(x) The methyl derivatives of Hg, Cd, Zn and Mg follows the order :

$$Hg > Cd > Zn > Mg$$
(as methyl derivatives)

This again, reflects the differences in electronegativities of these elements and carbon. The ionic character in these compounds increases in the opposite order to 9%, 15%, 18% and 35% respectively.

(ii) *Electron density effects in carbocations*

Due to presence of positive charge in carbocations, the protons in these ions get strongly deshielded.

Examples

1. **tert-Butyl carbocation :** The methyl protons resonate at δ 4.35 in tert-butyl carbocation.

$$CH_3$$

$$H_3C \quad CH_3$$

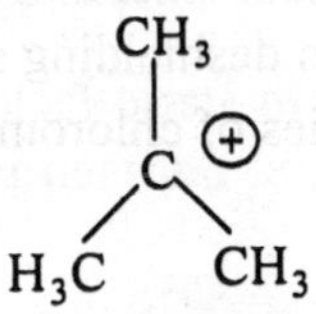

$$\delta = 4.35 \text{ ppm}$$

2. **Isopropyl carbocation :**

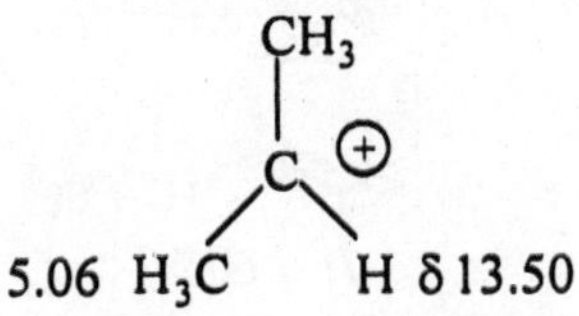

$$CH_3$$

$$5.06 \; H_3C \qquad H \; \delta \, 13.50$$

Isopropyl carbocation

Obviously, the proton directly attached to the carbon bearing the positive charge is so strongly deshielded that it absorbs at δ 13.5 ppm. As the distance of the proton from the carbon bearing the positive charge increases, the deshielding becomes relatively smaller.

3. **Cyclopropenylium carbocation :** The hydrogen present directly onto the ring is more deshielded as expected.

Compared to hydrogens present on the side chain attached to the ring as shown below.

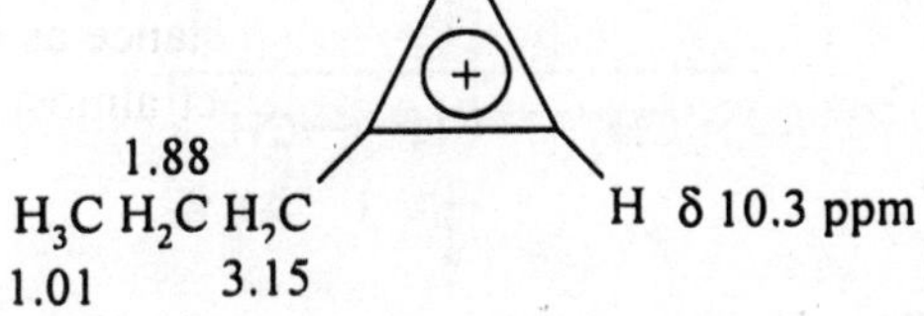

$$CH_2CH_2CH_3$$

$$1.88$$
$$H_3C \; H_2C \; H_2C \qquad \qquad H \; \delta \, 10.3 \text{ ppm}$$
$$1.01 \qquad 3.15$$

Deshielding of Protons in dipropyl cyclopropenylium carbocation

(iii) *Phenyl dimethyl methane carbocation*

The ortho and para hydrogens are deshielded compared to benzene protons (δ = 7.2 ppm). While the ortho protons resonate at δ 8.80 ppm, the para proton resonates at δ 8.45 ppm. The meta proton is also deshielded though to a smaller extent.

(iv) *Trimethyl anilinium carbocation*

Here, resonance can not play any role due to steric factors. Hence, only the substitution effect due to inductive effect (+ I) of positively charged nitrogen plays its role in deshielding the o, m and p protons.

(v) *Allyl carbocations*

The chemical shifts for the allyl carbocation are as under :

The Allyl carbocation

Evidently, the terminal protons are strongly deshielded and absorb at δ 8.97 ppm.

However, surprisingly, the proton at the central carbon is also and even more deshielded as it resonates at δ 9.64 ppm. This is unexpected if resonance or the Huckel Molecular Orbital Model is in action. This suggests the sharing and presence of sufficient positive charge on this carbon.

(vi) *Electron density effects in aliphatic carbanions*

If electron density effects play their role in deshielding the protons in carbocations, they must show the opposite effects in carbanions. Indeed it is so. The protons in carbanions get shielded to the extent that they appear on the upfield side of TMS! **That is they show negative chemical shifts as the electron density around the attached protons gets increased.**

Examples

1. **Methyl carbanion :** The methyl protons of methyl carbanion in methyl lithium resonate at $-\delta$ 1.3 ppm.

$$\overset{\ominus}{C}H_3 \overset{\oplus}{Li}$$

$$\delta -1.3 \text{ ppm}$$
Methyl carbanion

2. **Ethyl carbanion :** The methylene protons absorb at $\delta -0.99$ and the methyl protons resonate at $\delta +1.33$ in ethyl carbanion in ethyl lithium.

$$CH_3 \text{——} \overset{\ominus}{C}H_2 \quad \overset{+}{Li}$$
$$1.33 \qquad -0.99$$
Ethyl carbanion

Similar results are obtained in diethyl magnesium.

$$\left(\overset{1.26}{CH_3} \text{——} CH_2 \right)_2 Mg$$
$$\downarrow$$
$$-0.64$$

3. **Allyl carbanion :** The allyl carbanion occurs as a resonance hybrid.

$$\overset{\ominus}{C}H_2 \text{——} CH \text{===} CH_2 \longleftrightarrow CH_2 \text{===} CH \text{——} \overset{\ominus}{C}H_2$$

$$\text{\textbar\textbar\textbar}$$

$$CH_2 \text{----} CH \text{----} CH_2$$
$$2.46 \qquad\qquad 2.46$$
$$\downarrow$$
$$\delta \text{ 6.28 ppm}$$
Allyl carbanion

The terminal protons are shielded such that they resonate at 2.46 ppm. Proton at the middle carbon absorbs at δ 6.28 ppm showing it to be deshielded. In other words, the negative charge is localized on the terminal carbons.

(vii) *Electron density effects in aromatic carbanions*

The charge present on these anions gets delocalized on the ring positions due to **resonance.** Hence, as expected the ortho and para positions are shielded compared to insubstituted benzene protons that absorb at δ 7.27 ppm.

Examples

1. **Benzyl carbanion :**

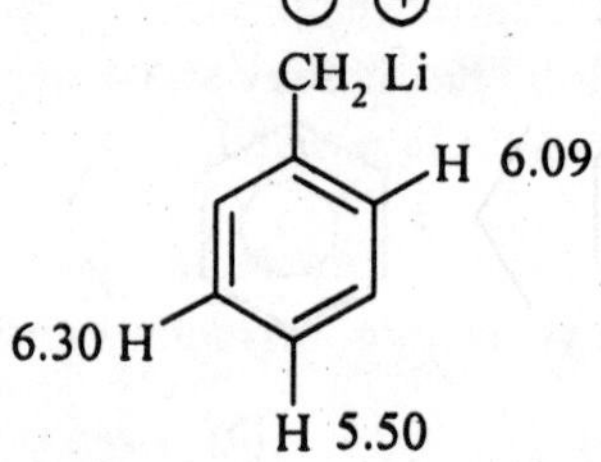

$$CH_2 \overset{\ominus}{} \overset{\oplus}{} Li$$

Benzyl carbanion in benzyl lithium

With ring positions labeled: H 6.09 (ortho), 6.30 H (meta), H 5.50 (para)

Thus, the ortho and para hydrogens absorbs at δ 6.09 and δ 5.50 respectively while the meta is also shielded and absorbs at δ 6.30 ppm.

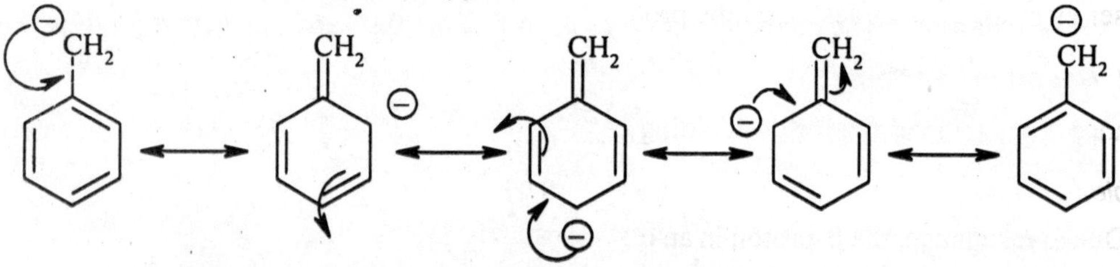

Resonance in benzyl carbanion

2. **Cyclopentadienyl carbanion :** The proton of the cyclopentadienyl carbanion is shielded and appears at δ 5.37 ppm in cyclopentadienyl lithium.

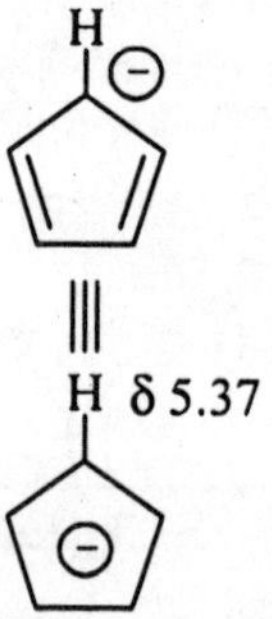

H δ 5.37

Cyclopentadienyl anion

(viii) π-Electron density influence on chemical shift in aromatic ions

A linear relationship between π-electron density and chemical shift in unsaturated compounds is observed. Thus, if π-electron density per carbon atom is less than that in benzene, the chemical shift of these aromatic compounds is found to be shielded compared to the hydrogen of benzene (δ 7.27 ppm). In case, it was more than that of the benzene carbon, the attached proton was deshielded.

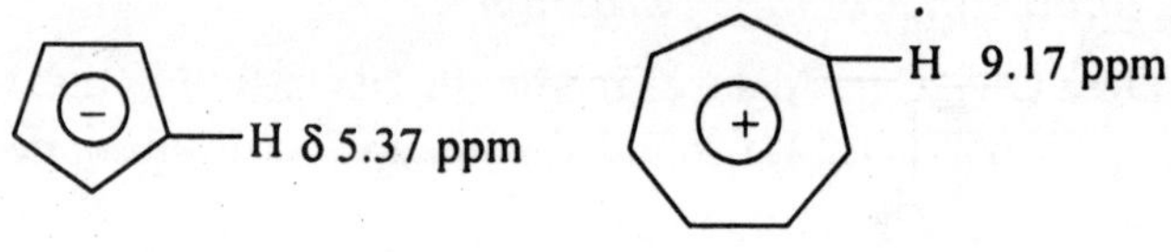

H δ 5.37 ppm   H 9.17 ppm

Thus, cyclopentadienyl anion protons resonate at δ 5.37 ppm as it has π electron density per carbon that is 20% more of an electron density per carbon of benzene. The reverse is true for tropylium cation whose proton resonate at δ 9.17 ppm.

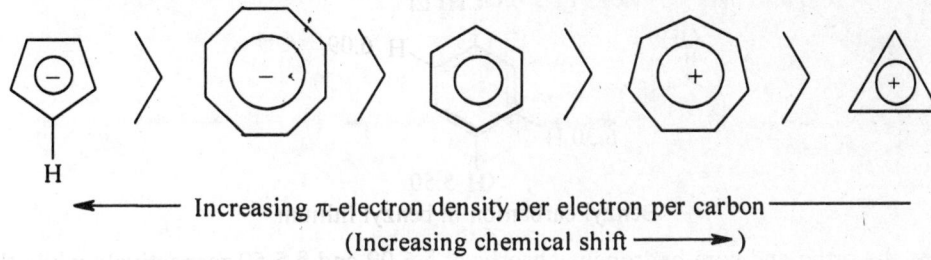

← ——— Increasing π-electron density per electron per carbon ———
(Increasing chemical shift ——→)

Obviously, more electron density at the carbon makes the proton of the C–H bond shielded while the lesser electron density deshields the proton.

2.5.2.2 *Resonance effects*

Resonance leads to shielding or deshielding effects.

Examples

(i) Due to resonance, the β-proton in an α, β-unsaturated ketone (i.e. vinyl hydrogen β to α carbonyl group) gets deshielded as shown below.

Obviously, the electron density gets removed from the β-carbon atom which develops some positive charge.

(ii) The aldehydic proton which in general absorbs in the range 9-10 ppm also show, deshielding in part due to resonance effect:

The electron density from between C–H bond is in turn pulled by the positively charged carbon. The proton thus gets deshielded.

(iii) The resonance effect is again visible in methyl propenyl ether in which the β-hydrogen is shielded.

Of course, the α-proton is deshielded due to inductive effect (–I) of the electronegative oxygen.

(iv) **Resonance effects in Phenols:** The ortho and para proton in phenols are shielded because of resonance. The OH group donates its electron pair to the ring as a result of which the electron density at ortho and para positions gets increased.

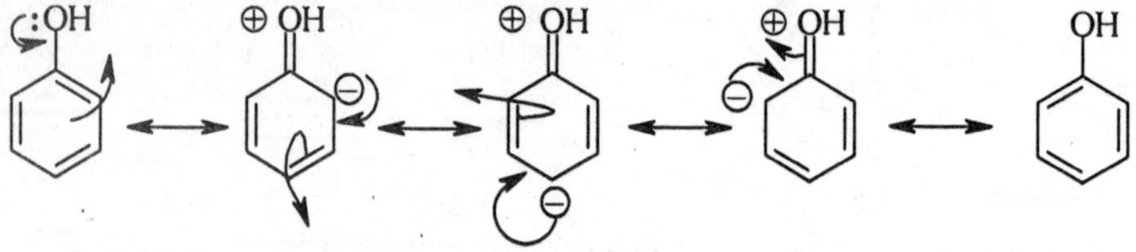

Resonance in Phenol

This proton gets shielded as electron density is increased at the carbon to which it is joined. Electron density is increased at ortho and para positions w.r. to OH group. This leads to an increase in the electron density in the C–H bond, consequently, increased electron density gives rise to increased induced secondary magnetic field that opposes the applied field. Hence, these protons are shielded.

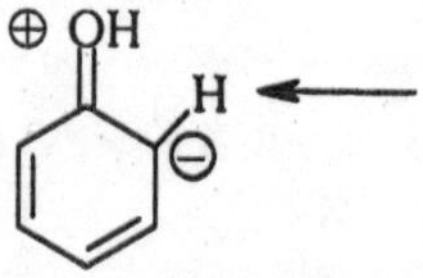

This proton gets shielded as electron density is increased at the carbon to which it is joined

(v) **Resonance effects in Nitrobenzene :** While resonance effects lead to shielding of O– and P– protons, they cause deshielding of these protons in nitrobenzene as shown below which the ortho protons resonate at δ 8.21 ppm, the para protons resonate at δ 7.60 ppm, as opposed to meta that absorbs at δ 7.47 ppm.

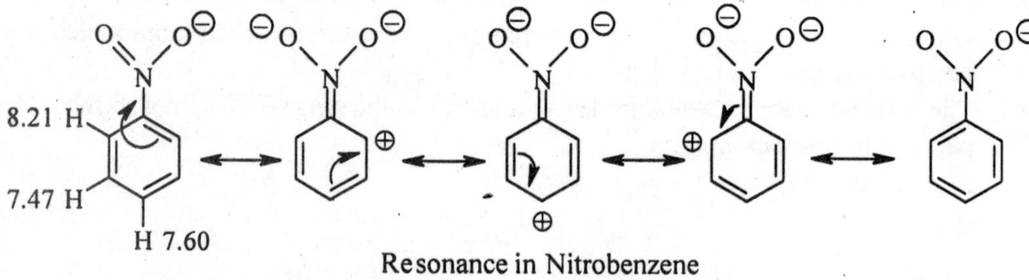

Resonance in Nitrobenzene

2.5.2.3 *Hybridization effects*

Hybridisation is an important basic effect in chemistry and therefore it is important to involve this concept with respect to changes in chemical shifts.

1. *sp³ protons*

The protons that are attached to sp^3 hybridised carbons absorb in the chemical shift range of 0-2 ppm. However, the upper range may increase if some groups that withdraw the electron density from around the protons are attached to the sp^3 carbon bearing the protons, which we have already discussed at length.

Among the protons attached to 3°, 2° and 1° (sp³)carbons, the decreasing order of chemical shifts is as follows :

δ ppm   1.5   1.3   0.9

The cyclopropyl protons are, of course, shielded and absorb in the range of upto 1 ppm from TMS.

2. sp² protons

The alkene protons which are attached to sp² hybridised carbons, resonate in the range of 4-6 ppm. Evidently, the sp² hydrogens appear at low field or we can say they are deshielded compared to the sp³ hydrogens. Why?

Let us try to find a suitable relationship here. We can think of one between the sp² hybridised carbon and electronegativity as we have already discussed as to how the later deshields a hydrogen.

The sp² carbon is more electronegative compared to a sp³ carbon. The reason is that there is more s-character (about 33%) in sp² carbon than in an sp³ carbon which has only 25% of s-character. In other words, we can say that sp² carbon has more ability to hold the electron-density on itself. So, the proton will be less shielded. Or we can also say that there is lower electron density around the proton in the C–H bond, and this deshields the proton. However, the deshielding observed is more than expected. Clearly, there is another factor – the dominant one called anisotropy which will be discussed next.

3. sp protons (Acetylenic Protons)

Going by the trend of deshielding that occurs when we shift from sp³ to sp² hydrogens, it can be easily concluded that the acetylenic hydrogens should be most deshielded. That is the order should be :

Increasing δ value from TMS (expected order)

This is to be anticipated as sp carbon is more electronegative (50% s character) than an sp^2 carbon which in turn is more electronegative than an sp carbon.

When we look at the chemical shifts of the acetylenic hydrogens, we find the situation to be the other way around as compared to olefinic protons. The acetylenic hydrogen absorbs in chemical shift range of 2-3 ppm compound to 4-6 ppm, that for olefinic protons.

$$R-C=C-H$$
4-6 ppm
Olefinic hydrogens

$$R-C\equiv C-H$$
2-3 ppm
Acetylenic hydrogens

Obviously, (sp)-character and the electronegativity factors are insufficient to explain the observed anomaly here. Then, what could be an alternative explanation here?

$$HC\equiv CH \qquad CH_2=CH_2$$
2.88 \qquad\qquad 5.84

Here, the idea of magnetic anisotropy was invoked to explain this anomaly away as shown in next section.

The idea of magnetic anisotropy was also required not only to explain the above anomaly but also to explain away the differences noted in chemical shifts of the axial and equatorial hydrogens in cyclohexane observed at − 90°C i.e. at low temperature studies. The equatorial hydrogens are shielded compared to axial hydrogens by 0.5 ppm (see Fig. 2.8).

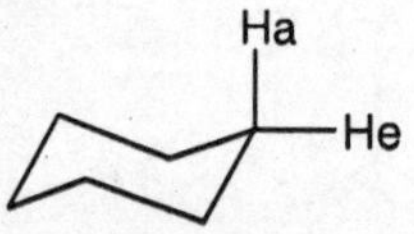

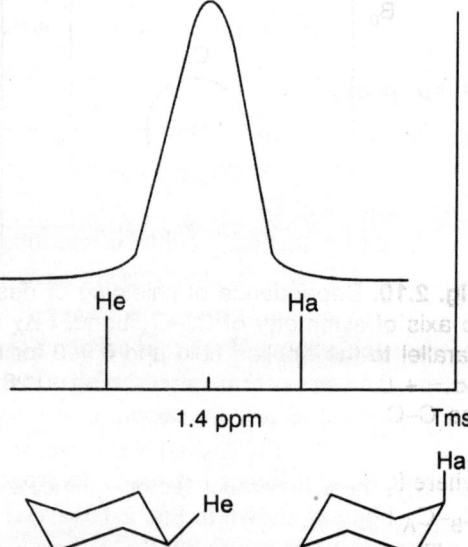

Fig. 2.8. The PMR of cyclohexane (a) at R–T, when a broad peak appears at δ 1.4 due to both equatorial and axial, (b) At − 90°C, when He is deshielded compared to Ha, due to magnetic anisotropy.

2.5.2.4 *Magnetic anisotropy*

Origin of magnetic anisotropy

Whether a proton attached to a C–C bond will be shielded or deshielded will depend upon its orientation with respect to the axis of symmetry of the C–C bond as shown in Fig. 2.9 in an applied magnetic field, B_0.

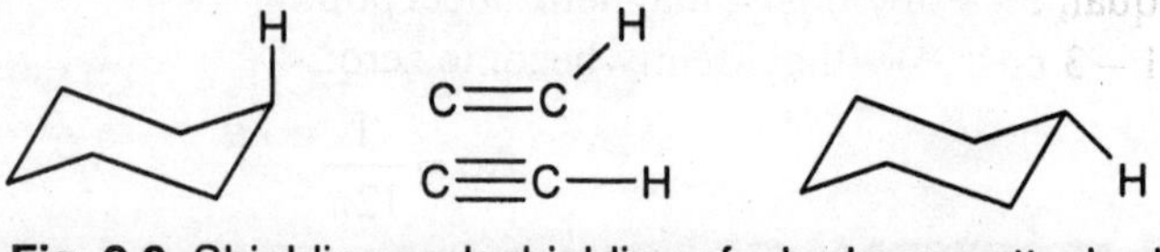

Consider a $C_{(B)}-C_{(A)}-H$ bond.

The dependence of shielding or deshielding of a proton on the orientation

Fig. 2.9. Shielding or deshielding of a hydrogen attached to a C–C bond will depend upon its orientation with respect to the axis of symmetry of this bond.

of the proton with respect to the axis of symmetry of the $C_{(B)}-C_{(A)}$ bond to which it is attached can be traced to the relation of the magnetic susceptibility $\Delta\chi$ of the $C_{(A)}-C_{(B)}$ bond. It is given by the relation

$$\Delta\sigma = \Delta\chi \ (1-3 \ \cos^2\theta)/12\pi R^3$$

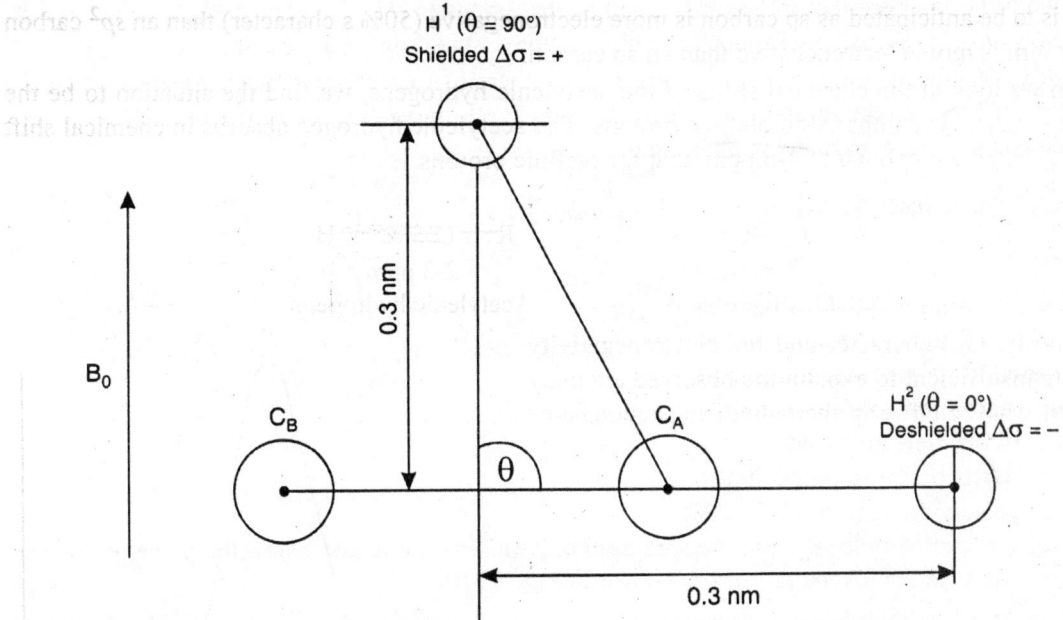

Fig. 2.10. Dependence of shielding or deshielding of a proton of C_B–C_A frame on its orientation w.r. to axis of symmetry of C_B–C_A bond. I $\Delta\chi$ C_B–C_A = 140 × 10^{-36} m^3 per molecule and θ = 90° for H^1 parallel to the applied field and θ = 0 for the H^2 along the axis of symmetry of $C_{(B)}$–$C_{(A)}$ bond, then, $\Delta\sigma$ = + 0.14 ppm for H^1 and Ds = – 0.28 ppm if the distance of the two protons from the centre of the C–C bond is 0.3 nm each.

where R is the distance between a hydrogen attached to $C_{(A)}$ of the C_B–C_A bond and the centre of the C_B–C_A bond as shown in Fig. 2.10.

The magnetic susceptibility is proportional to magnetic moment, μ, which is generated due to circulation of electrons on application of B_0. This $\mu c(A)$ will have three components $\mu A(x)$, $\mu A(y)$ and $\mu A(z)$ along the three cartesian coordinates. While H attached to the C_A experiences B_0 and B^1 when μ is along z-direction (μz) or when it is in y direction (μy), it is deshielded, it experiences lesser field B^0–B^1 (it is shielded) when μ is in the x direction. As the sample is in solution form, therefore, due to Brownian motion, the molecule undergoes tumbling and averaging is the result. It μx, μy, μz are all equal, then obviously, magnetic susceptibility will be zero as per the following equation in which case $(1 - 3\cos^2\theta)$ will evidently become zero:

$$\Delta\sigma = \frac{1}{12\pi} \sum_{i=x,y,z} \chi_A^i (1 - 3\cos^2\theta i)/R^3$$

where R symbolises the separation between the centres of the carbon and hydrogen atoms in the C_B–C_A–H bond.

Now, a question arises what will be the situation like when we consider hydrogens attached to multiply bonded carbons such as C=C, C=O, C≡C, C≡N etc. Obviously, these systems will show magnetic anisotropy and in fact more so, as due to π electrons circulation, they will have larger magnetic moments or succeptibilities.

It is worth noting here that in general, the chemical bonds to which hydrogen is attached are all magnetically anisotropic, otherwise no such shielding or deshielding would be observed.

In conclusion, magnetic anisotropy is a phenomenon wherein protons in different parts of the molecule experience different effective applied field ($B_{eff} = B_0 \pm \sigma$), depending upon the orientation of the molecular axis with respect to the applied field.

EXAMPLES OF ANISOTROPY

1. Alkenes

The alkene protons, in general, absorb in the range 4.5–6.0 ppm. The range is too high compared to sp^3 protons, and is hard to explain without the concept of aniso-tropic effect of the π-electrons. Maximum deshielding is to be anticipated if the alkene molecule is at right angle to the

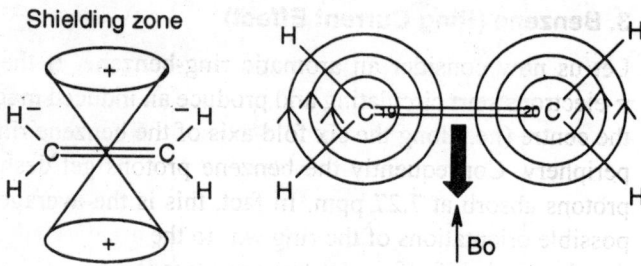

Fig. 2.11. Anisotropy in alkenes.

direction of the applied field, B_0. The induced field opposes Bo above and below the plane of the ring whereas it reinforces the alkene protons as shown in Fig. 2.11.

As the alkene molecule can align itself w.r. to *Bo* in many other orientations, obviously the observed range of chemical shift is averaged to 4.5–6.0 ppm.

Intext Exercise

1. While the circulated methyl protons in α-pinene absorb at 0.85 ppm, the corresponding protons in β-pinene absorb at 0.72 ppm. Explain.

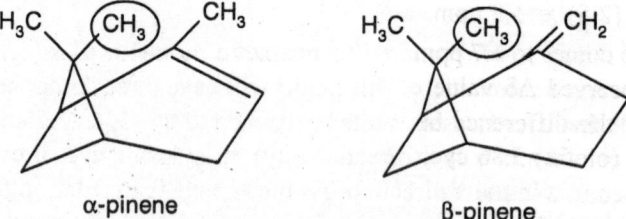

α-pinene   β-pinene

The reason for this observed fact is that the methyl protons in a-pinene are deshielded as they lie outside the shielding cone. On the other hand, the corresponding methyl protons lie in the shielding cone of the double bond in β-pinene.

---

2. Acetylene

If we take into account, the criterion of electronegativity, we would expect sp protons to be deshielded relative to sp^2 protons as sp carbon is more electronegative. However, it is found that the sp protons are rather shielded compared to sp^2 protons! On the other hand, if the acetylene molecule is held perpendicular to the applied field Bo, it is to be expected in view of the stronger induced field of the π-electrons which number four compared to two in C = C, the acetylenic protons would be more deshielded than alkene protons, the range will be more than 4.5–6.0. However, the range is rather smaller. So, what could be the best explanation?

The suggested explanation is that the acetylenic molecule holds itself mainly in a vertical axis orientation w.r. to B_0, the applied field. Consequently, the protons lie in the shielding zone and hence are shielded.

3. Benzene (Ring Current Effect)

Let us now consider an aromatic ring-benzene. If the benzene ring orients itself at 90° to B_0, the π-electrons start circulating and produce an induced magnetic field that opposes the applied field Bo in the centre (i.e. along the six fold axis of the benzene ring) but reinforces the protons of the ring at the periphery. Consequently the benzene protons get deshielded (low-field shift). That is why benzene protons absorb at 7.27 ppm. In fact, this is the average of the chemical shifts of these protons in all possible orientations of the ring w.r. to the applied field. One good formula that can be used to predict the chemical shift of the benzene protons is :

$$\Delta\delta = \mu(1-3\cos^2\theta)/r^3$$

where μ is the induced dipole, θ is the angle of the proton from the six fold axis ring and r is the distance of the proton from the centre of the ring as shown in Fig. 2.12. If the proton were to lie above or below the centre of the ring plane i.e. at 0°, $\Delta\delta$ will become negative which means the proton will be shielded or shifted upfield.

If $\theta = 90°$, $\Delta\delta$ will be positive at an angle of $\cos^{-1}\theta = 1/3$, $\Delta\delta$ will be zero which means there will be no shift. Now let us suppose, r in the above equation is equal to 2.5 Å, $\theta = 90°$ and $\mu = 27.0$, then as per the above equation :

$$\Delta\delta = 27\,(1-3\cos^2 90)\,(2.5)^3$$
$$= 27\,(2.5)^3 = 1.7 \text{ ppm}$$

Thus, calculated $\Delta\delta$ comes to 1.7 ppm. This is in close agreement with the observed $\Delta\delta$ value of 1.4 ppm. The latter value is actually the difference between the δ_H of benzene (7.27) and δ_H (olefin) 5.86 cyclohexadiene.

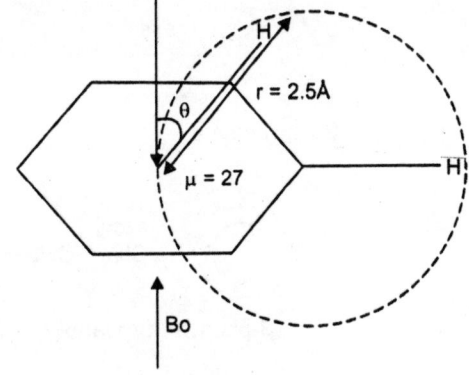

Fig. 2.12.

4. Benzyl protons

Anisotropy effect is also seen to occur on benzylic protons. The benzylic protons in toluene and p-xylene absorb at somewhat downfield δ 2.32 and δ 2.25 as compared to ordinary alkyl protons.

Toluene   p-xylene   Mesitylene

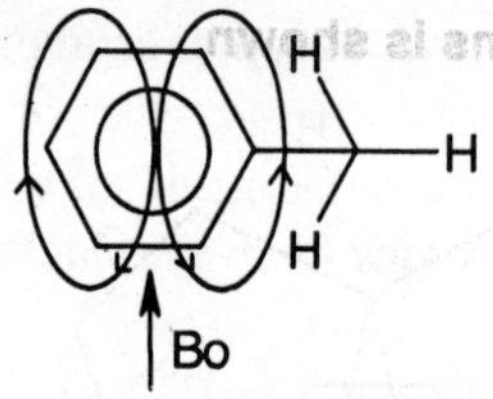

Anisotropy effect on CH_3 protons in Toluene

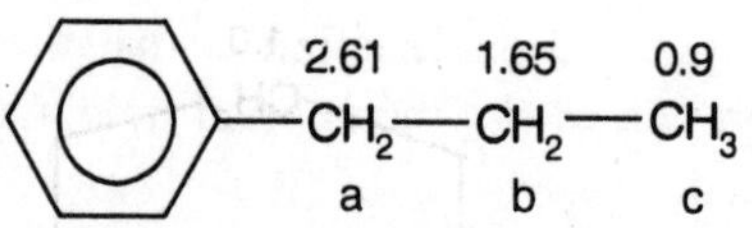

n-propyl benzene

This effect is more clear in *n*-propyl benzene. The benzylic protons (a) are more deshielded (δ 2.61) than the CH_2 protons (δ 1.65) attached to the methyl group (δ 0.9) which do not experience anisotropy effect being far removed from the nucleus.

More examples of deshielding effect on benzyl protons due to ring current anisotropy are shown below:

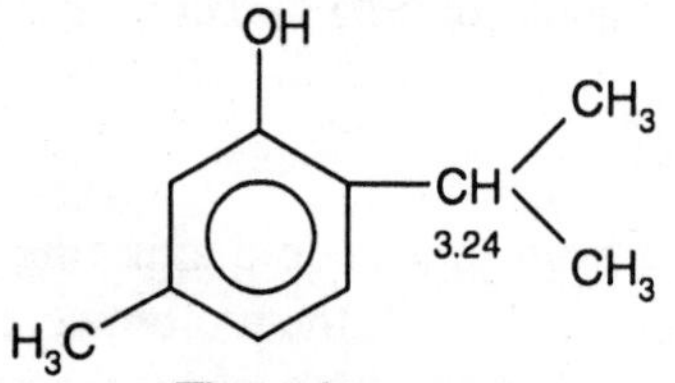

Thymol

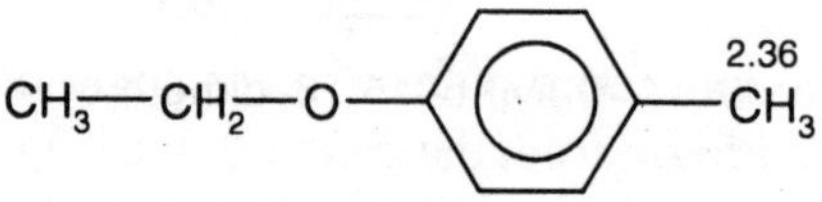

p-Methoxytoluene

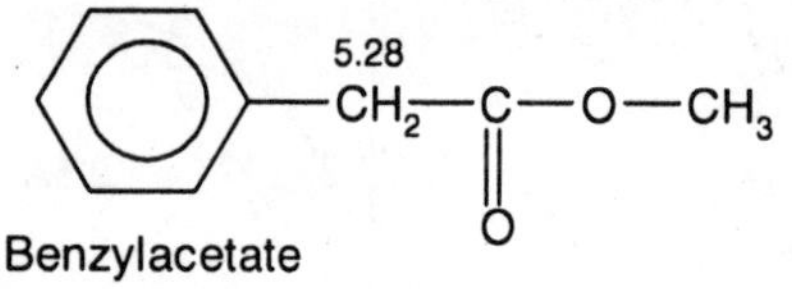

Benzylacetate

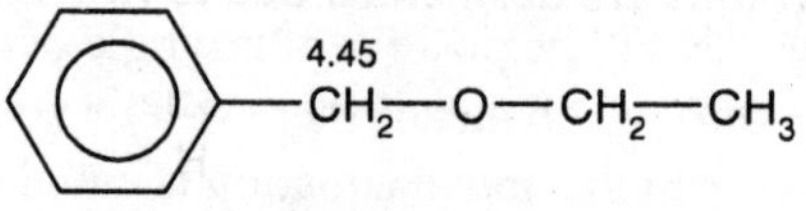

Benzyl ethyl ether

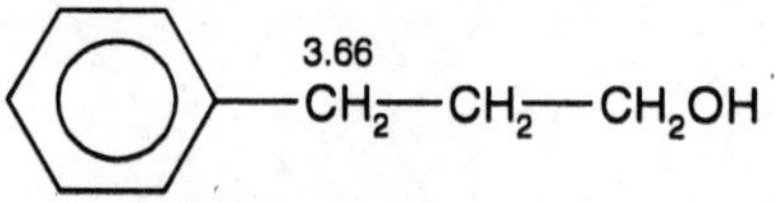

3-phenyl-1-propanol

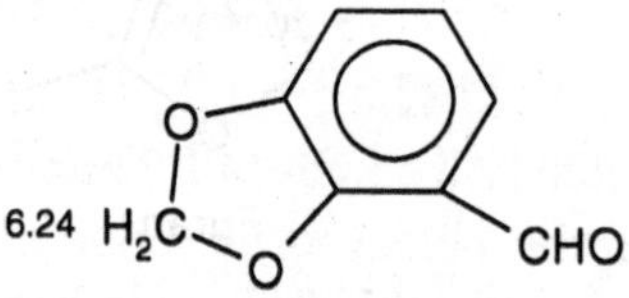

Piperonal

5. [10]–Paracyclophane

This is an example that elegantly demonstrates the ring current effect. As you can see, different methylene protons absorb at different chemical shift depending upon their position with reference to the benzene ring as shown herein.

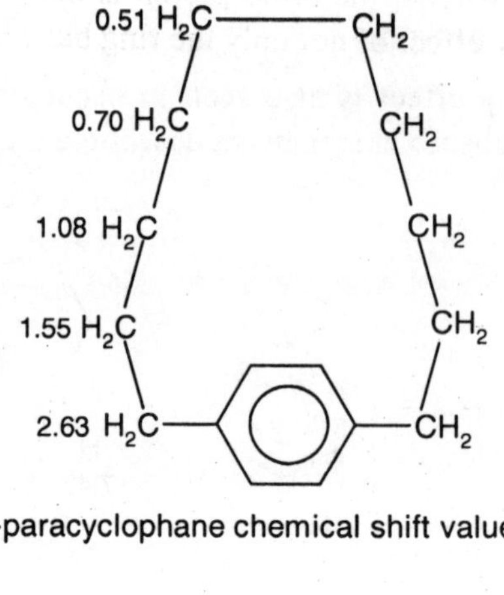

[10]-paracyclophane chemical shift values in ppm

6. Ring Current Anisotropy Effect in some more systems is shown.

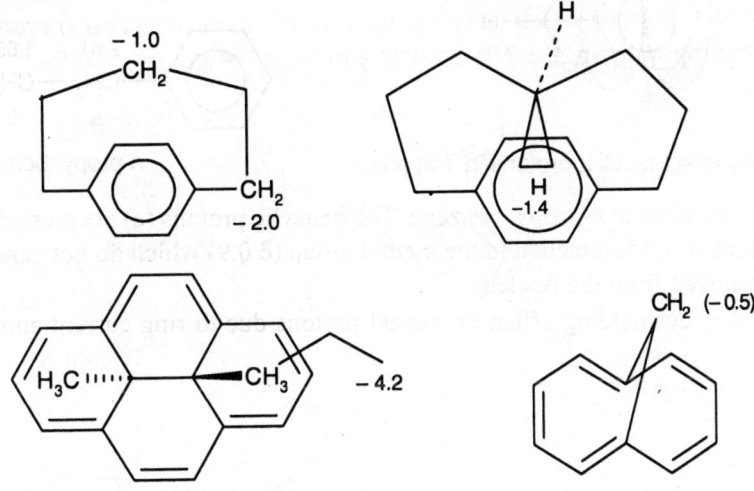

15,16–Dihydro–15,16–dimethylpyrene

7. Furan

The furan protons are deshielded due to ring current anisotropy effect by about 1 ppm :

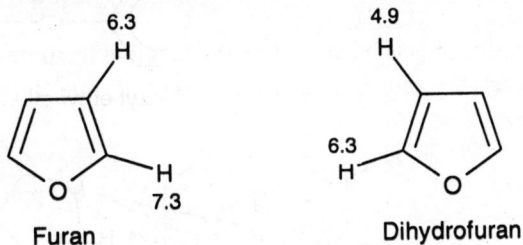

Furan

Dihydrofuran

8. Acetophenone

In acetophenone, the ortho-proton is most deshielded because it falls in the deshielding zone of the anisotropy effect of not only the ring but also the carbonyl group :

9. Porphyrins

In porphyrins, the N–H protons which lie within the ring are shielded and outer protons are deshielded. For example, in coproporphyrin, the NH protons absorb at -4 ppm, while the outer, meso protons, absorb at 10 ppm.

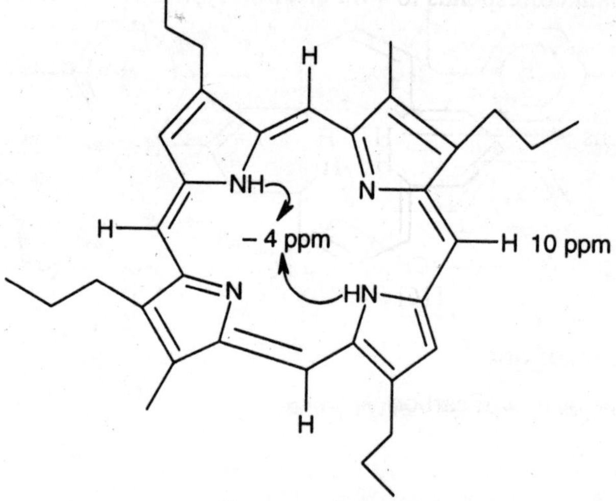

Coproporphyrin–1

10. Annulenes

(a) [14]–annulene is aromatic. This is borne out by the fact that the outer proton absorb at δ 7.6 ppm, while the inner ones are very much shielded as expected, due to ring current anisotropy effect and absorb at 0.0 ppm.

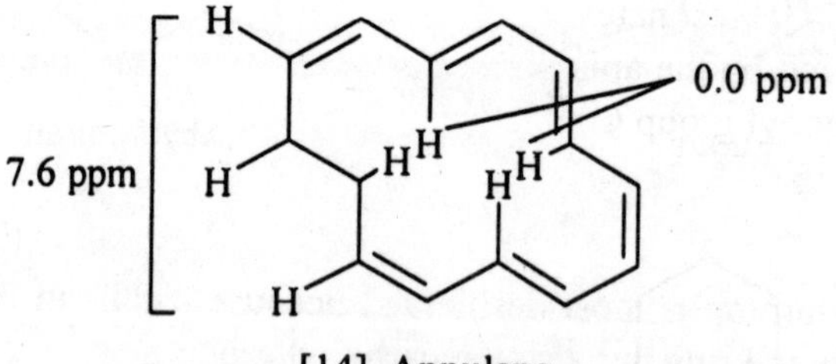

[14]–Annulene

(b) [18] annulene is aromatic. Proton NMR spectroscopy shows that while the outer twelve protons resonate at 9 ppm, the inner six protons are upfield at 3 ppm.

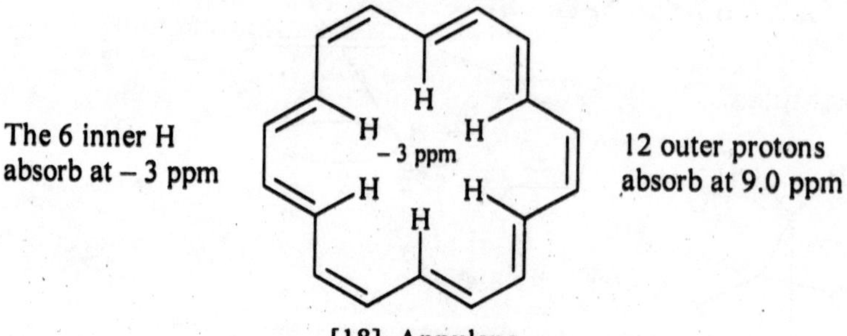

[18]–Annulene

(c) [16] annulene is not an aromatic compound. NMR spectrum of this molecule at – 130°C, shows two types of protons. The inner four protons absorb at 10.56 ppm, while the outer twelve protons absorb at + 5.35 (not – 5.35) ppm. This shows that the inner protons are not shielded. The [16] annulene system (that corresponds to 4 $n\pi$ electron system) is therefore not aromatic in nature.

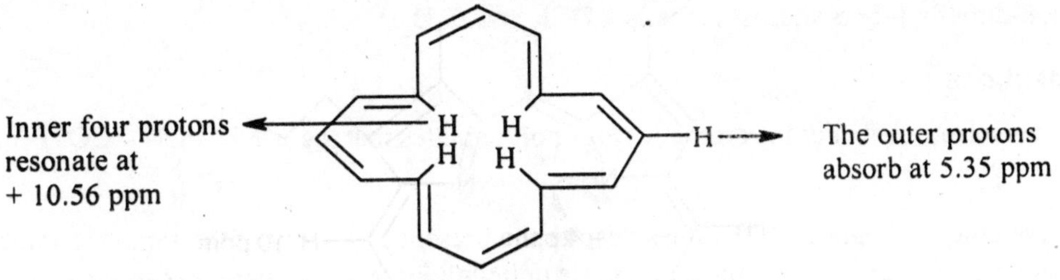

Inner four protons ⟵ resonate at + 10.56 ppm

The outer protons absorb at 5.35 ppm

[16] Annulene

11. 4,4–Dimethylcyclohexenone

This is an example of Anisotropy of carbonyl group on olefinic protons.

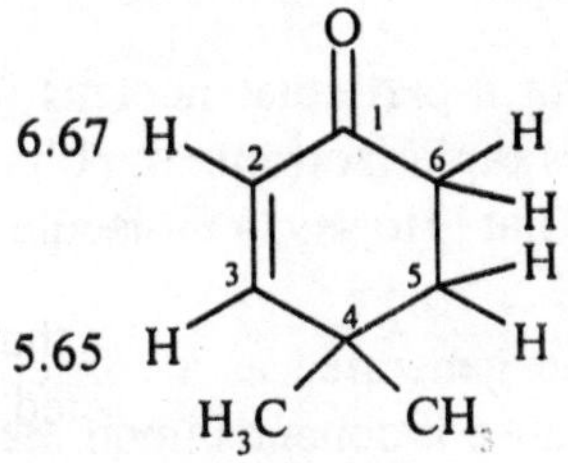

6.67 H
5.65 H
H
H
H
H
H_3C CH_3

In this molecule, while C–3H resonates at 5.65 ppm, the C–2H absorbs at δ 6.67 ppm. Evidently the last proton is being deshielded by the anisotropy of not only the double bond C=C, but also by the anisotropy effect of the carbonyl group C=O.

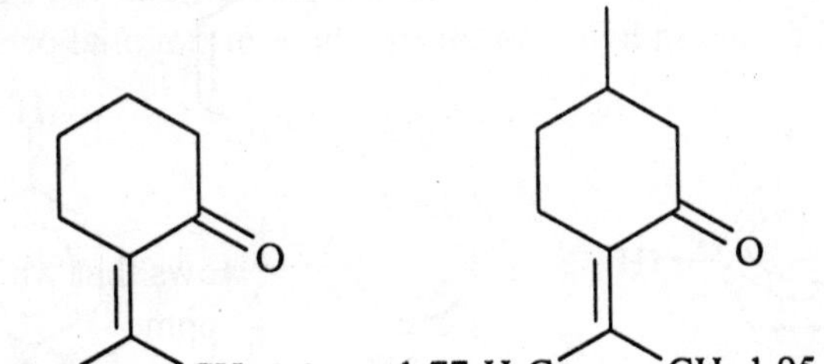

H_3C CH_3 1.0   1.77 H_3C CH_3 1.95

12. Some more examples

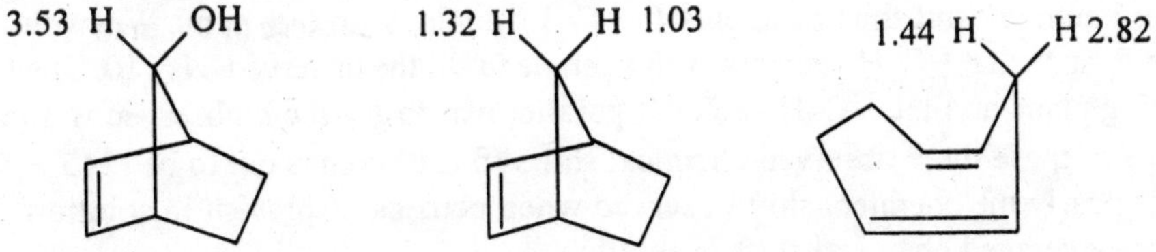

3.53 H   OH   1.32 H   H 1.03   1.44 H   H 2.82

13. Effect of Benzene as a solvent

When benzene (C_6D_6), C_6–benzene is used as solvent for recording of the NMR spectra of the natural products, overlapped chemical shifts get "spread out" by as much as 1 ppm. This is a consequence of the anisotropic effects of aromatic ring. This is sometimes called "Benzene trick". The effect is clearly seen for 4,4–dimethyl–5–α androstanone is $CDCl_3$ and C_6D_6.

14. Polypeptides

It is due to anisotropy effect of the aromatic rings polypeptides that the $(-NH-CH-CO-)$ monomeric

$$R$$

unit can have unique chemical shift values despite the presence of many of the same monomer units in the globular proteins. For instance, the monomeric unit with R = Me (i.e. alanine) can show five different δ values for the five methyl doublets in a polypeptide or protein (e.g. A5, A15, A28, A98). The main reason is that these monomeric units experience different inhomogeneous anisotropic effects of the aromatic rings present in the side chains of the nearby aromatic amino acids.

15. Chemical Shift Anisotropy (CSA)

The solution chemical shift reported for a particular nucleus is actually an average weighted value. This is because the molecule undergoes rapid isotropic tumbling. Its position w.r. to the applied field B_0, is not fixed and goes on changing. That is to say, a molecule orients itself w.r. to applied field in all possible orientations equally over time.

The intensity of the secondary field generated as a consequence of the electron circulation is a function of the orientation. This is because it depends upon the amount of electron circulation which depends upon the orientation of the molecule w.r. to the applied field B_0.

How do we know as to what will be the chemical shift of the nucleus of interest in a particular orientation w.r. to B_0? Clearly, this can not be done in a solution phase. However, it becomes possible to do that in solid state NMR wherein we can lock the molecule in the desired orientation. Thus, the chemical shifts of the C–13 nuclei in benzene for the three orthogonal orientation are shown below:

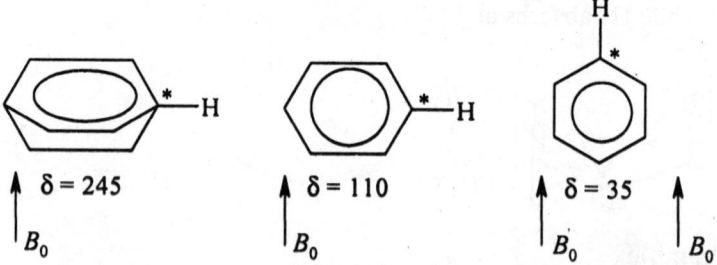

Obviously, the orientation of the ring plane at 90° to B_0 produces maximum electronic circulation and hence maximum B′ and thus deshields the C–13 nucleus to 245 ppm. When the ring plane is parallel w.r. to B_0 such that ^{13}C–H vector is at right angle to B_0, the observed δ is 110. The last orientation in which the ring plane and the ^{13}C–H vector is parallel w.r. to B_0, the δ observed is a mere 35.

The average of these three observed chemical shifts (δ is 0) comes out to be $(245 + 110 + 35) \div 3 = 130$ which is nearly the chemical shift observed when benzene is present in solution. Evidently, we observe the time-averaged chemical shift in solution.

The variation of the chemical shift with the orientation is known as Chemical Shift Anisotropy (CSA). However, this is mathematically defined as follows: CSA is equal to the difference between the smallest fixed-position chemical shift and the average of the remaining two principle fixed-position chemical shift values. Therefore, for benzene, CSA for ^{13}C is:

$$CSA = [(245 + 110) \div 2] - 35 = 142.5 \text{ ppm}$$

CSA does not influence chemical shifts in solution. However, it helps in relaxation. Further, CSA can be used in case of larger molecules like proteins to sharpen peaks. Normally, in these molecules the rate of molecular rumbling is less so that the CSA due to incomplete averaging broadens NMR lines.

Anisotropic effects of σ electrons : Not only π electrons by σ electrons of a C–C bond too show anisotropic effects. However, the effect is small. In cyclohexane, the equatorial protons are deshielded as compared to axial proton the same carbon $-C_1$. This is due to the anisotropy effect of the σ electrons of C_2–C_3 and C_5–C_6 bonds (Fig.).

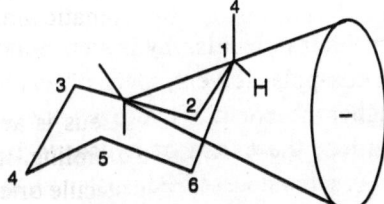

Anisotropic deshielding equatorial proton

2.5.3' Van der Waal's deshielding and steric shielding

If in molecules, the protons attached to different atoms are brought sufficiently close enough, then Vander Waal's repulsion results. The electron cloud around the proton is repelled by that of the bulky group. Thus, in the chair form of the rigid ring of *t*-butyl cyclohexane ring, H_A absorbs at lower field when R is a methyl group then when it is a hydrogen atom. Another example is 4–*t*-butyl 1–bromo cyclohexane in which H_a absorbs at 4.6 while H_a absorbs t 4.6 ppm due to Vanderwaal's repulsion with 3H and 5H protons while He absorbs at 3.83 ppm.

Steric shielding

In the above example, interestingly the chemical shift of the more sterically crowded proton H_{8x} is shielded (δ 0.98 ppm) compared to H_{8y} (δ 1.58 ppm). Similarly the F_{3x} is shielded (δ – 139.18 ppm, from internal $CFCl_3$) relative to F_{3y} (– 100.6 ppm relative to internal $CFCl_3$).

2.5.4 Hydrogen bonding

Protons of hydroxyl group and amino group show a wide range of absorption positions. For example, alcoholic proton absorbs in the range $\delta \sim$ 0.5 to 5.0. Phenolic O–H absorb in 4.0–7.0 amino proton (N–H) at 0.5 $\sim$ 5.0, protons of carboxylic acid resonate at 10.5 $\sim$ 12.0 ppm and enols at > 15 ppm. Further the range also depends upon the temperature and the nature of the solvent.

The reason for the wide absorption ranges of the above compounds is due to hydrogen bonding. A hydrogen bond is formed between two electronegative atoms and is represented as X–H$\cdots$Y (where X and Y are electronegative elements such as O, N, S or halides. The nature of the forces in a hydrogen bond is electrostatic (i.e. $\overset{\delta-}{X}$—$\overset{\delta+}{H}$$\cdots$$\overset{\delta-}{Y}$ The electron density around the proton gets reduced, so that the proton gets deshielded.

Since the amount or extent of intermolecular hydrogen bonding depends critically upon the concentration of the compound in a non-polar solvent, so the observed chemical shift shows a particular range. Higher the concentration, higher the extent of hydrogen bonding, greater the deshielding. As the concentration decreases upon dilution, the extent of hydrogen bonding also decreases and hence deshielding of the proton becomes lesser and lesser. For instance, the chemical shift of the OH proton which in neat ethanol is 5.28 ppm, becomes 0.78 in very dilute solution in aprotic carbontetrachloride. Intramolecular hydrogen bonding also results in the proton getting deshielded. For example, the OH proton in O-hydroxy acetophenone absorbs at δ 12.0 ppm. The OH proton in enols is greatly deshielded due to stronger hydrogen bonding in enols. For example the OH proton resonates at δ 12.1 in ethylacetoacetate. In acetyl acetone, the enolic proton absorbs at d 15.40 ppm.

o-hydroxyacetophenone   Phenol   Ethylacetoacetate

The carboxylic proton is also deshielded and occurs in the range δ 10–13.2 ppm. This is due to hydrogen bonding. The carboxylic acid occur as dimer due to stable hydrogen bonding.

Carboxylic acid dimer

2.5.4 Intramolecular H-bonding

What do you think, should be the likely situation w.r. to H bonding in phenols such as o-hydroxy-acetophenone.

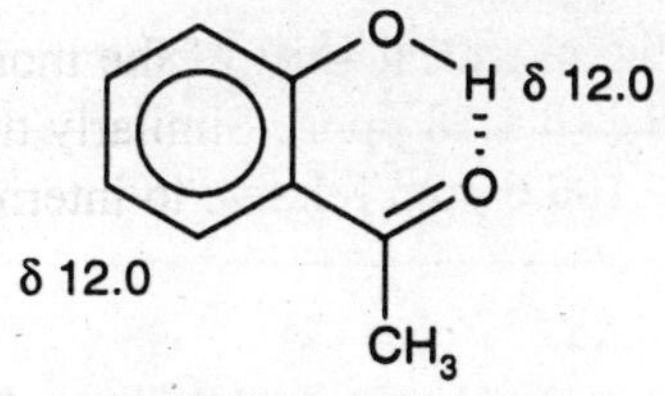

H δ 12.0

δ 12.0

CH₃

o-Hydroxyacetophenone

So, upon dilution, as anticipated, the effect will not be very much. For example, the H of OH in a hydroxy autophenone absorbs at δ 120, even upon dilution, δ 11.5. Not much difference.

Another example is o-hydroxy chlorobenzene. Salicylic acid and acetyl acetone also show intramolecular H-bonding.

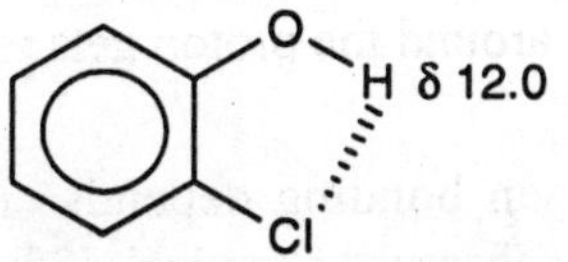

H δ 12.0   δ 6.3 ⟶ δ 5.6 (not much)

Cl   1 M   dilute

R

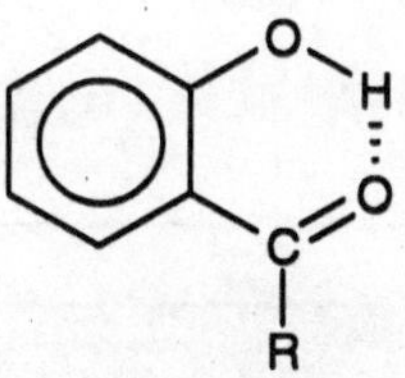

Salicylic acid

δ_{OH} 10–12 ppm

Acetyl acetone (β-diketone)

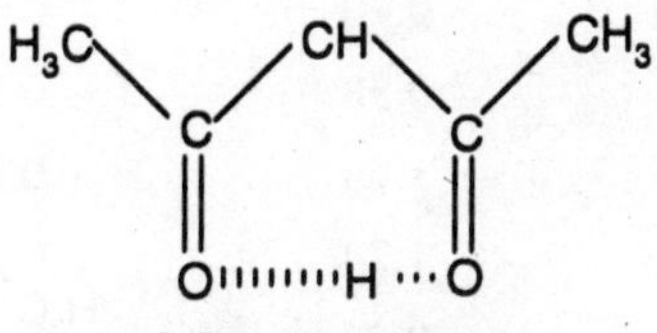

H₃C   CH   CH₃

C   C

Oıııııı.H ···O

δ OH 12–16 ppm

2.5.6 Substituent effects: Schoolery's Rules

(i) **Approximate chemical shifts for protons on carbon bearing more than one substituent :** These are the empirical rules which can be used to predict the chemical shifts of protons in X–CH₂–Y unit. What is to be done is to add the sum of the shielding constants for X and Y to 0.23, the chemical shift of methane. In fact, these are quite good for RCH₂R′, less good for RR′CHR″.

(ii) **Additive shielding increments for alkenes :** These are calculated using the following equation for the alkenes system shown:

$$\sigma_{alkyl} = 0.23 + \sum \sigma_{eff}$$

Group X or Y	σ_{eff}	Group X or Y	σ_{eff}	Group X or Y	σ_{eff}
Cl	2.53	$C \equiv CH$	1.44	SCN	2.30
Br	2.33	CN	1.70	NO_2	2.46
I	1.82	CH_3	0.47	OH	2.56
NRR′	1.57	CF_3	1.14	NCS	2.86
OR	2.36	COOR	1.55	OCOR	3.13
SR	1.64	C CAr	1.65	OPh	3.23
CRO	1.70	$CONR_2$	1.59		
$CR = CR'R''$	1.32	Ph	1.85		

$\sigma_H = 5.25 + Z_{gem} + Z_{cis} + Z_{trans}$ for

system.

Substituent R	Z_{gem}	Z_{cis}	Z_{trans}
H	0.0	0.0	0.0
Alkyl	0.45	− 0.22	− 0.28
Alkyl (cyclic)	0.69	− 0.25	− 0.28
CH_2OH	0.64	− 0.01	− 0.02
CH_2X (X = F, Cl, Br)	0.70	0.11	− 0.04
CH_2N	0.58	− 0.10	− 0.08
C = C (isolated)	1.00	− 0.09	− 0.23
C = C (conjugated)	1.24	0.02	− 0.05
$C \equiv N$	0.27	0.75	0.55
$C \equiv C$	0.47	0.38	0.12
C = O (isolated)	1.10	1.12	0.87
C = O (conjugated)	1.06	0.91	0.74
COOH (isolated)	0.97	1.41	0.71
COOH (conjugated)	0.80	0.98	0.32
CF_3	0.66	0.61	0.32
CHO	1.02	0.95	1.17
OR (R aliphatic)	1.22	− 1.07	− 1.21

(Contd.)

Substituent R	Z_{gem}	Z_{cis}	Z_{trans}
OR (R conjugated)	1.21	− 0.60	− 1.00
OCOR	2.11	− 0.35	− 0.64
CH_2AR	1.05	− 0.29	− 0.32
Cl	1.08	0.18	0.13
Br	1.07	0.45	0.55
I	1.14	0.81	0.88
Ar	1.38	0.36	− 0.07
Ar (o-substituents)	1.65	0.19	0.09

It needs to be noted that the increments 'R conjugated' are to be used instead of 'R isolated' when either of the substituent or the double bond is conjugated with further substituents. The increment alkyl (cyclic) is to be used when both the substituent and the double bond form part of a ring.

2.6 TYPICAL CHEMICAL SHIFTS

Typical chemical shifts for protons range from 0–13 ppm for organic compounds (Table 2.1).

Table 2.1. Typical δH for organic compounds

Proton		Chemical shift (ppm)
Cyclopropane		0.2
Primary	RCH_3	0.9
Secondary	R_2CH	1.3
Tertiory	R_3CH	1.5
Allylic	$C=C-CH_3$	1.7
Ester	CH_3COOR	2.0
Amide	CH_3CONR_2	2.0
Ketonealiph	CH_3COR	2.3
Alkyl-aryl	CH_3-Ar	2.3
Ketone-arom	CH_3COAr	2.6
Aromatic amine	$CH_3-NH-Ar$	3.0
Acetylenic	$C \equiv CH$	1.8–3.1
Vinylic	$CH = CH_2$	4.5–6.0
Aromatic		6.0–9.0
Aldehydic	$R-CHO$	9.4–10.5
Carboxylic	$RCOOH$	10.5–13.0

2.7 CHEMICAL SHIFTS FOR PROTONS OF SATURATED AND UNSATURATED HYDROCARBONS

Chemical shifts range for protons joined to saturated and unsaturated hydrocarbons are collected in Table 2.2 and Table 2.3 respectively.

Table 2.2. Chemical shifts values (ppm) for protons of methyl, methylene, and methine groups attached to various groups (X) shown

X	CH_3–X	RCH_2–X	RR'CH–X (R, R' alkyl)
Alkyl	0.9	1.25	1.5
R⌒⌒	1.69	1.95	2.6
RN = CH–	1.8	–	–
R–C ≡ C–	1.97	2.2	–
– COOR	2.0	2.1	–
– CN	2.0	2.48	2.7
– CONR$_2$	2.02	2.05	–
– COOH	2.07	2.34	2.57
– COR	2.10	2.40	2.5
– SR	2.10	2.40	3.1
– NR$_2$	2.15	2.50	2.87
– I	2.16	3.15	4.2
– CHO	2.17	2.2	2.4
– Ph	2.34	2.62	2.87
– COPh	2.62	–	3.58
– Br	2.65	3.34	4.1
– NRCOR	2.9	3.3	3.5
– Cl	3.02	3.44	4.02
– OR	3.3	3.36	3.8
– OH	3.38	3.56	3.85
– OCOR	3.65	4.15	5.01
– OPh	3.73	3.9	4.0
– OCOPh	3.9	4.23	5.12
– F	4.26	4.35	–
– NO$_2$	4.33	4.4	4.6

Table. 2.3. Chemical shift range for protons joined to saturated carbon i.e. methyl, methylene and methine groups

Chemical shift range (ppm)	Methyl groups	Typical ppm	Methyl groups[a]	Typical δ ppm	Methine groups	Typical δ ppm
< 1	CH_3C- (in sat. hydrocarbons)	0.9	Cyclopropane	0.3		
1–2	CH_3-C-Y	Depends on γ^b	$C-CH_2-C$ (in sat. hydrocarbons)	1.4	$C-CH-C$ (in sat. hydrocarbons)	1.5
	CH_3-C-C (in hydrocarbons)	1.6–2.0	$C-CH_2-C-Y$	Depends on γ^b	$C-CH-C-Y$	Depends on γ^b
2–3	$CH_3-CO-OR$	2.0	$C-CH_2-C=C-$ (in hydrocarbons)	2.0–2.2	$C-CH-CO-R$	2.7
	$CH_3-CO-NR$	2.0	$C-CH_2-CO-OR$	2.2	$C-CH-C\equiv N$	2.7
	CH_3-CO-R	2.2	$C-CH_2-CO-NR$	2.2	$C-CH-N-$	2.8
	CH_3-Ar	2.3	$C-CH_2C\equiv N$	2.3	$C-CH-Ar$	3.0
	CH_3-N-	2.3	$C-CH_2-CO-R$	2.4		
	$CH_3-CO-Ar$	2.6	$C-CH_2-N-$	2.5		
	CH_3-N-Ar	3.0	$C-CH_2-Ar$	2.6		
3–4	CH_3-O-R	3.3	$C-CH_2-I$	3.1	$C-CH-OR$	3.7
	$CH_3-O-CO-$	3.7	$C-CH_2-Br$	3.3	$C-CH-OH$	3.9
	CH_3-O-Ar	3.7	$C-CH_2-Cl$	3.4		
			$C-CH_2-OR$	3.4		
			$C-CH_2-OH$	3.6		
4–5			$C-CH_2-O-CO-$	4.2	$C-CH-I$	
			$C-CH_2-O-Ar$	4.3	$C-CH-Br$	4.1–4.4
			$C-CH_2-NO_2$	4.4	$C-CH-Cl$	
					$C-CH-NO_2$	4.7
					$C-CH-O-COR$	4.8

[a] It should be noted that further shifts to high frequency are caused upon attachment of additional deshielding groups to the carbon atom bearing the proton(s). For disubstituted methanes, Shoolery's rules may be applied to estimate the chemical shift of the CH_2 protons.

[b] Substituents on the β-carbon atom, relative to the given proton cause high frequency shifts of 0.1–1.0 ppm. Some important examples are: Y = –C = C, 0.1–0.2 ppm, Y = –C = 0, 0.2–0.3 ppm, Y = Ar, 0.35 ppm, Y = OR, 0.3–0.4 ppm.

Table. 2.4. Chemical shift values (ppm) for protons joined to unsaturated carbon: Acetylenic, Olefenic, aromatic and formyl protons. The chemical shift of such protons rises in the order discussed below (i.e. Table 2.4)

Range ppm	Unit	Comments
Acetylenic protons		
1.8–3.1	H–C≡C–	Conjugation, with C=C, Ar or C=O leads to absorption in the lower part of this range
Olefinic protons		
3.7–5.0	–HC=C–N– –HC=C–O–	β–H of enamines, enol-ethers etc.
4.5–6.0	–HC=C–	General range for olefinic hydrocarbons
5.7–7.0	–C=CH–N– –C=CH–O–	α-H of enamines, enol-ethers etc.
	–C=CH–CO– –C=CH–Ar	α-H of αβ-unsaturated carbonyl compounds
6.5–8.0	–HC=C–CO–	β-H of αβ-unsaturated carbonyl compounds; shifts are higher when proton is *cis*- to carbonyl compared to when it is *trans*
Aromatic protons		
6.0–9.0		Discussed in next section.
Formyl protons		
8.0–8.2	–O–CHO	Formates
	–N–CHO	Formamides
9.4–10.5	R–CHO	Aldehydes

2.8 CHEMICAL SHIFTS FOR AROMATIC PROTONS

The protons of benzene absorb at 7.37 ppm in $CDCl_3$. Substituents depending upon their nature may, however, cause shifts to high frequency or to low frequency. The shifts, for a given substituent, vary in magnitude with the position of the proton i.e. *o, m* or *p* relative to the substituent. The complete range of chemical shifts for *mono*-substituted benzenes is 6.–8.0 δ. In fact, the differential shielding of *ortho, meta* and *para*, protons is often useful in detecting the presence of strongly electron-releasing groups (NH_2, NR_2, OR). These groups cause the *ortho-* and *para*-proton signals to shift to low frequency with respect to those of the *meta*-protons. Strongly electron-withdrawing groups like NO_2, C=) etc. cause the *ortho*-proton signals to shift to high frequency relative to those of the *meta*- and *para*-protons. This is partly as a result of their magnetic anisotropies as shown for some representative substituents (Fig. 2.12).

The signals of protons adjacent to ring-junctions are shifted to high frequency in polycyclic benzenoid compounds. This is because they are influenced not only by the ring-current in the adjacent ring but by that in the ring to which they are attached.

The proton chemical shifts of aromatic heterocycles cover a wider range, *ca.* 6.0–9.0 δ compared to those of simple benzene derivatives. The protons joined to positions adjacent to the heteroatom generally

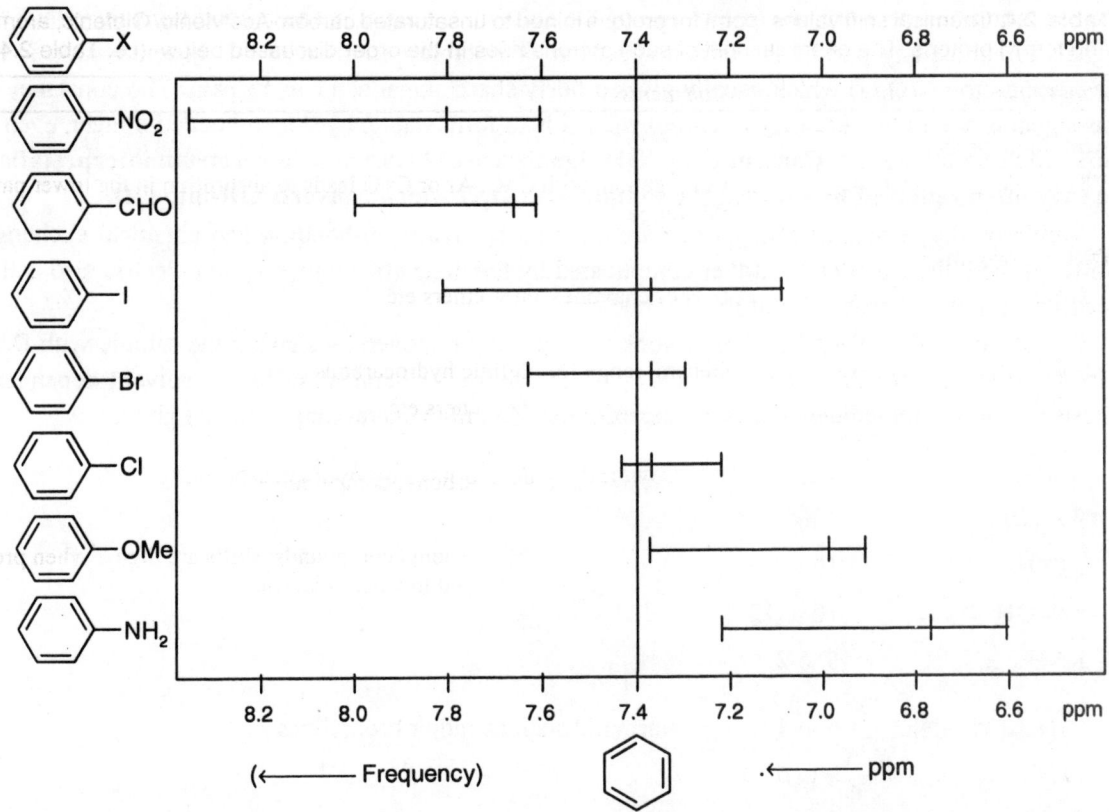

Fig. ^1H chemical shifts (ppm) of some *mono*-substituted benzenes while, the vertical lines represent the calculated chemical shifts, the actual signals are multiplets owing to spin-spin coupling.

give signals at higher chemical shift-values compared to other protons in the same ring due to the higher electronegativity of hetero atom relative to carbon.

2.9 PROTONS JOINED TO OXYGEN AND NITROGEN

The chemical shifts of protons joined to oxygen are very sensitive to the extent of hydrogen-bonding as well as to the extent of chemical exchange with other sources of mobile protons present in the medium. That is why the δ-values and line-widths of hydroxylic proton signals are strongly influenced by concentration, temperature, and the nature of the solvent. Changes in these conditions may shift the signals to almost any part of the proton spectrum. A notable exception to this generalisation is the *carboxyl* proton (CO_2H) which usually gives a fairly sharp signal at 11 to 13 ppm. The constancy of this signal is due to the tendency of carboxylic acids to form stable, hydrogen-bonded dimers, even in fairly dilute solution state. **Consequently, OH signals are of little value in spectrum interpretation, So they often removed by shaking the sample with D_2O which converts OH into OD.**

Similarly, the signals of NH protons are affected by hydrogen-bonding and chemical exchange. However, here the situation is further complicated by the magnetic (spin = 1) and electric also called quadrupole moment properties of the ^{14}N nucleus.

Signals for –OH, –NH, and –SH protons are normally removed by shaking the sample with D_2O, with D_2O/HCl for amines, or with D_2O/NaOD for amides. Chemical shifts are solvent dependent. These also vary with temperature and concentration. So only general ranges can be given :

R–OH	4 to 1	Lowered by upto 5 ppm by hydrogen-bonding
Ar–OH	5 to 4	
RCO–OH	10 to 13	
=N–OH	10 to 12	
RNH_2, RNHR	5 to 2	
$ArNH_2$, ArNHR	6 to 4	Normally seen as rather broad lines
$RCONH_2$	9 to 5	
R–SH	2 to 1	

Intext Exercise

1. How will you experimentally distinguish between carboxylic (acidic) and an aldehydic proton using NMR?

   Hint: In general, the acidic COOH appear in the range 10.5–13 ppm while the aldehydic proton range is to 10.5 ppm. In case of ambiguity, if the solution of the sample is prepared in D_2O or excess D_2O is put into the solution, then the COOH signal will disappear due to deuteration. Of course, DOH signal will also appear in the spectrum. On the other hand the aldehydic proton will not exchange with deuterium of D_2O.

   R–COOH + D_2O $\rightleftharpoons$ R–COOD + D–OH
   9–10.5   No signal
   ppm   in PMR

2.10 NMR SHIFTS OF CHEMICAL CLASSES

The chemical shifts along with involved coupling constants are collected in Table 2.5.

Table 2.5. Chemical shifts and involved coupling constants of various chemical classes

Class type	δ (ppm)	System	J (Hz)
1. Alkanes			
RCH_3	0.7–1.3		
R_2CH	1.2–1.4	–CH–CH– spin system	7–8 Hz
R_3C	1.4–1.7		12–15 Hz
2. Alkenes			
	4.5–6.5	$^3J_{cis}$	6–15
		$^3J_{trans}$	11–18
	1.6–2.6	$^4J_{(allylic)}$	0–3
		^2J	0–2
		$\overset{1}{CH}-\overset{2}{CH}=CH-CH$	$J_{1,2}=7$
3. Alkynes			
$-C\equiv C-H$	1.7–2.7		
	1.6–2.6		
		^4J	2–3
4. Alkyl halides			
$-CH-F$	4.2–4.8		
$-CH-Cl$	3.1–4.1		
$-CH-Br$	2.7–4.1	$H-\overset{\mid}{\underset{\mid}{C}}-F$	Ca 50
$-CH-I$	2.0–4.0	$H-\overset{\mid}{\underset{\mid}{C}}-\overset{\mid}{\underset{\mid}{C}}-F$	Ca 20

(Contd.)

Class type	δ (ppm)	System	J (Hz)
5. Nitriles			
—CH—CN	2.1–3.0		
6. Nitroalkanes			
H—C—NO$_2$	4.1–4.3		
7. Aromatic			
⬡—H	6.5–8.5	J$_0$	7–10
⬡—CH—	2.3–2.7	J$_m$	2–3
		J$_p$	0–1
8. Alcohols			
—C—OH	0.5–5.0		
H—C—OH	3.2–3.8		5
9. Ethers			
R—O—CH	3.2–3.8		
10. Amines			
R—N—H	0.5–4.0	—N—H	50
H—C—N—	2.2–2.9	—N—C—H	0 coupling not seen
Ph—NH	3.0–5.0	H—C—N—H	0 coupling not seen due to exchange
11. Aldehydes			
R—CHO	9.0–10.5		
R—C—CHO (with H)	2.1–2.4	—C—C=O (with H H)	1–3

(Contd.)

Class type	δ (ppm)	System	J (Hz)
12. **Ketones**			
H—C—C=O with R below	2.1–2.4		
13. **Carboxylic acids**			
— COOH	10.5–12.0		
H—C—COOH	2.1–2.5		
14. **Esters**			
H—C—COOR	2.1–2.5		
—C(=O)—O—C—H	3.5–4.8		
15. **Amides**			
—C(=O)—N—H	5.0–9.0	—C(=O)—N—H	~ 50
H—C—C(=O)—N—H	2.1–2.5		
—C(=O)—N—CH	2.2–2.9	—C(=O)—N—CH	~ 0
		—C(=O)—N(H)—C—H	~ 0

2.11 CHEMICAL SHIFT REFERENCE AND NMR SOLVENTS

TMS, tetramethyl silane is used as the reference because its protons of nearly all the organic compounds are the most upfield so that it is assigned a δ = 0 ppm.

$$H_3C—Si(CH_3)(CH_3)—CH_3 \quad \delta = 0 \text{ ppm}$$

Further advantages include :
- It gives a very sharp signal.
- The signal is very strong.
- TMS has low b.p. so that it can be easily removed from the sample, when required, thus making NMR technique a non-destructive technique.

Among the disadvantages, TMS is insoluble in deuterated water, D_2O. Hence it is replaced by a salt called sodium, 2, 2′, 3, 3′–d_4–3–trimethylsilyl propionate (TSP).

$$H_3C - \underset{\underset{CH_3}{|}}{\overset{\overset{CH_3}{|}}{Si}} - CD_2 - CD_2 - \overset{\ominus}{SO_3} \overset{\oplus}{Na}$$

D_2O is commonly used for recording NMR spectra of water-soluble organic compounds.

Further disadvantage of TMS is that TMS's carbon signal is generally very weak so that the solvent C–13 peak is usually used as C–13 chemical shift reference.

NMR Solvents

- **Deuterated chloroform, $CDCl_3$:**
  - Deuterated chloroform is the commonly used solvent as it can solubilize non-polar to polar solvents. As $CDCl_3$ contains a minute residual undeuterated chloroform ($CHCl_3$), a peak at ~ 7.27 ppm is seen in the spectrum. Further, because of its good volatility, it can be easily evaporated.

- **Deutero Dimethyl Sulfoxide DMSO-d_6, $(CH_3)_2S=O$:**
  - This solvent can solubilize relatively insoluble organic compounds (such as heterocyclics) as well as salts.
  - This can be used at high temperatures upto 140°C if required as it does not undergo decomposition.
  - The dual characteristics of high viscosity and the ability to cause some line-broadening, makes this solvent disadvantageous.
  - One of the major negative points about DMSO-d_6 is its strong affinity for water that makes it difficult to keep dry even when kept over molecular sieves. That is why a strong and a broad signal due to H_2O protons is seen at about 4.0 ppm that can hide the samples signals in this range.
  - This is a very expensive solvent.
  - As dimethyl sulfoxide is a mild oxidizing agent, it can sometimes cause oxidation of the test sample, more so when the sample solution has to be warmed up for achieving good solubility. Dewam (this author) noted that when O,O-diethyl monothiophosphoric acid was taken in DMSO for recording ^{31}P NMR spectrum, it was found that DMSO oxidized it to some extent to give an additional phosphorus signal due to formation of O,O-diethylphosphoric acid:

As DMSO-d_6 contains residual DMSO, CD_2HSOCD_3, it gives a signal at ~ 2.62 ppm.

Caution : DMSO-d_6 is hazardous as it is absorbed readily by skin. Take caution to immediately wash off the affected body parts with water.

Deutero Water, Water-d_2, D_2O

This is used for salts only. When the molecules are too non-polar for D_2O, CD_3CN is added as a co-solvent, otherwise poor solubility leads to broad NMR signals. The HOD signal appears as a strong signal at about 4.9 ppm. The cloudiness or turbidity of the D_2O solutions of samples can be eliminated by filtering off the solution through a tight cotton wool filter.

Other solvents that are used but not in routine include **deuteromethanol** MeOH-d_4 which is particularly used for salts and highly polar samples. The residual CD_2HOD appears at about 3.3–3.2 ppm.

Deutero benzene, Benzene-d_6 shows a residual C_6D_5H peak at about 7.27 ppm.

Trifluoroacetic acid, CF_3COOH is particularly used for amines and heterocyclic molecules. This shows a strong broad peak due to acidic proton at 11.0 ppm.

The chemical shift of residual protons in common deuterated solvents is given in Table 2.4.

Table 2.4. Residual protons in some common deuterated solvents

Solvent	δ	Solvent	δ
Acetic acid	2.05 (Me), 11.5 (OH)	Diethyl ether	1.2 (Me), 3.4 (CH_2)
Acetone	2.05	Dioxan	3.55
Benzene	7.27	Dimethyl sulphoxide	2.62
Chloroform	7.27	Ethanol	1.2 (Me), 3.6 (CH_2)
Cyclohexane	1.40	Methanol	3.3–3.2 (Me)
Deuterium oxide	4.9 (variable)	Pyridine	8.50, 7.35, 6.98

To conclude, while $CDCl_3$ is the best solvent for the lipophilic or "greasy" organic compounds, D_2O is the best one for hydrophilic compounds such as salts. For molecules having polarity in-between or having polar as well as non-polar parts like carboxylic acids, other solvents can be used. However, care needs to be taken to check the solubility of your sample in non-deuterated solvents first, rather than the deuterated solvents. The former are much cheaper than the latter. The cost of the deuterated solvents increases from acetone to THF :

Acetone-d_6 < Methanol-d_4 < Acetonitrile-d_3 < Benzene-d_6 < THF-d_4

$\longrightarrow$ Increasing cost $\longrightarrow$

2.12 SAMPLE SIZE AND SOLUTION

At this stage, you might be wondering about the sample size and nmr solution? About 5–10 mg sample size is required for medium-sized organic compounds (MW 40–400) for obtaining a PMR spectrum. For obtaining CMR spectra the amount needed is much higher, 30–40 mg as carbon–13 is about five thousands seven hundred times less sensitive than ^1H. Further, if the strength of the NMR instrument is high, then even lesser quantity of the sample is needed. Thus as low as 0.1 mg material size is enough for PMR at 500 MHz and about 2–3 mg is sufficient for CMR spectra.

2.12 PREPARATION OF SAMPLE SOLUTION

The volume of the sample needed is just 0.4 m in a standard NMR tube with 5 mm OD. Volumes smaller than this means that for proper shimming extra time will be required. On the other hand, volumes higher than the stated size contain smaller concentration of the sample and this will require more time for recording interpretable spectra and moreover spinning problems. The sample solution must not contain any solid residue, chunks or crystals. These should be filtered off through glass wool plug, otherwise line width goes degraded and also the spectrum obtained is not good. The solutions must be clear, not cloudy or turbid. Further, there should not be present any paramagnetic impurities in the solution as these lead to line-broadening in the spectrum. In fact, when relaxation times measurements are to be done, the paramagnetic dissolved oxygen has to be removed by passing nitrogen through it.

The sample is dissolved in a suitable solvent. A small amount of TMS reference (for ^{1}H and ^{13}C) is added. Only 0.4 ml of the sample solution is all that is needed for use in 5 mm outer diameter (OD). Volume less than this lead to poor resolution as well as spurious peaks as the vortex generated by spinning extends into the volume felt by the rf coil. The rate of spinning has to be such that it does not lead to spurious peaks and poor resolution. Suprious signals are always produced due to modulation of the signal by the spinning tube if it does not spin perfectly which is almost always the case. In fact, one can see small satellite peaks on either side of any large peak at a separation in Hz that is equal to the rate of spinning. You might wonder about this truth. All you got to do to verify this is to alter the rate of spinning and these satellite peaks position as well as intensity will change.

For obtaining spectra at temperatures up to 140°C, 1,1,2,2–tetrachloroethane is taken as the suitable solvent. Dimethylsulfoxide (DMSO) can be used for still higher temperatures. DMSO is a reactive substance and further disadvantage is that it can not be easily removed from the sample solution. 1,2,4–trichlorobenzene and nitrobenzene are also used.

Dichloromethane (–95°C), acetone (–95°C) and methanol (–98°C) are often used for low temperature investigation. A problem that is encountered under such conditions is the poor solubility of the sample. THF–CS$_2$ mixture is used down to –100°C.

PROBLEMS

1. Define chemical shift. What are its two types?
   Hint: See Sections 2.2 and 2.4.
2. Explain the theory and measurement of chemical shifts.
   Hint: See Section 2.3.
3. While hydrogen molecule shows chemical shift range of 1–10 ppm, other nuclei like carbon–13 show very large range of chemical shift. Why?
   Hint: See Section 2.4.
4. Enlist the parameters that affect chemical shift.
   Hint: See Section 2.5.
5. Explain electronegativity (electron density) effects in:
   (a) Neutral molecules
   (b) Carbocations
   (c) Carbanions

(d) Aromatic carbanions

Hint: See Section 2.5.2.1.

6. Discuss resonance effects on chemical shift.

Hint: See Section 2.5.2.

7. Discuss hybridization effects on chemical shift.

Hint: See Section 2.5.2.3.

8. What is magnetic anisotropy? Explain its origin.

9. Explain magnetic anisotropy in:

   (a) Porphyrins

   (b) p-cyclophanes

   (c) Annulenes

   (d) Benzene

10. Does ring anisotropy serve as a test for aromaticity? Explain with examples.

Hint: See Section 2.5.2.4.

11. Explain the reason for the decreasing order of proton chemical shifts for the following:

$$CH_3F > CH_3Cl > CH_3Br > CH_3I$$

12. Arrange the following in the decreasing order of proton chemical shift with suitable explanation:

$$(CH_3)_4C, (CH_3)_3N, (CH_3)_2O, CH_3F$$

Hint: See Section 2.5.2.1.

13. What would be the decreasing order of proton chemical shifts in these compounds? Give reasons.

   (i) CH_3Cl, $(CH_3)_2S$, $(CH_3)_3P$, $(CH_3)_4Si$

   (ii) R_3CH, R_2CH, RCH_3

Hint: See Setion 2.5.2.1.

14. The methyl derivatives of Hg, Cd, Zn and Mg show the following decreasing order for proton chemical shifts. Why?

$$Hg > Cd > Zn > Mg$$

Hint: See Section 2.5.2.1.

(13.50)

15. Explain the reason for the following observed proton chemical shifts CH_3 CH CH_3 (5.06 ppm). Or at what chemical shifts do different protons in isopropyl carbonium ions absorb and why?

16. Explain while ortho proton absorbs at δ 8.80 ppm, the para proton resonates at δ 8.45 ppm in phenyl dimethyl methane carbocation.

Hint: See Section 2.5.2.1 (electron density effects in carbocations).

17. What factor is responsible for causing deshielding of ortho, meta and para protons that absorbs at 7.98, 7.66 and 7.60 ppm respectively in trimethyl anilinium carbocation.

Hint: See Section 2.5.2.1: Electron density effects in carbocations.

18. While the terminal CH_2 protons absorb at δ 8.97, the central CH proton resonates at δ 9.64 ppm in allyl carbocation. Why?

Or Where do the protons in allyl carbocation absorb and why?

Hint: See Section 2.5.2.1: Electron effects in carbocations.

19. Why do the CH_3 protons in CH_3Li absorb at $\delta - 1.3$ ppm?
    Hint: See Section 2.5.2.1: Electron density effects in carbanions.

20. Explain while the CH_3 protons absorb at 1.26 ppm, the CH_2 protons absorb at $\delta - 0.64$ ppm in diethyl magnesium, $(CH_3CH_2)Mg$?
    Hint: See Section 2.5.2.1: Electron density effects in carbanions.

21. Give suitable explanation for the fact that while the CH_2 protons resonate at 2.46 ppm, the central CH proton absorbs at δ 6.28 ppm in the allyl carbanion. Why?
    Hint: See Section 2.5.2.1: Electron density effects in carbanions.

22. Explain while o- and p-protons absorb respectively at 6.09 and 5.50 ppm, the meta proton resonates 6.30 h in benzyl carbanion?
    Hint: See Section 2.5.2.1: Electron density effects in carbanions.

23. While the cyclopentadienyl anion protons resonate at δ 5.37, the tropylium cation protons absorb at δ 9.17 and that of benzene at δ 7.27. Explain.
    Hint: See Section 2.5.2.1: π-electron density influence on chemical shift in aromatic ions.

24. Besides anisotropy, there is another parameter that affects the chemical shift of the aldehydic proton. What is that?
    Hint: See Section 2.5.2.1: Resonance effects.

25. Explain while o- and p-protons absorb at δ 8.21 and δ 7.60 ppm, the meta absorbs at δ 7.47 ppm in nitrobenzene.
    Hint: See Section 2.5.2.1: Resonance effects.

26. In ethylpropenyl ether, α-proton is deshielded but the β-proton is shielded. Why?
    Hint: See Section 2.5.2.

27. What is the general range of olefinic protons chemical shift? What is the reason behind this small range of protons?
    Hint: See Section 2.5.3.

28. Why are acetylenic protons shielded compared to those of ethylene?

29. How will you distinguish between the axial and equatorial protons by NMR?

30. Explain that the ortho-proton is most deshielded in acetophenone.

31. Where do the inner and outer meso protons of porphyrins generally absorb in PMR spectra and why?

32. Show with the help of PMR spectroscopy that [14]–Annulene is aromatic while [16]–Annulene is not.
    Note: For answers to **Q. 28–32**, see Section 2.5.4.

33. Can we use ring current anisotropy effect as a test for aromaticity? Explain.
    Hint: Yes. See Section 2.5.4.

34. What is Chemical Shift Anisotropy (CSA)?
    Hint: See Section 2.5.2.5.

3

Spin-Spin Coupling, Spin Notation and ¹H NMR Interpretation

3.1 TYPICAL NMR SPECTRUM

An NMR spectrum that is a graph of Intensity Absorption (CW) or Emission (FT) versus Chemical shift looks as shown in Fig. 3.1.

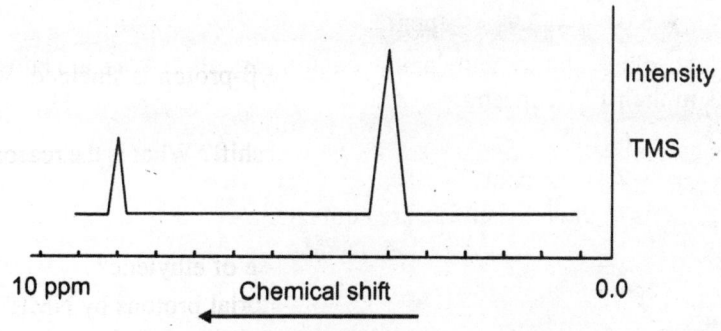

Fig. 3.1. A typical NMR spectrum.

What information does a NMR spectrum give to us? It gives us the following important messages about the structure of the compound it represents :

1. Number of signals
2. Position of signals
3. Intensities of signals

3.2 NUMBER OF SIGNALS, EQUIVALENT AND NONEQUIVALENT PROTONS

The number of signals in the NMR spectrum tells us the number of protons present in the sample molecule which are different from each other. Different in what sense? Different in that they are attached to different functional groups.

1. Chemically equivalent protons : Examples

(a) *Molecules containing all equivalent protons*

- **Methane, CH_4 :** In this compound, all the four hydrogens have the same chemical environment so that, it is not possible to distinguish one from another.

$$
\begin{array}{c}
H \\
| \\
C \\
H \diagup | \diagdown H \\
H
\end{array}
$$

- **Ethane, $CH_3–CH_3$:** Here, again all the three hydrogens within a methyl group are all equivalent. Since one methyl group is attached to the other methyl group, therefore, all the six hydrogens are equivalent and give a single peak in proton NMR spectrum at 0.26 ppm.

All the protons in the following monohalomethane compounds are equivalent as they give only peak in their PMR spectra:

- $\quad$ CH_3F $\quad$ CH_3Cl $\quad$ CH_3Br $\quad$ CH_3I
  $\quad$ 4.0 $\quad\quad$ 2.84 $\quad\quad$ 2.45 $\quad\quad$ 1.98 $\quad\quad$ ppm

- In the following dihalomethanes all protons are equivalent as indicated by single peaks in their NMR spectra:

  $\quad$ CH_2Cl_2 $\quad$ CH_2Br_2 $\quad$ CH_2I_2
  $\quad\quad$ 5.3 $\quad\quad\quad$ 5.0 $\quad\quad\quad$ 3.9 $\quad\quad$ ppm

- In trimethylphosphine and trimethylamine compounds all protons are equivalent as they give single peaks in their PMR spectra.

  $\quad$ $(CH_3)_3P$ $\quad$ $(CH_3)_3N$
  $\quad\quad$ 0.9 $\quad\quad\quad$ 2.1 $\quad\quad$ ppm

- All the six protons in dimethylsulfide are equivalent.

  $\quad$ $(CH_3)_2S$
  $\quad\quad$ 2.1 $\quad\quad$ ppm

- Dimethyl ether.

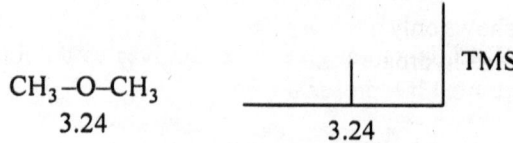

$\quad$ $CH_3–O–CH_3$ $\qquad\qquad\qquad\qquad$ TMS
$\qquad$ 3.24 $\qquad\qquad\qquad\qquad\qquad$ 3.24

- In dimethyl sulfoxide, all the six protons are equivalent and give only one signal at 2.60 ppm in the NMR spectrum.

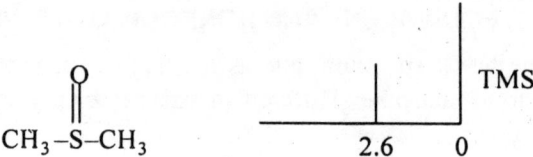

$$
\begin{array}{c}
O \\
\parallel \\
CH_3–S–CH_3
\end{array}
$$

$\qquad\qquad\qquad\qquad\qquad\qquad$ TMS
$\qquad\qquad\qquad\qquad\qquad$ 2.6 $\quad$ 0

- Acetone contains six equivalent protons as it shows only one signal in PMR spectrum at 2.5 ppm.

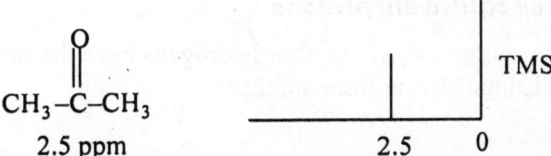

CH_3-C-CH_3
2.5 ppm

- In the spectrum of ethene we get only one signal as expected as it contains all equivalent protons.

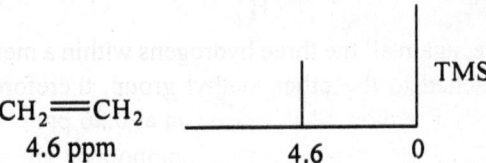

$CH_2=CH_2$
4.6 ppm

- Acetylene contains two equivalent protons.

$CH\equiv CH$
2.8 ppm

- Cyclopropane contains six equivalent protons as it gives a single peak at 0.2 ppm.

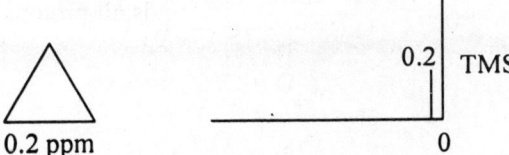

0.2 ppm

- Methyl carbanion shows a single peak as its PMR spectrum at –1.3 ppm.

$\overset{\ominus}{CH_3}$ $\overset{\oplus}{Li}$
–1.3 ppm

- tert-butylcarbocation shows only one signal in its spectrum which clearly indicates the chemical equivalence among these hydrogens.

CH_3 4.35

H_3C CH_3

- Cyclopentadienyl anion shows only one peak in its PMR spectrum.

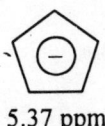

5.37 ppm

- Benzene, C_6H_6.

7.27 ppm

- Formaldehyde, CH_2O.

- Urea.

- Thiourea.

- Dimethylacetylene.

$$H_3C—C\equiv C—CH_3$$

- Biacetyl.

- Acetic anhydride.

- Acetyl chloride.

- Trimethylphosphate.

- Zinc O,O–diethyldithiophosphate.

- Phosphoric acid, H_3PO_4.

$$\underset{HO}{\overset{HO}{>}}P\underset{OH}{\overset{O}{<}}$$

- Thiophosphoric acid.

$$\underset{HO}{\overset{HO}{>}}P\underset{OH}{\overset{S}{<}}$$

Examples of non-equivalent protons

- $CH_3^a{-}C{-}O{-}CH_3^b$

  with $\overset{||}{O}$ below the C

  Methyl acetate contains two sets (a, b) of non-equivalent protons, the CH_3^aC and OCH_3^b protons.

- $H_3^aC{-}\langle\text{ring } b\ b/b\ b\rangle{-}CH_3^a$

  p-xylene contains two sets (a, b) of non-equivalent protons, the six methyl protons and four aromatic protons.

- Mesitylene structure with H_3C (a), H (b), CH_3 (a) substituents

  Mesitylene contains two sets (a, b) of non-equivalent protons.

- $H_3^aC{-}\underset{O}{\overset{||}{C}}{-}H^b$

  Acetaldehyde contains two types (a, b) of protons, the three non-equivalent methyl protons and the single aldehydic proton.

- $H_3^aC{-}\underset{O}{\overset{||}{C}}{-}OH^b$

  Acetic acid contains two sets (a, b) of non-equivalent protons.

- $H_3^aC{-}NH^b{-}\underset{O}{\overset{||}{C}}{-}NH^b{-}CH_3^a$

N,N–Dimethyl urea contains two (a, b) sets of non-equivalent protons.

- $\overset{a}{CH_3O}\diagdown \overset{S}{\diagup}$
  $\underset{\overset{|}{CH_3O}}{}P\diagdown \overset{}{OH}^b$
  $\overset{a}{CH_3O}\diagup \quad OH^b$

O,O–Dimethyl thiophosphoric acid contains two types (a, b) of protons in the ratio of 6:1.

- $\overset{a}{CH_3O}\diagdown \overset{S}{\diagup}$
  P
  $\overset{a}{CH_3O}\diagup \quad SH^b$

O,O–Dimethyldithiophosphoric acid contains two sets (a, b) of non-equivalent protons in the ratio of 6:1.

- $\overset{a}{CH_3}\overset{b}{NH_2}$

  Methylamine contains two sets (a, b) of non-equivalent protons.

- $\overset{a}{CH_3}\overset{b}{OH}$

  Methyl alcohol contains two sets of (a, b) of protons.

- $Br—\overset{a}{CH_2}—\overset{b}{CH_2}—Cl$

  1–Bromo–2–chloro contains two sets (a, b) of protons.

Some more examples of molecules containing many sets of non-equivalent protons are as follows:

- $\overset{a}{CH_3}\overset{b}{CH_2}\overset{c}{OH}$

- $\overset{a}{CH_3}\overset{b}{CH_2}\overset{c}{CH_2}Cl$

- $\overset{a}{CH_3}\overset{b}{CH_2}O\diagdown \overset{S}{\diagup}$
  P
  $\overset{a}{CH_3}\overset{b}{CH_2}O\diagup \quad S—H^c$

- $\overset{a}{CH_3}—\overset{b}{CH_2}—O\diagdown \overset{S}{\diagup}$
  P
  $\underset{a\quad b}{CH_3—CH_2—O}\diagup \quad S—\underset{c}{CH_3}$

- $\overset{a}{CH_3}\overset{b}{CH_2}—O\diagdown \overset{S}{\diagup}$
  P
  $\underset{a\quad b}{CH_3—CH_2—O}\diagup \quad S—\overset{c}{CH_2}—\overset{d}{CH_3}$

  (4 sets a, b, c, d)

- $Cl—\overset{a}{CH_2}—\overset{\overset{O}{\|}}{C}—O—\overset{b}{CH_2}—\overset{c}{CH_3}$

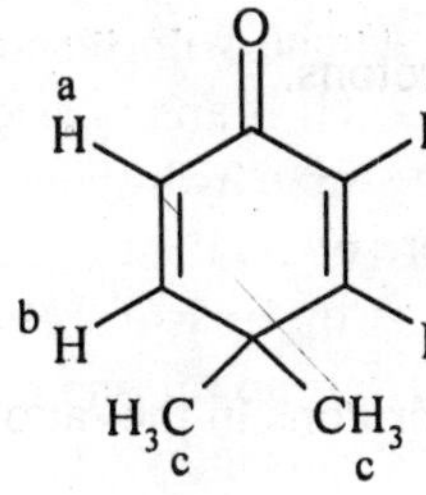

(3 sets a, b, c)

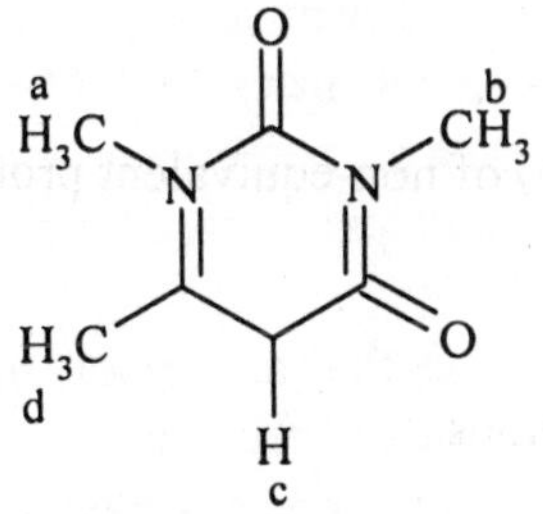

(4 sets a, b, c, d)

- **Ethyl bromide, C_2H_5Br** : Ethyl bromide is

$$CH_3-CH_2-Br$$

Here, there are two different types of protons on each carbon i.e. the methyl and methylene protons are chemically non-equivalent. CH_3 group is attached only to $-CH_2-$ while CH_2 is attached to CH_3 and Br.

How can we say that the three protons of the methyl group in CH_3CH_2Br, ethyl bromide are all equivalent? On the basis of analysis, it can be shown that these are different or non-equivalent. But, we will first of all analyse, as to how the three methyl protons are different or non-equivalent and then we will discuss why do they behave as chemically equivalent.

3.3 EQUIVALENT OR NON-EQUIVALENT PROTONS – HOW TO DECIDE?

Equivalent protons are the protons which have the same chemical environment and hence they resonate at the same chemical shift. If their chemical environments are different, they will be called non-equivalent protons and will resonate at different chemical shifts.

- **Deciding Ethyl bromide :** Ethyl bromide can exist in the following conformations (1–3).

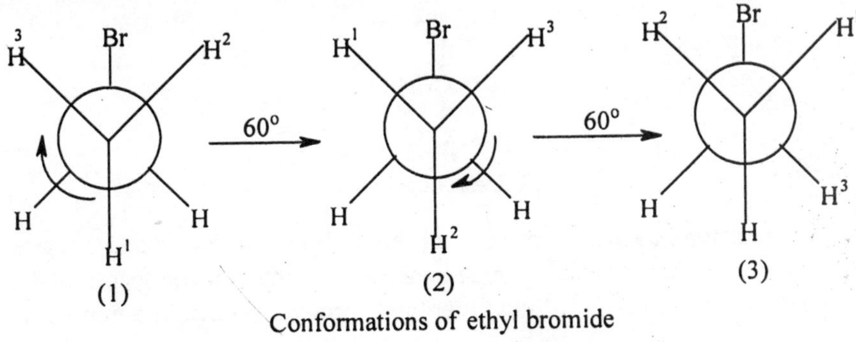

Conformations of ethyl bromide

As can be seen in conformation (1), H^1 is anti while H^2 and H^3 are gauche with respect to Br. Obviously, H^1 is chemically non-equivalent to H^2 and H^3. In conformation 2, H^2 is anti w.r. to Br, and in conformation 3, it is H^3 that is anti w.r. to Br. It is clear, therefore, that the three hydrogens – H^1, H^2 and H^3 are non-equivalent. Yet all the three protons behave as if they were equivalent in the proton NMR. That is they resonate at the same chemical shift! Therefore what is the reason behind their equivalence? In all the three conformations (1–3) CH_2 protons have a CH_3 group on one side and a bromine atom on the other side. Hence, as the chemical environments of both the methyl as well as the methylene protons are different, therefore, they absorb at different positions. In fact, their multiplicities are also different, while CH_3 group appears as a triplet, the $-CH_2-$ group appears as a quartet.

Is there a formula with the help of which we could indicate with clear cut surity that indeed all the protons on a carbon are the same? Yes, if we could replace one proton on a carbon by a new group, N, on and if the substituted products are the same, as the original protons are identical. In case the substituted products are different, the protons are non-equivalent.

Here, the three conformations are of equal stability. Because of this reason, they are equally populated as well (~ 33.33% each). They exist in equilibrium with each other. The rate of their interconversion is fast on the NMR time scale. Hence, NMR "instrumental camera" sees them in an average environment, so that they behave as an equivalent set of three protons.

Let us see these two operations on the Fischer's projection formulas of ethyl bromide :

$$
\begin{array}{ccc}
\text{CH}_3 & & \text{CH}_3 \\
\text{H}\!-\!\!\!\!+\!\!\!\!-\text{H} & \xrightarrow[+\,N]{-\,Hb} & \text{H}\!-\!\!\!\!+\!\!\!\!-\text{N} \\
\text{Br} & & \text{Br}
\end{array}
$$

$$
\begin{array}{ccc}
\text{CH}_3 & & \text{CH}_3 \\
\text{H}\!-\!\!\!\!+\!\!\!\!-\text{H} & \xrightarrow[+\,N]{-\,Ha} & \text{N}\!-\!\!\!\!+\!\!\!\!-\text{H} \\
\text{Br} & & \text{Br}
\end{array}
$$

Now, the two substituted products are actually mirror images and form an enantiomeric pair (pairs of protons like this are called **enantiotopic pairs**) of each other. Hence, they do not absorb at different chemical shifts in NMR spectrum. They absorb at identical chemical shifts. So, we can say enantiotopic protons absorb at identical chemical shifts.

We will discuss a new molecule, 1,2-Dibromopropane.

$$
\begin{array}{l}
c\ \ \text{CH}_2\text{Br} \\
\ \ \ \ \ | \\
b\ \ \text{CHBr} \\
\ \ \ \ \ | \\
a\ \ \text{CH}_3
\end{array}
$$

1,2–Dibronopropane

This contains three different kinds of protons as shown by number a, b and c. Here, the casually expected spectrum would be the presence of three peaks in the proton NMR spectrum due to a, b and c protons in the ratio 2:1:3. However, it is found that the C protons behave in a non-equivalent manner and absorb at different positions, giving a total of four signals. In fact, the protons should be expected to behave in a non-equivalent chemical manner. This can be shown on the basis of the formula we have already mentioned (isomer number).

$$
\begin{array}{c}
\text{CH}_3 \\
| \\
\text{H}-\text{C}-\text{Br} \\
| \\
\text{H}-\!\!\!\!-\text{H} \\
| \\
\text{Br}
\end{array}
$$

1,2–Dibromopropane

$$
\begin{array}{c|c}
\text{Imaginative} & -\text{H} \\
\text{replacement} & +\text{N}
\end{array}
$$

↓

$$
\begin{array}{cc}
\text{CH}_3 & \qquad \text{CH}_3 \\
\text{H}-\!\!\!\!-\text{Br} & \qquad \text{H}-\!\!\!\!-\text{Br} \\
\text{H}-\!\!\!\!-\text{N} & \qquad \text{N}-\!\!\!\!-\text{H} \\
\text{Br} & \qquad \text{Br}
\end{array}
$$

As can be seen, the replacement of both the C protons, one at a time, gives two diastereomers, which are definitely different compounds. So, two C protons are non-equivalent and hence they resonate at different chemical shifts. Hence, these pairs of protons are also called **diastereotopic protons**. Any amount of rotation can not make them equivalent at all. Let us consider, one more example, that of vinyl protons of 2-chloro propane are the two protons equivalent or non-equivalent.

$$
\begin{array}{c}
\text{CH}_3 \diagdown \qquad \diagup \text{Hb} \\
\text{C}=\text{C} \\
\text{Cl} \diagup \qquad \diagdown \text{Ha}
\end{array}
$$

2-chloropropane

If we apply the same formula as applied above, the substituted products are diastereomeric products. Hence, these two protons are non-equivalent and therefore, they should absorb at different chemical shifts in NMR spectrum. Indeed, they do so.

$$
\begin{array}{c}
\text{CH}_3 \diagdown \qquad \diagup \text{Hb} \\
\text{C}=\text{C} \\
\text{Cl} \diagup \qquad \diagdown \text{Ha}
\end{array}
$$

$$
\begin{array}{c}
-\text{H} \\
+\text{N}
\end{array}
$$

↓

$$
\begin{array}{cc}
\text{CH}_3 \diagdown \qquad \diagup \text{N} & \qquad \text{CH}_3 \diagdown \qquad \diagup \text{H} \\
\text{C}=\text{C} & \qquad \text{C}=\text{C} \\
\text{Cl} \diagup \qquad \diagdown \text{H} & \qquad \text{Cl} \diagup \qquad \diagdown \text{N}
\end{array}
$$

Diastereomors

Predict, whether the C-protons of 1,2-dibromo-1-phenyl ethane are equivalent or non-equivalent.

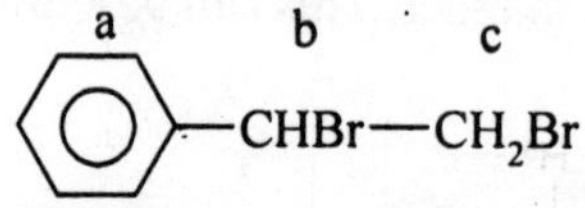

$$\overset{a}{\underset{}{\bigcirc}} - \overset{b}{CHBr} - \overset{c}{CH_2Br}$$

1,2–Dibromo-1-phenyl ethane

Let us write it in a Fischer projection formula and apply the isomer no formula at C-2.

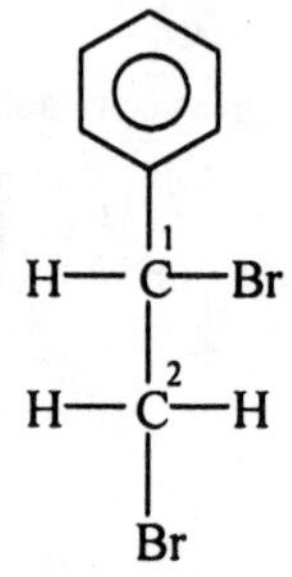

H—C¹—Br
H—C²—H
Br

1,2–Dibromo-1-phenyl ethane

$$\downarrow \quad \begin{matrix} -H \\ +N \end{matrix} \left(\begin{matrix} \text{at } C-2 \\ \text{one at a time} \end{matrix} \right)$$

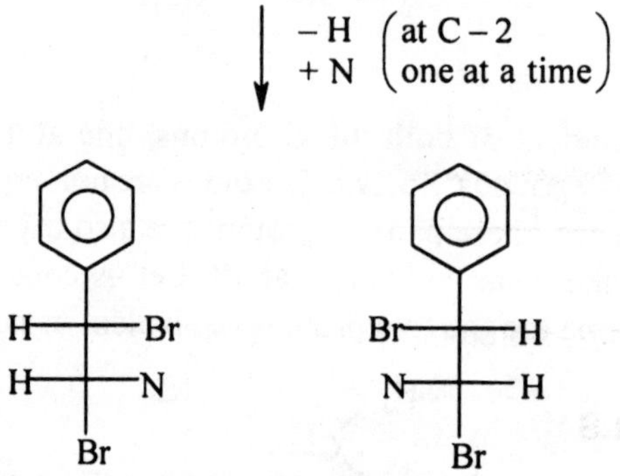

Here, we find the products obtained are diastereomers. So, the two C-protons are different. They must absorb at different shifts. Indeed, they do in the proton NMR spectrum shown in Fig. 3.2a. No amount of rotation around the C–C bond can make them equivalent i.e. interconvert them. This can be easily seen by considering the three conformations shown below.

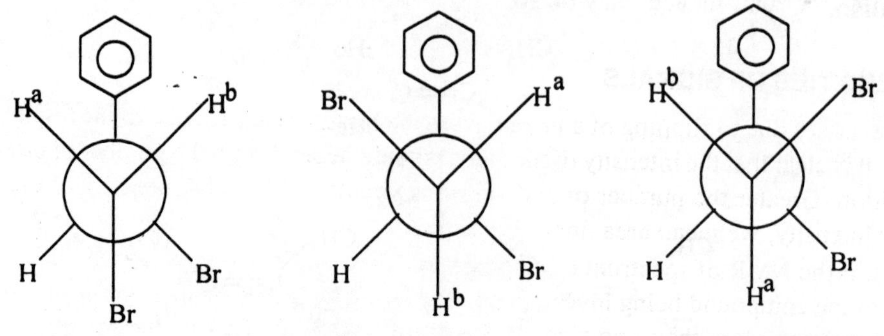

Conformations of 1,2–dibromo–1–phenyl ethane in Newman's projections

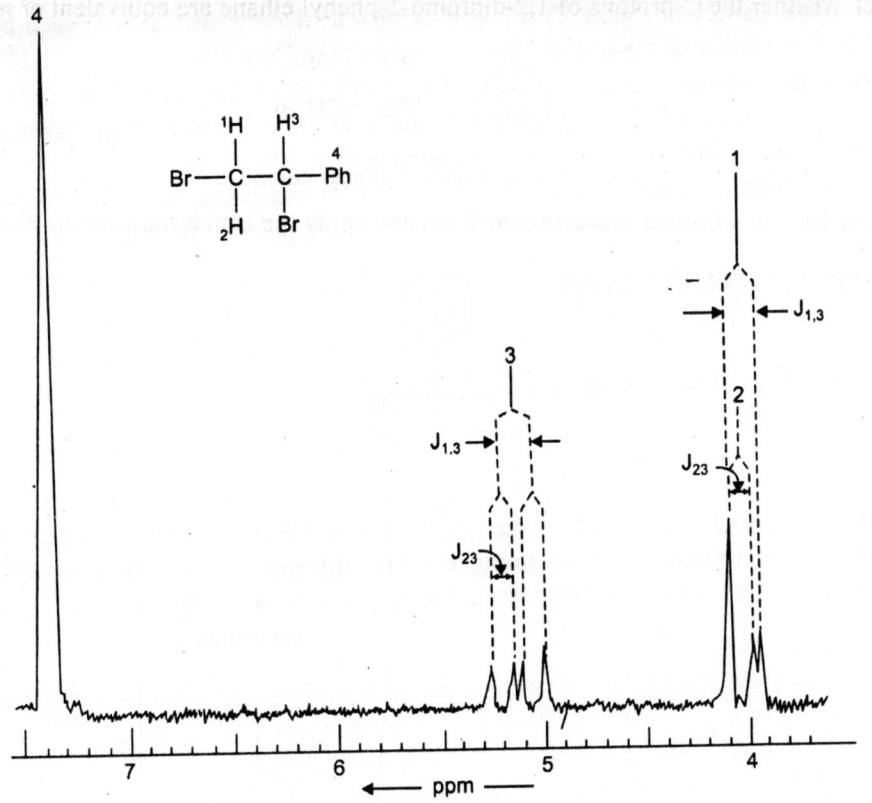

Fig. 3.2a. PMR spectrum of 1,2–dibromo–1–phenylethane. No peaks before 3.9 ppm and after 7.5 ppm.

3.4 POSITION OF SIGNALS

The position of a peak is also very valuable as it gives us the message as to the kind of the proton, what kind of functional group does it make a part of. For example, it tells us whether the signal is due to proton of a–COOH group or an–OH group or a CH$_3$ group or a–CH=CH$_2$ group or a–C≡C–H group or an aromatic proton etc. This is because different protons appear at different positions, chemical shifts. So, we get a clue regarding the type of the functional unit present in the molecule under consideration.

3.5 INTENSITIES OF SIGNALS

As a signal arises due to flipping of a proton from the lower energy α-state to the higher energy β-state, therefore, it is clear that the intensity of the signal should depend upon the number of protons undergoing the transition. Greater the number of such protons, greater will be the intensity of the signal and vice versa. By intensity, we mean area under the signal.

In fact, if the NMR of spectrum of a compound shows only one signal, then this tells us the simple structure of the compound being investigated. The intensity factor assumes great significance when the spectrum contains more than one signal. The NMR spectrum gives us the relative number of nuclei contributing to that particular signal. This is self-evident as the intensity area of each peak is directly contributed by the number of the nuclei of that type as already explained.

Indeed, it is this relative number of protons that gives us the ability to find out the structure of the compound. In some cases, it is even possible with the NMR data alone to assign the exact structure of the compound. That is to say we can tell the exact number of protons present in the compound. However, this is not a very common situation. We will now consider some examples which will prove the utility of the relative number of protons seen in NMR spectra of organic compounds.

3.6 SOME SIMPLE NMR SPECTRA

Example 1

The NMR spectrum of Methylmethanoate:

$$H-\underset{\underset{O}{\|}}{C}-OCH_3$$

The NMR spectrum of methyl methanoate (methyl formate, $C_2H_4O_2$ shows two signals at 8.1 and at 3.6 ppm in the integral ratio of 1:3, conforming to a total of four protons. The signal at 8.1 is the HCO proton and the other signal is due to the three methoxy protons (see Fig. 3.2b).

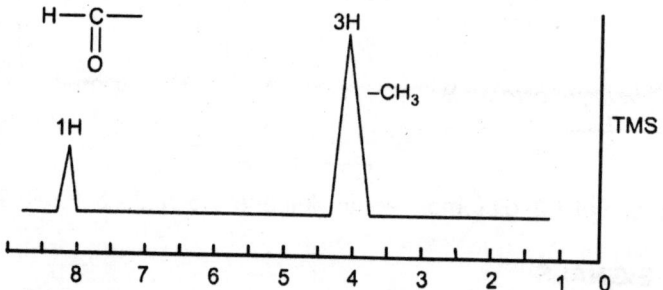

Fig. 3.2b. NMR spectrum of methyl methanoate.

Example 2

NMR spectrum of Phenylacetic acid, $C_8H_8O_2$ has the following structure which can be confirmed from its NMR spectrum shown in Fig. 3.2a and b.

COOH
|
CH$_2$

Phenylacetic acid

The spectrum shows three singlets at 12, 7.21 and at 3.58 ppm in the integral ratio of 1:5:2 making a total of eight protons. As the singlet at 12 ppm is due to 1H, obviously the aromatic protons correspond to 5H and the 2H protons indicate a CH$_2$ group, that is the benzylic protons at 3.58 ppm.

Thus, the structure of this compound is confirmed as shown.

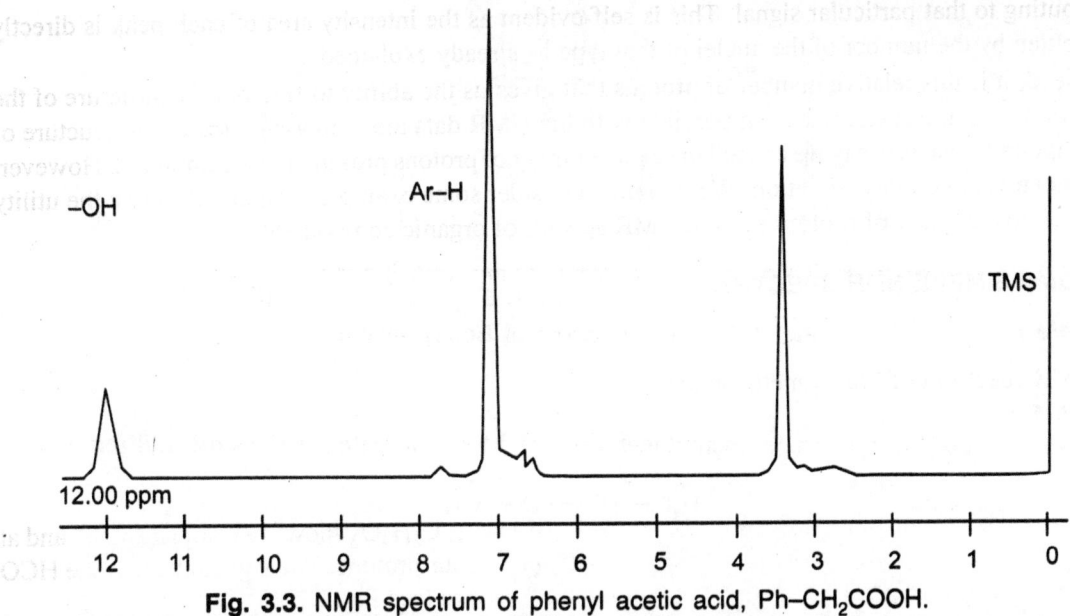

-OH

Ar-H

TMS

12.00 ppm

12 11 10 9 8 7 6 5 4 3 2 1 0

Fig. 3.3. NMR spectrum of phenyl acetic acid, Ph–CH₂COOH.

Example 3

The NMR spectrum of benzyl acetate : Benzyl acetate or Benzyl ethanoate $C_9H_{10}O_2$ has the structure :

$$\text{Ph}-CH_2-O-\overset{\displaystyle O}{\overset{\|}{C}}-CH_3$$

Benzyl acetate

The PMR of Benzyl ethanoate shows three peaks at 7.20, 5.0 and 2.0 ppm (Fig. 3.4). Their intensities as given by the electronic integrator are in the ratio 5:2:3. These signals arise from the aromatic (Ph), methylene (–CH₂–) and methyl (–CH₃) signals respectively. As the molecular formula of this compound contains 10 protons, therefore, these are accounted for without any iota of doubt (5 + 2 + 3 = 10). As the –CH₂– protons resonate at S 5.0 ppm, it is clear that these are the benzylic methylene protons. Therefore, the structure of Benzyl acetate is confirmed.

Example 4

The NMR spectrum of Methyl benzoate:

$$C_6H_5-\overset{\displaystyle}{\underset{\displaystyle O}{\overset{\|}{C}}}-OCH_3$$

$C_6H_5 : OCH_3$
5:3
1.66:1

The NMR spectrum of this molecule is shown in Fig. 3.4. There are two singlets, one at 3.80 ppm and another at 7.05 ppm. The integrals as given by the NMR machine are in the ratio of 1.66:1. As the molecule contains one phenyl and one methyl group, therefore, the expected relative integral ratio of the phenyl and methyl ratio 5:3 is clearly satisfied. Hence, the structure of the molecule is as shown.

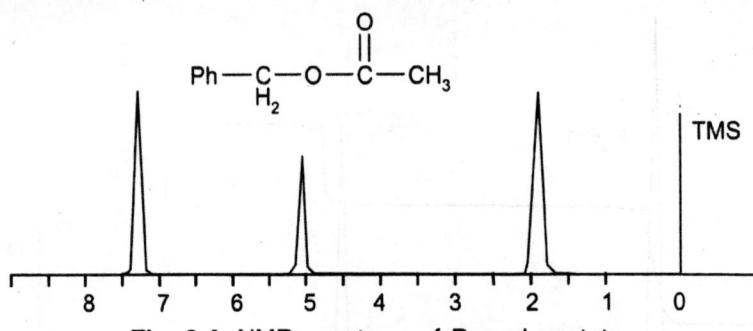

Fig. 3.4. NMR spectrum of Benzyl acetate.

Example 5

NMR spectrum of Methyl acetate (methyl methanoate). Methyl acetate has the structural formula :

$$H_3C—O—\underset{\underset{O}{\|}}{C}—CH_3$$

The NMR spectrum is shown in Fig. 3.6. The spectrum contains two singlets at 3.65 and 2.0 ppm. The ratio of their integrals comes out to 1:1, as expected. As the OCH_3 protons are deshielded due to electron withdrawl by oxygen compared to $COCH_3$, so the signal at 3.65 ppm is due to OCH_3. Obviously, the signal at 2.0 ppm is due to $COCH_3$.

Example 6 : NMR spectrum of Phenyl acetate

Phenyl acetate has got the structural formula

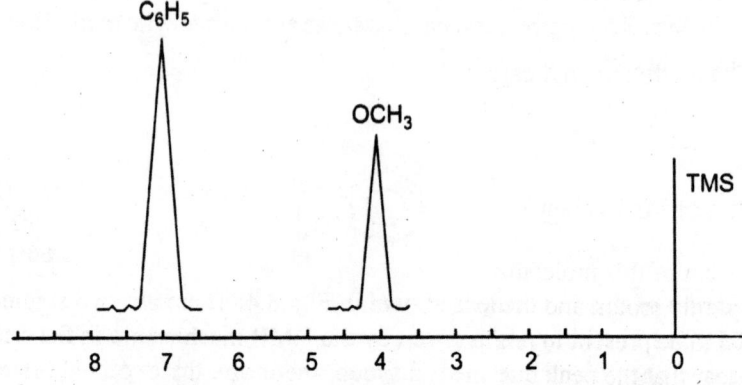

Fig. 3.5. NMR spectrum of Methyl benzoate at 60 MHz.

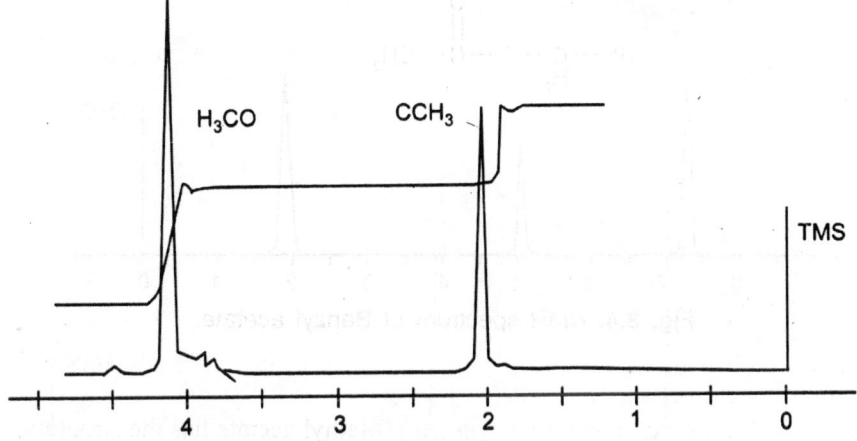

Fig. 3.6. NMR spectrum of methyl acetate.

The NMR spectra of phenyl acetate is shown in Fig. 3.7. The spectrum shows two singlets, one at 2.2 ppm and another 1.5 ppm. The ratio of their integrals 1:1.66. As the molecule contains CH_3 and C_6H_5 units, therefore their ratio should be 3:5 or 1:1.66.

It should be noted that the methyl protons absorb at 2.2 ppm rather than at 3.8 ppm, therefore it is clear that CH_3 group is a CH_3CO group rather than being due to a $-COOCH_3$ group.

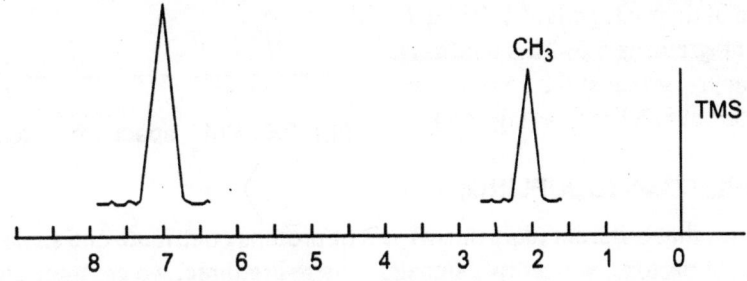

Fig. 3.7. NMR spectrum of phenyl acetate at 60 MHz.

Example 7

NMR spectrum of Dimethyiethynyl carbinol, M.F C_5H_8O has the structure:

$$HC\equiv C-\underset{\underset{OH}{|}}{\overset{\overset{CH_3}{|}}{C}}-CH_3$$

The PMR spectrum of this molecule (Fig. 3.8) shows three singlet peaks at 3.78 due to OH proton, at 2.41 due to acetylenic proton and the largest signal at 1.48 ppm due to methyl protons ($2 \times CH_3$). The integral shows them to be present in relative 1:1:6 ratio. Thus, if acetylenic and OH protons account for two protons, it is clear that the peak due to 6H protons must correspond to $2CH_3$ group protons. Hence, NMR alone has proved sufficient enough in elucidating the structure of this molecule.

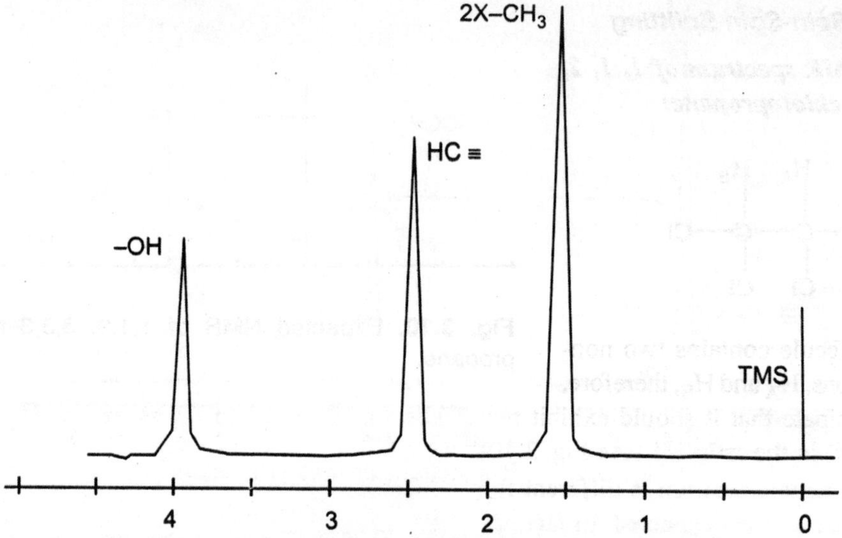

2X–CH₃

HC ≡

–OH

TMS

4   3   2   1   0

Fig. 3.8. NMR spectrum of Dimethylethynylcarbinol.

Example 8

The NMR spectrum of toluene : Toluene shows two peaks – one at δ 2.35 ppm and the other at 7.17 ppm. The ratio of their integrals as calculated by the electronic integrator is 5:3. This confirms the presence of a methyl group at δ 2.35 ppm and five aromatic protons at δ 7.17 ppm (Fig. 3.9).

TMS

7.17   2.35   0

Fig. 3.9. PMR spectrum of toluene at 60 MHz.

3.7 SPIN-SPIN SPLITTING (COUPLING)

So far, we have learnt that different (equivalent) sets of protons contribute one signal each. If there are two sets of equivalent protons, we get two signals, if there are three, we get three signals and so on.

For example :

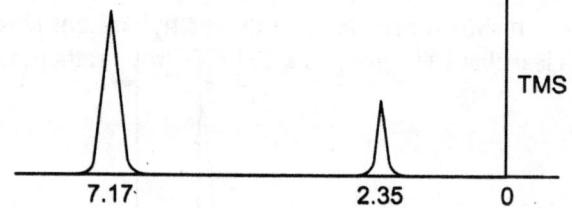

Compounds	No. of signals in the NMR spectrum
CH₃—O—CH₂—Cl	2
CH₃—C(=O)—O—CH₃	2
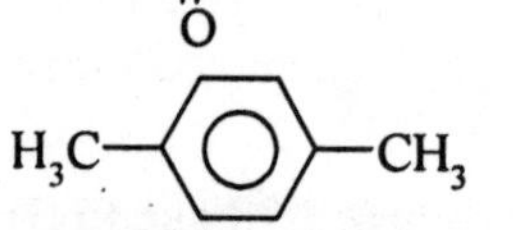 H₃C—⟨C₆H₄⟩—CH₃	2
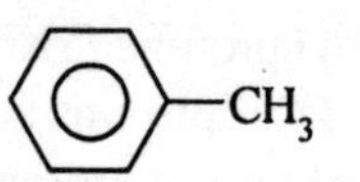 ⟨C₆H₅⟩—CH₃	2

However, it is not always so, as is shown below in examples.

Examples of Spin-Spin Splitting

Example 1: NMR spectrum of 1, 1, 2, 3, 3, 3, – hexa chloropropane:

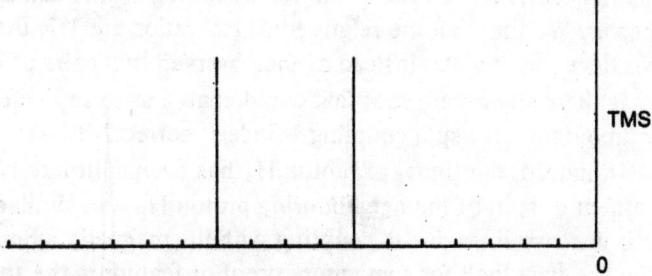

Fig. 3.10. Expected NMR of 1,1,2, 3,3,3–hexochloropropane.

$$Cl_3C—\overset{\overset{\displaystyle H_A}{|}}{\underset{\underset{\displaystyle Cl}{|}}{C}}—\overset{\overset{\displaystyle H_B}{|}}{\underset{\underset{\displaystyle Cl}{|}}{C}}—Cl$$

As this molecule contains two non-equivalent protons, H_A and H_B, therefore, we would anticipate that it should exhibit two peaks one each due to H_A as well as H_B at different positions (shifts) in the ratio 1:1 (see Fig. 3.10).

However, the real spectrum is different from that predicted as shown in Fig. 3.11. That is to say, there are more peaks than expected. In fact, there are four peaks instead of two only. This is exciting. Therefore, the NMR game we were playing does not now seem to be a very simple and straightforward game. The important question is how to interpret the four line spectrum of the molecule in hand?

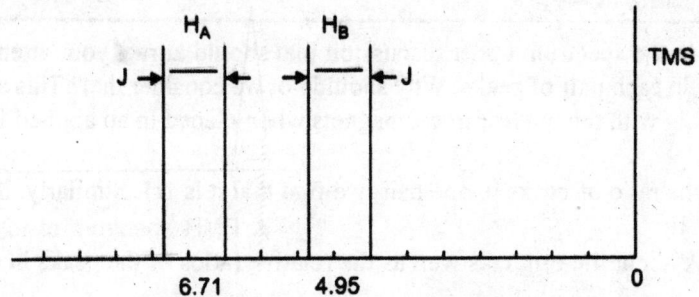

Fig. 3.11. NMR spectrum of 1,1,2,3,3,3–hexachloropropane.

If we look very carefully at the spectrum, it becomes clear that the four lines are not equally spaced, the distance between the inner two lines being much larger than the distance between the other two lines at the two extremes. We can say that there are two pairs of lines. As we had expected two singlets, one due to each proton being separated from each other, therefore, it seems that each proton is giving two lines, instead of one. That is to say if one pair of closely spaced lines is due to H_A, the other pair of lines is due to H_B. If that is so, we can conclude that H_A is showing one line more than the number of protons on the adjacent or the neighbouring carbons (i.e. $1 + 1 = 2$). Similarly, we can conclude that H_B is also showing one line more than the number of protons on the adjacent or the neighbouring carbon (i.e. $1 + 1 = 2$).

The preceding discussion leads us to conclude that there is some mutual interaction or coupling of the magnetic moments or the spins of both these types of neighbouring or the vicinal protons between each other – **magnetic moment–magnetic moment coupling or spin-spin coupling. ¶**

We also need to answer as to what is the proof that one pair of lines at one extreme is due to one proton and the other pair of lines is due to the other proton. Let us re-examine the NMR spectrum of this molecule. If we look at the relative integral intensities of both the pairs of lines, therein lies the answer. We find that the relative integral ratios are 1:1, the same as would be expected if these were two lines (or singlets) instead of the observed two pairs of lines if this interaction were not to occur.

Is there any other proof that could enable us to say with certainty that what we have concluded so far about the spin-spin coupling is indeed correct?

If, indeed, the signal of proton H_A has been split into two lines due to coupling with the magnetic moment or spin of the neighbouring proton H_B and similarly if the signal due to proton H_B has been split into two lines due to coupling with the magnetic moment or spin of the neighbouring proton H_A, then we must look for some more proof or feature in the spectrum. What could be that?

We should also look at the distances between the lines in each pair. We should expect to see the distance as we measure it in Hertz (Hz) in one pair being equal to the distance in Hertz between the lines in the other pair, if the theory we have advanced for the reciprocal interaction between the two neighbouring protons is correct. And indeed you would be surprised to learn that the two distances are equal in magnitude in both the pairs of lines lending strong support to the idea of mutual spin-spin coupling.

Intext Exercise

1. What further feature is left in the above spectrum which we have not talked about as yet? Think.

The other feature in the spectrum under discussion that should attract your attention is the relative ratio of the peaks within each pair of peaks. Why should not we consider that? This also forms a part of the game we are playing with the nuclear micromagnets when placed in an applied field and irradiated with radiowaves.

When we look at the ratio of peaks in one pair, we find that it is 1:1. Similarly, it is found to be 1:1 in the other pair as well.

Can you now think about the origin as well as the relative ratios of the peaks in each pair? What is it possibly due to?

Well, we have seen that the NMR is basically a game based upon interaction of magnetic moments of nuclei in an applied magnetic field (B_0).

A proton that is α with the respect to the applied field has its own magnetic moment. When a suitable radiofrequency is applied, it gets flipped from α-state into the β-spin state, thereby producing a signal for that proton.

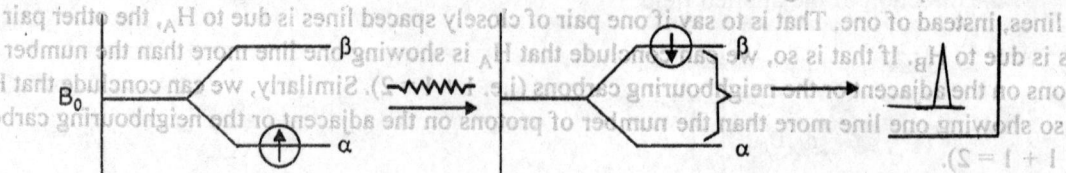

Now, as H_A is giving instead of a singlet signal, a pair of peaks (doublet), it is crystal-clear that this proton instead of [facing the applied field B_0 – its own induced field due to circulating of its electrons], must face two different effective B (instead of B_0), so that it could give two different peaks.

How can we think of two different B_{eff} fields for H_A?

Two different B_{eff} fields could result from the following possibilities or interactions.

(i) The proton, H_B in 50% of the molecules will have its magnetic moment aligned with the direction of the applied field, B_0 and will give one peak. We represent this situation as follows:

$$B_0 \uparrow \quad \uparrow \quad Cl_3C\overset{H_A}{\underset{Cl}{-C-}}\overset{H_B}{\underset{Cl}{-C-}}Cl \quad \uparrow B_0$$

50% molecules

(ii) The proton H_B may have its magnetic moment aligned against the direction of the applied field B_0 in the remaining 50% of the molecules. This situation can be represented as :

$$B_0 \downarrow \quad \downarrow \quad Cl_3C\overset{H_A}{\underset{Cl}{-C-}}\overset{H_B\downarrow}{\underset{Cl}{-C-}}Cl \quad \uparrow B_0$$

50% molecules

Consequently, the spin of H_A is coupled to the spin of H_B such that the uncoupled signal of H_A we can say is split into a doublet, the ratio between the component peaks being 1:1 as statistically in some 50% of molecules the spin of H_B is in $\downarrow$ and in other 50% molecules, it it $\uparrow$ with respect to the applied field, B_0. This can be illustrated with the Fig. 3.12.

Let us now analyse the corresponding situation w.r. to the other proton H_B. This proton must also experience two different $B_{effective}$ magnetic fields, due to two spin states proton H_A :

(i) The proton, H_A, in 50% of the molecules will have its magnetic moment aligned with the direction of the applied field, B_0. So it will give one (deshielded) signal.

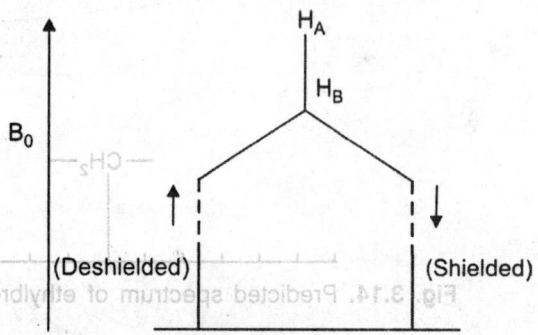

Fig. 3.12. Origin of doublet of H_A due to coupling with H_B.

$$B_0 \uparrow \quad \uparrow \quad Cl_3C\overset{H_A}{\underset{Cl}{-C-}}\overset{H_B}{\underset{Cl}{-C-}}Cl \quad \uparrow B_0$$

50%

(ii) The proton in the remaining 50% of the molecules will have its magnetic moment aligned with the direction of the applied field B_0. Therefore, it will contribute one (shielded) signal.

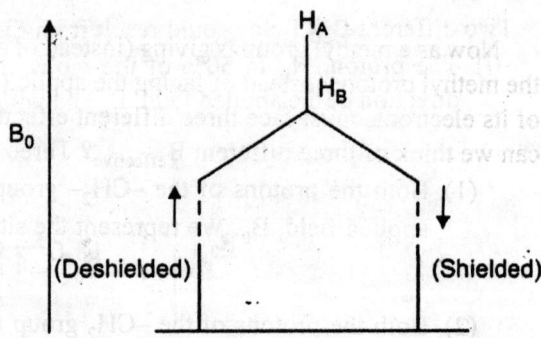

$$B_0 \qquad Cl_3C—\overset{\underset{\displaystyle Cl}{|}}{\underset{}{C}}—\overset{\underset{\displaystyle Cl}{|}}{\underset{}{C}}—Cl \qquad B_0$$

50%

As a result, the spin of proton H_B is coupled to the spin of proton H_A such that the uncoupled signal of H_B is split into a pair of lines (a doublet), the ratio between the component peaks being 1:1 as statistically in some 50% of molecules, the spin of H_B is ↑ and in other 50% of molecules, it is ↓ with respect to the applied field, B_0. This is shown in Fig. 3.13.

(Deshielded)   (Shielded)

Fig. 3.13. Origin of doublet from H_B due to coupling with H_A.

Example 2 : The NMR spectrum of Ethylbromide

$$CH_3—CH_2—Br$$

This molecule contains two sets of non-equivalent protons. Hence, it is expected to show two peaks only, one due to each set, in the ratio of 2:3 (CH_2 : CH_3), as shown in Fig. 3.14.

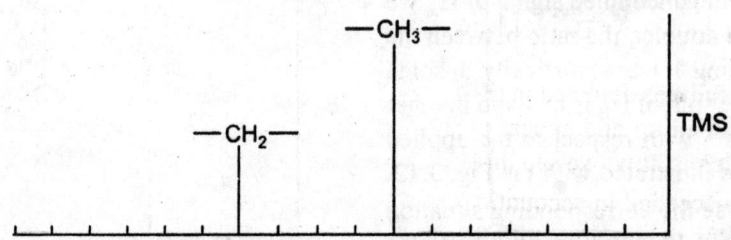

Fig. 3.14. Predicted spectrum of ethylbromide without taking coupling into account.

However, when we look at its spectrum, we find that in this example also, there are more peaks than expected as shown in Fig. 3.15. There are seven peaks instead of two peaks.

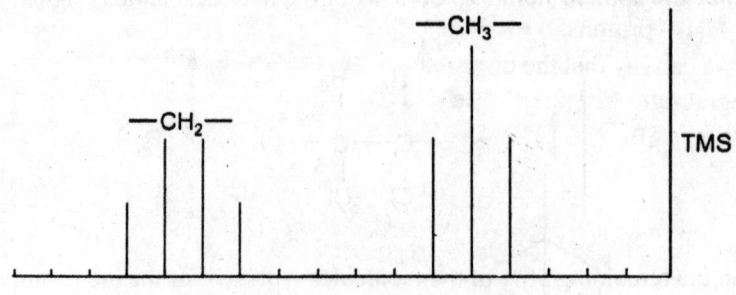

Fig. 3.15. NMR spectrum of ethylbromide.

Now as a methyl group is giving (instead of a singlet), a triplet i.e. three peaks, it is crystal-clear that the methyl protons instead of facing the applied field B_0 minus its own induced field due to circulation of its electrons, must face three different effective B_0 so that it could give three different peaks. How can we think of three different $B_{effective}$? Three possible B_{eff} could result from following situations.

(1) Both the protons of the $-CH_2-$ group may have their magnetic moments aligned with the applied field, B_0. We represent the situation as

$$B_0\uparrow \quad \uparrow\uparrow \quad CH_3CH_2Br$$
$$\uparrow\uparrow$$

(2) Both the protons of the $-CH_2$ group may have their magnetic moments aligned against the applied field, B_0 we represent this possibility as :

$$B_0\uparrow \quad \downarrow\downarrow \quad CH_3 CH_2 Br$$
$$\downarrow\downarrow$$

Due to this arrangement, the methyl protons will give most shielded peak.

(3) (a) One proton (say H_1) of the $-CH_2-$ group may have its magnetic moment aligned with while, the other one (call it, H_2) may have its magnetic moment aligned against the applied field B_0.

$$B_0\uparrow \quad \uparrow\downarrow \quad CH_3 CH_2 Br \text{ (25\% molecules)}$$
$$\uparrow\downarrow$$

(b) While proton H_1 may have its magnetic moment aligned against B_0, the proton H_2 may have its magnetic moment aligned with B_0, the possibility being depicted as :

$$B_0\uparrow \quad \downarrow\uparrow \quad CH_3 CH_2 Br \text{ (25\% molecules)}$$
$$\downarrow\uparrow$$

The possibilities depicted in (a) and (b) in point (3) will have equal energies. So, their signals will be added up and appear at one and the same position, somewhere in between the two peaks. This is how, we see three different magnetic fields in operation for the CH_3 protons.

OK, we have succeeded in accounting for or "creating" three different B_{eff} magnetic moments for the $-CH_3$ protons due to coupling with the $-CH_2$ protons.

But, we are still left with an important question to answer and that is about the relative ratios of these three peaks which is observed to be 1:2:1.

All we can say about this is that this is now merely a question of statistics. At any moment, of the total molecules in the sample, 25% of molecules will have $\uparrow\uparrow$ combination, 25% of molecules will have $\downarrow\downarrow$ combination and 50% of molecules will have $\uparrow\downarrow$ or $\downarrow\uparrow$ (25% each) combination of magnetic moments of their $-CH_2-$ protons.

In conclusion, we can say that the uncoupled $-CH_3$ proton signal is split into 3-equally spaces lines, a triplet in the integral ratio of 1:2:1.

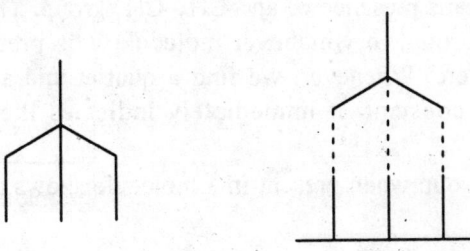

Similarly, we can have the following four B_{eff} for the $-CH_2-$ protons arising from the CH_3 protons.

$CH_3 CH_2Br$ (12.5%)
↑↑↑

$CH_3 CH_2Br$ (12.5%)
↑↑↑

$CH_3 CH_2Br$ (12.5%)
↑↑↑

↑↑↑   ↓↑↑ ↑↓↑ ↑↑↓   ↓↓↑ ↓↑↓ ↑↓↓   ↓↓↓

$CH_3 CH_2Br$ (12.5%)
↑↓↑

(i)   (ii)   (iii)   (iv)

Expected ratio :

$CH_3 CH_2Br$ (12.5%)
↑↑↓

1   :   3   :   3   :   1

$CH_3 CH_2Br$ (12.5%)
↓↓↑

$CH_3 CH_2Br$ (12.5%)
↓↑↓

$CH_3 CH_2Br$ (12.5%)
↓↓↓

As arrangements (ii) and (iii) both have three possibilities, therefore, their signals are expected to be three times that of arrangement (i) or (iv). This comes to the ratio 1:3:3:1, which is indeed what it is. Statistically speaking, of the total molecules in the sample, 1/8 molecules will have the possibility (i), 3/8 molecules will have possibility no (ii) and another 3/8 molecules will have possibility shown in (iii) and the remaining 1/8 molecules have possibility (iv) of alignment of magnetic moments of their $-CH_3$ protons.

In conclusion, we can say that the signal from the uncoupled $-CH_3$ protons is split into four equally spaced lines i.e. a quartet.

As I indicated in the beginning, if in reality the spin of one set of protons is splitted by the spin of second set of protons in the molecule, it must be a reciprocal affair and that the distances between the peaks in multiplets of both the sets must be identical. Indeed, the distance (Hz) between the peaks of CH_2 quartet and those of CH_3 quartets are found to be equal i.e. 7 Hz.

Now, there arises an important question, still untouched in the above discussion and that is how do we know whether the peaks in a multiplet are indeed component peaks of the multiplet or do they arise from non-equivalent protons?

We still require some more proof to confirm that. Fortunately, it was discovered that the coupling constant J did not change (increase or decrease) but the distance in Hz between the chemical shift in Hz (not in ppm) of both the multiplets increased, as the power of the NMR spectrometer was increased as shown in Fig. 3.16.

Triplet quartet pattern means presence of an $-CH_2-CH_3$ group. The example of ethyl bromide is representative of the ethyl group, in whichever molecule it is present, such as in $CH_3CH_2NH_2$, CH_3CH_2OH, CH_3CH_2COCl etc. Whenever, we find a quartet and a triplet, each having the same magnitude of the coupling constant, it immediately indicates the presence of an ethyl group, $-CH_2CH_3$.

In conclusion, the ethyl group when present in a molecule shows the characteristic triplet-quartet multiplicity pattern.

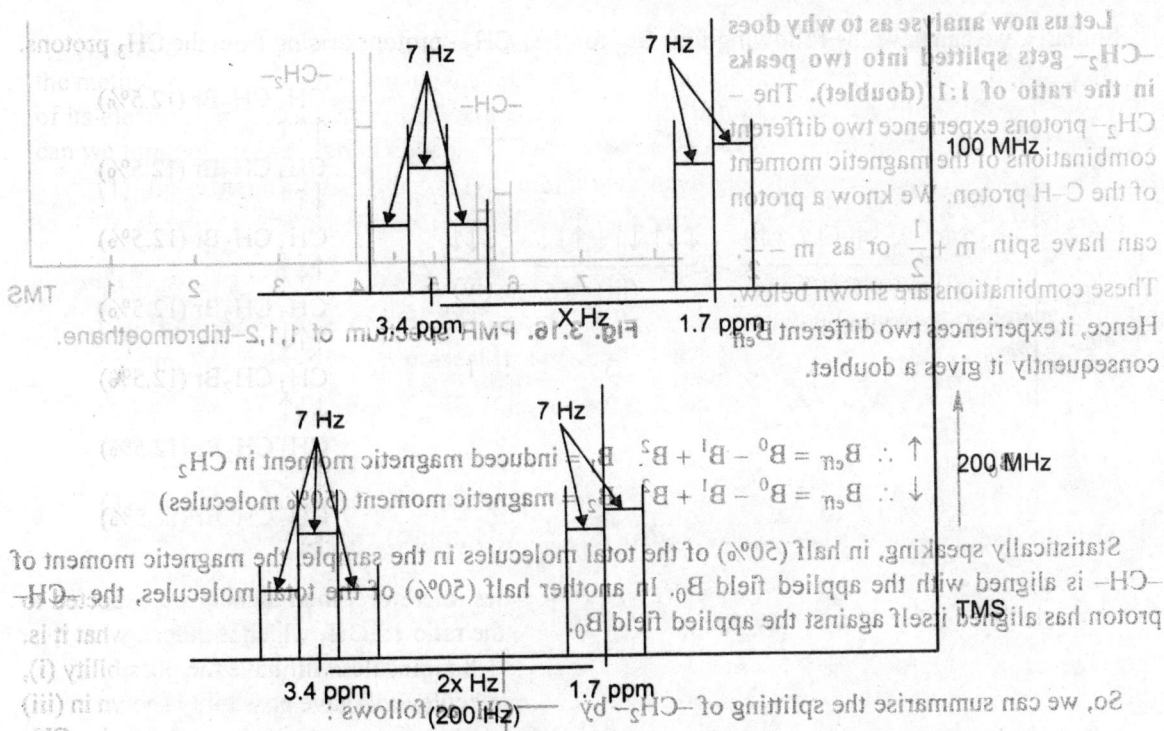

Fig. 3.16. Effect of high resolution power on chemical shift and J (in Hz).

Example 3 : NMR spectrum of 1,1,2-tribromoethane

We have discussed above a representative example (Example 1) a 3° and a 3° proton and of coupling between secondary (–CH₂–) and primary protons (–CH₃) (Example 2). Let us now discuss the coupling

between a tertiary $\left(\diagup_{\diagdown} CH- \right)$ and secondary protons as shown herein.

$$\underset{3°}{-HC}-\overset{\overset{\displaystyle H}{|}}{\underset{\underset{\displaystyle H}{|}}{C}}-\quad 2°$$

We will consider the example of 1,1,2-tribromoethane, whose structural formula is :

$$\underset{3°}{CHBr_2} - \underset{2°}{CH_2Br}$$

The NMR spectrum of this molecule is shown in the Fig. 3.16. This shows a multiplet and a doublet instead of two singlets, at 5.75 and 4.5 ppm, in the ratio of 1:2. This again shows spin-spin coupling between the two sets of non-equivalent protons. The –CH– proton is split into a triplet (1:2) due to coupling with –CH₂– protons and the –CH₂– protons are split into a doublet (1:1).

Let us now analyse as to why does –CH$_2$– gets splitted into two peaks in the ratio of 1:1 (doublet). The –CH$_2$– protons experience two different combinations of the magnetic moment of the C–H proton. We know a proton can have spin $m + \dfrac{1}{2}$ **or as** $m - \dfrac{1}{2}$. **These combinations are shown below. Hence, it experiences two different B$_{eff}$ consequently it gives a doublet.**

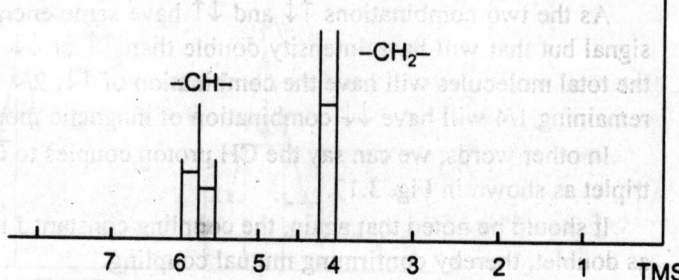

Fig. 3.16. PMR spectrum of 1,1,2–tribromoethane.

$$B_0 \quad \uparrow \therefore B_{eff} = B^0 - B^1 + B^2 \quad B_1 = \text{induced magnetic moment in CH}_2$$
$$\downarrow \therefore B_{eff} = B^0 - B^1 + B^2 \quad B_2 = \text{magnetic moment (50\% molecules)}$$

Statistically speaking, in half (50%) of the total molecules in the sample, the magnetic moment of –CH– is aligned with the applied field B$_0$. In another half (50%) of the total molecules, the –CH– proton has aligned itself against the applied field B$_0$.

So, we can summarise the splitting of –CH$_2$– by $-\overset{|}{\underset{|}{C}}H$ as follows :

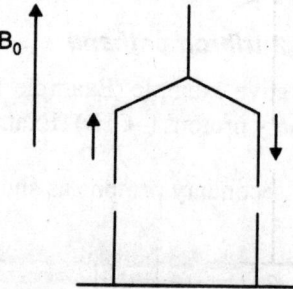

How can we analyse splitting of $-\overset{|}{\underset{|}{C}}H$ by –CH$_2$ protons? The triplet shown by CH arises due to following combinations of magnetic moments of the two CH$_2$ protons.

$$B_0 \quad \begin{array}{l} \uparrow\uparrow \\ \uparrow\downarrow \quad \uparrow\downarrow \\ \downarrow\downarrow \end{array}$$

Different combination of
magnetic moments of CH$_2$ protons

As the two combinations ↑↓ and ↓↑ have same energy, therefore, they will give rise only to one signal but that will have intensity double than ↑↑ or ↓↓ arrangement. Statistically speaking, 1/4th of the total molecules will have the combination of ↑↓, 2/4 will have combination of ↑↓ and ↓↑ and the remaining 1/4 will have ↓↓ combination of magnetic moments of CH_2 protons.

In other words, we can say the CH proton couples to CH_2 protons such that its signal is split into a triplet as shown in Fig. 3.17.

It should be noted that again, the coupling constant J is found to be equal in both the triplet as well as doublet, thereby confirming mutual coupling.

The proton of a double–triplet pattern means presence in the molecule $-CH_2-CH-$ Unit.

The doublet–triplet splitting pattern is a characteristic splitting pattern for the presence of the $-CH_2-CH-$ unit in the molecule.

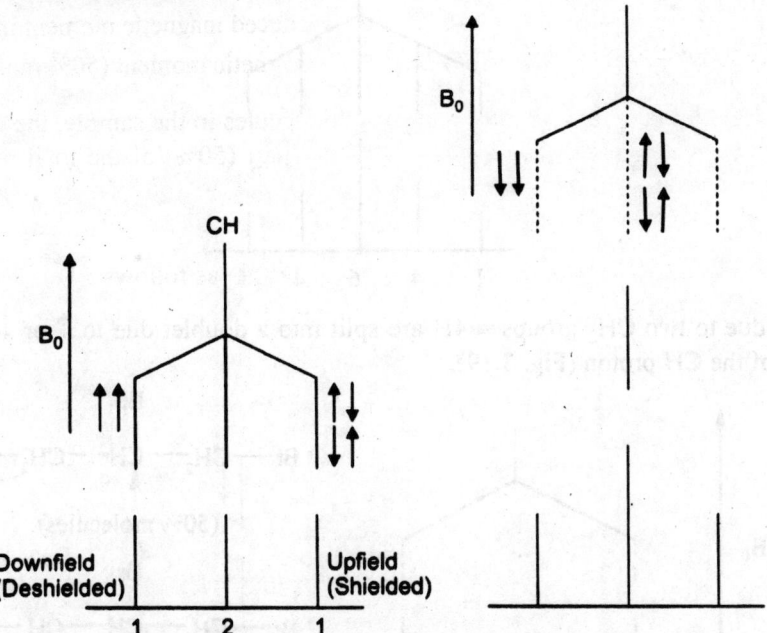

Fig. 3.17. Splitting of CH signal by CH_2 signal into a triplet (1:2:1).

Example 4 : NMR spectrum of 1,2,3–Tribromopropane

Let us now consider a new situation in which a proton has more than 3 equivalent adjacent protons, say four equivalent adjacent protons such as in the molecule of 1,2,3-tribromopropane.

$$\overset{3}{\text{Br}}-\overset{}{\underset{}{\text{CH}_2}}-\overset{2}{\underset{\underset{\text{Br}}{|}}{\text{CH}}}-\overset{1}{\text{CH}_2}-\text{Br}$$

1,2,3–tribromopropane

The spectrum shows a quintet and a doublet. Evidently, the multiplet is due to coupling of CH proton to four equivalent methylene group, magnetic moments five combinations :

As the two combinations ↑↓ and ↓↑ have same energy, therefore they will give rise only to one signal but that will have intensity double than ↑↑ or ↓↓ arrangement. Statistically speaking, 1/4th of the total molecules will have the combination of ↑↑, 2/4 will have combination of ↑↓ and ↓↑ and the remaining 1/4 will have ↓↓ combination of magnetic moments of CH_2 protons.

In other words, we can say two equivalent CH_2 protons couples with another CH proton such that its signal is split into a triplet as shown in Fig. 3.17, expected.

It should be noted that again, the coupling constant J is found to be equal in both the triplet as well as doublet, thereby confirming mutual coupling.

To give five peaks in the ratio 1:4:6:4:1. Hence, we can say the singlet due to uncoupled proton is split into a quintet.

The doublet–triplet splitting pattern is a characteristic splitting pattern for the presence of the –CH_2–CH– unit in the molecule.

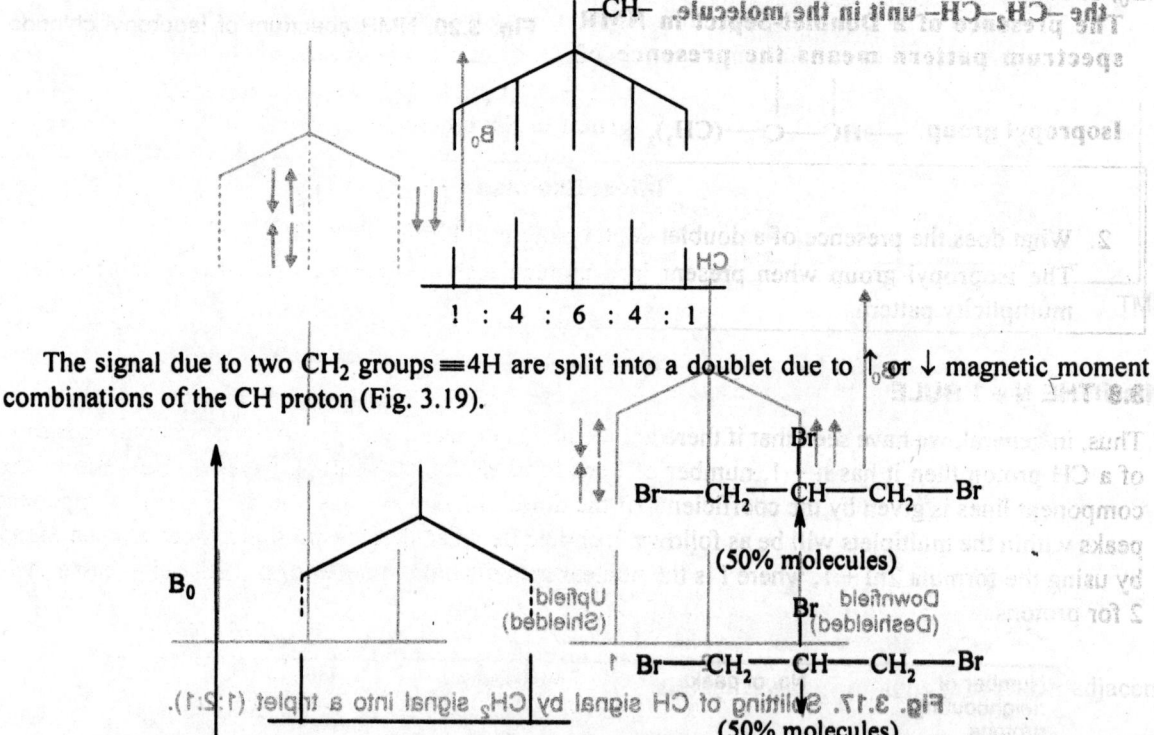

The signal due to two CH_2 groups ≡ 4H are split into a doublet due to ↑ or ↓ magnetic moment combinations of the CH proton (Fig. 3.19).

$$Br—CH_2—CH—CH_2—Br$$
(50% molecules)

$$Br—CH_2—CH—CH_2—Br$$
(50% molecules)

Fig. 3.19. Coupling of (CH_2 × 2) protons with CH protons two combinations.

Fig. 3.17. Splitting of CH signal by CH_3 signal into a triplet (1:2:1).

The presence of a doublet-quintet pattern in the NMR spectrum means the presence of a – CH_2–CH–CH_2– unit in the molecule.

Example 5 : NMR spectrum of Isopropylchloride

Let us consider Isopropyl chloride which contains two sets of protons, –CH– and 6H due to two equivalent methyl groups (2 × CH_3).

$$Cl—CH—CH_3$$
$$CH_3$$

The spectrum shows a quintet and a triplet. Evidently, the multiplet is due to coupling of CH proton to four equivalent methylene group, magnetic moments five combinations :

The spectrum is shown in Fig. 3.20, which shows a septet for –CH– due to coupling with the 6 methyl protons (2 × CH_3). This is to be expected on the basis of spin-spin coupling between these two sets of equivalent protons. The ratio of the peaks in the doublet is 1:1 as expected. The ratio of the peaks in the septet is 1:6:15:20:15:6:1 due to various combinations, the first and the last combination of spins of 6 methyl protons being all aligned with and all aligned against the applied field B_0, of course.

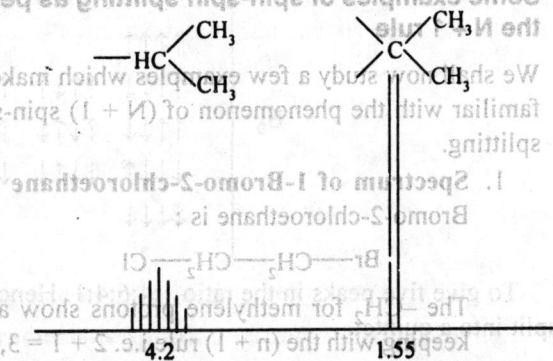

Fig. 3.20. NMR spectrum of Isopropyl chloride.

The presence of a Doublet-Septet in NMR spectrum pattern means the presence of

Isopropyl group   —HC—C—(CH₃)₂ group in the molecule.

Intext Exercise

2. What does the presence of a doublet-septet pattern in PMR (NMR) indicate?

The Isopropyl group when present in a molecule shows the characteristic doublet-septet multiplicity pattern.

3.8 THE N + 1 RULE

Thus, in general, we have seen that if there are n equivalent nuclei attached to the neighbouring carbon of a CH proton then it has n + 1, number of lines in its multiplet (splitting pattern). The ratio of the component lines is given by the coefficients of the times of $(g + 1)^n$. Thus, the ratios of the component peaks within the multiplets will be as follows. It should be noted that the multiplicity can also be found by using the formula 2nI + 1, where I is the nuclear spin quantum number of proton, being equal to 1/2 for protons.

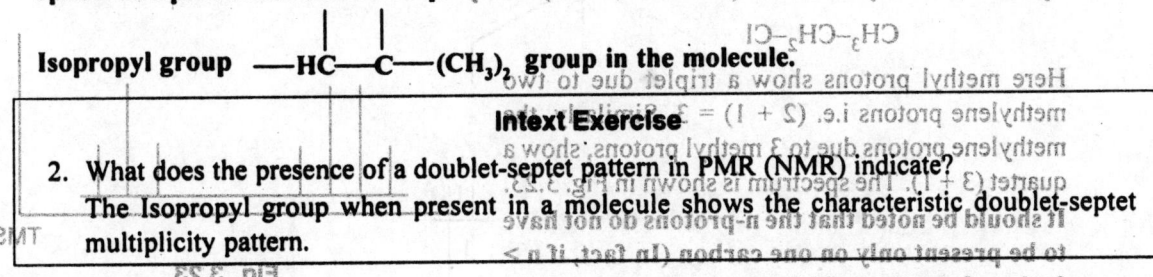

Number of neighbouring protons	No. of peaks n + 1	Multiplicity	Ratio of component peaks
1	1 + 1	doublet (d)	1 : 1
2	2 + 1	triplet (t)	1 : 2 : 1
3	3 + 1	quartet (q)	1 : 3 : 3 : 1
4	4 + 1	quintet	1 : 4 : 6 : 4 : 1
5	5 + 1	sextet	1 : 5 : 10 : 10 : 5 : 1
6	6 + 1	septet	1 : 6 : 15 : 20 : 15 : 6 : 1
7	7 + 1	octet	1 : 7 : 21 : 35 : 21 : 7 : 1

Fig. 3.21. N + 1 rule in action.

Some examples of spin-spin splitting as per the N + 1 rule

We shall now study a few examples which make us familiar with the phenomenon of (N + 1) spin-spin splitting.

1. **Spectrum of 1-Bromo-2-chloroethane :** 1-Bromo-2-chloroethane is :

$$Br\text{—}CH_2\text{—}CH_2\text{—}Cl$$

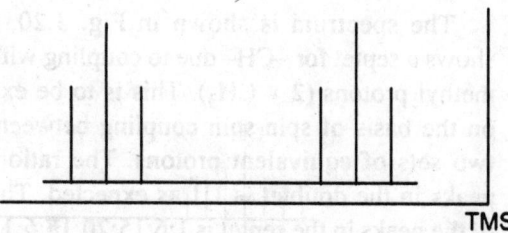

Fig. 3.22. Spectrum of 1-Bromo-2-chloroethane.

The $-CH_2$ for methylene protons show a triplet due to two protons of the CH_2Cl. This is in keeping with the (n + 1) rule i.e. 2 + 1 = 3, triplet. The spectrum is shown in Fig. 3.22. Similarly, the CH_2Cl protons show a triplet due to coupling with $-CH_2Br$.

2. **Spectrum of ethyl chloride (1-chloroethane) :** Ethyl chloride or 1-chloroethane is :

$$CH_3\text{–}CH_2\text{–}Cl$$

Here methyl protons show a triplet due to two methylene protons i.e. (2 + 1) = 3. Similarly, the methylene protons due to 3 methyl protons, show a quartet (3 + 1). The spectrum is shown in Fig. 3.23. **It should be noted that the n-protons do not have to be present only on one carbon (In fact, if n > 3, therefore, they will be present on more than**

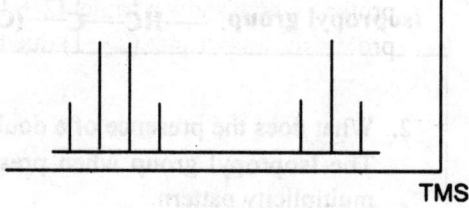

Fig. 3.23.

one carbon). They may be present on different carbons as well but they must be magnetically equivalent.

Example 1 : Spectrum of 2-Bromopropane :

$$\overset{1}{CH_3}\text{—}\overset{2}{\underset{\underset{Br}{|}}{CH}}\text{—}\overset{3}{CH_3}$$

The spectrum of 2-bromopropane is shown in Fig. 3.24.

So, here the $-CH-$ proton shows a septet due to coupling with 6 protons present on adjacent methyl groups that are magnetically equivalent.

Example 2 : Spectrum of 2-Methylpropane. The structural formula of 2-methyl propane is :

$$CH_3\text{—}\overset{\overset{\displaystyle CH_3}{|}}{\underset{\underset{H}{|}}{C}}\text{—}CH_3$$

As per the (n + 1) rule, the $-CH-$ proton shows a multiplet containing ten lines as per the formula (9 + 1) = 10. The three methyl protons give a doublet due to coupling with the $-CH-$ proton.

If a set of equivalent protons is joined to two sets of non-equivalent protons say na and nb, then the number of lines in its multiplet will be equal to the formula (na + 1)·(nb + 1).

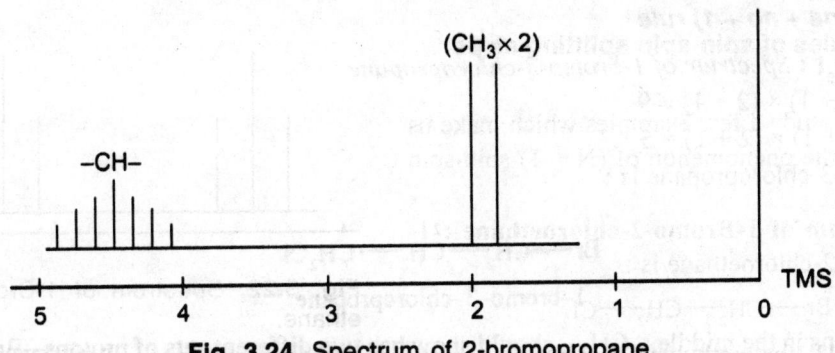

Fig. 3.24. Spectrum of 2-bromopropane.

Example 1 : *Spectrum of ultra-pure ethanol* : The PMR of ethanol is shown in Fig. 3.25. The $-CH_2-$, methylene protons have two neighbouring sets of non-equivalent protons, the CH_3 protons and the O–H protons. It shows an octet i.e. eight lines. While (n + 1) rule is followed by the $-CH_3$ protons which show a triplet (2 + 1) due to coupling with the CH_2- protons. Similarly, the –OH proton shows a triplet (2 + 1) due to coupling with the two $-CH_2$ protons.

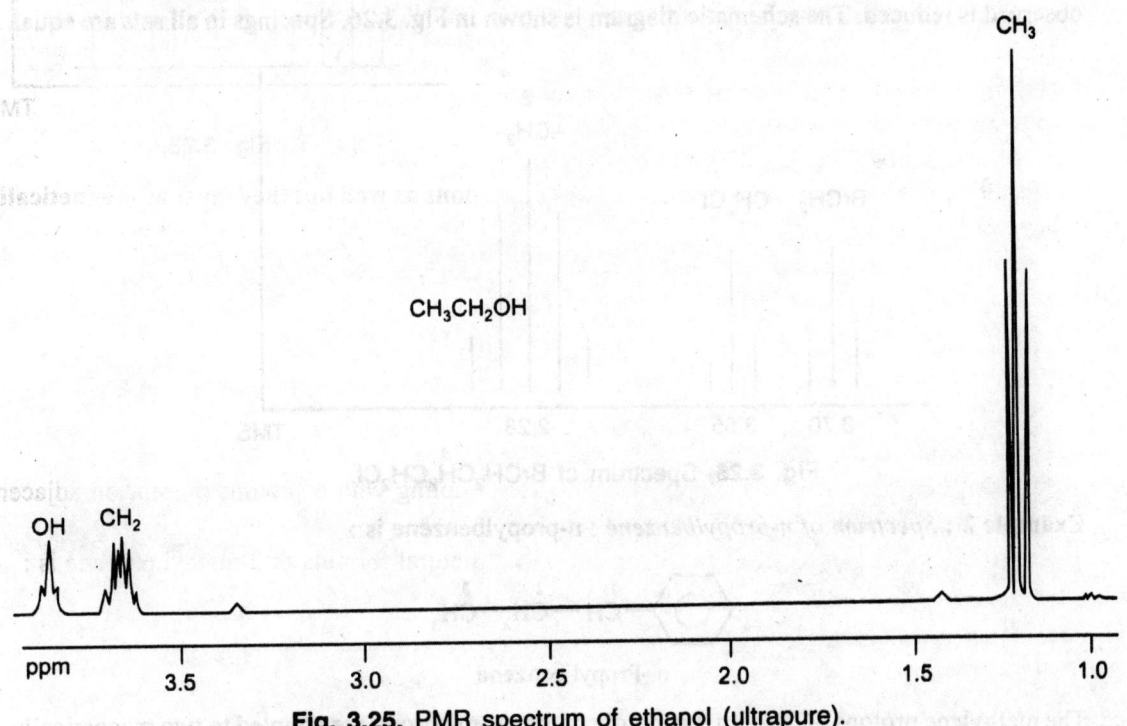

Fig. 3.25. PMR spectrum of ethanol (ultrapure).

Note : Sometimes, the formula (na + 1) (nb + 1) may turn out to be equal to (na + nb + 1) i.e. the expected number of lines may get reduced to fewer lines. This is seen when the size of the involved coupling constants is equal.

Examples of (na + nb + 1) rule

Example 1 : *Spectrum of 1-bromo-3-chloropropane :*
where $(2 + 1) \times (2 + 1) \neq 9$
rather $(2 + 1) \times (2 + 1) = 5$
1-Bromo-3-chloropropane is :

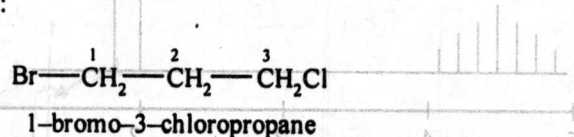

$$\overset{1}{Br—CH_2}—\overset{2}{CH_2}—\overset{3}{CH_2Cl}$$

1–bromo–3–chloropropane

The protons in the middle, $-CH_2-$, should show has two different sets of protons $-BrCH_2-$ and $-CH_2Cl$. So, as per the simple formula $(na + 1)(nb + 1)$ should show $(2 + 1)(2 + 1) = 3 \times 3 = 9$ lines. But, it shows five lines in its multiplet in the ratio 1:4:6:4:1 (i.e. a pentet). Although both these sets of protons are magnetically equivalent, yet we find that these are behaving as if they were equivalent w.r. to $-CH_2-$ protons as per the formula $(na + nb + 1)$. We can say the observed number of lines is lesser than that expected from the simple rule $(na + 1)(nb + 1)$. This has so happened as the coupling constraints between the $BrCH_2$ protons and the $-^2CH_2-$ protons are of equal magnitude (~ 6Hz), so that due to overlapping of some peak, the number of lines actually observed is reduced. The schematic diagram is shown in Fig. 3.26. Spacings in all sets are equal.

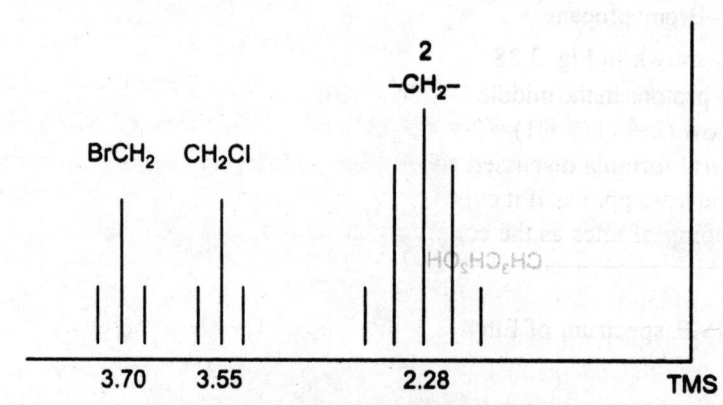

Fig. 3.26. Spectrum of $BrCH_2CH_2CH_2Cl$.

Example 2 : *Spectrum of n-propylbenzene :* n-propylbenzene is :

$$\overset{1}{CH_2}—\overset{2}{CH_2}—\overset{3}{CH_3}$$

n–Propyl benzene

The methylene protons $-CH_2-$, in the middle of the propyl group are coupled to two magnetically non-equivalent sets of protons, the benzylic methylene CH_2 and the methyl CH_3 protons. Therefore, as per the formula, it is expected to show $(2 + 1)(3 + 1) = 3 \times 4 = 12$ lines. But in the spectrum, it shows only 6 lines. This number of lines corresponds to the formula $(na + nb + 1) = 5 + 1 = 6$. Again, this happens as $J_{1, 2}$ is equal to $J_{2, 3}$ (Fig. 3.27).

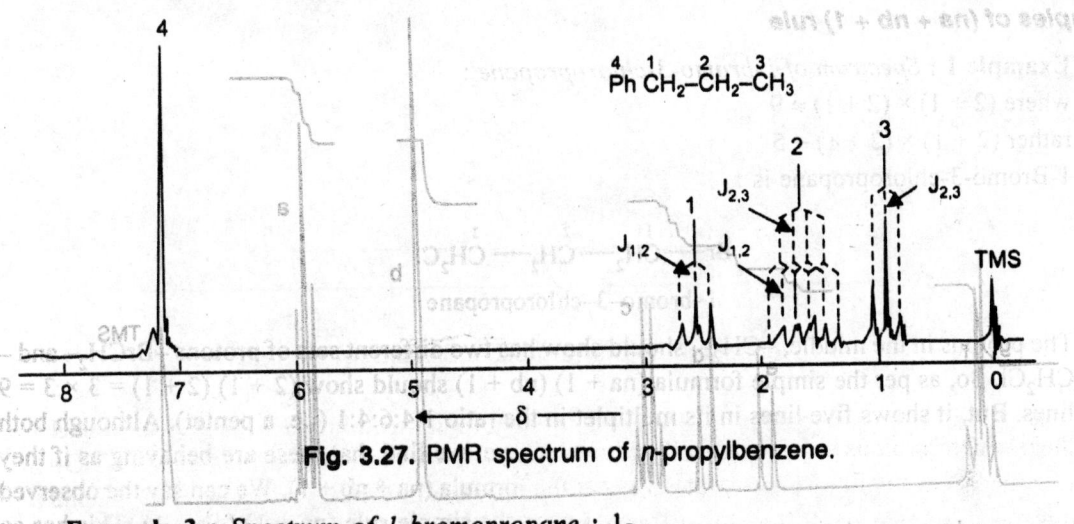

Fig. 3.27. PMR spectrum of *n*-propylbenzene.

Example 3 : *Spectrum of 1-bromopropane* : 1-Bromopropane also called n-propyl bromide is :

$$Br\overset{1}{-}CH_2\overset{2}{-}CH_2\overset{3}{-}CH_3$$

1–Bromopropane

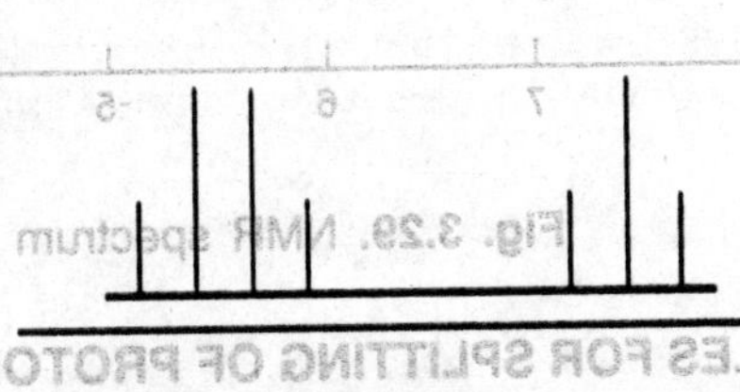

Its spectrum is shown in Fig. 3.28.

The methylene protons in the middle ($-^2CH_2-$) were expected to show $(2+1)(3+1) = 3 \times 4 = 12$ lines as per the general formula discussed above $(na+1)(nb+1)$ but the observed spectrum shows it to be a sextet, at 1.95 ppm as if it corresponds to $(na+nb+1)$ formula. Again this has happened due to overlapping of lines as the coupling constants $J_{1,2}$ is equal in magnitude to $J_{2,3}$.

Fig. 3.28. PMR spectrum of 1-bromopropane.

Intext Exercise

3. Explain the NMR spectrum of Ethyl 2,3–dibromo–3–(p-tolyl)propionate $C_{12}H_{14}Br_2O_2$ shown in Fig. 3.29.

Hint:

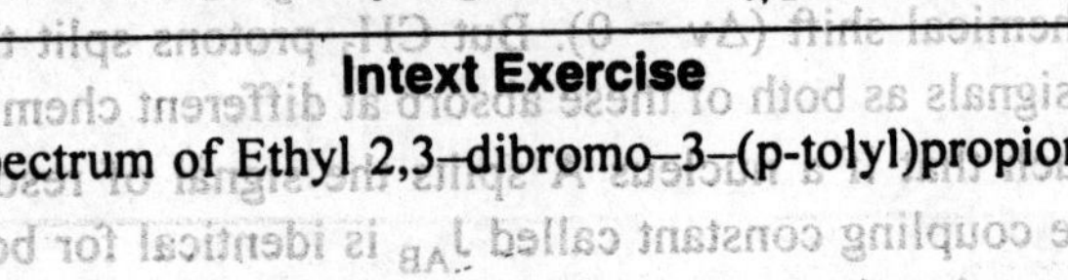

$$H_3C\overset{b}{-}\underset{g}{\bigcirc}\overset{f}{-}\underset{\underset{H_e}{|}}{\overset{\overset{Br}{|}}{C}}\overset{d}{-}\underset{\underset{Br}{|}}{\overset{\overset{H_d}{|}}{C}}\overset{c}{-}\overset{\overset{O}{||}}{C}-O\overset{a}{-}CH_2CH_3$$

The NMR of this compound is shown in Fig. 3.29. It shows a multiplet at 7.1 ppm, a doublet at 5.37 ppm, a doublet at 4.80 ppm, a quartet at 4.31 ppm, a singlet at 2.45 ppm and a triplet at 1.32 ppm in the integral ratio 4:1:1:2:3:3. This ratio corresponds to a total of exactly 14 protons. Thus, it is clear that it has the structure as shown. The singlet at 2.35 ppm is due to CH_3 group. The benzylic proton H_e appears as a doublet due to coupling with the adjacent proton H_d at 5.37 ppm. The doublet at 4.80 is due to H_d as a result of coupling with H_e. The quartet at 4.31 ppm and the triplet at 1.32 ppm indicate them to be present together as an ethyl group as OCH_2CH_3.

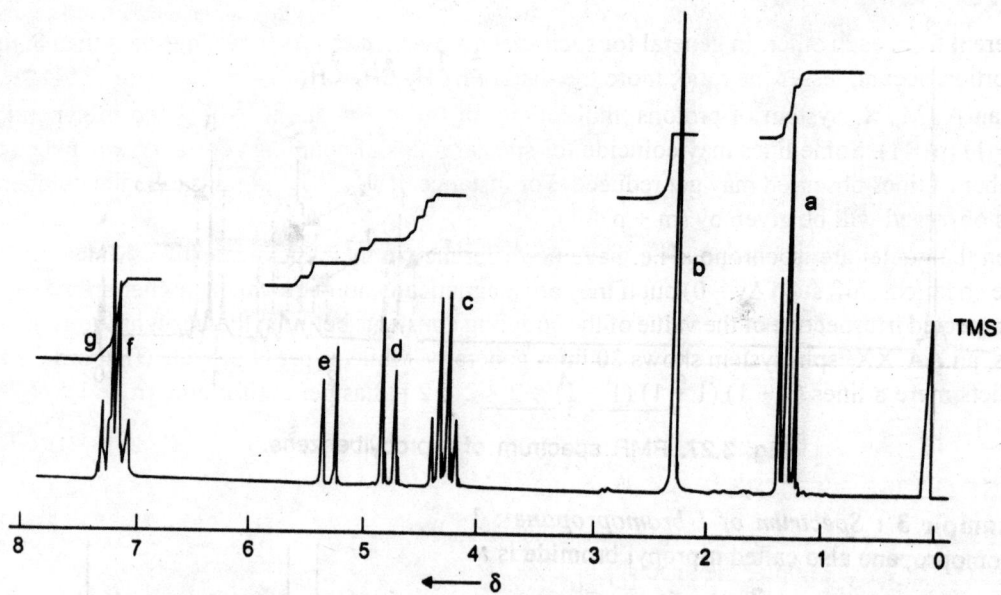

Fig. 3.29. NMR spectrum of Ethyl 2,3-dibromo-3-(p-tolyl)propionate.

3.9 RULES FOR SPLITTING OF PROTON SIGNALS

1. Splitting is not caused due to equivalent protons as they absorb at the same chemical shift. Thus CH_3 protons do not couple to each other as there is no difference in their chemical shifts.

2. Splitting is caused by the neighbouring protons which are non-equivalent i.e. which absorb at a different chemical shifts. Thus, in CH_3CH_2Br, CH_3 protons all have same chemical shift ($\Delta v = 0$), hence they do not split each other. Similarly CH_2 signals do not split each other as they also have the same chemical shift ($\Delta v = 0$). But CH_3 protons split the CH_2 signals and CH_2 protons split the CH_3 signals as both of these absorb at different chemical shifts.

3. Coupling is mutual such that if a nucleus A splits the signal of resonance of nucleus B, the reverse is true, and the coupling constant called J_{AB} is identical for both the multiplet patterns ($J_{AB} = J_{BA}$). This is to say that the coupling constants in a multiplet are equal and are also equal to the coupling constants arising from reciprocal coupling in another multiplet.

4. Coupling of H–nuclei bonded to oxygen or nitrogen is not always visible and usually just a broad peak is seen.

5. Coupling is not usually observed between protons that are separated by more than three bonds.

6. For more than two non-equivalent H-nuclei, coupling becomes more complicated i.e. complicated splitting patterns are obtained.

7. The absolute magnitude of coupling constant (in Hz) is independent of the external applied field or the radiofrequency (note that this is opposite to what we see in case of chemical shift).

8. The appearance of the multiplicities (i.e. splitting pattern) depends upon the size of the coupling constant J (in Hz) and Δv, the difference in chemical shift (in Hz).

9. Simple "first-order" spectra are obtained only when all the protons in the given molecule are very

different from each other. In general for such spectra $\Delta v/J > 8$. As $\Delta v/J$ becomes less than 8, then distortion occurs, lesser the ratio, more the distortion.

10. For an $A_n\ M_n\ X_p$ system of protons. multiplicity of the signal due to A is given in general by $(m + 1)\ (p + 1)$. Some lines may coincide for special ratios of coupling constants, and hence the number of lines observed may get reduced. For instance, if $J_{AM} = J_{AX}$, in this case the number of lines observed will be given by $(m + p + 1)$.

When the nuclei are isochronous i.e. have no difference in their chemical shift (these absorb at same chemical shift such $\Delta v = 0$) but if they are magnetically non-equivalent, higher order spectra are expected irrespective of the value of the coupling constants between these isochronous nuclei. Thus, an $AA'XX'$ spin system shows 20 lines generally, while as per $N + 1$ rule (first order rule) predicts mere 8 lines $(1 + 1)\ (1 + 1)\ (1 + 1) = 2 \times 2 \times 2 = 8$ as per the formula $(n_a + 1)\ (n_b + 1)$ $(n_c + 1)$.

3.10a FIRST-ORDER SPECTRA

The spectra which follows the "N + 1" rule are called first-order spectra. The spin-multiplicities can be readily interpreted. For example, the spectrum of ethylbromide, CH_3CH_2Br shows a clear-cut quartet due to CH_2 protons and a triplet due to CH_3 protons. There is no overlapping of any peaks as there is large difference in their chemical shifts and the coupling constant, J between them is small compared to the difference in the chemical shifts, Δv.

In fact, it has been found that the spin-multiplicities stand our clearly and the spectrum is worth ready interpretation if $\Delta v/J > 5$. If it is less than that, then the spectra are no longer first-order spectra.

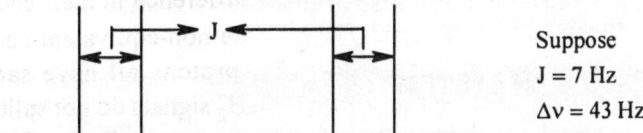

Suppose

J = 7 Hz

$\Delta v = 43$ Hz

As $\dfrac{\Delta v}{J} > 5$ so, it is a first-order spectrum.

How do we calculate $\Delta v/J$, is shown in the following Intext Exercise for the molecule of 1–bromo–3–chloropropane whose spectrum is given in Fig. 3.26.

Intext Exercise

4. From the given data at 40 MHz for 1–bromo–3--chloropropane, predict whether the NMR spectrum of this molecule will be of first or second order.

$$\overset{3}{C}H_2\!\!-\!\!\overset{2}{C}H_2\!\!-\!\!\overset{1}{C}H_2$$
$$\quad|\qquad\qquad\quad|$$
$$\ \ Cl\qquad\qquad\ Br$$

δ–CH_2Br = 3.70 ppm

–CH_2– = 2.28 ppm

–CH_2Cl = 3.55 ppm

J for CH_2Br–CH_2 = 6.2 Hz

J for CH_2Cl–CH_2 = 6.2 Hz

Solution

Here we need to find out $\Delta v/J$. If it is more than 6, spectrum is of first order, otherwise it will be different.

Now let consider the pair:

CH_2–CH_{23}

$\Delta v = ?$ $J = 6.2$, $\delta = 3.70$

We know δ ppm $= \dfrac{\Delta v(Hz) \times 10^6}{rf\ (Hz)}$

or $\Delta v\ (Hz) = d \times r.f. \times 10^6$

$= (3.70 - 2.28) \times 40 \times 10^6$

$= 1.42 \times 40 \times 10^6 = 57$ Hz

$\therefore$ $\Delta v/J = \dfrac{57}{6.2} = 9.2$

For the pair CH_2Cl–CH_2

$\Delta v = (3.55 - 2.28) \times 40 \times 10^6$

$\therefore$ $\Delta v/J = \dfrac{51}{6.2} = 8.2$

$= 1.27 \times 40 \times 10^6 = 51$

As $\Delta v/J$ is 76 for both pairs, so, it is a case of first-order spectra.

3.10B ANALYSIS OF TWO SPIN SYSTEM

Energy Level Diagram and Possible Transitions

Let us consider the coupling between vicinal protons A and X where, $J_{AX} << v_A - v_x$.

$$\overset{\displaystyle H_A \quad H_X}{\underset{\displaystyle |\quad\ |}{-C-C-}}$$

Energy of a transition is given by the relation :

$$\text{Energy} = - (m_A v_A + m_X v_X) + m_A m_X J_{AX}$$

where m_A means magnetic quantum number of proton A. m_X is the magnetic quantum number of Proton X, V_A and V_X are chemical shift in Hz of proton A and X respectively, J_{AX} represents coupling constant between protons A and X.

For H_A, there are two possible orientations of X (α and β), which split its signal. Similarly, for H_X there are also two (α and β) possible orientations of H_A that split its signal. Thus, in all, there are four energy states. These are shown in Fig. 3.30.

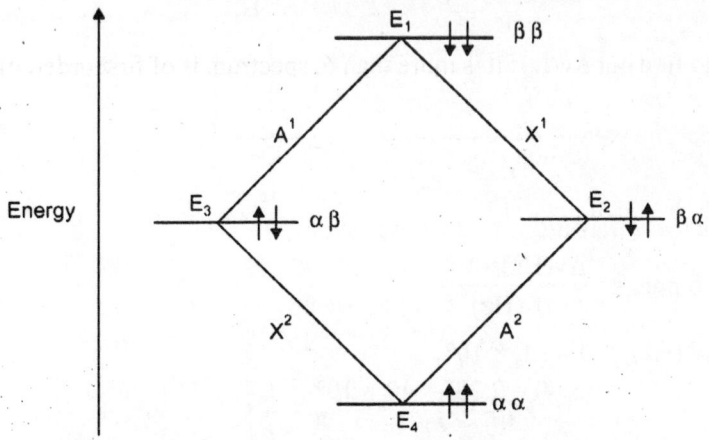

Fig. 3.30. Energy level diagram for coupled protons H_A and H_X.

For proton H_A as per selection rule, $\Delta m_A = -1$ for absorption of energy and $\Delta m_X = 0$. Consequently, only two transitions A^1 and A^2 are possible:

$$A^1 \text{ from } \uparrow\downarrow (\alpha\beta) \text{ to } \downarrow\downarrow (\beta\beta) \text{ Transition energy } V_A + \frac{1}{2}$$

$$A^2 \text{ from } \uparrow\uparrow (\alpha\alpha) \text{ to } \downarrow\uparrow (\beta\alpha) \text{ Transition energy } V_A - \frac{1}{2}$$

Similarly, for proton H_X, selection rule demands $\Delta m_X = -1$ and $\Delta m_A = 0$. In consequence, only two transitions X^1 and X^2 are possible:

$$X^1 \text{ from } \downarrow\uparrow (\beta\alpha) \text{ to } \downarrow\downarrow (\beta\beta)$$

$$X^2 \text{ from } \uparrow\uparrow (\alpha\alpha) \text{ to } \uparrow\downarrow (\alpha\beta)$$

On the basis of the fundamental energy equation given above, the energies for these states are as follows :

State	A	X	Energy
1	β	β	$\frac{1}{2}(V_A + V_X) + J/4$
2	β	α	$\frac{1}{2}(V_A - V_X) - J/4$
3	α	β	$\frac{1}{2}(-V_A + V_X) - J/4$
4	α	α	$-\frac{1}{2}(V_A + V_X) + J/4$

The spectrum for the coupling between H_A and H_X gives two doublets, having the integral ratio 1:1:1:1.

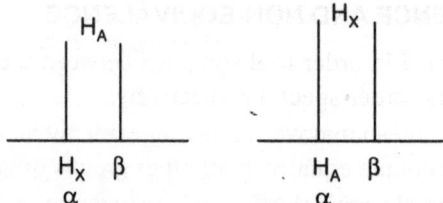

Let us now assign these transitions to the observed lines :

A^1	A^2	X^1	X^2
$\beta\beta$	$\beta\alpha$	$\beta\beta$	$\alpha\beta$
$\alpha\alpha$	$\alpha\alpha$	$\beta\alpha$	$\alpha\alpha$
$\left(V_A + \dfrac{1}{2}\right)$	$\left(V_A - \dfrac{1}{2}\right)$	$\left(V_B - \dfrac{1}{2}\right)$	$\left(V_B + \dfrac{1}{2}\right)$ Transition energy

As the spectrum is run in increasing frequency units from right to left (as opposed to magnetic field), therefore, it is clear from the above analysis that the frequency separation between the transitions A^1 and A^2 equals the frequency separation between transition X^1 and X^2. It should be noted that the lower field proton is labelled as proton A. Further when $J_{AX} > 0$, A^1 transition is to low field of A^2 and X^1 transition is to low field of X_2. The situation reverses when $J_{AX} < 0$.

3.11A SECOND ORDER SPECTRA

When the difference in Hertz in chemical shift of two groups of protons coupled to each other is large as compared to the coupling constant linking them, so that $\Delta v/J$ is large (more than 5), the spectra can be analysed by the N + 1 rule or simple graphical analysis based upon the diagrams. However, if the difference (in Hertz) in the chemical shifts of protons is similar to the coupling constant (i.e. $\Delta v/J$ is nearly one), the spectra cannot be analysed by the N + 1 rule and are called non-first order or second-order spectra. In other words, the coupled nuclei have **nearly equivalent chemical shifts** in second order spectra while they have **wide difference** in their chemical shifts in first order spectra. We can conclude that compared to first-order spectra, the second-order spectra are reflective of stronger coupling. **Thus, while the first-order spectra are weakly coupled, the second order spectra are strongly coupled.**

$$J_{AB}$$

$$\frac{\delta_A - \delta_B\ (\Delta v)}{J_{AB}} > 5$$

δ_A δ_B

First – order coupling (case of **weak** coupling)

$$\frac{\delta_A - \delta_B\ (\Delta v)}{J_{AB}} < 5$$

Second – order coupling (case of **strong** coupling)

Fig. 3.31. First-order versus second-order spectra.

3.11B MAGNETIC EQUIVALENCE AND NON-EQUIVALENCE

These two terms have been framed in order to distinguish between the necessary basic conditions for obtaining first-order and non-first-order spectra respectively.

By magnetic equivalence, we mean that we are dealing with nuclei which have same chemical shift (isochronous) nuclei and which couple equally to all other groups of nuclei in the molecule.

In general, we can show magnetic equivalence between two protons A and B with respect to another proton C in the molecules :

$$H_A \!-\! \overset{\displaystyle |}{\underset{\displaystyle |}{C}} \!-\! \overset{\displaystyle |}{\underset{\displaystyle |}{C}} \!-\! \qquad \begin{array}{l} \delta_A = \delta_B \\ J_A = J_B \end{array}$$
$$\underset{\displaystyle H_B \;\; H_C}{}$$

Example : The two protons in $-CH_2-$ group in CH_3CH_2 group are magnetically equivalent. This is because, they absorb at the same chemical shift and also couple equally with the CH_3 protons. Similarly, all the three CH_3 protons absorb at the same chemical shift and also couple equally with the methylene, $-CH_2-$ protons. The result of this magnetic equivalence is that if the difference in their chemical shifts is wide i.e. much larger than their coupling constants ($\Delta V/J = 5$) the spectra are called first order spectra. So, this is the basic condition which gives rise first order spectra.

Magnetically nonequivalent protons

$$CH_3 \!-\!\! CH_2 \!-\!\! O \!-\!\! CH_2CH_3$$

Magnetically
equivalent protons

By **magnetic non-equivalence,** we mean nuclei which behave in an opposite manner to equivalent nuclei. That is they do not absorb at the same chemical shift and also do not couple equally to all other groups of nuclei in the molecule. We can represent this as follows in which proton H_A and H_B do not absorb at the same chemical shift (i.e. $\delta_A \neq \delta_B$) and do not couple equally to another proton H_C ($J_{AC} \neq J_{BC}$).

Example 1: Styrene oxide :

$$\begin{array}{l} J_{BC} = 4.0 \, Hz \\ J_{AC} = 2.6 \, Hz \\ \delta_{HA} \neq \delta_{HB} \end{array}$$

The spectrum of this compound shows that the two methylene protons H_B and H_A are not magnetically equivalent as they resonate at different chemical shifts, at δ 3.09 and 2.75 respectively (i.e. $\delta H_A \neq \delta H_B$). Further, they also couple to H_C differently such that J_{AC} is different from J_{BC}. While J_{AC} is 2.6 Hz, J_{BC} is 4.0 Hz. Both H_A and H_B show a doublet of doublet. This can not be explained by $N+1$ rule established for first order spectra.

Example 2: Now let us consider the spectrum of 1,1–difluoroethene, $CH_2 = CF_2$:

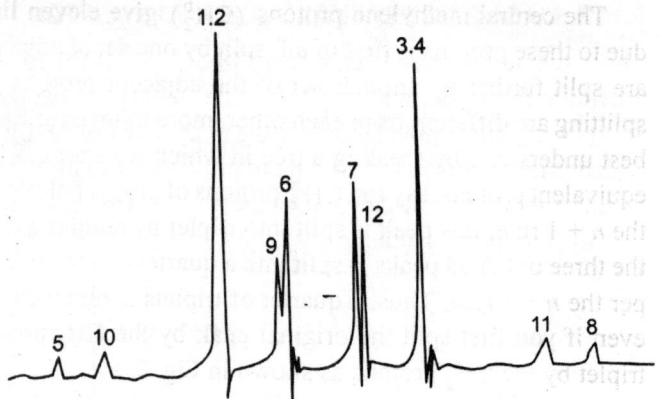

$$\delta H^1 \neq \delta H^2$$
$$J_{1,4} \neq J_{2,4}$$

Fig. 3.31. The NMR spectrum of 1,1–difluoroethylene.

In the PMR spectrum of this compound we see twelve lines (Fig. 3.31). We find that H^1 and H^2 absorb at different chemical shifts, well separated from each other (i.e. $\delta H^1 \neq \delta H^2$). Further, $J_{1,4}$ due to coupling between *cis* H^1 and F^4 is not equal to $J_{2,4}$, due to coupling between *trans* H^2 and F^4. So, the $N+1$ rule established for first-order spectra is not followed. In fact, the spectrum is complex and consists of twelve lines. Thus H^1 and H^2 are magnetically non-equivalent.

Similarly, the spectrum of acrylonitrile is a non-first-order compli-cated spectrum that consists of fifteen lines (Fig. 3.32), more than expected on the basis of $N + 1$ rule. Here, H_a, H_b absorb at different chemical shifts and their couplings to H_c are also different i.e. :

$$J_{AC} \neq J_{BC}$$
$$\delta H_A \neq \delta H_B$$

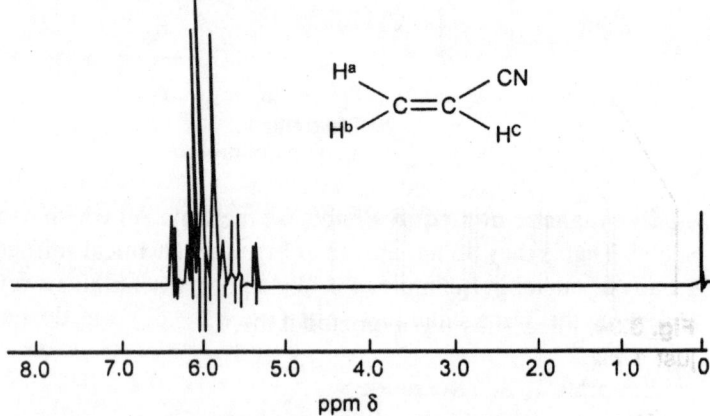

Acrylonitrile

Fig. 3.32. ^{1}H-NMR spectrum of acrylonitrile at 60 MHz.

3.12A CHEMICAL SHIFT: LANTHANIDE SHIFT REAGENTS

Simplification of spectra by creating a tree diagram and determination of J. When the spin-spin coupling is simple, the $N + 1$ rule follows and the spectral interpre-tation is easier. However, the spin-spin coupling becomes complicated when there are two adjacent sets of non-equivalent protons around a proton. In such cases, multiple splittings complicate the spectrum. For instance in propyl chloride:

$$\overset{c}{C}H_3 \overset{b}{C}H_2 \overset{a}{C}H_2 - Cl$$

The central methylene protons (CH_2^b) give eleven lines. What happens is that the original signal due to these protons is first of all, split by one set of adjacent protons and then the signals thus obtained are split further by another set of the adjacent protons. As the coupling constants involved in each splitting are different from each other, more number of lines are obtained. This multiple splitting can be best understood by creating a tree in which we start off with a single original peak due to one type of equivalent protons, say for CH_2^b protons of propyl chloride at its chemical shift value. Then by following the $n + 1$ rule, this peak is split into triplet by coupling due to the adjacent CH_2 protons. Next, each of the three obtained peaks is split into a quartet due to coupling with three protons of the methyl group as per the $n + 1$ rule. Thus, a quartet of triplets is obtained in the end as shown. It makes the same sense even if you first split the original peak by the CH_3 protons into a quartet and then each peak into a triplet by the CH_2 protons as shown in Fig. 3.34.

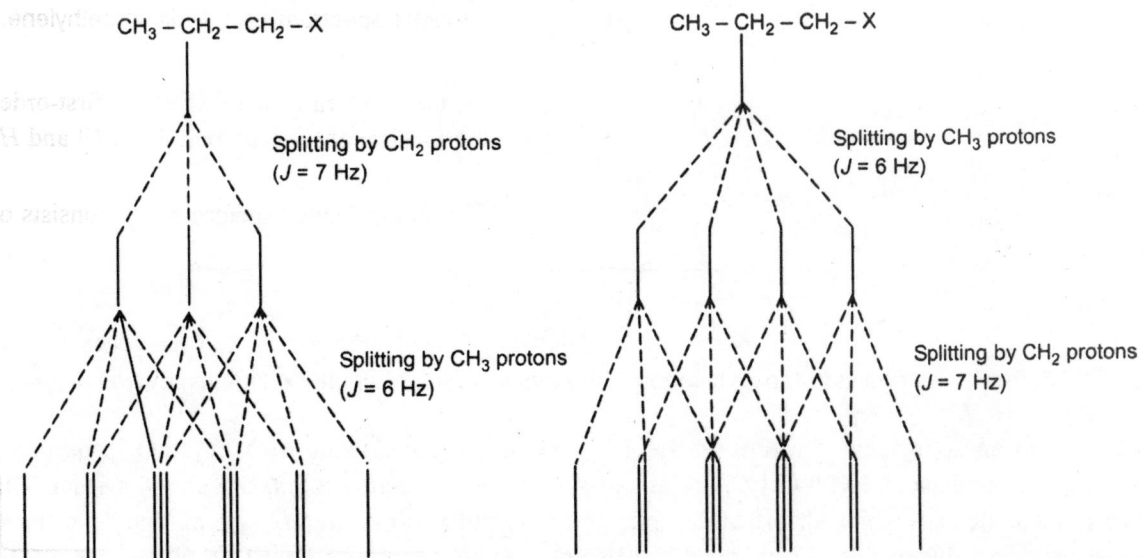

Fig. 3.34. More lines are expected if the difference between the two coupling constants were less say just 1 Hz.

However, if the J value difference between $J_{CH_3CH_2}$ (6 Hz) and $J_{CH_2CH_2}$ (7 Hz) were less, then the number of lines obtained may be even lesser and the peaks may appear to be broader on closer look as shown for the central CH_2 protons for the compound butanoyl chloride, $CH_3CH_2CH_2COCl$ in Fig. 3.35.

3.12B SPIN SYSTEM NOMENCLATURE

A_n system (one isolated set of nuclei)

When all the magnetically active nuclei in a system have the same chemical shift, they absorb as a single peak (singlet). Such spin systems are notated by A_n system where n means the number of magnetically active nuclei having same chemical shift. For example, the protons of methyl iodide,

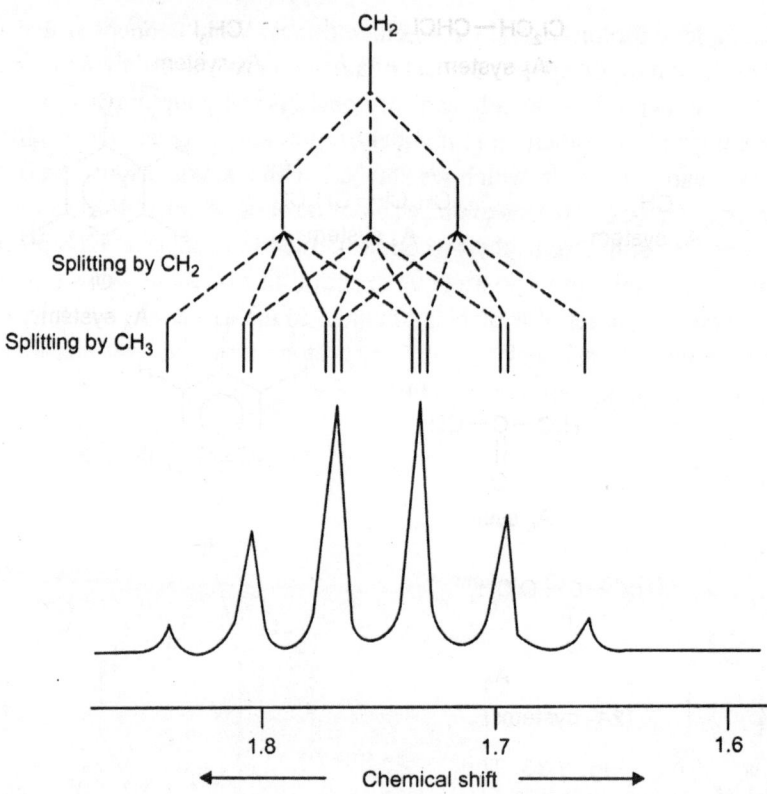

Fig. 3.35. PMR spectrum of butanoyl chloride in the region 1.6–1.85 ppm. Explanation by tree diagram.

CH_3I form an A_3 system. Protons of 1,1,22–tetrachloroethane form an A_2 system, protons of 1,2–dichloromethane, $CH_2Cl–CH_2Cl$ are an A4 system, the benzene protons are an A6 system. The protons in molecules which absorb at different chemical shifts form different systems and hence have to be considered independently and notated differently. Methyl acetate, $CH_3–COOCH_3$ has two sets of methyl groups which appear as two independent singlets at different chemical shifts. So, it contains two A_3 systems. Ethyl acetate, $CH_3COOCH_2CH_3$ contains two A_3 systems and one A_2 system. Similarly, p-dichlorobenzene contains A_4 system.

The above systems are shown in Fig. 3.35.

Two spin system (AB, AX system)

Intext Exercise

5. Show with the help of diagrams, under what conditions does the AX pattern reduce to A_2 pattern.

   Ans. Draw the diagram shown in Fig. 3.36.

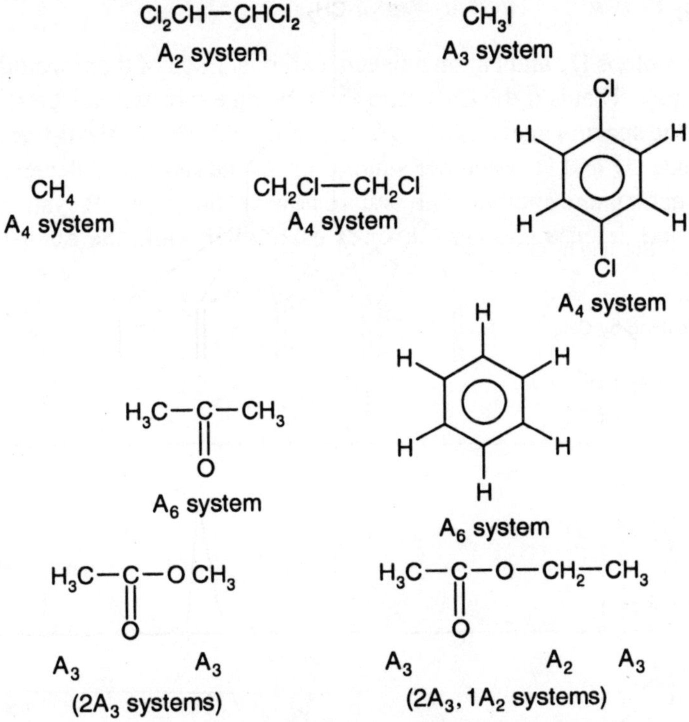

$Cl_2CH—CHCl_2$

A_2 system

CH_3I

A_3 system

CH_4

A_4 system

$CH_2Cl—CH_2Cl$

A_4 system

A_4 system

$H_3C—\overset{\overset{\displaystyle }{|}}{\underset{\underset{\displaystyle O}{||}}{C}}—CH_3$

A_6 system

A_6 system

$H_3C—\underset{\underset{\displaystyle O}{||}}{C}—O\;CH_3$

A_3 A_3

(2A_3 systems)

$H_3C—\underset{\underset{\displaystyle O}{||}}{C}—O—CH_2—CH_3$

A_3 A_2 A_3

(2A_3, 1A_2 systems)

Fig. 3.36. The various A_2, A_3, 2A_3, A_4, A_6, etc.

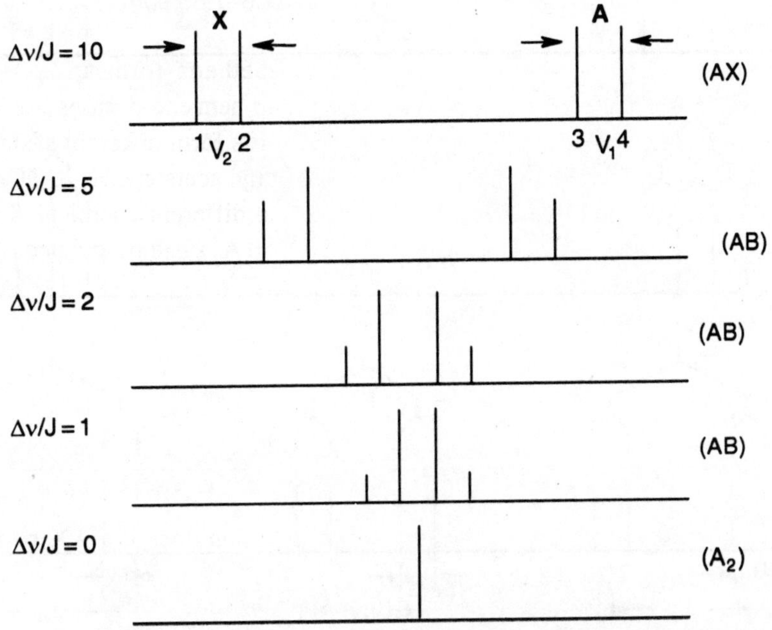

Fig. 3.37. Breakdown of first-order or (approximation). AX pattern reducing to A_2.

(i) *AX–AB system*

Let us consider two protons H_A and H_X on adjacent carbons. Each of them would appear as a doublet if it follows the N + 1 rule. That is if the $\Delta v/J$ ratio (both being expressed in Hertz) will be more than 6, it has been noticed in the spectral analysis of organic compounds that as the difference in chemical shifts of the coupled protons H_A and H_X becomes smaller i.e. as the ratio $\Delta v/J$ decreases (see Fig. 3.38), the doublets start approaching one another. The system now becomes an AB system. The inner two peaks (2 and 3) become more intense and **lean** towards each other while the outer two peaks decrease in

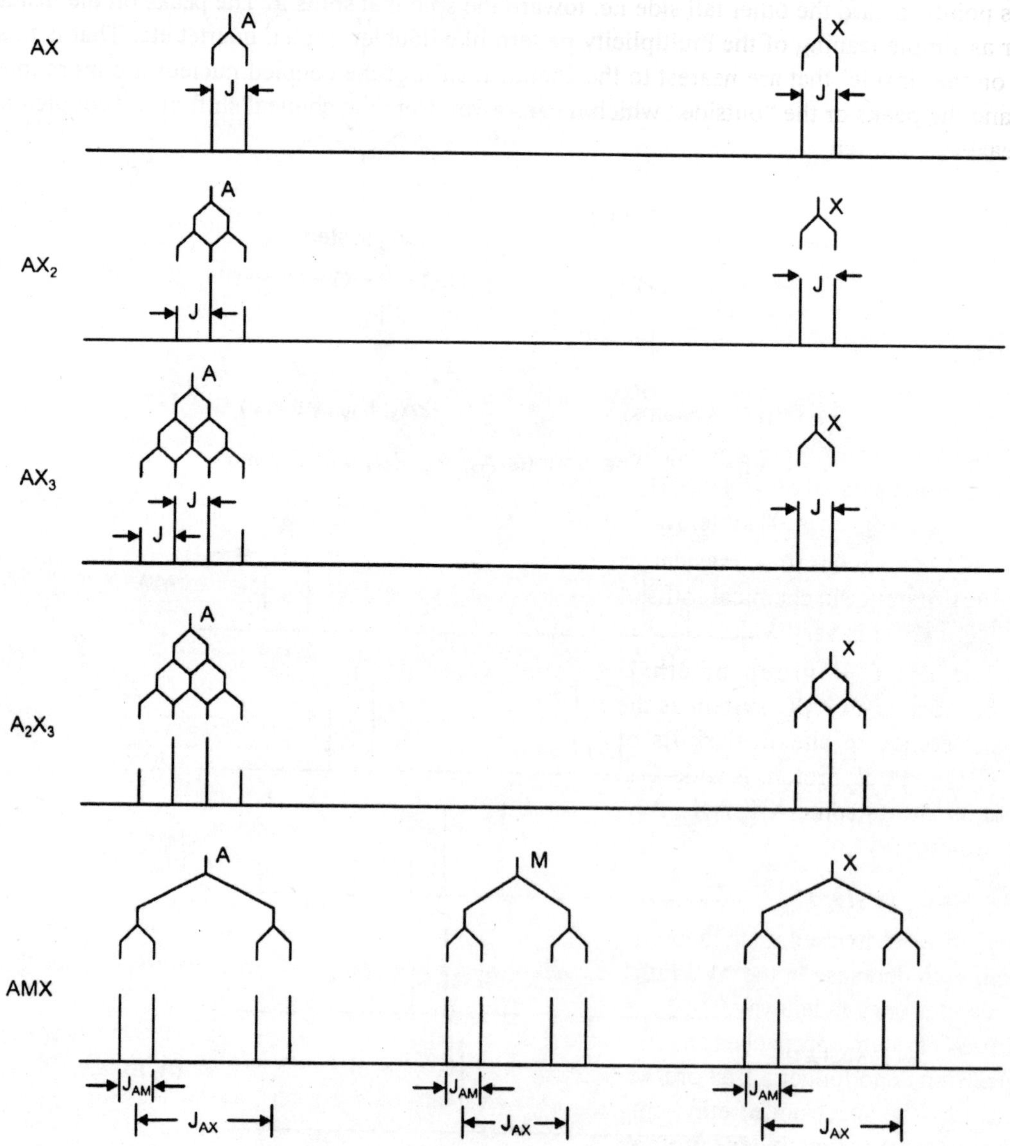

Fig. 3.38. AX, AX_2, AX_3, A_2X_3, AMX systems.

intensity correspondingly. If careful attention is not paid to the smaller outer peaks, one is likely to interpret the spectrum as being a doublet. As the difference in the chemical shifts becomes zero (that is as $\delta_{HA} = \delta_{HX}$), the middle lines (2 and 3) of the coupled protons merge to become a single peak. The difference in chemical shifts of the two protons is determined by using the formula,

$$\Delta v = \sqrt{(\delta_1 - \delta_4)(\delta_2 - \delta_3)}$$

where δ_1, δ_2, δ_3 and δ_4 respectively are the chemical shift positions of the four lines. In general, the second order multiplets show what is called as the **roofing effect** i.e. the tall side of the leaning multiplet always points toward the other tall side i.e. toward the spin that splits it. The peaks on the inside often appear as simple leaning of the multiplicity pattern like doublet, triplet, quartet etc. That is to say the peaks on the 'inside' that are nearest to the chemical shift of the coupled nucleus are more intense or taller and the peaks or the "outside" which means away from the chmical shift of the coupled nucleus are weaker or shorter.

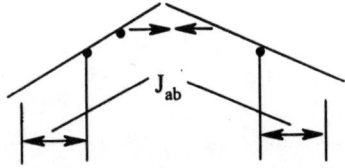

Roofing effect in AB system

- $^{13}CH_3Br$ is an AX_3 system as the difference in chemical shifts of ^{13}C and ^1H is very wide. The isopropyl side chain $-CH-(CH_3)_2$ of cumene is an A_6X system.
- $ClCH_2CF_3$ is an A_2X_3 system as the difference in chemical shifts of ^{13}C and ^1H is very wide.
- The CH_3CH_2 group of ethylbenzene is an A_3X_2 system as the difference in chemical shifts of CH_3 and CH_2 protons is wide. Fig. 3.39 shows some AX, AX_2, AX_3 systems.

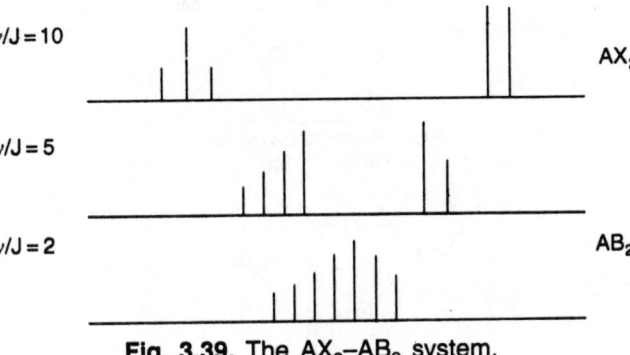

Fig. 3.39. The AX_2–AB_2 system.

(ii) AX₂–AB₂ system

Calculated spectra based upon theoretical analysis by computer are shown in Fig. 3.39 and 3.40. As can be seen, with decrease in the $\Delta v/J$ ratio, the peaks move closer, extra lines appear, the inner lines grow and the outer ones fade away.

An AX_2 system approaches an AB_2 system as the ratio $\Delta v/J$ falls (see Fig. 3.39). In such a situation, the spectrum is no longer a first order spectrum, rather it gets distorted. An example of A_3X_2 system is provided by the spectrum of ethyl chloride, CH_3CH_2Cl which shows a triplet for the methyl protons and a quartet for the methylene protons. $\Delta v/J$ for this system is about 14. β-chlorophenetole, $C_6H_5-O-CH_2-CH_2-Cl$ is an example of A_2B_2 system, while phenyl ethyl acetate $C_6H_5-CH_2-CH_2-OO-CXCH_3$

is an A_2X_2 system for the coupling between the two adjacent methylene protons (Fig. 3.40b). The 2–chloroethanol, $ClCH_2$–CH_2–OH is an A_2B_2 system.

CH_2Cl–CH_3 is an A_2B_2 system.

AA´XX´ spin system

1–bromo–4–chlorobenzene and 1,2–dichlorobenzene are some examples of AA^1XX^1 spin systems in which J_{AX} is not identical to $J_{A·X·}$ (Fig. 3.41)

Another example of AA^1XX^1 system is provided by 1–bromo–2–chloroethane, in which the two methylene sets are non-equivalent.

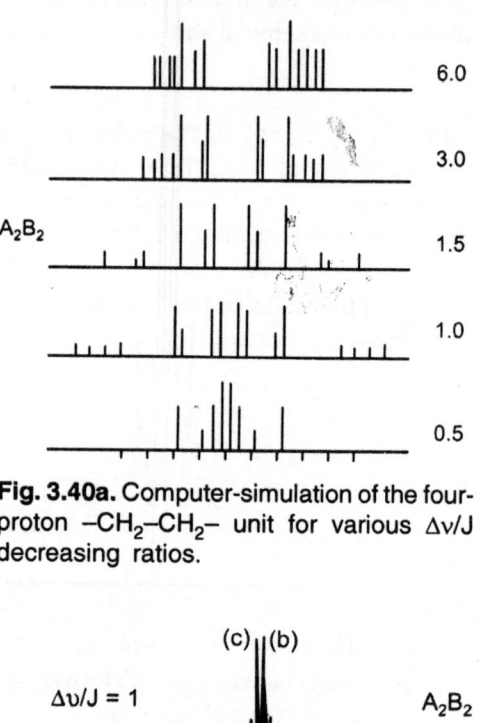

Fig. 3.40a. Computer-simulation of the four-proton –CH_2–CH_2– unit for various $\Delta v/J$ decreasing ratios.

1,2–dichlorobenzene   1–bromo–4–chlorobenzene

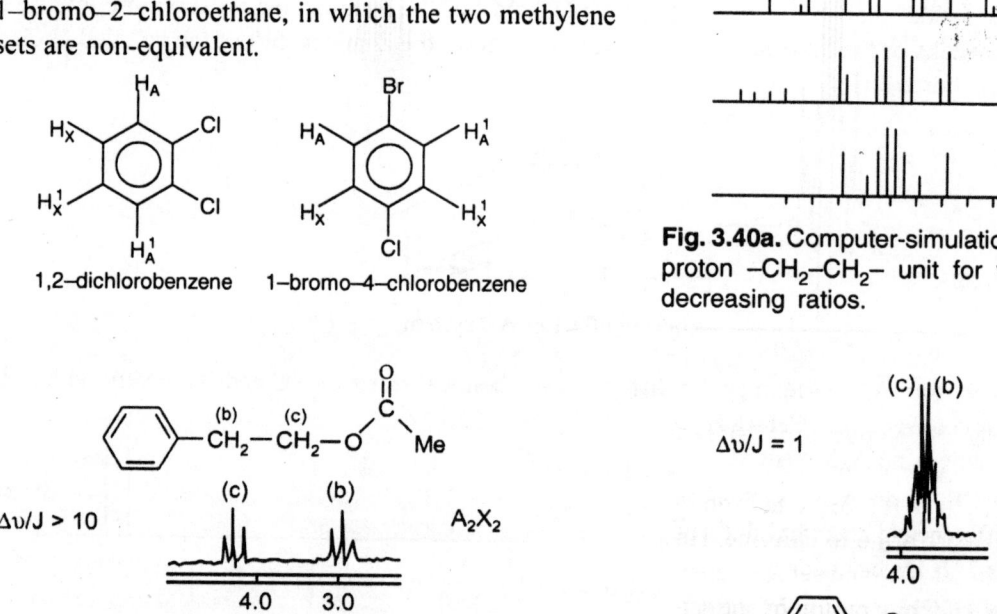

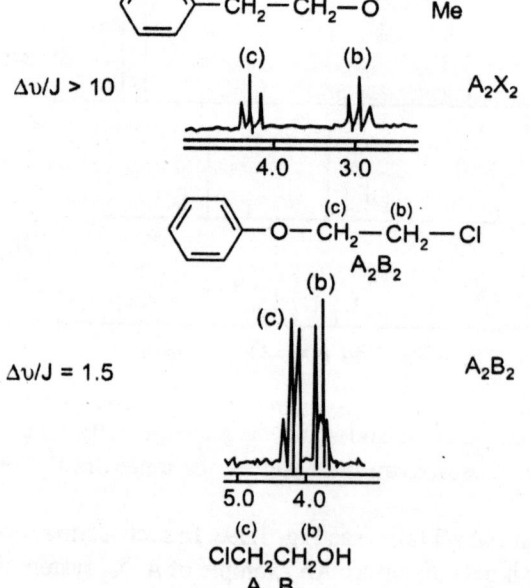

Fig. 3.40b. Examples of –CH_2–CH_2– (four protons) (A_2X_2, A_2B_2) containing compounds in which $\Delta v/J$ goes on decreasing from 10 to almost zero.

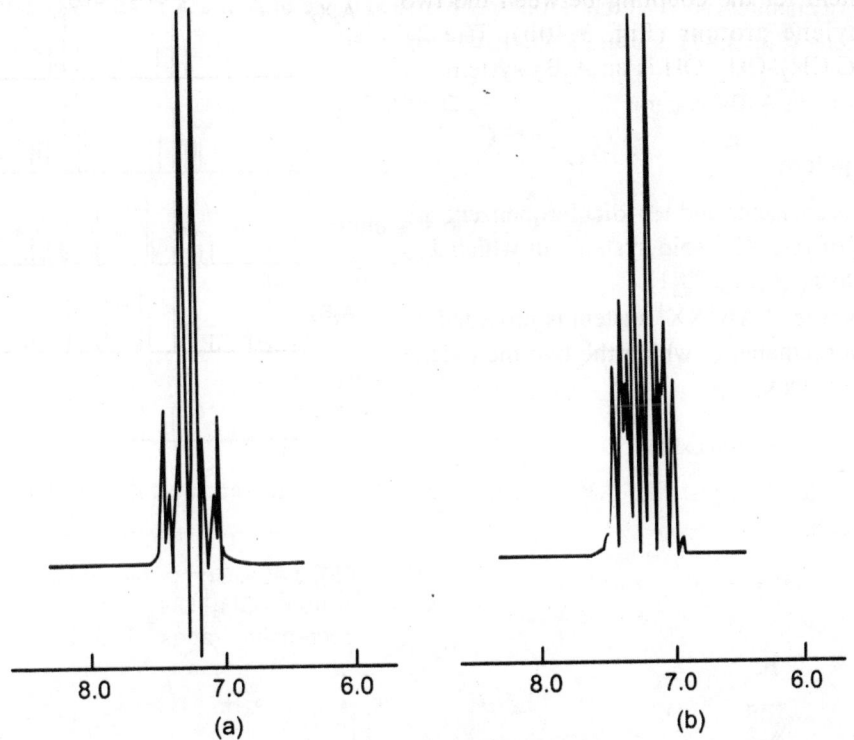

Fig. 3.41. PMR spectra of (a) 1–bromo–2 chloro-benzene and (b) 1,2–dichlorobenzene.

The protons H_A, H_A^1 ortho to bromine have the same chemical shift. So, do the other two protons H_X, H_X^1 which are ortho to chlorine. However, the coupling constants between the two magnetically active nuclei in set AA^1 and set XX^1 are not identical. So, the two sets are magnetically non-equivalent. This is because, for any proton in one set, there is a proton in the other set ortho to it and one, proton in the other set para to it. Further, ortho usually has higher magnitude then J_{para}. In other words, proton H_A is coupled differently to protons, HX and HX′. Hence the two sets of protons H_X and H_X^1 form AA^1XX^1 spin system.

AA′BB′ spin system

As the difference in the chemical shifts of protons AA^1 and XX^1 becomes smaller, the system becomes what is called as AA^1BB^1 system. The middle peaks approach each other while the outer peaks either grow weaker or fade away. Eventually, when Δv, the difference in the chemical shifts becomes zero, the two peaks merge to give a single peak as is observed in p-dichlorobenzene or p-xylene.

Three spin system (AMX, ABC, ABX systems)

● AMX system

A system in which the three sets of protons differ widely in their chemical shifts, is notated as an AMX system ($\Delta v/J$ is about 5). Actually an AMX system is a type of an AX system. M, which is in the middle of the system, has a chemical shift which is midway between those of A and X (Fig. 3.42). For example, vinyl acetate styrene (Fig. 3.43), Furan–2–aldehyde (Fig. 3.44).

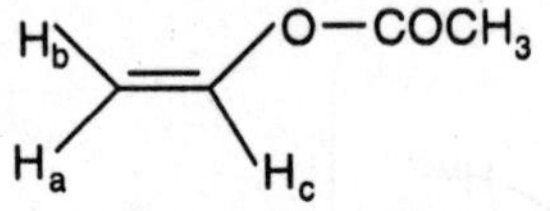

Fig. 3.42. Vinyl acetate.

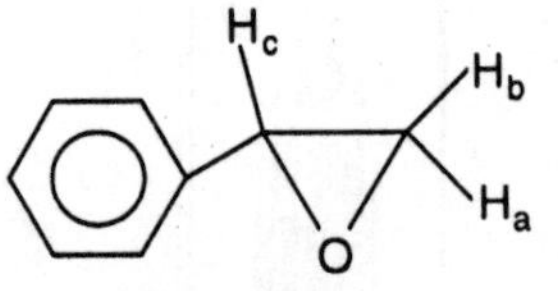

Styrene oxide

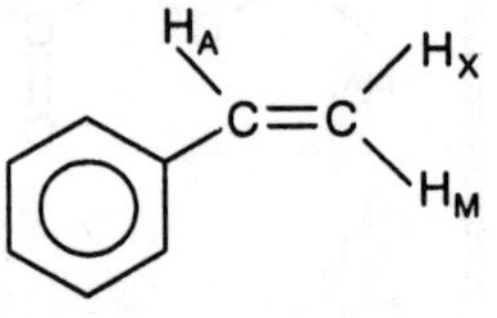

Styrene

It should be noted that just like AX systems, the AMX systems are also first-order in analysis, although complicated.

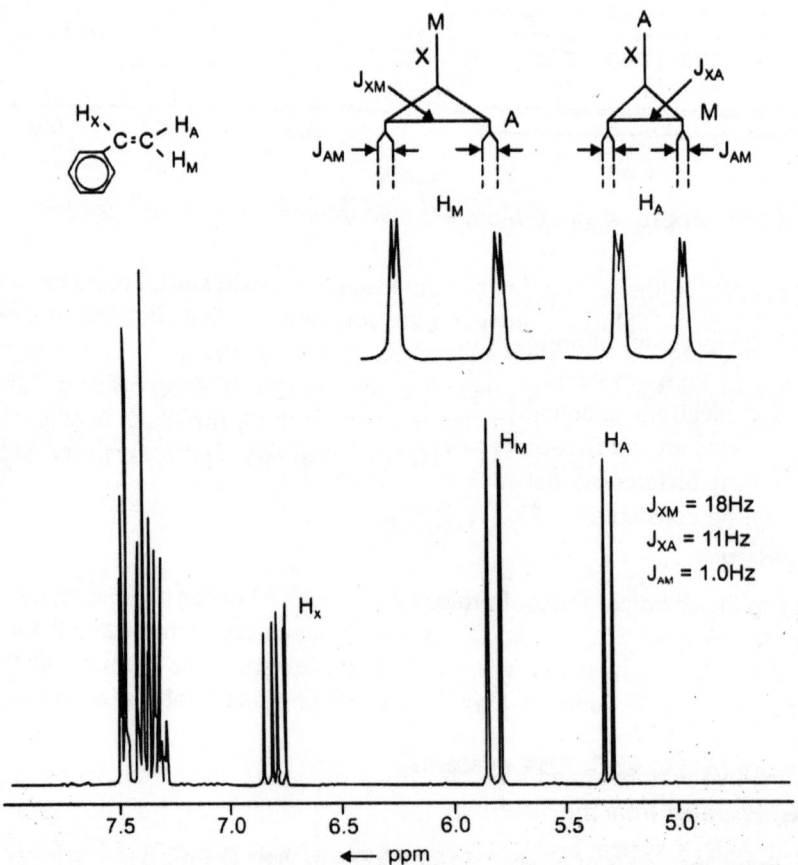

$J_{XM} = 18Hz$

$J_{XA} = 11Hz$

$J_{AM} = 1.0Hz$

Fig. 3.43. AMX system: coupling constants $J_{AX} > J_{MX} > J_{AM}$ in styrene.

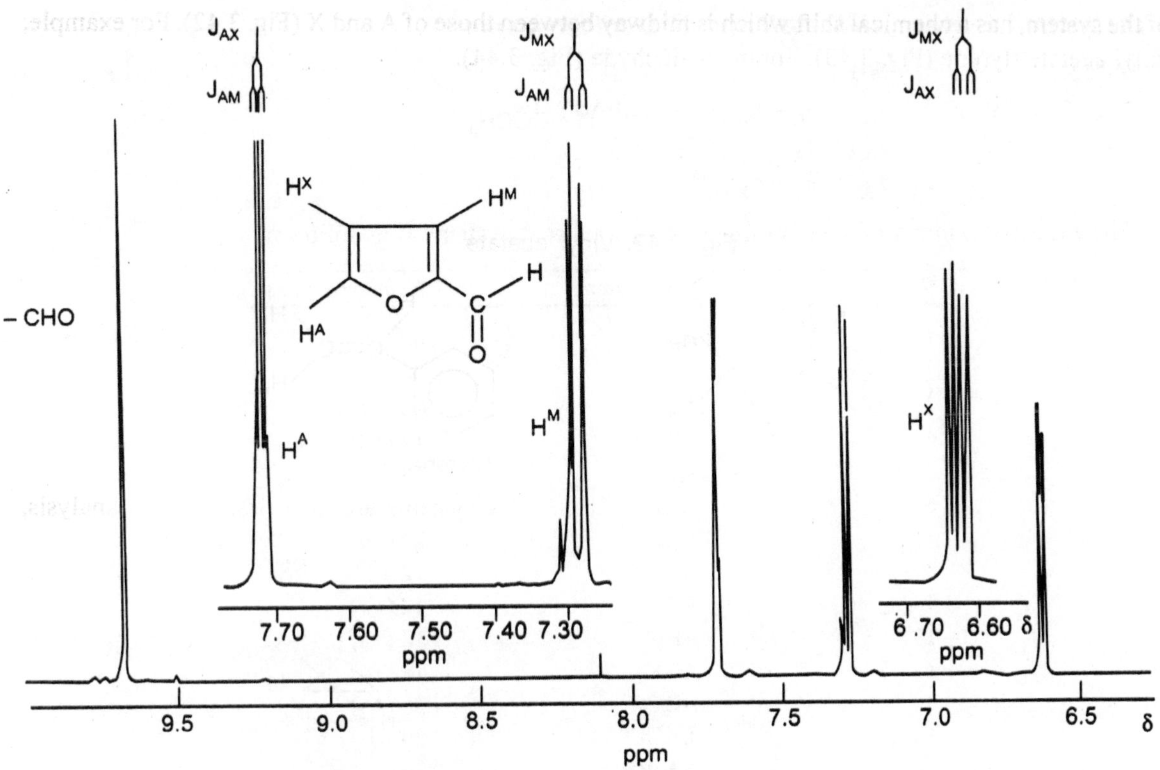

Fig. 3.44. PMR spectrum of furan–2–aldehyde.

• ABC system

A system in which the three sets of protons differ only slightly in their chemical shifts, is called an ABC system. An example of such a system is acrylonatrile. While N + 1 rule predicts three pairs of doublets in its spectrum, the spectrum is actually complex and contains a total of fifteen lines (Fig. 3.38). Obviously, ABC systems are not first-order and so can not be analysed by the N + 1 rule. The reason is that the chemical shift differences between the three involved protons are large compared to the corresponding coupling constants.

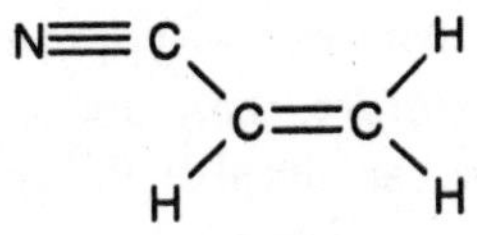

Acrylonitrile.

• ABX system

In such systems, the two protons A and B are separated from each other by a small difference while the third proton, C is separated from the other two by a large difference.

CH_3CH_2F is an A_3B_2X system because the difference in chemical shifts of the protons of CH_3 and CH_2 sets is small while the difference in the chemical shifts of protons of CH_2 and F is very large.

- ## Distinction between AMX, ABX and ABC spin systems

AMX	ABX	ABC
$J_{AM} < \delta_A - d_B$	$J_{AB} \geq \delta_A - d_B$	All $\Delta d < J$'s
$J_{XM} < \delta_M - d_X$	$J_{AX} < \delta_A - d_X$	
	$J_{BX} < \delta_B - d_X$	

The expected number of spectral lines for various spin systems is as follows:

S. No.	Spin system	Number of lines
1	AX	04
2	AB	04
3	AB_2	08 (+1)
4	AB_3	14 (+2)
5	A_2X_2	06
6	A_2B_2	14 (+4)
7	A_3B_2	25 (+9)
8	AMX	12
9	ABX	12 (+2)
10	ABC	12 (+3)
11	ABX_2	18 (+4)
12	ABC_2	28 (+6)
13	AA'XX'	20
14	AA'BB'	24
15	ABCX	32 (+18)
16	ABCD	32 (+24)

Note: The number of lines within brackets corresponds to weaker combination bonds which might though not necessarily be observed in the spectrum.

3.13 SECOND ORDER-SPECTRA BECOMING FIRST ORDER SPECTRA AT HIGHER FIELD STRENGTH (SIMPLIFICATION OF SECOND ORDER SPECTRA)

In case of bigger molecules, it is found that the ^1H–NMR spectra are quite complicated. This is because of overlapping of the resonances of the various protons. This would not have been the case if the range for protons resonances were larger rather than just 0–10 ppm which is the actual range in general. As all protons mostly absorb in this range, therefore, there are more probabilities of the overlappings to occur. The question arises as to whether we can simplify the spectra? Can we be in a position to know which protons are overlapping in reality?

Yes, it seems possible to simplify the complicated spectra at least by one strategy—if we can increase the difference in the chemical shifts (Δv) of the coupled protons but at the same time, we do not allow the distance or the separation between the peaks of multiplets (called coupling constant). As for the first point is concerned, we know that the larmor precession frequency v_0 is dependent upon the applied field strength, B_0. So do we not imagine the difference in the chemical shifts of the coupled protons to widen as we use a spectrometer having higher field strengths?

$$\nu_0 = y \cdot \frac{B_0}{2\pi}$$

The protons are expected to precess at higher speed as the strength of B_0 is enhanced thereby leading to higher $\Delta\nu$.

However, this approach will fail if the distances between the peaks of multiplets also increased proportionately. Fortunately, nature favours us in these experiments. It was discovered that while $\Delta\nu$, the difference in the chemical shifts of the coupled protons, increased considerably, the coupling constants (J) remained constant! So, the multiplets that overlapped at low field strength, separated out at higher field strength and therefore could be easily interpreted.

The distorted N + 1 rule spectra or the second-order spectra usually get simplified to "first-order" appearance at higher field strengths of the NMR instrument e.g. 300 MHz or even higher. Evidently, the reason behind this simplification is that while chemical shift depends upon the field strength, the magnitude of the coupling constant, J, does not. Consequently as $\Delta\nu$, the difference in chemical shifts of the coupled protons increases, the ratio $\Delta\nu/J$ in Hertz increases. The second-order complexities are, therefore, reduced and the spectra are now "first-order" in appearance. That is why, it is always better to get the spectra of complicated molecules on a high-resolution NMR instrument. The spectra n-butylvinyl ether (Fig. 3.46), 9–methoxyphenanthrene (Fig. 3.47) and statin units (Fig. 3.48) clarify the effects of the higher field strengths.

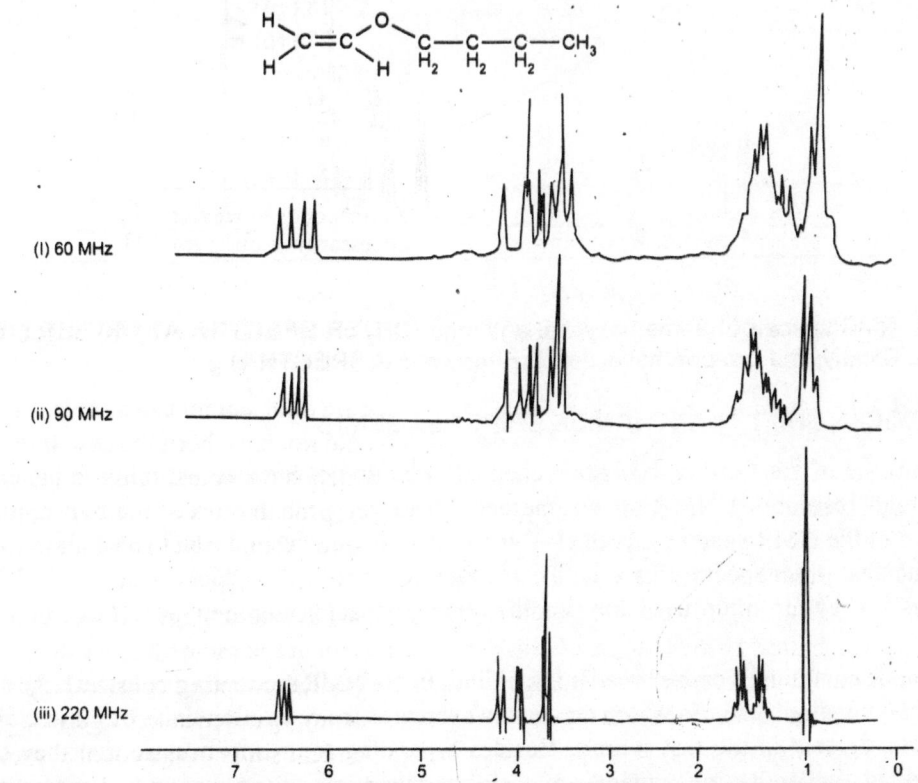

Fig. 3.46. ¹H-NMR spectra of *n*-butylvinylether in CDCl₃ at (i) 60 MHz, (ii) 90 MHz and (iii) 220 MHz.

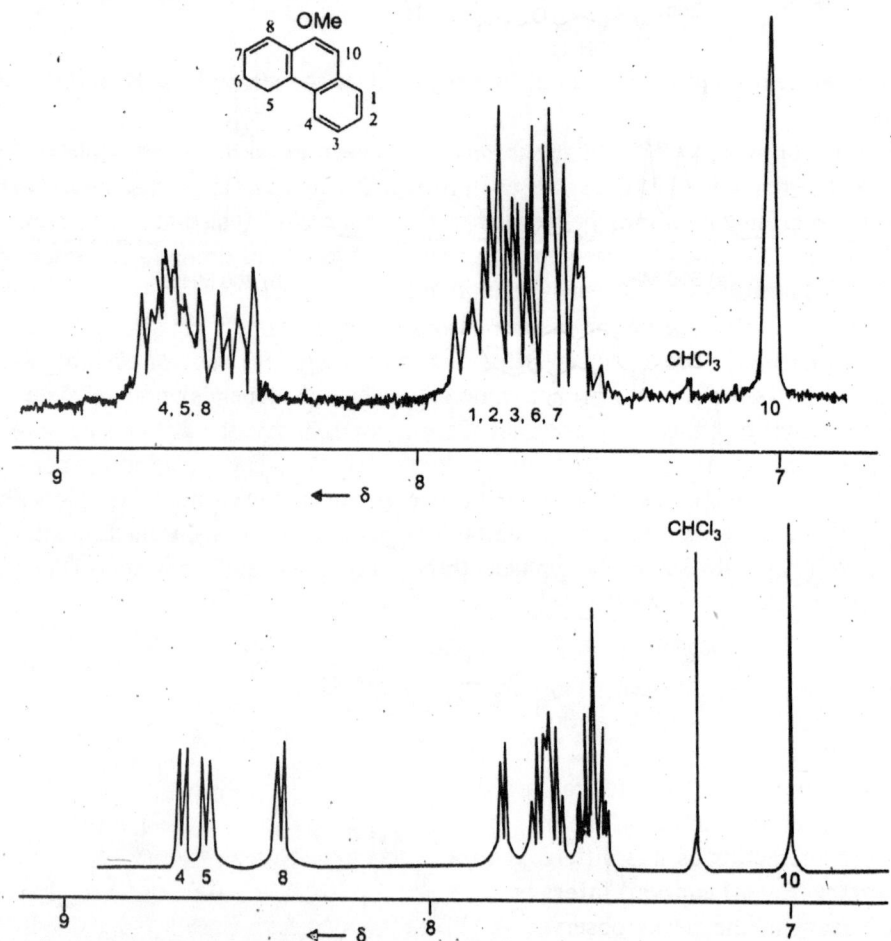

Fig. 3.47. ^{1}H-NMR spectra of 9–methoxyphenanthrene (CH$_3$ protons not shown) (a) at 100 MHz, (b) at 360 MHz. Clearly, the protons have become resolved at higher strength.

3.13A CHEMICAL SHIFT : LANTHANIDE SHIFT REAGENTS

These reagents are of great utility to organic chemists who do not have accessibility to the expensive high field (high resolution) NMR spectrometers. These reagents are used in small amounts for simplification of the NMR spectra – both H–1 and C–13. In fact, second order spectra are frequently converted into first order spectra this way. That is why, they are called "poor man's high field NMR spectrometers". They are often used for simplification of spectra recorded at 60 MHz or 100 MHz resolution.

Paramagnetic compounds cause broadening of lines in the NMR spectrum due to the large magnetic moment of their unpaired electron which drastically decreases the relaxation times of the nuclei such as H–1, C–13 etc. present in the test sample. Besides separating the resonances so that they could be easily interpreted, the lanthanide reagents are useful in determining the structure and configuration of molecules in solution. Most commonly used examples are the β-diketone complexes of the lanthanide

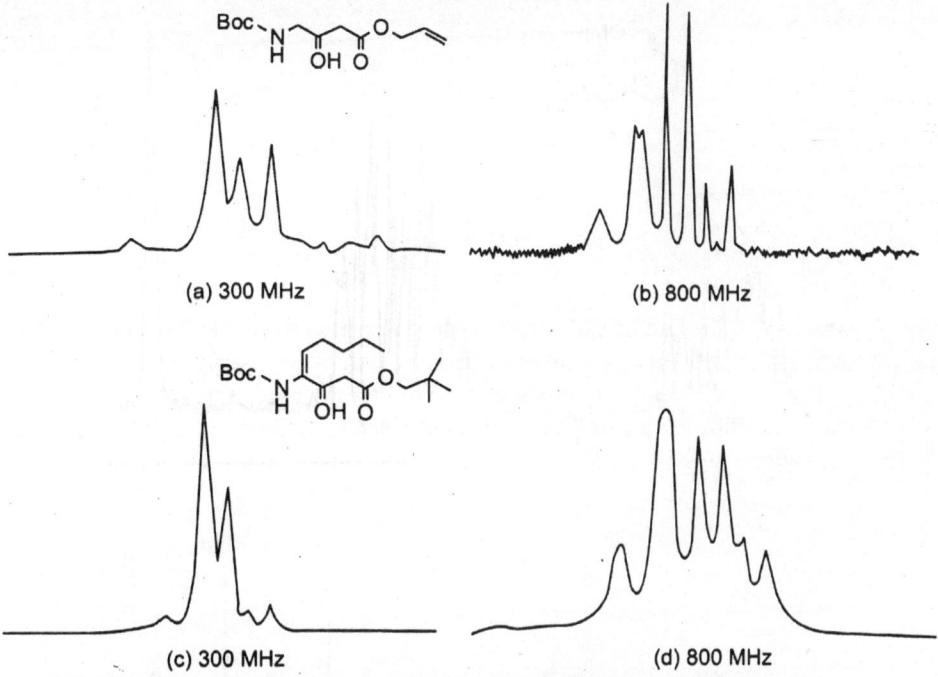

Fig. 3.48. Expansion of the AB pattern for H₂–2 in the ¹H NMR spectra of Statin units: (a) 10b at 300 MHz, (b) 10b at 800 MHz, (c) 16b at 300 MHz, and (d) 16b at 800 MHz.

metals such as +3 europium (Eu) and praseodymium (Pr) by an unpaired electron of the lanthanide ion. This through – space interaction of the magnetic field with the sample (substrate) nuclei is called a **pseudo-contact** interaction as it is different from the through – bonds interaction of nuclei, which is called the **contact (Fermi contact) interaction.** As the test sample is involved in a rapid equilibrium with the shift reagent, the peaks observed in mixtures with shift reagent are indeed the averaged environments of the nuclei in the substrate plus its complex formed with the shift reagent. This averaging of the chemical shifts is quite common with rapidly exchanging systems. Because the shift reagents are hard Lewis acids, the functional group $L^- + nS = L\ Sn$ that complex to shift reagents are hard Lewis bases, for example alcohols (ROH) amines (RNH₂). It needs to be noted that the position of a given peak in a mixture with a shift reagent depends upon many factors such as the stability of the formed complex, the quantity of shift reagent used, as well as the distance between the Lanthanide metal centre, the nucleus being observed. For a given molecule the Lanthanide-induced shift (Δv_i) are known to be inversely proportional to the cube of the internuclear distance r_i^3 between the lanthanide metal, and the nucleus under consideration. Eu(fod)₃ reagent has a greater solubility in common organic solvents. It has higher Lewis acidity because of the electron withdrawing ability of the Fluorine atoms. Most Europium derivatives induce shifts to high frequency. On the other hand, complexes of Pr(III) cause shifts to low frequency.

The large changes observed in chemical shift produced by the paramagnetic reagents, are due to the coordination of the sample molecule to the paramagnetic lanthanide ion. The bound organic substrate protons experiences changes in the effective magnetic field because of the magnetic field produced.

$$\Delta v_i = \frac{X(3 \cos^2 \theta - 1)}{r_i^3}$$

X is a constant.

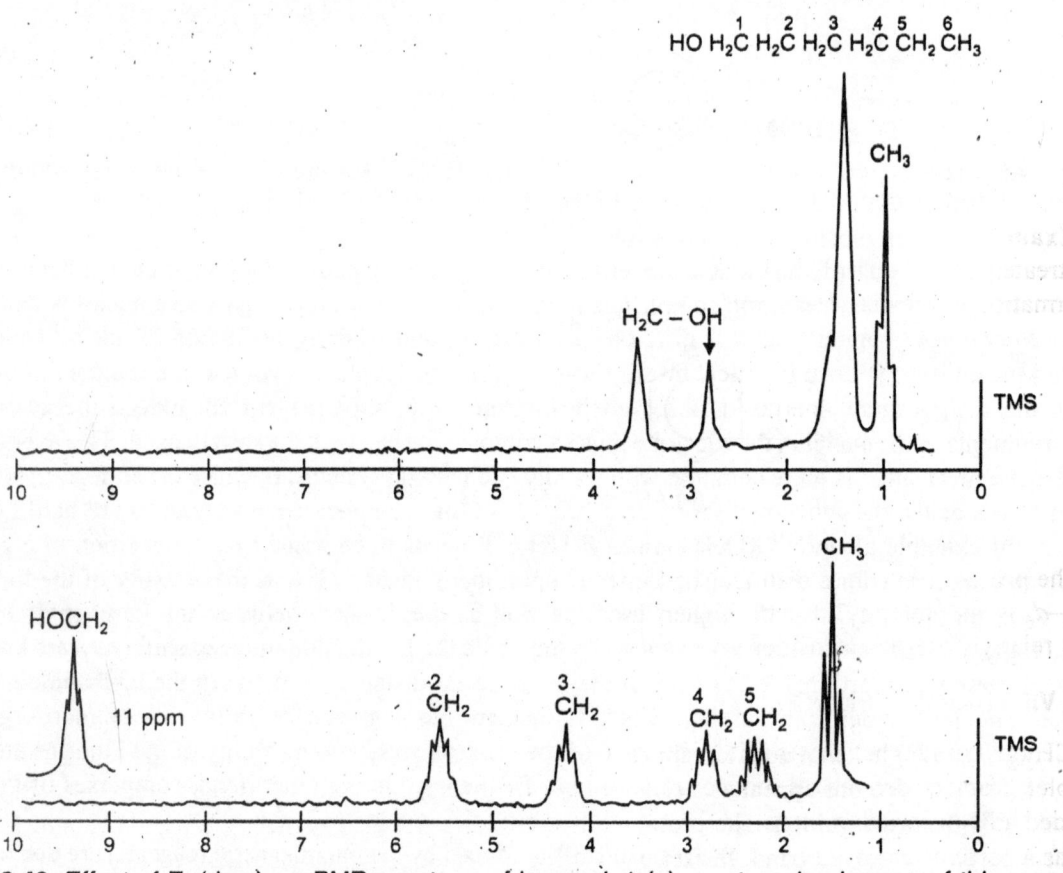

Example : Hexanol–1 : The use of Eu(dpm)$_3$ is elegantly illustrated by the example of hexanol–1, whose spectrum recorded at 100 MHz is shown in Fig.. As can be seen only the triplet due to the only methyl group and that due to CH$_2$OH are resolved. The remaining methylene protons occur as a broad overlapping multiplet. Addition of a small amount of Eu (dpm) (0.29 mole equivalent) separates the overlapping four methylene signals as shown in Fig. 3.49, thus making the spectrum, a first order spectrum.

Fig. 3.49. Effect of Eu(dpm)$_3$ or PMR spectrum of hexanol–1 (a) spectrum in absence of this reagent (b) spectrum in presence of this reagent (0.29 mol equivalent).

3.13B CHIRAL RESOLVING AGENTS

Enantiomers cannot be differentiated by proton NMR spectra, that is to say, they have identical chemical shifts for the groups attached to a chiral carbon atom. However, if they can be converted into diastereomers by treatment with a chiral resolving agent such as **the chiral lanthanide shift reagent** or compounds like (−)2,2,2−trifluoro−1−(9−anthryl) ethanol (−) TFAE.

(−) TFAE

Example : When racemic 2−amino−1−phenyl ethanol (APE) which contains an asymmetric carbon was treated with (−) TFAE, the following spectral changes were observed in the ^{1}H NMR spectra due to formation of the diastereomeric complexes :

(−) APE + (−) TFAE + (+) APE + (+) TFAE
Diastereomeric complexes

The proton−2 becomes distinguished in (−) TFAE, the overlapping triplets become more so when C_6H_6−d_6 is added (Fig. 3.50). At higher field strength, the two triplets become quite distinguishable. Their relative integral intensities give us their % in the diastereomeric mixture.

3.14 VIRTUAL COUPLING

The CH_3 group of 1−hexanol does not appear as a simple triplet. Rather it appears as a broadened, filled in triplet. The CH_2 protons appear as a clear-cut triplet as expected (Fig. 3.49). The CH_2 (2) protons are recorded as a distorted quintet. The protons on carbon 3 to 5 which have similar chemical shifts are seen as a partially resolved band. In fact, their spins act as a conglomerate of spins and couple of the methyl group. This effect is called virtual coupling. Although the CH_3 group protons do not couple to the CH_2 (3) protons or CH_2 (3 protons) (J = 0), yet their spin is effected by these protons.

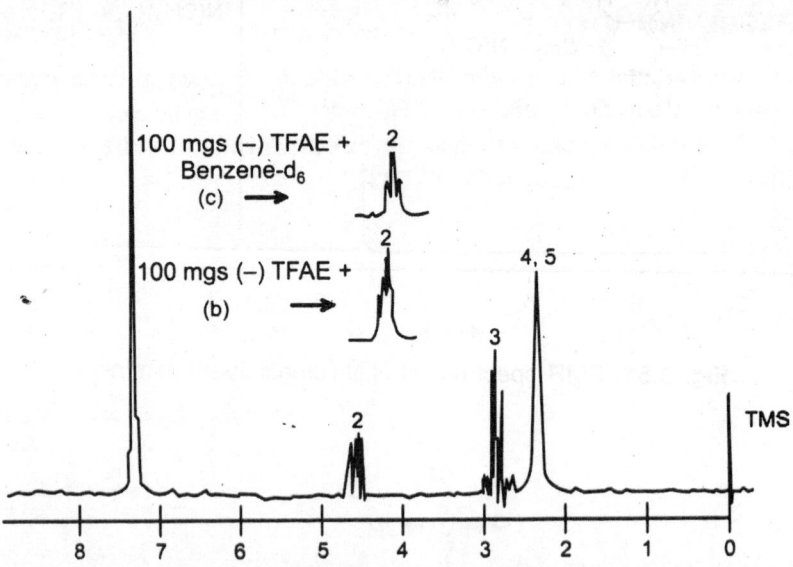

Fig. 3.50. Differentiating between enantiomeric 2–amino–1–phenyl ethanol (APE) by (–) TFAE. (a) The lowermost spectrum is due to racemic APE, (b) Upon addition of (–) TFAE (100 mgs), we see now two overlapping triplets middle trace which become more differentiated when we add some (0.2 mL) $C_6H_6d_6$ into the sample solution as shown in the top portion.

3.15 ANALYSIS OF AROMATIC COMPOUNDS

(i) Monosubstituted Benzenes

The chemical shift of the protons in benzene rings depends upon the nature of the substituent. Sometimes, the five ring protons although chemically non-equivalent appear as a singlet when the chemical shifts of the protons are very similar as in alkyl benzene at 60 MHz. This happens when the substituent is neither a strongly electron donating or a strongly electron withdrawing group. The reason for this observation is that the induced π-electrons ring current has a tendency to equalize the small differences in the chemical shifts of the ring protons.

Examples :

1. N,N-Dimethylbenzylamine (Fig. 3.51).
2. Ethylbenzene (Fig. 3.52).
3. Toluene (Fig. 3.53).

• When the substituent is strongly electron-donating in nature, it enhances the electron density at o- and p-positions. This leads to shielding of these protons relative to m-position. This is how these protons absorb at different chemical shift positions. Consequently, the spectrum is complicated.

Example : Anisole.

The PMR of anisole is shown in Fig. 3.54. While the two meta protons are slightly deshielded, the three o- and p-protons get shielded.

When the substituent is electron-withdrawing in nature, the o- and p-protons get deshielded as the electron-density from around these positions gets lowered down, while the meta protons get shielded.

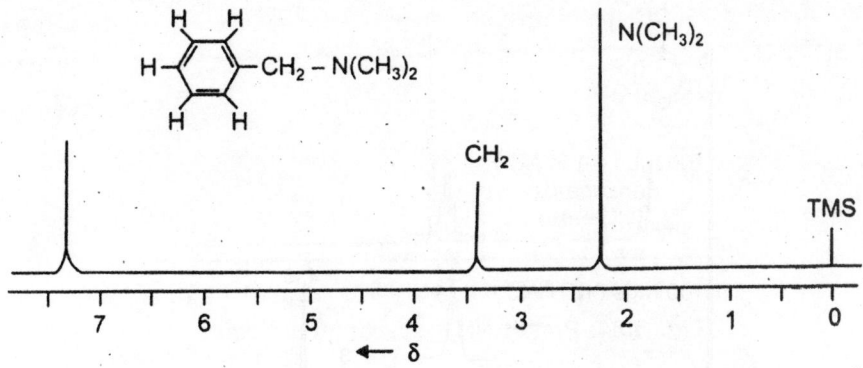

Fig. 3.51. PMR spectrum of N,N-Dimethylbenzylamine.

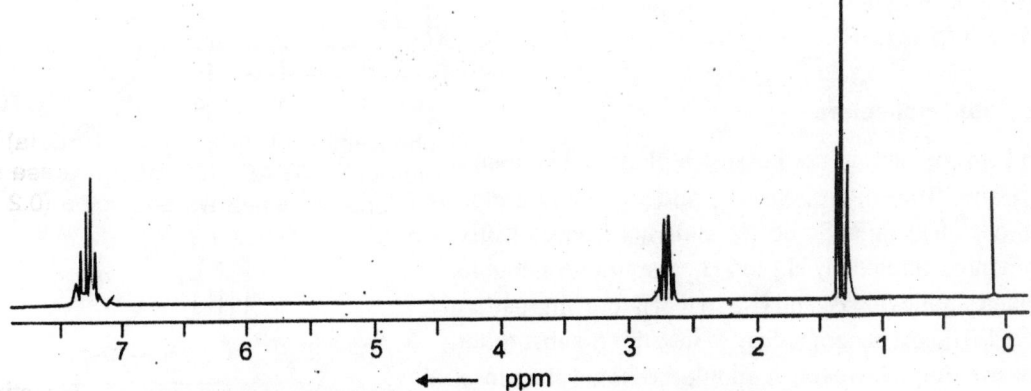

Fig. 3.52. PMR spectrum of Ethylbenzene.

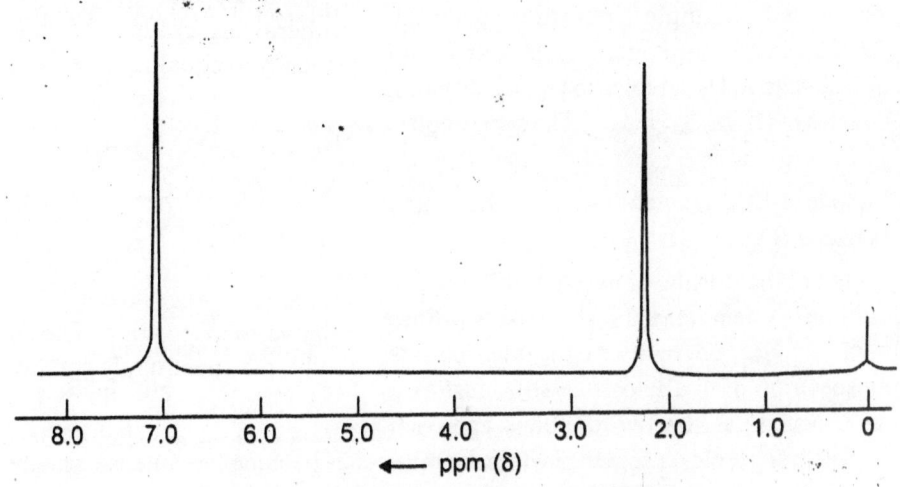

Fig. 3.53. PMR spectrum of Toluene.

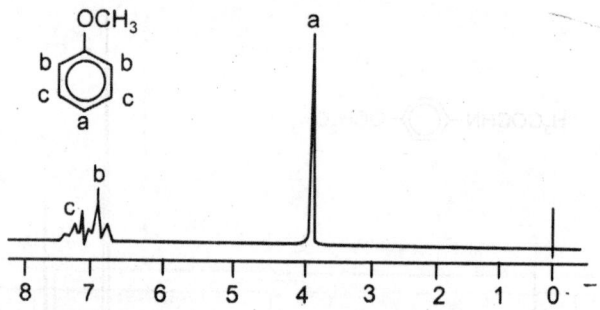

Fig. 3.54. Proton NMR spectrum of anisole.

Examples :

Benzaldehyde (Fig. 3.55).

Styrene (Fig. 3.45).

Disubstituted Benzenes

As such benzene derivatives possess a plane of symmetry, therefore the ortho-hydrogens H_A and $H_{A'}$ have almost identical chemical shift. So do H_B and $H_{B'}$. Consequently, H_A is split into a doublet by H_B and H_B is split into a doublet by H_A. Same applies to $H_{A'}$ and $H_{B'}$ so that a four-line pattern is observed. Thus, it becomes easy to identify p-substitution in a benzene ring. However, it should be noted the closer examination by expansion reveals that the four-line pattern is actually a AA'BB' system (Fig. 3.56). That is to say it is a second-order rather than a simple first-order spectrum. Although H_A is chemically equivalent to $H_{A'}$, it is not magnetically equivalent to it. H_A couples to H_B in a different manner than it couples to $H_{B'}$ i.e. $J_{AB} \neq J_{AB'}$. The same applies to $J_{BA} \neq J_{BA'}$.

Examples include p-Ethoxacetanilide (Fig. 3.57) and p-Chloronitro benzene (Fig. 3.58).

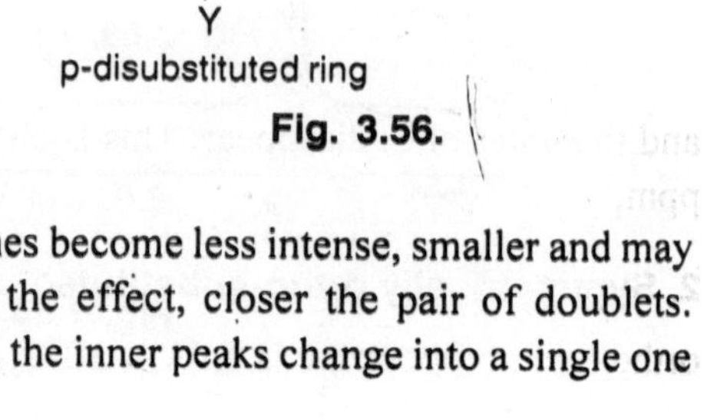

It needs to be noted that for the above AA'BB' system, the observed four lines system takes the shape of two-lines pattern if $\Delta\delta = \delta_{H_A} - \delta_{H_B}$ becomes negligible. This is borne out by the spectrum of 4–allyloxy-anisole. Just as it happens in an AX system, as the two doublets approach each other, the inner lines get closer together while the outer ones become less intense, smaller and may even become conspicuous by their absence. In fact, greater the effect, closer the pair of doublets. When the chemical shifts of H_A and H_B are just about the same, the inner peaks change into a single one

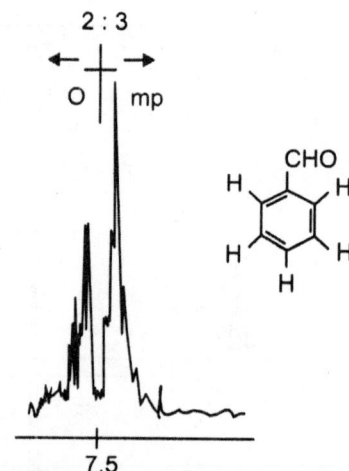

Fig. 3.55. PMR spectrum of benzaldehyde in aromatic region.

X

H_A ⟶ $H_{A'}$ ⟶ Plane of symmetry

H_B ⟶ $H_{B'}$

Y

p-disubstituted ring

Fig. 3.56.

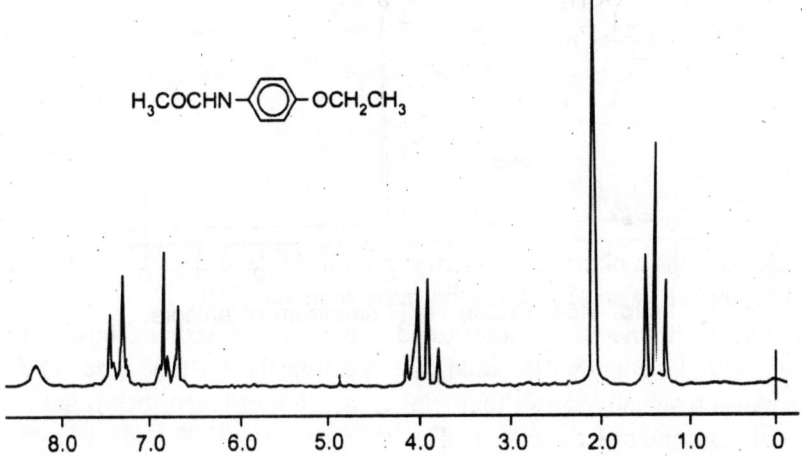

Fig. 3.57. PMR spectrum of p-ethoxyacetanilide (phenacetin).

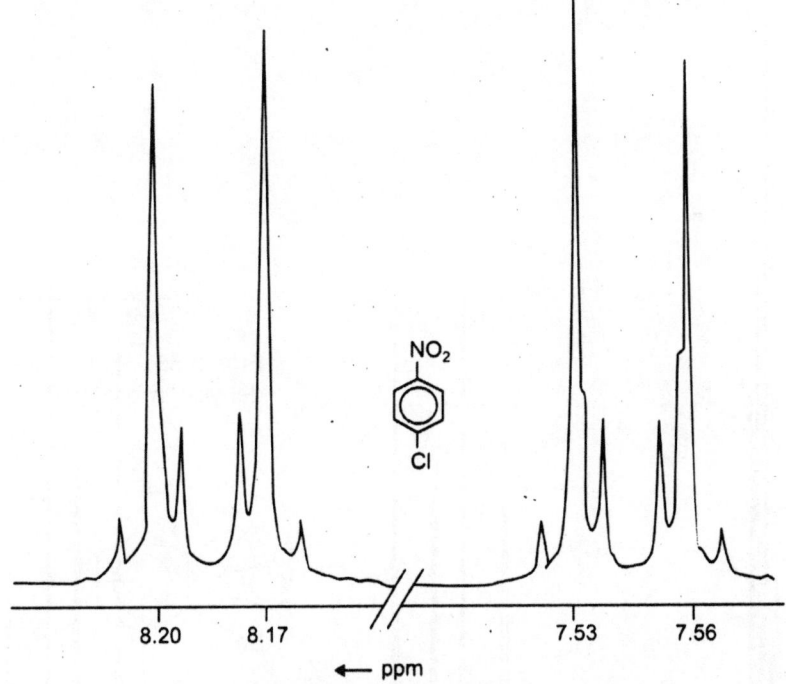

Fig. 3.58. PMR spectrum of p-chloronitrobenzene.

and the outer ones disappear. This is clear from the spectrum of p-xylene with a single peak about 7.0 ppm.

2. Symmetrically ortho-substituted benzene

ortho-Dichlorobenzene is an AA′BB′ spin system as shown in Fig. 3.59

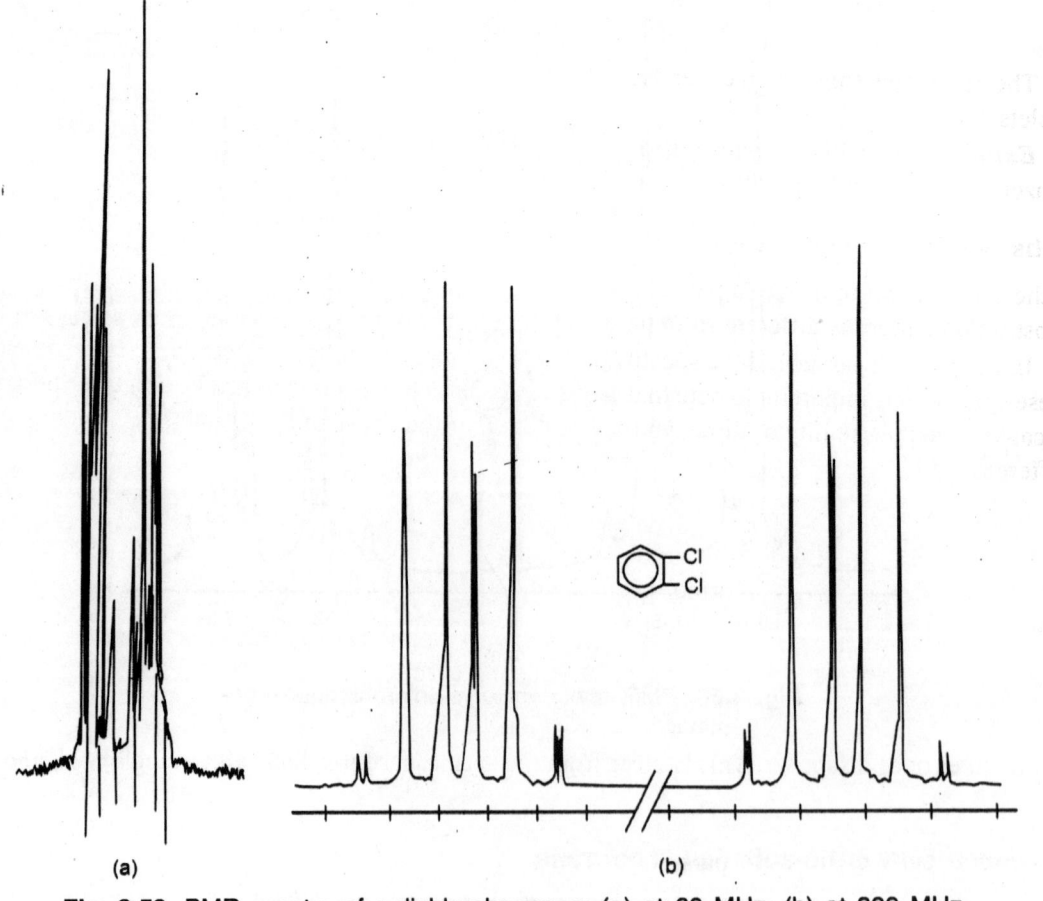

As the molecule contains a plane of symmetry, protons H_A and $H_{A'}$ have identical chemical shift. Similarly protons H_B and $H_{B'}$ also absorbs at the same chemical shift.

The case is identical with that of p-disubstituted ring discussed earlier. Thus, a characteristic four-line pattern is obtained. As already discussed, the spectrum is AA'BB' type. The aromatic region spectrum upon expansion actually shows four triplets which means the spectrum is not a simple first order rather a complex second order spectrum. The PMR spectrum (300 MHz) of o-dichlorobenzene is shown in Fig. 3.59.

Fig. 3.59. PMR spectra of o-dichlorobenzene: (a) at 60 MHz, (b) at 300 MHz.

ABB'MM' Spin System

Such spectra are shown by benzene rings substituted with a highly electronegative group. Examples include bromo-benzene, fluorobenzene etc. The PMR spectrum of bromobenzene is shown in Fig. 3.60. The protons that are α, w.r. to bromine behave like M and M' protons. The remaining three protons act as ABB' protons. The spectrum is a complex second order spectrum with the J values being 0.5–8 Hz and chemical shifts being just about 0.5 ppm.

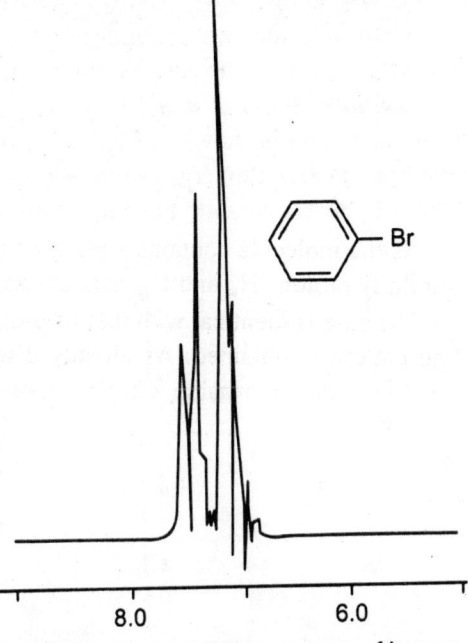

Fig. 3.60. Proton NMR spectrum of bromo-benzene.

The above spectrum when expanded appears as four triplets.

Example: The PMR spectrum of p-chloronitro-benzene is shown in Fig. 3.60.

Substitution at Other Positions

If the symmetrical four line (a pair of doublet) is not seen in the aromatic region, it clearly means the substitution pattern is different from para one.

In fact, the appearance of the spectra will depend upon the mode of substitution. Before we discuss these spectra, it is important to note that the complexity in the spectra noticed in aromatic regions arises because of the possibility of three types of coupling : ortho, meta and para and the J_o, J_m and J_p are all different.

J	Hz
ortho, ^3J	7–10
meta, ^4J	1–3
para, ^5J	0–1

In general, the para-coupling is normally not observed.

When only the two couplings ortho and meta are observed, the spectrum is relatively easier to interpret relative to the case exhibiting all the three couplings.

Example: *3–Nitro, 4–hydroxy acetophenone*: The spectrum of this compound (Fig. 3.61) in the aromatic region is shown in Fig. 12. Of the eight lines seen, the most deshielded doublet at 8.4 ppm corresponds to proton H_2, the doublet of doublet arises from H_6 while the doublet at 6.9 ppm is due to proton H_C as shown with the help of tree-diagram.

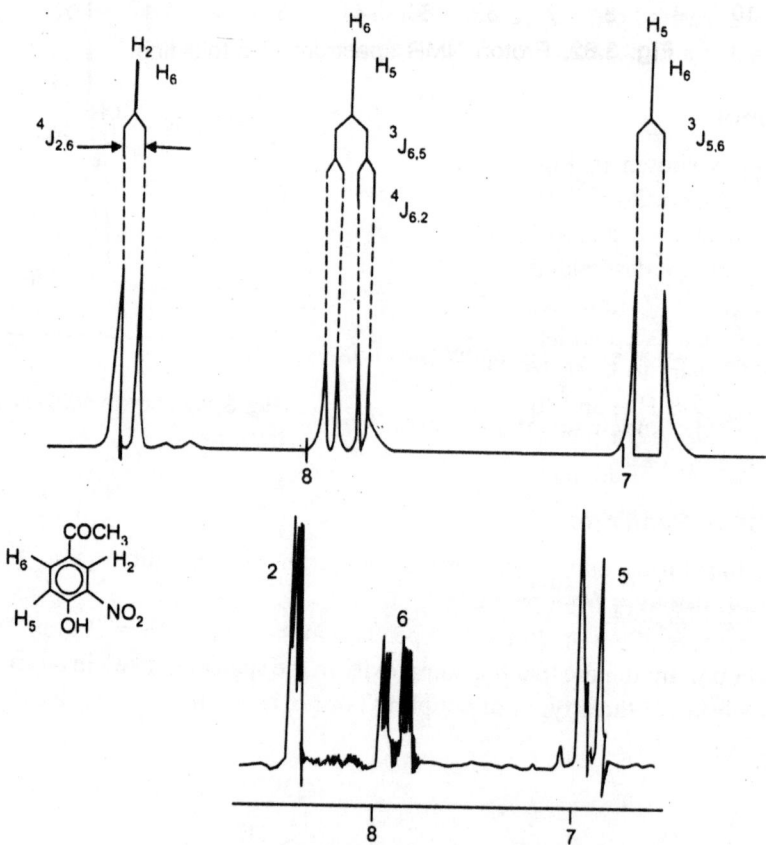

Fig. 3.61. PMR spectrum of 3–nitro–4–hydroxy acetophenone.

The proton NMR spectra of some typical aromatic molecules:

1. p-Toluidine

The PMR spectrum of p-toluidine is shown in Fig. 3.62. As is evident, the characteristic four-lined (a pair of doublets) of p-disubstitution is visible in the aromatic region. The proton meta to amino group are most deshielded at δ 6.79 Hz while the protons at 6.37 are relatively shielded. Evidently, this is the effect of electron-donating NH_2 group. Of course, the singlet at δ 3.23 arises from the amino protons and corresponds to 2H, while the singlet at δ 2.17 is due to CH_3 protons and integrates to 3H.

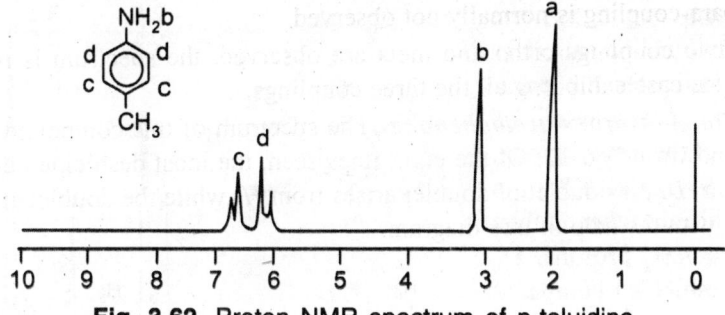

Fig. 3.62. Proton NMR spectrum of p-toluidine.

2. 2,4–Dinitrophenol

The PMR spectrum is shown in Fig. 3.63. H_a the proton, being ortho to both NO_2 groups is most deshielded, followed by H_b which in turn is more deshielded than H_c. H_a is coupled via J_{ab} (2.8 Hz) to H_b, meta to it and appear as a doublet. It is not coupled to H_c, para to it. H_b is coupled to H_a via J_{ba} (2.8 Hz) and to proton H_c, ortho to it via J_{bc} (9.1 Hz). So, it appears as a doublet of doublet. Proton H_c is split only by H_b via J_{cb} (9.1 Hz).

 p-Nitrotoluene: The PMR of this compound is shown in Fig. 3.64.

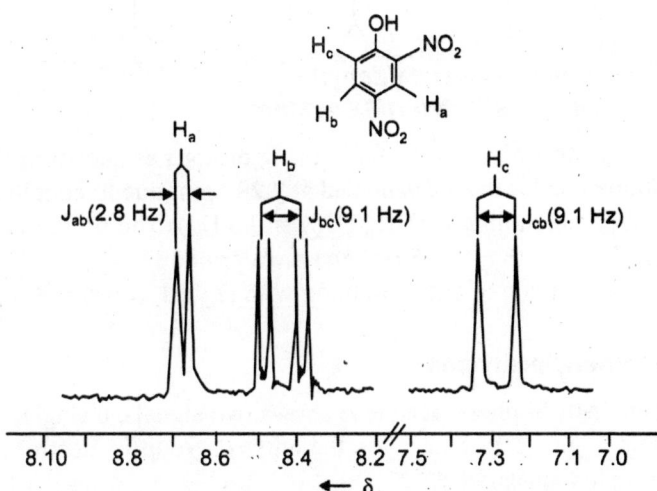

Fig. 3.63. ¹H NMR spectrum of 2,4-dinitrophenol.

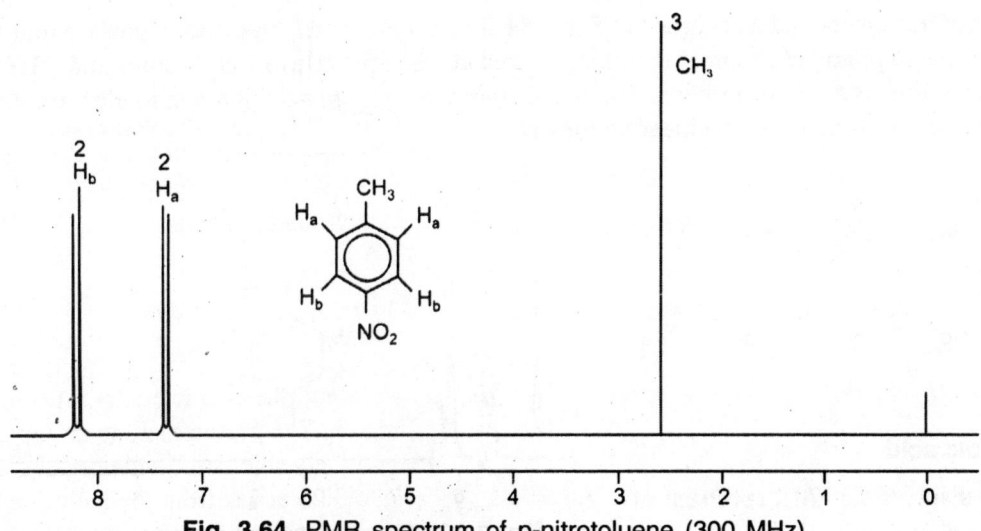

Fig. 3.64. PMR spectrum of p-nitrotoluene (300 MHz).

As is clear from Fig. 3.64, the aromatic region, the four-line pattern (a pair of doublet), indicates the para-disubstitution pattern. The singlet at δ 2.5 corresponds to 3–H of the methyl group. The doublet (J = 9 Hz) at 8.2 ppm corresponds to H_b while the other doublet at δ 7.40 arises from H_a protons. H_b protons are more deshielded compared to H_a protons due to anisotropy effect of the NO_2 group.

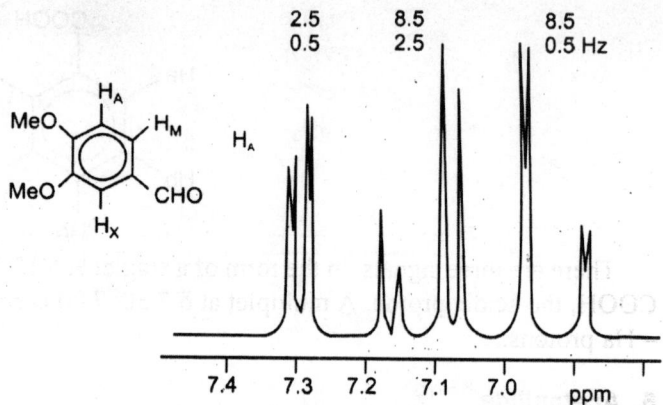

Fig. 3.65. NMR spectrum of 3,4–dimethoxybenzaldehyde.

3,4–Dimethoxy benzaldehyde (1,2,4–trisubstituted AMX system)

This is an AMX system for the ring protons as shown in Fig. 3.65. The X proton shows a doublet of doublet and is most deshielded at 7.29 ppm, due to coupling with the meta proton H_M ($^4J_{XM}$ = 2.5 Hz) and para-coupling with H_A ($^5J_{XA}$ = 0.5 Hz). The proton H_M shows a doublet of doublet, due to ortho proton, H_A ($^3J_{MA}$ = 8.5 Hz) and meta proton H_X ($^4J_{MX}$ = 2.5 Hz). The proton H_A also shows a doublet of doublet due to ortho coupling with H_M ($^3J_{AM}$ = 8.5 Hz) and para proton H_X ($^5J_{AX}$ = 0.5 Hz).

3. Phenylacetylene

The PMR of phenylacetylene shows two signals, a singlet at 2.99 ppm and a multiplet centred at 7.40 ppm in the ratio of 1:5. As the ethynyl group is electronegative in nature, aromatic region shows a complex appearance.

4. Anisole

The PMR of this compound is recorded in Fig. 3.54. There are present three clear signals, a multiplet at 7.15 ppm, due to proton H_b, another multiplet centred at 6.85 ppm due to 3 H_a protons and a 3H singlet at 3.70 ppm, due to methoxy protons. The o and p-protons, H_a are shielded due to electron-donating nature of methoxy group than the meta protons H_b.

5. Benzoic acid

Fig. 3.66 displays the PMR spectrum of benzoic acid.

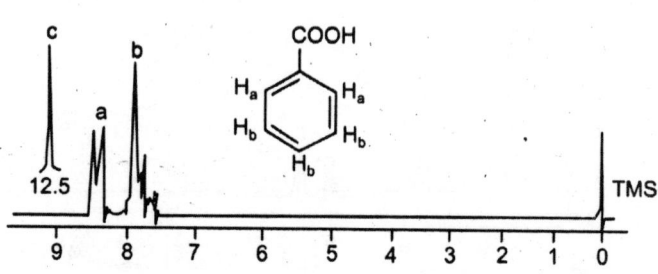

Fig. 3.66. Proton NMR spectrum of benzoic acid.

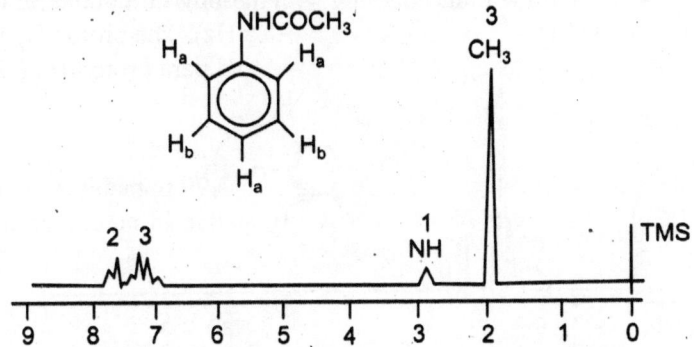

There are three signals, in the form of a singlet at δ 12.50 ppm which corresponds to 1H arises from COOH, the acidic proton. A multiplet at δ 7.50–7.70 corresponds to 2H and arises from the two ortho – Ha protons.

6. Acetanilide

As can be seen from Fig. 3.67, the acetanilide molecule shows a 3H singlet at 2.08 ppm due to $COCH_3$ group. The NH proton appears as a broad singlet at 3.08 ppm and has intensity equal to ^1H. The aromatic region shows a multiplet corresponding to $2H$, due to two meta protons, Hb and another multiplet centred at d 7.27 ppm of intensity $3H$.

Fig. 3.67. Proton NMR spectrum of acetanilide.

7. Acetophenone

The proton NMR spectrum of acetophenone is shown in Fig. 3.68.

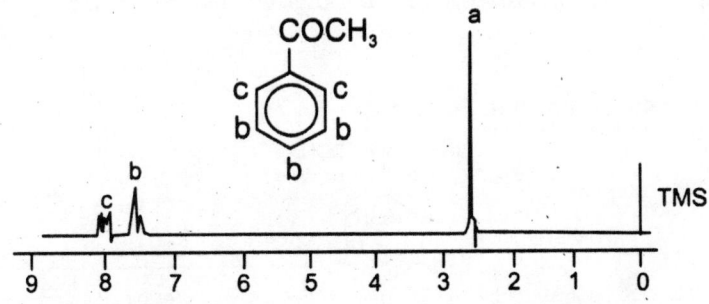

Fig. 3.68. Proton NMR spectrum of acetophenone.

This compound shows a 3*H* singlet at 2.47 ppm due to the CH_3 group. The aromatic region shows a multiplet at 7.90 ppm equivalent to 2*H*, the ortho protons and another multiplet due to the remaining three protons, two ortho and a meta proton. Notice that the ortho protons are more deshielded due to anisotropy effect of the carboxyl group.

8. Cinnamaldehyde

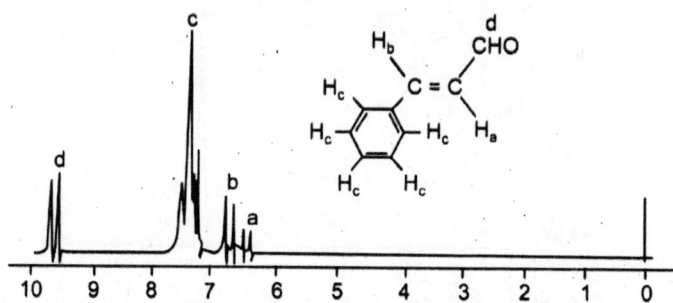

The PMR of cinnamaldehyde is shown in Fig. 3.69. The doublet (with *J* = 7.4 Hz) centred at 9.67 ppm, corresponding to 1*H* is due to the aldehydic proton. CHO proton gets splitted due to coupling with the proton H_A. The aromatic region shows a complex multiplet at 7.40 ppm equivalent 5*H*. A doublet of doublet due to H_B, positioned at δ 6.62 ppm integrating to 1*H* arises due to coupling with the aldehydic proton (*J* = 7.4 Hz) and the trans coupling with the proton H_A (*J* = 16.3 Hz).

Fig. 3.69. Proton NMR spectrum of cinnamaldehyde.

9. Benzaldehyde

The PMR of benzaldehyde shown in Fig. 3.55 contains the following peaks : a singlet at δ 8.50 ppm due to the formyl proton and the multiplet due to 5*H* protons at 7.50 ppm. The multiplet actually consists of two groups – the more deshielded 2*H* ortho group and the 3*H* meta/para group.

10. Phenacetin

The spectrum of phenacetin is shown in Fig. 3.57.

In the aromatic region, phenacetin shows a symmetrical four line pattern characteristic of *p*-disubstitution, a pair centred at 8.05 ppm and 7.41 ppm. $COCH_3$ methyl appears as a singlet at 2.10 ppm. The ethyl group CH_2 appears as a quartet at 3.95 ppm, while the methyl at 1.25 ppm as a triplet.

11. Aspirin

o-acetyl salicylic acid is called aspirin that is an important analgesic widely used the world over. Its PMR is shown in Fig. 3.70. It shows a multiplet that consists of two groups in the aromatic region. The –COOH– group appears at 11.9 ppm. The $COCH_3$ protons resonate at 2.4 ppm as a singlet.

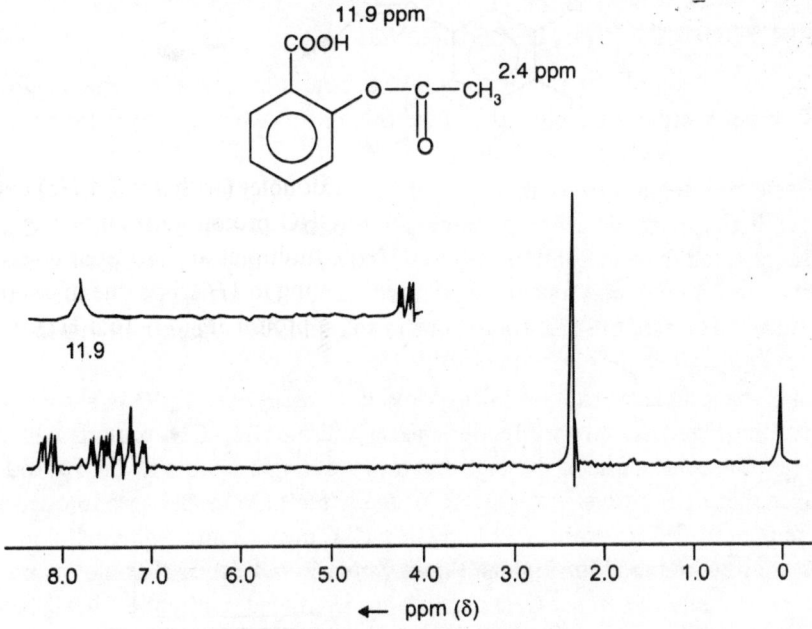

Fig. 3.70. PMR spectrum of aspirin.

12. 2–Nitrophenol

This compound shows all the three coupling constants as can be seen in Fig. 3.71. The 3–H proton is most deshielded as expected because of its closeness to nitro group – an electron withdrawing group.

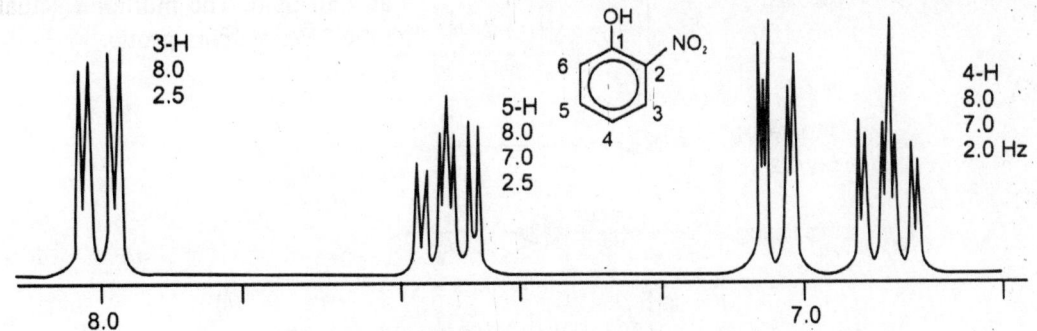

Fig. 3.71. PMR spectrum of 2–nitrophenol.

This shows a doublet of doublet at δ 7.95 as a result of coupling with 4–H ($J = 8$ Hz) and 5–H ($J = 2.5$ Hz). p-coupling is not seen. The next deshielded proton is 5–H as it is positioned para to the NO_2 group as well as it is meta (and not ortho or para) releasing group, –OH. It shows a three fold doublet at δ 7.5 and shows three couplings, $J = 8.0$ with one ortho proton, 6–H and $J = 7.0$ Hz with 4 –H, another ortho proton and the last $J = 2.5$ Hz with the 3–H meta proton. The next less deshielded proton 6–H shows a doublet of doublet at 7.35 due to splitting with ortho proton 5–H ($J = 8.0$ Hz) and the meta proton 4–H ($J = 2.0$ Hz). The most upfield 4–H proton shows a three fold doublet at d 6.87 due to three couplings $J_{ortho} = 8$ Hz with 3–H, $J_{ortho} = 7$ Hz with 5–H and $J_{meta} = 2.0$ with 6–H.

3.16 DOUBLE RESONANCE (SPIN DECOUPLING)

This technique is used for simplification of complex spectra. It tells us as to which spin-spin multiplets are correlated. In other words, it enables us to determine as to which protons are spin coupled to one another.

What is done in this technique is that one of the two coupled spins is irradiated by a second radiofrequency while the spectrum is being scanned in routine. As a result the selected proton(s) spin is magnetically disconnected from the proton spin to which it was coupled. This magic happens due to the fact that the second radiofrequencies forces the selected proton to undergo very rapid transitions between its α and β spin states. The rate of these transitions is so rapid, that the proton to which it was coupled is unable to see its spin and so gets decoupled.

Let us consider the simplest example of n-propyl chloride whose PMR is shown in Fig. a. When CH_2Cl protons are irradiated, its own triplet disappears and the CH_2–CH_3 protons which earlier gave a hextet, now appear as a quartet due to the fact that they no longer couple to $ClCH_2$ and only couple to CH_3 protons under these conditions. No change in the triplet due to CH_3 group occurs which shows that it was not coupled to $ClCH_2$ protons. When CH_2–CH_3 protons are irradiated, both the $ClCH_2$ and the CH_3 protons are now reduced to singlets, thereby clearly indicating that they were coupled to the central CH_2 protons. Finally, when the CH_3 protons are irradiated, while the $ClCH_2$ protons appear as a triplet, the CH_2CH_3 protons also appear as a triplet as they are not able to spin couple to the CH_3 protons. Further, it should be noted that the irradiating power, I_0 required to spin-decouple a nucleus completely from a nucleus to which it is spin coupled is given by $I_0 > 2\pi J/Y$ where Y is the gyromagneto ratio that represents the nuclear strength.

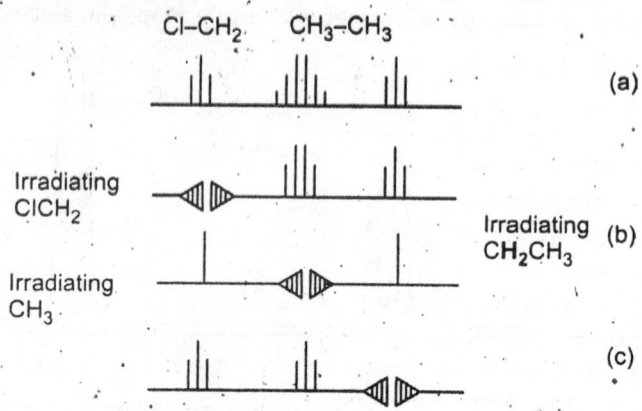

Thus, it is clear from the above simple example that the double irradiation technique has great potential in simplifying the complex spectra even at low resolution spectrometers operating at 60 MHz.

Finally below is shown the role of double resonance in CH_3CHO which shows a doublet for methyl and δ 2.05 and a quartet for CHO proton at δ 9.75. If CHO proton is irradiated, the methyl signal becomes a singlet for CHO. When methyl protons are irradiated, the CHO proton gives a singlet.

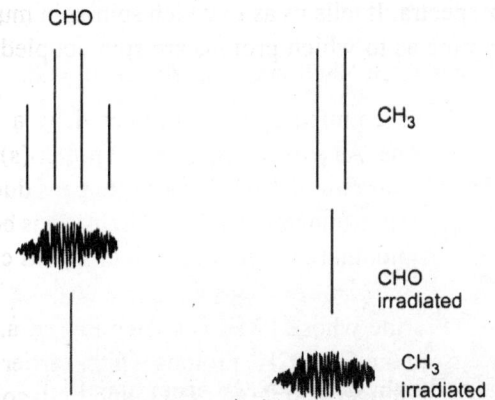

3.17 DEUTERATION – DEUTERIUM EXCHANGE

The acidic hydrogens such as the protons of $-COOH$, $-OH$, $-SH$, $-NH_2$ groups are exchangeable with deuterated water, D_2O. These groups exchange protons very rapidly. For carboxylic and phenols, basic catalysts are very effective while acidic catalysts are required for the alcoholic and amines.

$$RCOOH + D_2O \rightleftharpoons RCOOD + DOH$$
$$RNH_2 + D_2O \rightleftharpoons RND_2 + ROH$$

In general,
$$R–XH + D_2O \rightleftharpoons R—XD + HDO$$

The deuterium exchange is so rapid on the nmr time scale that the signals due to the exchanged protons disappear from their PMR spectra. However, a new signal at about 4.5–5.0 ppm due to DOH protons that are generated during the exchange appear in the spectra. The signals arising from the introduced deuterium are not seen as deuterium will require a frequency about 1/7th of that of protons.

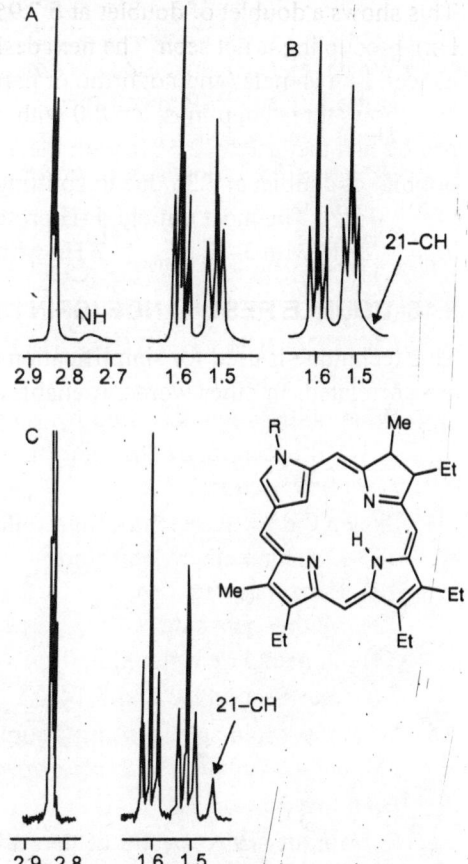

Fig. 3.72. Partial 400 MHz proton NMR spectra of N-methyl NCP in $CDCl_3$. (A) Upfield region showing the broad NH peak at 2.75 ppm; the 21–CH overlaps with the triplet at 1.5 ppm. (B) Proton NMR spectrum run at a slightly different concentration showing the 21–CH as a broad shoulder. (C) Proton NMR spectrum for the same NMR solution as A after a D_2O shake. The NH peak has been lost and the 21–CH resonance sharpens up and shifts slightly upfield.

PMR spectrum (Fig. 3.72) of the following porphyrin recently reported by Lash and Ruden shows 21–H proton at about 1.5 ppm and the NH as a broad peak at 2.75 ppm. When D_2O is added, the N–H broad peak disappeared due to exchange as expected. In the process, however, the 21–CH that earlier overlapped with the triplet at 1.5 ppm now became sharp and also got shifted slightly upfield as shown in Fig. below. This example shows the additional benefit of deuteration.

PROBLEMS

1. What is an NMR spectrum? Is it an absorption or an emission spectrum? Enlist the three messages carried by an NMR spectrum.

   Hind: See Section 3.1.

2. Which of the following protons are equivalent and which are non-equivalent?

		$\overset{\ominus}{CH_3Li}$	
CH_3SCH_3	CH_2Cl_2	CH_3Li	$(HO)_3PO$
CH_3COOCH_3	CH_3CHO	$CH_3NHCONHCH_3$	
$(CH_3O)_2P(S)OH$	CH_3OH	CH_2BrCH_2Cl	
$ClCH_2COOCH_2CH_3$	$(CH_3CH_2O)_2P(S)SH$		

   Hint: See Section 3.2.

3. What information is carried by intensities of signals in an NMR spectrum? Explain with the aid of NMR spectrum of phenylacetic acid.

   Hint: See Section 3.3.

4. Sketch the NMR spectra of the following molecules:
   (1) Dimethyl ethynyl carbinol
   (2) Benzyl acetate
   (3) Methyl benzoate
   (4) Dimethyl benzylamine

   Hint: See Section 3.3 and 3.14.

5. What is the spin-spin splitting (coupling)? Explain with the help of NMR spectrum of 1,1,2,3,3,3–hexachloropropane.

   Hint: See Section 3.5

6. Explain the NMR spectra of the following:
   (1) CH_3CH_2Br
   (2) 1,1,2–tribromoethane
   (3) 1,2,3–tribromopropane
   (4) $(CH_3)_2CHCl$

   Hint: See Section 3.5.

7. What is N + 1 rule? Explain this rule with the help of NMR spectra of the following compounds.
   (1) $BrCH_2CH_2Cl$
   (2) CH_3CH_2Cl
   (3) $CH_3CHBrCH_3$
   (4) $(CH_3)_3CH$
   (5) Ethyl 2,3–dibromo–3–(p-tolyl) propionate

   Hint: See Sectin 3.6.

8. Give an example of NMR spectrum that corresponds to $(na + 1)(nb + 1)$ multiplicities.

   Hint: See Section 3.6, example of NMR spectrum of ultra-pure ethanol.

9. Give two examples of NMR spectra where multiplicities are given by the formula $(na + nb + 1)$ rule rather than by $(na + 1)(nb + 1)$ rule.

   Hint: Give examples of $BrCH_2CH_2CH_2Cl$, $PhCH_2CH_2CH_3$, $BrCH_2CH_2CH_3$. See Section 3.6.

10. Sketch and explain the NMR spectrum of Ethyl 2,3–dibromo–3–(p-tolyl) propionate.
    Hint: See Section 3.6 (Intext Exercise).
11. Explain the spin rotation AMX and give one example.
12. Explain the following spin notations: (i) ABX system, (ii) ABC system, (iii) AMX system.
13. What are the rules for splitting of proton signals?
    Hint: See Section 3.7.
14. What are first-order spectra? Show the breakdown of first-order spectra.
    Hint: See Section 3.8 and Section 3.10 (two spin system).
15. Explain second order or non-first order Spectra? How do they differ from first order spectra? What is roofing effect?
    Hint: See Sections 3.8 and 3.9.
16. Explain the following spin notations with examples.
    (1) An system
    (2) AB system
    (3) AX system
    (4) AX-AB system
    (5) AX_2–AB_2 system
    (6) AA'XX' system
    (7) AA'BB' system
    Hint: See Section 3.10.
17. Illustrate the following with two examples each: Magnetic non-equivalence and Magnetic equivalence.
    Hint: See Section 3.11A.
18. Second order spectra become first-order spectra at higher field strength. Why? Give reasons.
19. Illustrate the use of chemical shift reagents.
    Hint: See Section 3.12.
20. Explain double resonance.
    Hint: See Section 3.17.
21. Illustrate deuteration-deuterium exchange.
    Hint: See Section 3.18.
22. How will you determine coupling constant for a double doublet and a double triplet?
    Hint: See Section 3.16.
23. Whether the methylene protons in the following pyrrolic molecule are equivalent or non-equivalent.

Hint: The methylene protons are non-equivalent and form an AB system as they are adjacent to a chiral centre.

24. Tell whether in the following sulfoxide compound, the methylene groups are equivalent or non-equivalent.

Hint: The methylene protons are non-equivalent due to their different spatial disposition w.r. to S = O group. In fact, they form an AB system.

25. How would the ¹H spectrum of the following compound look like for the CH_3—CH_2 part?

Hint: As the CH_3—CH_2 unit is joined to a chiral centre C–5, therefore, the CH_2 protons would behave as magnetically different. Hence, they would absorb at different chemical shifts. Therefore, the spectrum of the ethyl group would appear as a ABM_3 spin system.

One H of the CH_2 group appears as a multiplet (due to coupling with the another H of the CH_2 group and the three methyl protons) at δ 1.43 ppm, the other appears as a multiplet (due to similar reasons) at d 1.60 ppm. The CH_3 appears as a triplet at δ 0.77 ppm.

26. Explain whether the two methylene hydrogens of the ethyl group are equivalent?

Hint: The two hydrogens in question are non-equivalent because of their spatial disposition as shown.

In fact, these are **diastereotopic** hydrogens. While H¹ is on the side of the ring CH₃ group H² is on the side of the ring proton at C–4 shown. Thus, they have different chemical environments and hence absorbs at different chemical shifts.

27. Explain whether the two ethyl groups in the following compound are non-equivalent.

• *Hint*: Both the ethyl groups are magnetically non-equivalent. They are chemically equivalent. The ring as a whole is chiral. In fact, a mirror plane divides the molecule into two equal halves.

This plane passes through the nitrogen and the CH_3—CH group, perpendicular to the plane of the $C=C$ double bonds.

— mirror plane

28. An organic compound with MF $C_5H_8O_2$ gave the following PMR spectrum at 100 MHz. What is the probable structure of the compound?

Solution: We can clearly confirm the presence of an ethyl group - CH_2CH_3 because of he presence of a triplet (at 1.30 ppm) and a quartet. As the quartet is present at 4.19 ppm, the CH_2 is group is deshielded. This means the CH_2 group is attached to oxygen i.e. it is a $–OCH_2CH_3$ group. The remaining peaks in the region 5.7 to 6.6 correspond to three protons. As these peaks are present in the olefinic region, so they must be alkene protons. The *dd* at 6.40 has J = 13 Hz which indicates coupling between the protons trans to each other i.e. H_C w.r. to H_B and a coupling of 2 Hz indicates splitting of the signals of H_C with genital proton H_B ($J_{AB} \neq 2$ Hz). Similarly, a *dd* is clearly seen at δ 5.75. As one J = 8 Hz and another 2 Hz this indicates the coupling of proton H_B with proton H_A that is cis to it and further splitting of the doublet obtained with the geminal proton H_A ($J_{AC} = 2$ Hz). The remaining peaks in this region represent the proton H_A. Clearly, the *dd* of H_A has been affected by the roofing effects of protons AB and protons BC. The compound is therefore, assigned the structure corresponding to ethyl acrylate.

Ethylacrylate

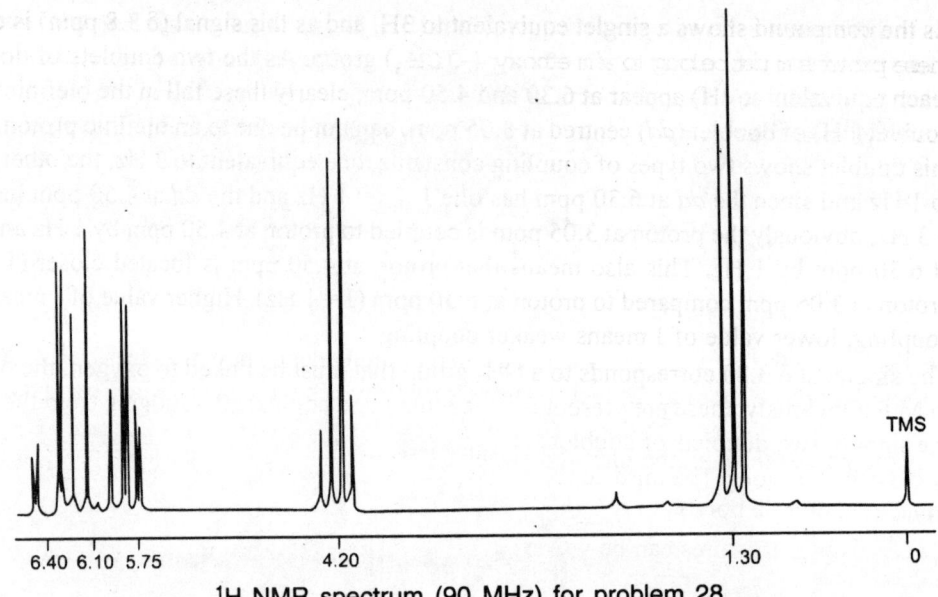

¹H NMR spectrum (90 .MHz) for problem 28.

29. A compound with molecular formula, C_5H_6O shows the following PMR spectrum with relative intensities and coupling constants as shown. What could be the possible structure of this compound.

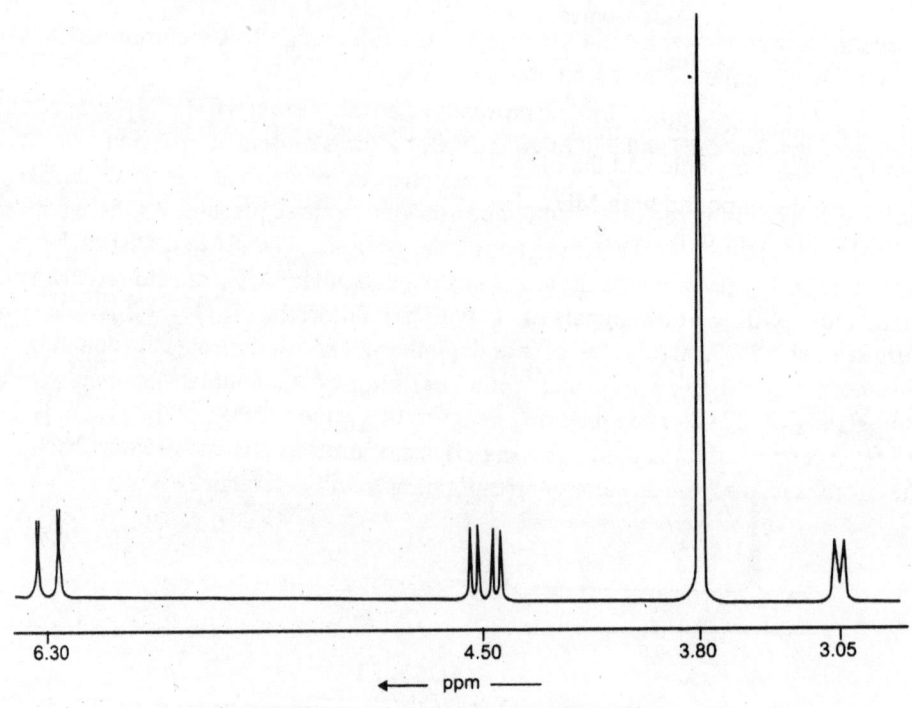

¹H NMR (90 MHz) for problem 29.

As the compound shows a singlet equivalent to 3H, and as this signal (δ 3.8 ppm) is deshielded, these protons must belong to a methoxy ($-OCH_3$) group. As the two doublets of doublets (*dd*) (each equivalent to ¹H) appear at 6.30 and 4.50 ppm, clearly these fall in the olefinic range. The doublet (¹H) of doublet (*dd*) centred at 3.05 ppm, can not be due to an olefinic proton. Further as this doublet shows two types of coupling constants, one equivalent to 3 Hz, the other equivalent to 1 Hz and since the *dd* at 6.30 ppm has one J_{value} = 1 Hz and the *dd* at 4.50 ppm has one J_{value} = 3 Hz, obviously the proton at 3.05 ppm is coupled to proton at 4.50 ppm by 1 Hz and to proton at 6.30 ppm by 1 Hz. This also means that proton at 4.50 ppm is located closer (J = 3 Hz) to proton at 3.05 ppm compared to proton at 6.30 ppm (J = 1 Hz). Higher value of J means stronger coupling, lower value of J means weaker coupling.

The singlet at δ 3.80 corresponds to a CH_3 group that must be linked to oxygen, the only oxygen in M.F. Obviously, these are present three double bond equivalents. Judging from the position of the signals, two doublets of doublets at 6.30 ppm and at 4.50 ppm, it is clear that these belong to two olefinic protons. The third doublet of doublet that absorbs at δ 3.05, must clearly be acetylenic in nature.

Two possible structures can be written as:

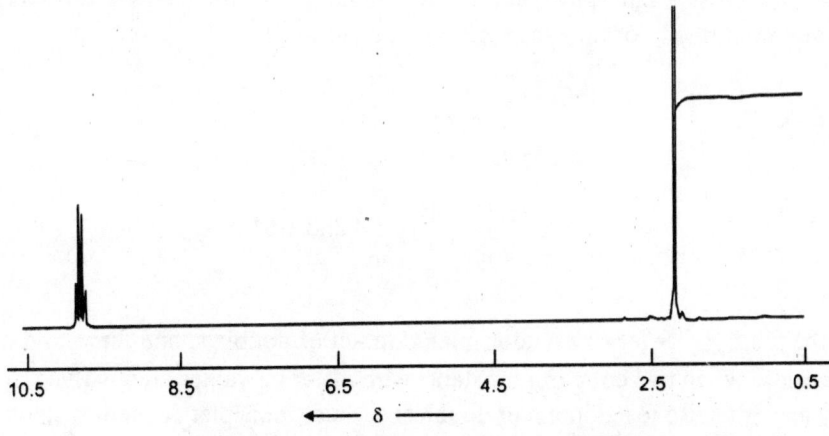

cis-isomer   trans-isomer

Now, whether the alkene is cis or trans can be readily deduced by looking at the J_{values}. As the J value is 8 Hz, evidently, we are dealing with the cis isomer. If it were higher in the range 11–18 Hz, the isomer would be trans. Further, we can also see the presence of long range coupling between the acetylenic and the olefinic proton H_X J_{AX} = 1 Hz, J_{AM} being 3 Hz.

30. An organic compound with MF C_2H_4O shows the following ¹H NMR spectrum. Assign a most suitable structure to it.

¹H NMR for problem 30 (Hint: CH_3CHO)

31. Assign the various peaks seen in the ^1H spectrum of the following pyrrolic compound at 60 MHz.

2.15 (s, 3H), 2.31 (t, 2H), 2.78 (t, 2H), 3.38 (s, 3H), 5.18 (s, 2H), 7.18 (s, 5H), 9.58 (s, 1H).

Hint: 2.15 (s, 3–Me), 2.31 (t, CH_2–ring), 2.78 (t, CH_2COO), 3.38 (s, OMe), 5.18 (s, $CH_2C_6H_5$), 7.18 (s, C_6H_5), 9.58 (s, CHO).

32. Assign the various peaks obtained in the following spectrum to the pyrrolic compound shown:

2.31 (s, 3H), 2.62 (t, 2H), 2.85 (t, 2H), 5.69 (s, 2H), 6.73 (s, 1H), 7.29–7.26 (m,, 5H), 9.2 (s, 1H).

Hint: δ 2.31 (s, CH_3), 2.62 (t, CH_2–CH_2), 2.85 (t, CH_2–CH_2), 5.69 ($CH_2C_6H_5$), 6.73 (1H, C–5), 7.29–7.45 (C_6H_5), 9.2 (COOH).

33. Predict the multiplicity of CH_2 protons in 3–methyl–2–pentanone.

Hint: The –CH_2– protons form an AB system being adjacent to a chiral carbon. These appear at 1.4 and 1.67 ppm as a multiplet each due to coupling with the CH and CH_3CH_2 protons. The position and multiplicity of the other protons is as follows:

34. Explain the multiplicity terms pseudotriplet, doublet of doublets, and three fold doublet.

Multiplicities: When two coupling constants with different values are involved in a spin system, then they may give rise to a doublet of doublets or a pseudotriplet depending upon the amount of difference in their size.

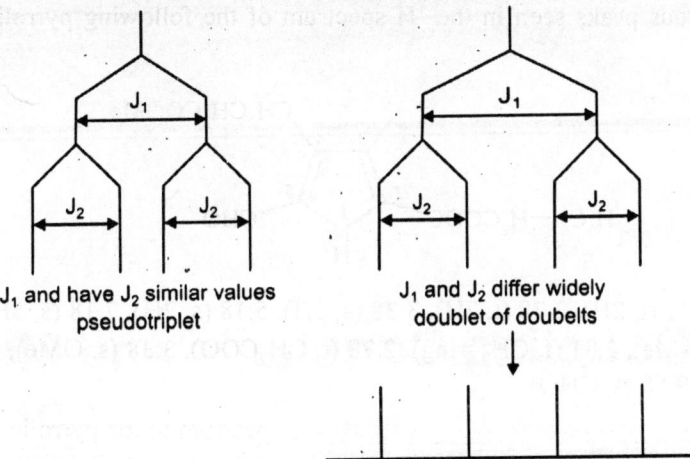

J_1 and have J_2 similar values
pseudotriplet

J_1 and J_2 differ widely
doublet of doubelts

When three coupling constants which differ widely in their size are present in a system, then the multiplet formed via their interaction is called a three fold doublet.

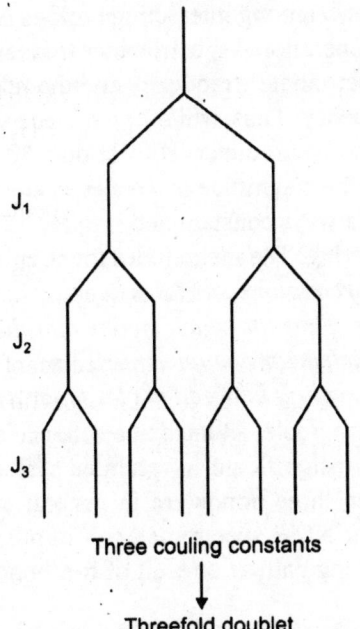

Three couling constants

Threefold doublet

Three coupling constants $\longrightarrow$ Three fold doublet.

4

Coupling Constants and Mechanism of Coupling

4.1 INTRODUCTION

The magnitude of coupling constant, J among interacting protons is always constant, irrespective of the strength of the applied field or the operational spectrometer frequency. The value of J can be found out by knowing the strength of the spectrometer frequency and the relationship between 1 ppm and Hertz (Hz) at the strength of the radiofrequency. Thus, while 1 ppm is equal to 60 Hz on a 60 MHz spectrometer, it is equal to 100 Hz on a 100 MHz spectrometer, 800 Hz on a 800 MHz spectrometer and so on. The magnitude of J is very variable, but the magnitude of J between any two interacting nuclei in a particular chemical setting or environment is always constant and is in fact, a characteristic of the nuclei between which spin-spin interaction is occurring. The magnitudes for coupling constant between different types of protons are different. *The value of coupling constants depends upon the distance between the coupled nuclei and decreases with distance. Thus ^1J, which means that there is only one bond separating the coupled nuclei is higher than ^2J which means coupled nuclei are separated by two bonds, which in turn is higher than ^3J, that represents coupling between nuclei separated by three bonds and so on.*

The coupling that occurs between nuclei situated at a distance of over four or more bonds is called **long-range coupling.** It is usually insignificant in saturated systems but is significant in unsaturated systems. Couplings over more than three bonds are in general quite small, less than 3 Hz and are usually not resolved with the routine NMR spectrometers. Coupling may be enhanced due to presence of an unsaturated bond in the coupling path as a result of σ-π bond configuration interaction :

$^4J = 0\text{-}3$ Hz

$^4J = 0\text{-}3$ Hz

$^4J = 0\text{-}3$ Hz

and may be resolved over up to even nine bonds. An example is $H_3C–(C≡C)_3–CH_2OH$, whence $^9J_{H–H}$ is equal to 0.4 Hz between the hydrocarbon hydrogens.

$$H_2\overset{2}{C}\overset{}{—}\overset{3}{C}≡\overset{4}{C}\underset{^9J}{—}\overset{5}{C}≡\overset{6}{C}—\overset{7}{C}≡\overset{8}{C}—\overset{}{C}H—OH$$

^9J coupling between hydrocarbon protons through 9 bonds

$$^9J_{HH} = 0.4 \text{ Hz}$$

$$C\overset{1}{———}H \qquad ^1J$$

One bond coupling

$$H\overset{1}{———}\overset{}{C}\overset{2}{———}H \quad ≡ \quad \overset{}{C}\big\langle\, \overset{H}{_H} \qquad ^2J\,(6\text{–}12\text{ Hz})$$

Two bonds geminal coupling

$$H\overset{1}{—}\overset{}{C}\overset{2}{—}\overset{}{C}\overset{3}{—}H \qquad ^3J\,(6\text{–}8\text{ Hz})$$

Three bonds vicinal coupling

$$H\overset{1}{—}\overset{}{C}\overset{2}{—}\overset{}{C}\overset{3}{—}\overset{}{C}\overset{4}{—}H \qquad ^4J$$
$$H\overset{1}{—}\overset{}{C}\overset{2}{—}\overset{}{C}\overset{3}{—}\overset{}{C}\overset{4}{—}\overset{}{C}\overset{5}{—}H \qquad ^5J$$
$$\left.\right\}\text{ insignificant}$$

Long range coupling

Further, **the magnitude of J can also tell us about the stereochemical disposition of the coupled protons with respect to each other in** saturated as well as unsaturated systems. Thus, while the ^3J value for cis protons is 6–15 Hz, it is 6-12 Hz for vicinal protons, 12-18 Hz for trans protons.

It should be noted that the coupling is a reciprocal affair. It is characterized by the presence of adjacent pairs of features (Fig. 4.1) which would have exactly the same value of coupling constants. Thus for CH_3CH_2 group, there are two multiplets – a triplet for CH_3 and a quartet for CH_2 which have identical value of J. But if we do not find pairs of features rather we find only one pair of feature (Fig. 4.2), it shows that it is not a H–H coupling, rather it is the coupling of a proton with some nearby NMR-active nucleus like ^{31}P, ^{19}F etc.

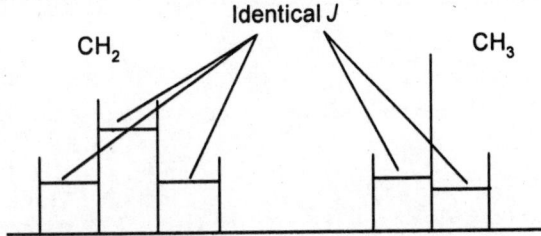

Fig. 4.1. Pairs of features in CH_3CH_2 group containing molecules.

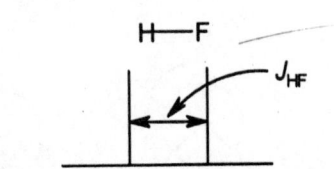

Fig. 4.2. Only one pair (doublet) feature in H–X containing molecules.

4.2 FACTORS THAT AFFECT MAGNITUDE OF J

The magnitude of coupling constant J is variable from 5 Hz to several thousand Hz and depends upon:
  (1) The number of bonds between the coupled nuclei.
  (2) The bond order of the bonds between the coupled nuclei.
  (3) Angle between the bonds i.e. the stereochemical disposition of the coupled nuclei w.r. to each other in the molecule.

Before we discuss these factors, it is important to note that the magnitude of J which gives us the relevant information about the bonding systems is obscured due to contributions of γ_A and γ_B, the gyromagneto ratios of the coupled nuclei. That is why often the reduced coupling constant, called K, equal to $4\pi^2 J/(h \gamma_A \gamma_B)$ is used for correlating bonding system with spin-spin coupling.

Further, noteworthy point about coupling constants is that they can be either positive or negative, the sign depends upon the bonding system as well as on the product of γ_A and γ_B. The signs are noted for theoretical considerations.

We will show the dependence of J upon above factors as we discuss the following important HH couplings :
  1. Vicinal couplings ($^3J_{HH}$)
  2. Geminal HH couplings
  3. Longe-range H–H couplings.

4.2.1 Vicinal Couplings

This is the coupling between protons linked through three intervening bonds ($^3J_{HH}$). This occurs in both saturated as well as unsaturated systems. In both these systems, the coupling is transmitted by σ-electrons and is always positive. We will consider $^3J_{HH}$ in saturated, unsaturated olefinic and in aromatic systems separately.

4.2.2.1 *Saturated Systems*

Let us consider the system in which two non-equivalent protons are shown as H_A and H_X.

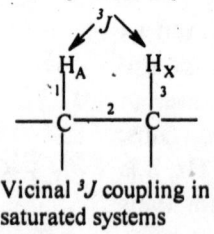

Vicinal ^3J coupling in
saturated systems

The coupling constant, $^3J_{HH}$ is found to be dependent upon the dihedral angle ϕ (Fig. 4.3) between the two C–H bonds both for cyclic and acyclic systems.

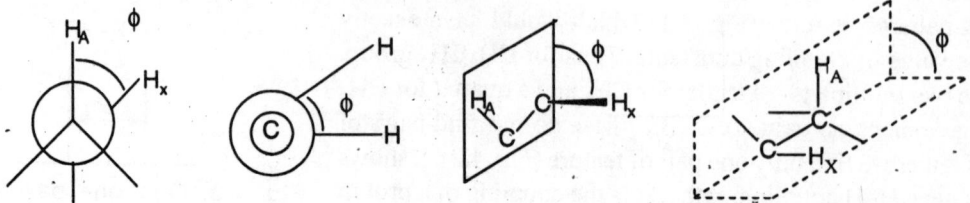

Fig. 4.3. The directional angle between two C–H bonds is called ϕ, the dihedral angle.

The magnitude of $^3J_{HH}$ is maximum at 0° (eclipsed conformation) and 180° (staggered conformation) although ^3J 180° is always larger than ^3J 0° in practice as predicted as well. It is minimum at 90° i.e. to say when the two carbon-hydrogen bonds are orthogonal to each other (Fig. 4.4).

Thus ^3J for the trans-vicinal protons in cyclopentanes is 0 Hz as the dihedral angle, ϕ is 90°. The $^3J_{HH}$ for the cis vicinal protons in these systems is 8 Hz as the $\phi = 0$.

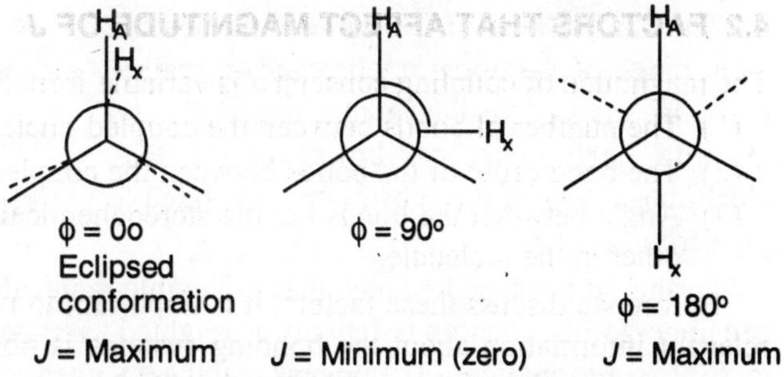

$\phi = 0o$
Eclipsed
conformation

$\phi = 90°$

$\phi = 180°$

J = Maximum   J = Minimum (zero)   J = Maximum

Fig. 4.4. Variation of J_{HH} with dihedral angle ϕ.

$^3J_{cis} \sim 8\,Hz$
$\phi = 0°$

$^3J_{trans} \sim 0\,Hz$
$(\phi = 90°)$

Karplus gave an equation to represent the relationship between $^3J_{HH}$ and ϕ.

$$^3J_{HH} = A + B\,Cos\,\phi + C\,Cos\,2\phi \quad \text{where } A = 7, B = -1, C = 5$$

or

$$^3J_{HH} = 7 - Cos\,\phi + 5\,Cos\,2\phi$$

The dependence of $^3J_{HH}$ on ϕ is shown in the **Karplus equation.** The curve obtained is called **Karplus curve.**

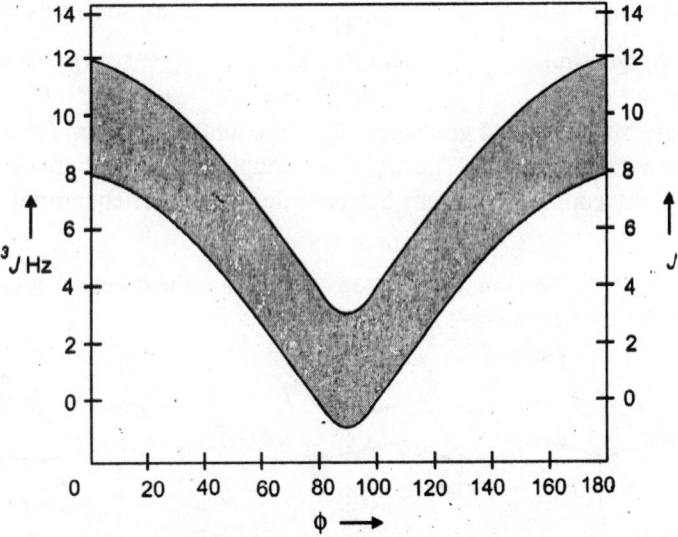

Fig. 4.5. The Karplus curve.

The shaded area in the curve indicates the wide range of variation as observed in reality. Other factors such as the valence angles Q_1 and Q_2 and carbon-carbon bond length R_{cc}, electronegativity of the substituent X bonded to the carbon atoms.

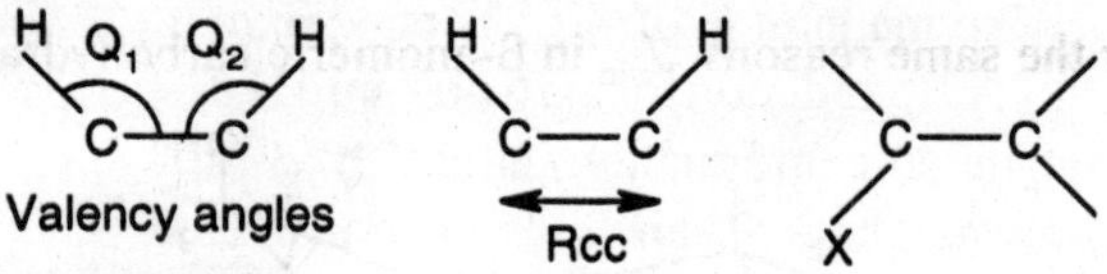

Valency angles

Fig. 4.6. Q, R_{CC} and electronegativity factors that affect J.

Further, it needs to be noted that in flexible molecules, the $^3J_{HH}$ coupling across a C—C bond that can undergo free rotation is actually a weighted average of the values expected for each of the possible multiple conformations. That means that the J values are weighted by the percent of time spent in each conformation. Thus, the $^3J_{HH}$ around a free rotating C—C bond determined as 7 Hz is indeed an average value of the three staggered conformations (the coupling protons pass twice through syn configuration and once through anti-configuration).

ϕ	J Hz
60°	4
−60°	4
180°	13 Hz

$J_{average} = 4 + 4 + 13 = 21/3 = 7$ Hz

$J_{determined} = 7$ Hz

This conformational averaging is not observed in case of rigid molecules like steroids.

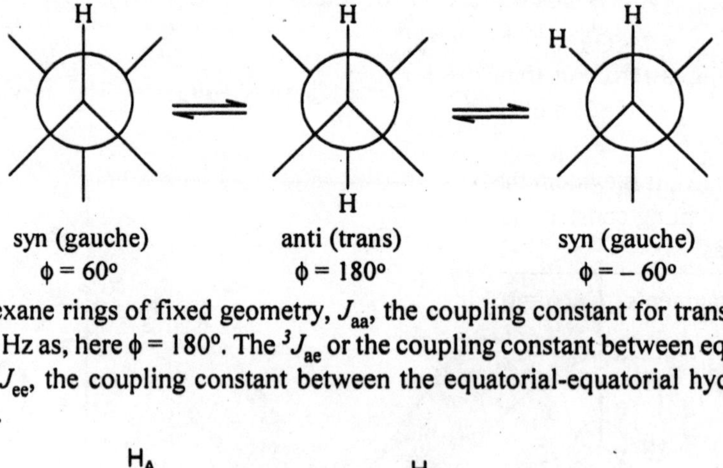

syn (gauche)	anti (trans)	syn (gauche)
$\phi = 60°$	$\phi = 180°$	$\phi = -60°$

For the cyclohexane rings of fixed geometry, J_{aa}, the coupling constant for trans di-axial coupling, is equal to 10 to 14 Hz as, here $\phi = 180°$. The $^3J_{ae}$ or the coupling constant between equatorial-equatorial hydrogens or the $^3J_{ee}$, the coupling constant between the equatorial-equatorial hydrogens is equal to 4–5 Hz as $\alpha = 60°$.

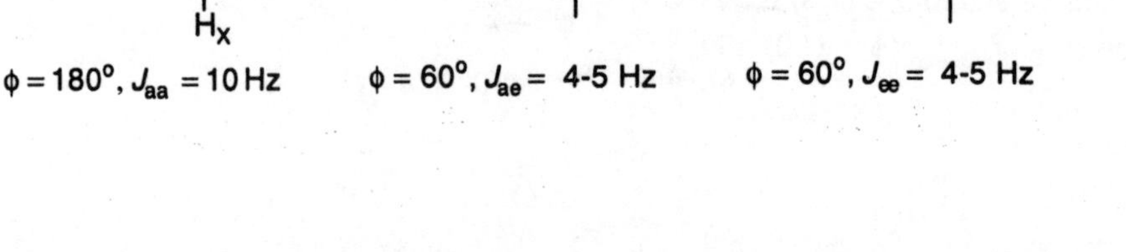

| $\phi = 180°$, $J_{aa} = 10$ Hz | $\phi = 60°$, $J_{ae} = 4$–5 Hz | $\phi = 60°$, $J_{ee} = 4$–5 Hz |

For the same reasons, J_{vic} in β-anomeric carbohydrates is larger than J_{vic} in α-anomer.

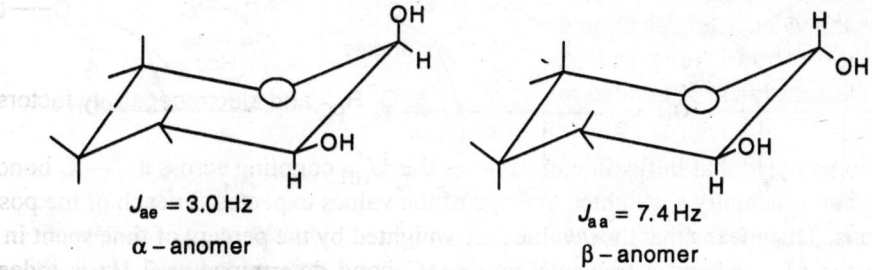

$J_{ae} = 3.0$ Hz

α – anomer

$J_{aa} = 7.4$ Hz

β – anomer

Karplus's original relationships were :

$$J_{vic} = 8.5 \cos^2 \phi - 0.28 \, (0° < \phi < 90°)$$
$$9.5 \cos^2 \phi - 0.28 \, (90° < \phi < 180°)$$

Subsequently, Karplus gave a better form :

$$J_{vic} = 4.22 - 0.5 \cos\phi + 4.2 \cos^2\phi$$

Much simpler Karplus equations based on original theoretical predictions were given by Williamson and Johnson approximately written as :

$$^3J_{CHCH} = 10 \cos^2\phi \, (0 < \phi < 90°) \quad\quad ...1$$
$$16 \cos^2\phi \, (90 < \phi < 180°) \quad\quad ...2$$

For $\phi = 90°$, the coupling is zero. For trans diaxial coupling J_{aa}, equal for $\phi = 180°$, the coupling should be ~ 10 Hz. For $^3J_{ea}$ or $^3J_{ee}$ ($\phi = 60°$) should be ~ 2.5 Hz. These results are in agreement with the experimental values.

From equations (1) and (2), it is evident that stereochemistry around the double bond should affect the magnitude of the coupling constant. Hence, it (J) enables us to distinguish between trans and cis disubstituted alkenes.

In planar or eclipsed fragments, J_{cis} ($\phi = 0°$) is ~ 10 Hz while J_{trans} ($\phi = 120°$) is ~ 2.5 Hz.

$\phi = 0°, J_{cis} = 10$ Hz $\phi = 120°, J_{trans} = 2.5$ Hz

These results are in line with those predicted on the basis of the equation :

$$^3J_{CHCH} = 10 \cos^2\phi$$

Thus the predicted values of J_{cis} ($J_{0°}$) is 10 Hz and J_{trans} (120°) is ~ 2.5 Hz.

In the camphene ring, $J_{exo\text{-}exo}$ ($\phi = 180$) and $J_{endo\text{-}endo}$ ($\phi = 0$), $J \sim 8$ to 9 Hz while $J_{exo\text{-}exo}$ ($\phi = 120$) is 2.3 Hz.

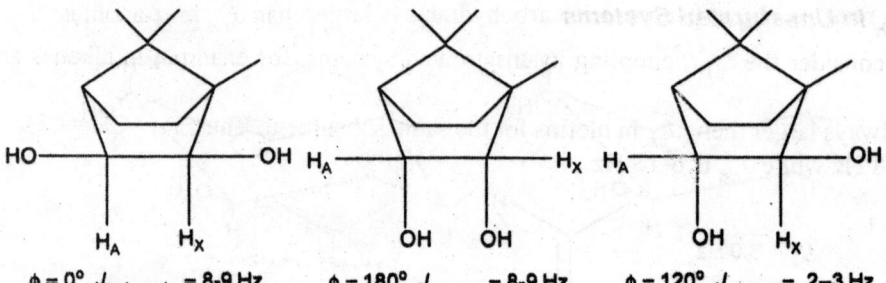

$\phi = 0°$, $J_{endo\text{-}endo} = 8\text{-}9$ Hz $\phi = 180°$, $J_{exo\text{-}exo} = 8\text{-}9$ Hz $\phi = 120°$, $J_{exo\text{-}exo} = 2\text{-}3$ Hz

Similarly, for the rigid cyclopropane derivatives 2-3 Hz J_{cis} is 10-12 Hz ($\phi = 0°$) and J_{trans} is 7-8 Hz ($\phi = 120°$).

$\phi = 0°$, $J_{cis} = 10\text{-}12$ Hz $\phi = 120°$, $J_{trans} = 7\text{-}8$ Hz

Further, this effect is also illustrated in following cyclopropanes :

$J_{cis} = 11.2$
$J_{trans} = 8.0$

$J_{cis} = 8.4$

$J_{trans} = 3.8$

Some more examples are shown in Table 4.1.

Table 6.1. Examples of $^3J_{HH}$ in saturated bonds

Compound	Coupling constant ^3J	Compound	Coupling constant ^3J
Acetaldehyde	2.9 Hz	$^3J_{cis}$	7.3 Hz
Ethyl alcohol	7.0 Hz	$^3J_{trans}$	6.0 Hz
	8.0 Hz	$Br\text{---}CH\text{---}CH\text{---}CH_2Cl$	6.30 Hz

4.2.1.2 $^3J_{HH}$ in Unsaturated Systems

Let us now consider the $^3J_{HH}$ coupling in unsaturated systems, for example in alkenes and aromatic compounds.

J_{trans} is always larger then $^3J_{cis}$ in olefins for the same substituent. Thus, for $-CH=CH_2-$ system, the J_{trans} is 11-18 Hz while J_{cis} is 6-15 Hz.

6–15 Hz   11–18 Hz

Of course, the nature of the substituent has great effect on these couplings. The magnitude of the vicinal coupling also depends upon C–C–H angles. For example, the $^3J_{cis}$ depends upon the ring size in cis alkenes (see Fig.4.7), this also applies to aromatic system. The $^3J_{cis}$ increases from 2.7 Hz in cyclopropene to 10.8 Hz in cycloheptene. Of course, there is no further increase in the magnitude of $^3J_{cis}$ with increase in ring size as the internal angles become almost strainess. This is shown in Fig. 4.7.

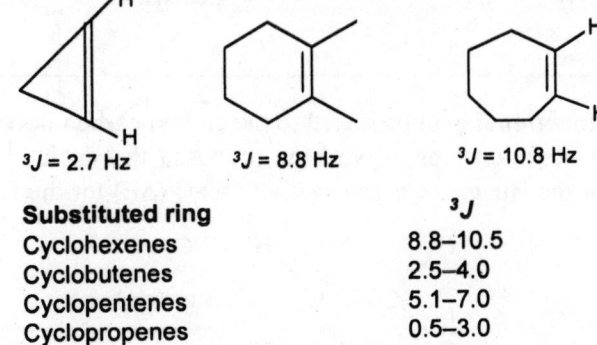

^3J = 2.7 Hz ^3J = 8.8 Hz ^3J = 10.8 Hz

Substituted ring	^3J
Cyclohexenes	8.8–10.5
Cyclobutenes	2.5–4.0
Cyclopentenes	5.1–7.0
Cyclopropenes	0.5–3.0

Fig. 4.7. Decrease of $^3J_{HH\ cis}$ with decreasing ring size or increasing bond angle

Such an effect is also seen in aromatic systems like azulene, benzene etc. Similarly, J varies from 2 to 5 Hz in furan, pyrrole and thiophene heterocyclic ring systems. Of course, the electronegativity of the hetero-atom and the varying nature of the double bond also exert their influence besides the ring size factor (also see Section 4.2.3.4).

Azulene
J = 4.0 Hz

Benzene
J = 7.5 Hz

Naphthalene
J_{12} = 8.6 Hz
J_{23} = 6.0 Hz

Azulene
J = 10.3 Hz

Some more examples of $^3J_{HH}$ are collected in Table 4.2.

Table 4.2. Examples of $^3J_{HH}$ in unsaturated systems

Molecule		Coupling constant (Hz)
$^3J_{cis}$		6–15
$^3J_{trans}$		11–18
Allylic		0–2
^5J Homo-allylic		0–2
Geminal		0–3

Electronegativity of the functional groups linked to the carbon-carbon double bonds affects the size of the coupling constant. Relationships hagve been proposed that include either the Pauling's electronegativity scale (ΔX) or the Huggins electronegativity scale (ΔE) for the following system.

$J_{trans} = 19.1 - 3.3 \, (\Delta E)$

$J_{cis} = 11.7 - 4.0 \, (\Delta E)$

$J_{gem} = 2.5 - 3.2 \, (\Delta E)$

Relationships based upon Huggin's electronegativity scale (ΔE)

$J_{gem} = 2.5 \, (1 - 0.056 \, (\Delta X))$

$J_{trans} = 19.1 \, (1 - 0.18) \, (\Delta x)$

$J_{cis} = 11.6 \, (1 - 0.34 \, (\Delta x))$

Relationships based upon Pauling's electronegativity scale (ΔX)

The electronegativity effects are clearly seen in the following series :

Compound	^3J
$CH_3-CH_2-SiR_3$	8.0 Hz
CH_3-CH_2-CN	7.6 Hz
CH_3-CH_2-Cl	7.2 Hz
$CH_3-CH_2-OCH_2CH_3$	7.0 Hz
$CH_3-CH_2-OR_2$	4.7 Hz

In naphthalene, J_{12} is much higher then J_{23}. This is because, the C_1–C_2 bond length is shorter and therefore, leads to more interaction through the σ-bonds. This is not due to the increase in the π-electrons contribution.

4.2.2 Geminal Protons Coupling $^2J_{HH}$

These have the range –20 to +40 Hz. Note that unlike ^3J vicinal coupling, ^2J coupling can be either sign. The variation of the $^2J_{HH}$ depends upon the environment i.e. the bond angle H–C–H ϕ and nature of the groups attached to CH_2.

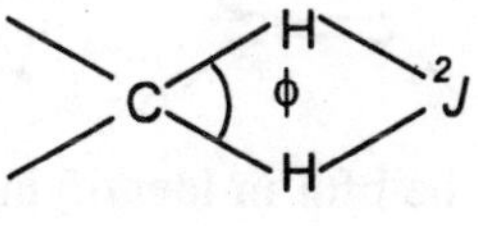

$^2J_{HH}$

Electronegative groups lead to reduction in ^2J.

Thus ^2J for CH_3OH is –10.8 Hz and while –9.6 Hz in CH_3F and CH_3Cl, ^2J is –10.8 Hz.

The unsaturated substituents lead to an increase in the magnitude of ^2J :

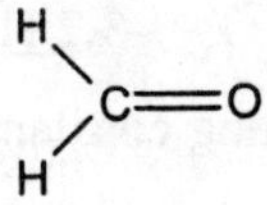

$^2J = + 41$ Hz

$$CH_2\!=\!\!=\!CH_2 \qquad ^2J = + 2.5 \text{ Hz}$$

A substituent that withdraws electrondensity from the anti-symmetric molecular orbitals leads to a negative contribution. This effect can be called as **hyperconjugative effect** :

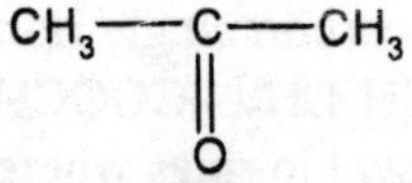

$^2J = –14.9$ Hz

Acetone

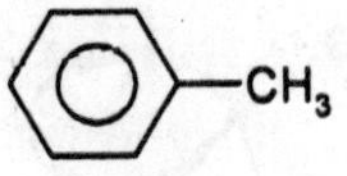

$^2J = –14.4$ Hz

Toluene

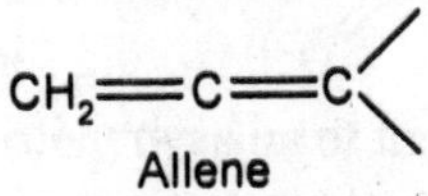

$^2J = –9$ Hz

Allene

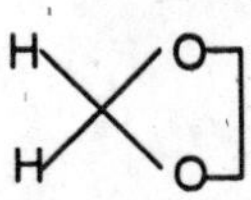

$^2J = \sim 0$ Hz

$^2J_{HH}$ for the five-membered dixolane ring is ~ 0 Hz due to hyperconjugative overlapping if oxygen lone-pair is taken as electron donating π system.

^2J increases, becomes more positive or we can say less negative with increases in the **H–C–H** ϕ angle. In other words, it occurs due to increase in s-character of the orbitals :

$$CH_4 \qquad ^2J = -12.4 \text{ Hz}$$
Methane

Cyclopropane $\qquad ^2J = -4.5 \text{ Hz}$

$\qquad ^2J = +2.5 \text{ Hz}$

The bond angle relationship is helpful in identifying $-CH_2-$ in various systems. Thus, in fused cyclohexane ring system, $^2J_{HH}$ is 12-18 Hz.

In cyclopropane, it is 5 Hz. It should be noted that $^2J_{HH}$ is 0–3 Hz for a terminal methylene (= CH_2).

· Effect of β-substituents

The presence of an electronegative element in a β-position decreases $^2J_{HH}$.

$$CH_2\text{=}CH.F \quad ^2J = -3.2 \text{ Hz}$$

So, we find that compared to $^3J_{HH}$ vicinal coupling constant, the $^2J_{HH}$ depends upon a number of factors.

Intext Exercise

When do geminal protons of $-CH_2-$ group show coupling?

Geminal protons are often equivalent. Why?

That is due to rapid rotation about carbon–carbon single bonds so that the coupling is not seen because of the resultant equivalence as in $C_6H_5CH_2$—$COOCH_3$, Methyl benzoate ($^2J = 0$ Hz). So, ^2J will be seen when the $-CH_2-$ group is present in rings wherein free rotation around C—C single bond is inhibited.

^2J is also seen when $-CH_2-$ is present adjacent to an asymmetric centre as the free rotation around the C—C single bond does not lead to resultant magnetic equivalence in this case.

4.2.3 Long Range Coupling

Coupling between hydrogens separated by more than three intervening bonds is called long range coupling. This is seen in alkenes, alkynes, allylic and homoallylic systems and in aromatic systems.

4.2.3.1 *Alkynes*

σ–H interaction leads to couplings that can be transmitted over many conjugated bonds. $^4J_{HH}$ is found to be in the range 2-3 Hz in the systems given below :

(a)

$$\overset{1}{H}-\overset{2}{C}-\overset{3}{C}\equiv\overset{4}{C}-H \qquad ^4J = \text{2-3 Hz}$$

^4J

(b) ^4J is found to be 2 Hz in the following example :

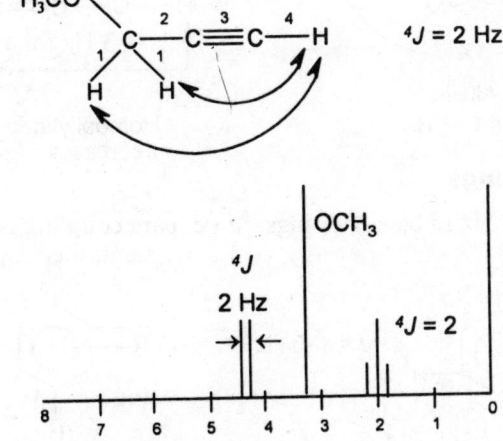

(c) ^4J is equal to 2.5 Hz in the following molecule :

$$^5J = 1 \text{ Hz, } \quad ^4J = 2.5 \text{ Hz}$$

(d) As the number of intervening bonds increases, J decreases. Thus in the example given in point (c), the ^5J is found to be 1.3 Hz. Similarly, ^7J is found to be 1.3 Hz in this molecule.

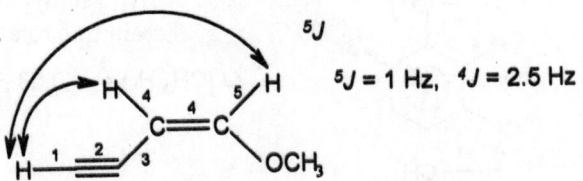

$^7J = 1.3$ Hz

^9J has even lesser magnitude of 0.4 Hz as expected.

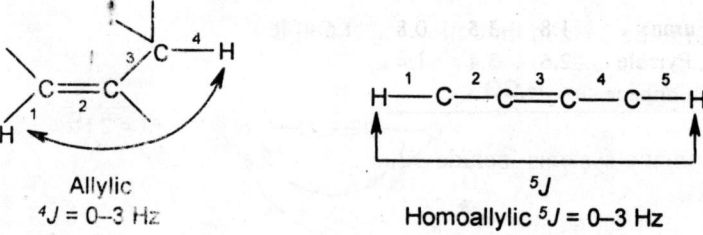

$$^9J = 0.4 \text{ Hz}$$

4.2.3.2 Allylic and Homoallylic Systems

Here, the coupling constant $^4J_{HH}$ is of the size of 0–3 Hz in allylic and $^5J_{HH}$ is also in the same range of 0–3 Hz.

Allylic
$^4J = 0\text{–}3 \text{ Hz}$

$5J$
Homoallylic $^5J = 0\text{–}1 \text{ Hz}$

4.2.3.3 Aromatic Couplings

^4J, meta coupling is ~ 1-3 Hz in benzene rings. ^5J i.e. para coupling is about 0-1 Hz.

$^4J = 1\text{–}3 \text{ Hz}$

$^5J = 0\text{–}1 \text{ Hz}$

The magnitude of ^4J, ^5J and ^6J in the following molecule are –0.63, +0.40 and –0.58 Hz respectively.

$^4J \, (CH_3\text{-}H_6) = -0.63 \text{ Hz}$

$^5J \, (CH_3\text{-}H_3) = +0.40 \text{ Hz}$

$^6J \, (CH_3\text{-}H_6) = -0.58 \text{ Hz}$

4.2.3.4 Heteroaromatics

Long-range coupling is also seen in heteroaromatics such as Furans, thiophenes, pyrroles, pyridines etc.

The values of ^4J and ^5J are shown below along with those of ^3J.

Molecule	$^3J_{23}$	$^3J_{34}$	$^4J_{24}$	$^5J_{25}$
X = O, Furan	1.8	3.5	0.8	1.6
X = NH, Pyrrole	2.6	3.4	1.4	2.1
X = S, Thiophene				

Other aromatic systems include quinolines (see Fig. 6.8).

$^5J_{48} = 0.8$ Hz

Quinoline

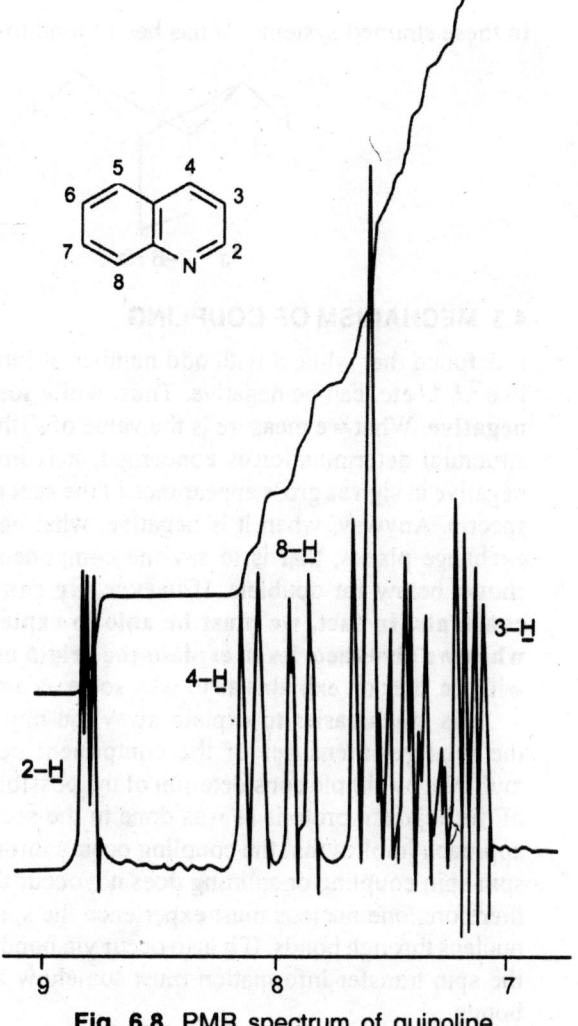

Similarly, long-range coupling is also noticeable in coumarins:

$$^4J_{45} = -0.31 \text{ Hz}$$
$$^5J_{35} = +0.32 \text{ Hz}$$
$$^5J_{48} = +0.65 \text{ Hz}$$
$$^7J_{37} = +0.34 \text{ Hz}$$

4.2.3.5 Saturated Cyclic Systems

Although these systems do not contain π bond for interaction with σ electrons, yet ^4J long-range coupling has been observed in these molecules, via what is called a W type (or a planar zig-zag type) arrangement of atoms :

Fig. 6.8. PMR spectrum of quinoline.

W type arrangement

In non-strained systems it is of 1–2 Hz :

^4J = 1–2 Hz ^4J = 1–1.5 Hz ^4J = 1 Hz

Dark lines show W-type arranged coupled protons

4.2.3.6 Saturated Bicyclic Systems

In these strained systems, ^4J has been found to be of large magnitude of about 7–8 Hz.

^4J = 7–8 Hz ^4J = 7 Hz

4.3 MECHANISM OF COUPLING

It is found that while J with odd number of intervening bonds like ^1J, ^3J are positive, even number Js like ^2J, ^4J etc. can be negative. Thus, **while some coupling constants can be positive, others can be negative.** What we measure is the value of J, that is actually the absolute value of J. In any case, as for structural determination is concerned, it is immaterial whether the coupling constant is positive or negative in sign as gross appearance of the spectrum remains unaffected except in case of more complex spectra. Anyway, when it is negative, what happens is that the upfield and the downfield peaks just exchange places, that is to say the component peaks in a multiplet assume opposite definitions as shown below for doublets. **However, we can not just ignore the negative sign of same coupling constants. In fact, we must be able to explain as to why some coupling constants are negative, when we give theories to explain the origin or mechanism of coupling.** Dirac vector approach as we will see later on explains as to why some Js are negative while others are positive.

It is much easier to explain away the multiplicities and the relative intensities of the component peaks within a multiplet by simple consideration of the possible orientations of the adjacent protons as was done in the section 3.5. That approach implies that the coupling occurs through space. As spin-spin coupling or splitting does not occur through space, therefore, one nucleus must experience the spin of the other nucleus through bonds. If it is to occur via bonds, then clearly the spin transfer information must somehow travel through bonds.

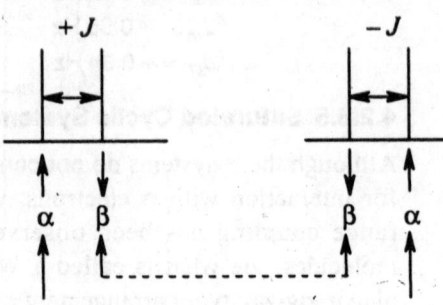

Spin-spin splitting occurs through the intervening bonds in three ways. Since a bond is made up of electrons, we can implicate electrons in the process. That is to say spin-spin splitting occurs between the coupled nuclei through bonding electrons:

(i) A nucleus senses or experiences the spin of the other nucleus with which it couples through bonding electrons. What happens is that the interaction or the contact between magnetic moment of one nucleus and its s electrons spin causes a perturbation in the electronic orbitals around the atom. This perturbation transmits information about the nuclear energy of that nucleus to the nuclei located at closer distances in the molecule, which perturbs their nuclear frequency. This perturbation through bonding electrons is a reciprocal process. This interaction between nuclear spins and s-orbitals is called **contact term**. This contact term is the major process for coupling between the hydrogen nuclei.

(ii) The nuclear moments interact with the electronic currents generated through electrons circulating in the orbits.

(iii) The nuclear moments interact with the electronic magnetic moments via a dipolar interaction. Whereas, for protons, contact term is the major contributing process, for other nuclei such as C⋯C, C⋯F, F⋯F couplings, the other two terms contribute equally along with the contact term.

4.3.1 Two-Bond Coupling (^2J) (Geminal Coupling)

Geminal coupling constants (Fig. 4.8a) vary from -10 to -18 Hz. They are usually negative. Application of Dirac's model leads to the preferred arrangement (b) shown in Fig. 4.8. The two hydrogen spins are anti-parallel as a result of the intermediacy of the carbon-12 atom which is itself NMR-inactive ($I = 0$).

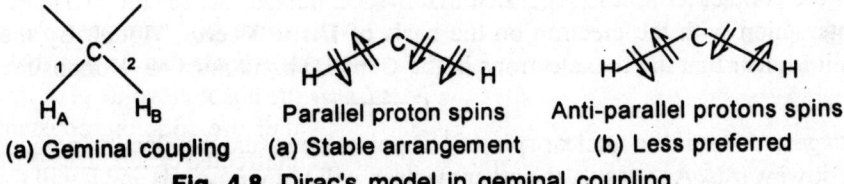

H_A $\quad$ H_B	Parallel proton spins	Anti-parallel protons spins
(a) Geminal coupling	(a) Stable arrangement	(b) Less preferred

Fig. 4.8. Dirac's model in geminal coupling.

This model also explains as to why ^2J inreases with decrease in HCH angle θ, there occurs more electronic interaction (see Fig. 4.9).

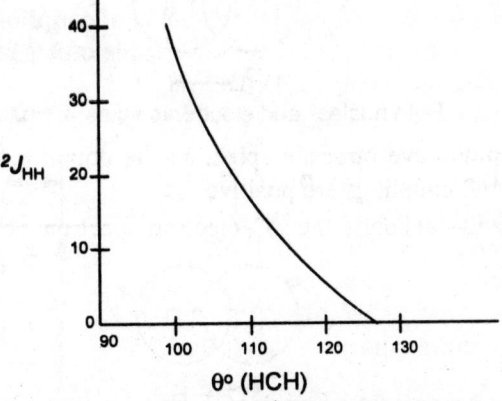

Fig. 4.9. $^2J_{HH}$ versus $\theta°$, HCH angle.

The dependence of $^2J_{HH}$ on HCH angle θ is clear from the following examples :

System	θ	$^2J_{HH}$		θ
Cyclohexane	109°	–12-18 Hz	H / H	109°
Cyclopropane	118°	– 5 Hz	H	118°
Terminal methylene (= CH$_2$)	120°	+ 0-3 Hz	H	120°

Let us now see exactly how does the Dirac Vector Model explains the origin of coupling.

4.3.2 One Bond Coupling $^{13}C-^1H$ (^1J)

Recall the principle we used to explain away the appearance of a doublet for each of the two vicinal protons. We explained this saying that each hydrogen sees or senses or experiences an α (m + 1/2) or a β (m – 1/2) spin of the other proton and is therefore, split into a doublet. In a similar manner, exactly, the spin of a ^{13}C nucleus directly bonded to hydrogen is a split into doublet as it senses two spins m + 1/2 (or α) and m – 1/2 (or β) of the hydrogen.

As per the contact term, it is suggested that the ^{13}C nucleus senses the two spin states of hydrogen via the interaction with the electron on the basis of **Dirac Vector Model.** By the Pauli's exclusion principle, it is clear that the two electrons in the C—●●—H bond must have opposite spins.

$$C-\uparrow\downarrow-H$$

It is suggested that if the nuclear spin of ^{13}C points upwards, the electron adjacent to it in the bond will point downwards. As a result, the other electron will point upwards and it will force the proton spin to align downwards. This is the preferred, low energy ground state, which undergoes transition w.r. to ^{13}C spin.

$$\Uparrow\downarrow \quad \uparrow\Downarrow$$

$$^{13}C-H$$

Both nuclear and electronic spins are paired

As the ^{13}C and ^1H spins have opposite spins, so the coupling is positive – all directly bonded $^{13}C-H$ as well as $^{13}C-^{13}C$ couplings are positive.

In the other 50% of the C—H bonds, the ^{13}C–electron–electron–proton spins are in this arrangement.

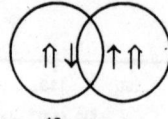

$$^{13}C-H$$

Nuclear spins opposed, electron spins paired

This is how the ^{13}C nuclear spin is split into a doublet.

Further, since in the above model, there occurs an interaction between the nuclear moments and the electronic spins in the s-orbitals, therefore, ^1J couplings should be stronger as the percentage of s-character of the bonds increases or the hybridisation state changes from sp^3 to sp. Indeed, it is so. Thus, while ^1J for ethane, $CH_3—CH_3$ (sp^3) is 125 Hz, for ethene, $CH_2═CH_2$ (sp^2), it is 156 Hz and it is 249 Hz in ethyne $CH≡CH$, which has carbons in sp hybridisation state :

|← 125 Hz →| |← 156 Hz →| |← 249 Hz →|

$$H_3C—CH_3 \qquad H_2C═CH_2 \qquad HC≡CH$$

The following relationship is found to hold good for hybridisation, Sp^n :

$$^1J_{CH} = 500 \text{ Hz} \cdot \left(\frac{1}{n+1}\right)$$

where, n can be   3,   2,   or   1
           (sp^3) (sp^2) (sp)

4.3.3 Three-Bond Coupling $^3J_{HH}$ (The Dirac's Vector Model)

How does the spin of proton sense the spin of the proton vicinal to it that is three bonds away to it? This is particularly important as the intervening two carbon–12 nuclei cannot be involved in the transfer of the spin information between the vicinal protons as they are spin inactive (I = 0).

The spin information transfer as shown herein
is not possible as the C–12 are NMR inactive

Therefore, the spin information transfer must be a business of the two protons and the two pairs of electrons, present in the two C—H sigma bonds. How can that occur? It is suggested that the orbitals involved in C—H bond formation must overlap with each other or else, it is impossible to explain the splitting phenomenon origin in three bond coupling. Greater the overlapping, greater will be the coupling.

Obviously, for the maximum overlap between the orbitals involved, the dihedral angle between them must be zero as shown below in the side view. In this mode, the spins of H_A and H_X are paired, so are the electronic spins in both the C—H bonds.

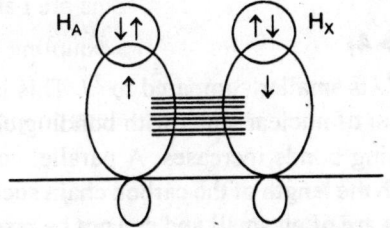

Expected $^3J_{H-H}$ = maximum
$\phi = 0°$: Maximum overlap

As the dihedral angle increases, the $^3J_{HH}$ should decrease because the extent of overlapping shall decrease such that at 90°, the overlap being almost zero or minimum, therefore, the $^3J_{HH}$ should be zero or minimal accordingly :

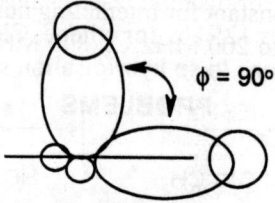

Expected $^2J_{HH} = 0$
Zero or minimum overlap

Then as the dihedral angle increases, the overlapping increases. Consequently $^3J_{HH}$ should increase as well. This is truly so in practice. Karplus discovered that indeed at 90° dihedral angle, $^3J_{HH}$ was zero. This is shown in the graph in Fig. 6.5. From the **Karplus curve**, it can also be seen that the $^3J_{HH}$ is also maximum at a dihedral angle of 180°. This is surprising, as it is impossible for the front orbital lobes to overlap and consequently it also makes the spin information transfer impossible as well. Hence, how can the maximum value of $^3J_{HH}$ then be explained away. The only way to do that will be to implicate the back lobes of the orbitals involved in overlapping with the front lobes as shown in the side view:

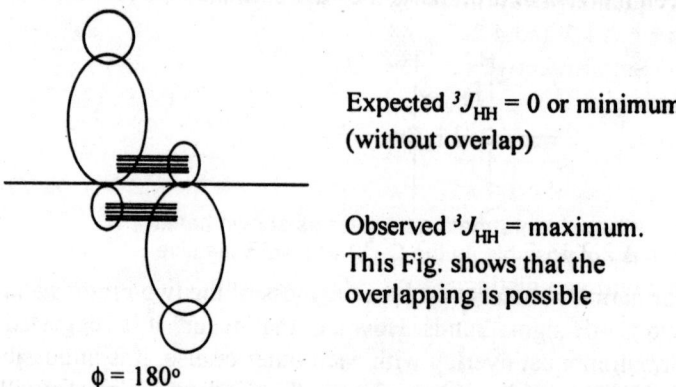

Expected $^3J_{HH} = 0$ or minimum
(without overlap)

Observed $^3J_{HH}$ = maximum.
This Fig. shows that the
overlapping is possible

$\phi = 180°$

This is how, in the above model, H_A senses the spin of H_X oriented against the applied field.

When the proton H_A sees the spin of H_X in the orientation parallel to it, in the remaining 50% of the molecules. That is how H_A gives a doublet. Similarly H_X also gives a doublet due to two spins of H_A in a reciprocal manner.

4.3.4 Long Range Coupling ^nJ (n > 4)

The magnitude of ^nJ i.e. ^4J, ^5J, ^6J, ... ^9J is smaller compared to ^3J. This is to be expected. Because the spin-spin coupling occurs by interaction of nuclear spins with bonding electrons, therefore, it is likely to diminish as the number of intervening bonds increases. A parallel can be seen with the inductive effect in this context which falls off with the length of the carbon chain such that it becomes insignificant at carbon–3 in the chain. The couplings are often small and can not be resolved with the common NMR machines so that the peaks then appear as broad, closely spaced rather than as lines.

In conclusion, the spin-spin coupling occurs with the aid of bonding electrons spins which is to be expected in the presence of magnetic field. We have also seen that this nuclear-electronic spins sensing depends upon the structure and geometry of the molecules, so, that is why, it is independent of the applied field strength i.e. J is always constant for interacting nuclei and does not vary as the strength of the field is altered from say 100 MHz to 200 MHz, ... 800 MHz.

PROBLEMS

1. What are coupling constants?
   Hint: See Section 4.1.

2. What is the decreasing order among following and why so?
   $^1J, \,^2J, \,^3J, \,^4J, \,^5J$
   Hint: See Section 4.1.

3. What is the relation between coupling constant and Bo, the applied field?

4. What are the factors that affect magnitude of J?
   Hint: See Section 4.2.

5. Discuss the factors that affect vicinal couplings in details with examples.
   Hint: See Section 4.2.2.1.

6. Illustrate the factors that affect vicinal couplings in unsaturated systems.
   Hint: See Section 4.2.1.2.

7. What is Karplus equation? Draw the Karplus curve for saturated and unsaturated vicinal couplings.
   Hint: See Section 6.2.1.2 and 4.2.2.1.

8. How will you distinguish between the following on the basis of NMR.

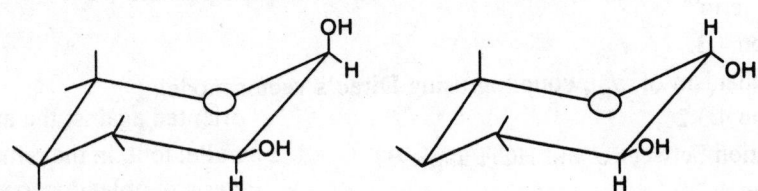

Hint: See Section 4.2.2.1

9. Using NMR how will you distinguish between the following anomers.

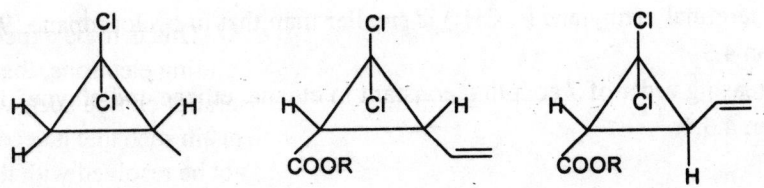

Hint: See Section 4.2.2.1.

10. How will you distinguish among these three using NMR.

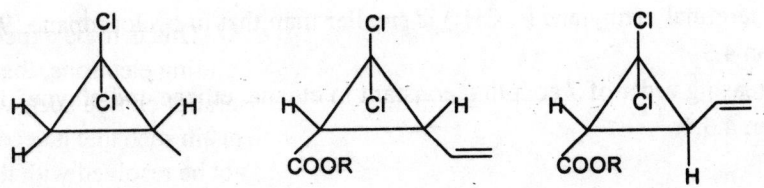

Hint: See Section 4.2.2.1.

11. Can you distinguish between the following three on the basis of NMR. If yes, how?

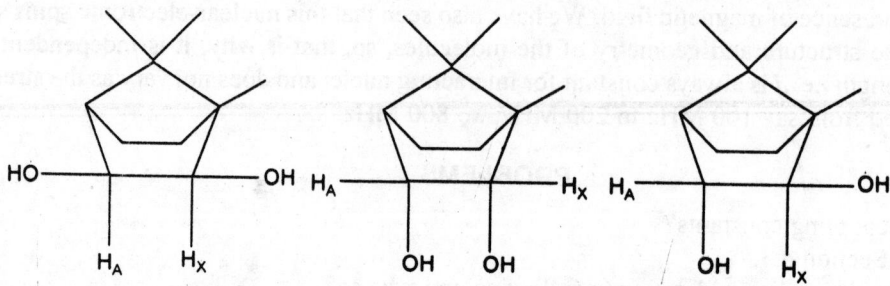

Hint: See Section 4.2.2.1.

12. How can we distinguish between the following olefins.

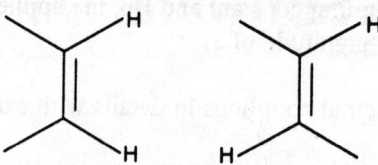

Hint: See Section 4.2.1.2.

13. In naphthalene, J_{12} is much higher than J_{23}. Why?
    Hint: See Section 4.2.2.1 (last para).

14. What factors affect coupling in geminal protons? Illustrate with examples.

15. Sketch and explain the PMR spectrum of $CH_3OCH_2C \equiv CH$.
    Hint: See Fig. 4.8.

16. What is the usual range for J_o, J_m and J_p protons in benzene systems? Explain the difference in their magnitude.

17. Give an example of ^4J long-range coupling via a W-type arrangement of atoms.
    Hint: See Section 4.2.3.5.

18. What is contact term?
    Hint: See Section 4.3.

19. Explain the mechanism of $^3J_{HH}$ coupling using Dirac's vector model.
    Hint: See Section 4.3.2.

20. What is the relation between J and HCH angle θ?
    Hint: See Section 4.3.

21. $^2J_{HH}$ in cyclohexane is higher than $^2J_{HH}$ in cyclopropane. Why?
    Hint: See Section 4.3.

22. Explain $^2J_{HH}$ in terminal methylene ($= CH_2$) is smaller than that in cyclopropane. Why?
    Hint: See Section 4.3.

23. What is the decreasing order of J coupling constant in ethane, ethene and ethyne? Explain.
    Hint: See Section 4.3.1.

156 Organic Spectroscopy

11. Can you distinguish between the following three on the basis of NMR. If yes, how?

5

Fourier Transform (FT) NMR: Hardware and Software: Data Processing

5.1 THE NMR HARDWARE

The NMR hardware for the NMR instrumentation (Fig. 5.1 and 5.3) consists of:
- Superconducting magnet
- The deuterium lock feedback loop
- The shim system
- Probe
- Timing and matching the probe
- Radiotransmitter
- Radioreceiver
- Analogue-to-digital converter (ADC)
- Computer

Superconducting magnet

The required magnetic field is provided by a solenoid (a closed loop) of superconducting niobium/titanium alloy. This is kept immersed in liquid helium. A strong current flows around this solenoid that generates a strong continuous magnetic field. No external power supply is required. In order to obtain a homogeneous stable magnetic field, the helium bath is equipped with a vacuum jacket. The helium bath is kept cooled by an outer bath of liquid nitrogen. It is very important to achieve a homogeneous field throughout the length and breadth of the sample. The magnet is cryostatically controlled even though the sample lies at room temperature due to the thermal isolation.

The deuterium lock feedback loop

The stability of magnetic fields is a very important parameter whether the magnet is electromagnet or a superconducting solenoid. Despite insulation of the superconducting solenoids, the field strength drifts after an FID. Consequently, as succeeding FIDs would have different frequencies, it will not be possible to sum the FIDs. Hence, it is necessary that the homogeneity of the magnetic field is maintained by a control mechanism. This is best done by another spectrometer within the spectrometer i.e. by using the NMR signal of another nucleus usually deuterium that operates at a different frequency. A separate channel called lock channel is used to detect the deuterium signal of the deuterated solvent as well as to monitor its chemical shift. This is linked to a feedback loop that ensures that the deuterium frequency remains constant.

The Shim System

The purpose of shim system is to cancel out the inhomogeneities of the magnetic field is three dimensions within the sample volume. This is very important as a variation of 1 ppm in the field strength gives rise to a peak having 1 ppm line width that means 800 Hz on a 800 MHz spectrometer. These days, that is best done by autoshimming.

The probe is a coil of wire that surrounds the sample tube. It has a small vertical hole which holds the NMR sample tube and also contains the radiotransmitter and the radio receiver coils around the sample. These coils are aligned with the centre of the superconducting solenoid magnet. The probe coil acts as a radio transmitter antenna and radio receiver antenna during the application of the pulse and FID acquisition respectively.

Ideally, NMR spectrometers possess probes that are optimized for different purposes. They contain for C-13 spectra a direct C-13 probe (this means C-13 coil inside, H-1 coil outside). For exotic nuclei such as Si-29, Fe-57 and Se-77, a direct broad band probe is also present. For heteronuclear 2D experiments, an inverse C-13 probe with H-1 coil inside and C-13 coil outside is used. For carrying out biological work, special probe known as "HCN" or "tripple-resonance" probe having H-1 coil inside, double tuned C-13/N-15 coil outside is provided. A "water-suppression" probe is also provided for use with the biological sample that are often prepared in 90% H_2O/10% D_2O solvent system. The shielded wires that come from the probe prevent the very strong water (H_2O) protons from being recorded by these wires.

Many probes have the ability to detect more than one nucleus. These are called double-tuned. Nuclei like F-19, H-1, C-13 and P-31 and C-13 and N-15 can be paired together with such probes. Some of the double-tuned probes have about eight tuning knobs at the probe head that indicates the difficulties that can be encountered in obtaining a good compromise between the two nuclei. On the other hand, the "broadband" probes can be used to detect almost all the nuclei in a single probe coil.

The probes have to be properly tuned and matched otherwise the exciting pulse will be reflected off and comes back to the amplifier instead of reaching its target – the sample solution.

Timing and Matching the Probe

The purpost of tuning is to make sure that there is no difference between the resonant frequency of the coil and the radiofrequency used. Matching the probe aims at matching the probe coil as a load to the internal electrical resistance, the impedence of the amplifiers which maximizes the transfer of the power to the load. This is best done by a trained NMR spectroscopist and not left to the new contrained people as the involved capacities positioned at the top of the probe can get damaged and their repairing is a very expensive affair.

The computer controls the radiotransmitter and the receiver i.e. it not only instructs the transmitter for sending a high power pulse having a short duration to the probe but also the receiver for receiving the voltage generated. The computer also processes the digital information data coming out of the ADC and then carries out fourier transformation and eventually displays the NMR spectrum. Therefore, computer plays a very significant role in giving us the finger-print of the suspected sample.

As for the cost of NMR spectrometers is concerned, in general, the latest estimates put it as about $ 1000 per MHz of field strength at strengths upto 600 MHz. The cost rises exponentially above 600 MHz strength to about $ 5 million for a 900 MHz NMR spectrometer. In conclusion, it lies in the range of $ 120,000–$ 5000,000 for NMR spectrometers with the magnetic field strength of 200–900 MHz.

5.2 INSTRUMENTATION

These are of two types :
1. Continuous wave (CW) NMR spectrometers
2. Pulsed Fourier Transform NMR spectrometers

5.3 CONTINUOUS WAVE (CW) NMR SPECTROMETERS

These are also known as 'Conventional' NMR spectrometers. These are the instruments in which the radiofrequency (v_o) is held constant and the magnetic field (B_1) is varied continuously, hence the name. The resonance lines or the Larmor frequencies are observed one at a time in sequence method called continuous wave method. A schematic CW spectrometer is shown in Fig. 5.1.

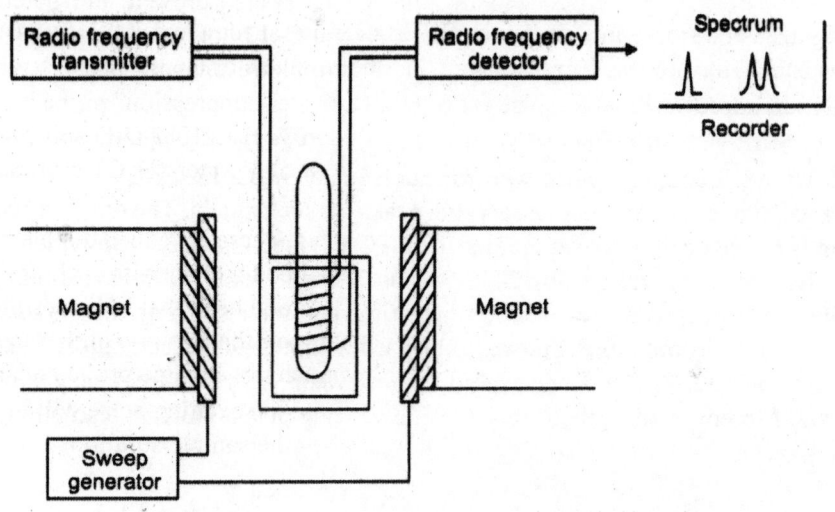

Fig. 5.1. A schematic CW NMR spectrometer.

Frequency v and B_1 is varied over the appropriate range (for protons this is ~ 1000 Hz at 100 MHz and pen traces value of M_y. This is zero if v does not correspond to a resonant v_x in the sample.

Field of B_1, usually fairly low. ~ 0.01 m Gauss. Sweep rate is 2 Hz/second. Sweep time is ~ 500s.

In continuous wave spectrometers, a weak, an infinitely long and an infinitely selective pulse is used as a continuous wave.

The continuous wave causes the precession of the spins at one point only in the spectrum. The frequency B_1 is swept slowly and the magnetization M_{xy} transverse to the Z-axis is detected as it produces current much the same way a generator produces an electric current. The *XY* recorder records the spectrum as absorption versus frequency. That is why it is also called Frequency Domain Spectrum. The X-axis of the recorder is swept synchronously with the frequency B_1.

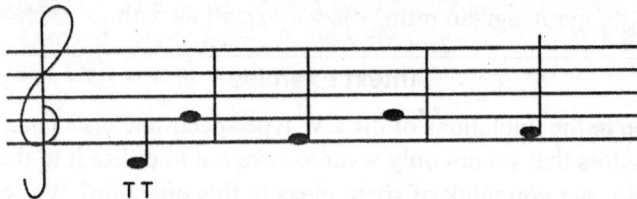

The CW spectrometers do not require a computer or other expensive parts unlike modern FT NMR spectrometers (to be discussed later). The technique is less sensitive. It requires more time as major part of the sweep time is lost in searching areas where no resonances occur.

The level of the field B_1 to be used as decided on the basis of some important parameters. These include the relaxation time (T_1) of the protons as well as the time required to traverse the lines and the sweep rate. The signal-to-noise ratio problem arises as the transmitter that supplies B_1 field has to be kept on all the time.

Spectral Accumulation

Spectrum is digitized and stored in a computer. The successive spectra and similarly treated and added to the previous ones. This process increases signal at the response of the noise.

N accumulation improve signal to noise ratio by $\sqrt{N}$.

This technique works well for nuclei such as H–1, F–19 and P–31 which have very high natural abundance. However, it does not work well for nucleu such as C–13, Si–29, N–15 which have low natural abundance. It does not produce observable peaks for such nuclei. The only way to obtain a good C–13 spectrum is to use computer average transients (CAT) (see Fig. 5.2) or to enrich the compounds with the C–13 isotope. Furthermore, for C–13, the usual range being 5000 Hz (200 ppm), each 1 Hz wide resonance line is observed $\rightleftharpoons$ 1/5000 of the time and the remaining time is used in observing other peaks and for finding out more rf power to be used without causing saturation. Therefore, the rate of sweep has to be increased. But despite rapid rate of sweep, only one frequency is observed at one particular instant. Moreover, the enhanced rates of sweeping puts a limit on resolution, and results in broadening of signals.

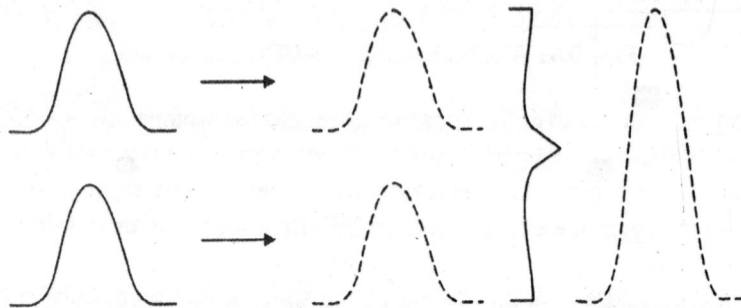

Fig. 5.2. CATing : Signals are added up while noise goes down.

5.4 PULSE FOURIER TRANSFORM NMR SPECTROMETERS

We have learnt that the CW NMR spectrometers require considerable time to obtain a single spectrum. Further, it is very difficult to get a good spectrum for nuclei whose natural abundance is low and whose nuclear magnetic strength, gyromagneto ratio, γ is very small as with C–13, N–15 etc.

Intext Exercise

Can we find a solution to the limitations of the CW type spectrometers? Today, time is also one of the most important factors that we not only want to save but to utilise it to the best of our abilities if we could do that. So, can you think of some ideas in this direction? We want to record greater number of NMR spectra in as short a time as possible.

Hint: See below.

It is possible to find a solution to the time consumption problem. The major limitation of CW spectrometers is that only one frequency is irradiated at a time that records only one particular kind of nucleus. What if we irradiated all the Larmor frequencies corresponding to all the nuclei together simultaneously? Of course, all the resonance signals will have to be detected at once as well. Fortunately, we were able to do that by what is called pulsed fourier transformation. A schematic, FT NMR spectrometer is shown in Fig. 5.3a. In this technique a powerful but short pulse called a RF pulse is applied that simultaneously excites all the nuclei of one type present in the sample. The technique is analogous to playing chord on the piano (Fig. 5.3b) as well as recording the decaying sound signal coming out of a microphone!

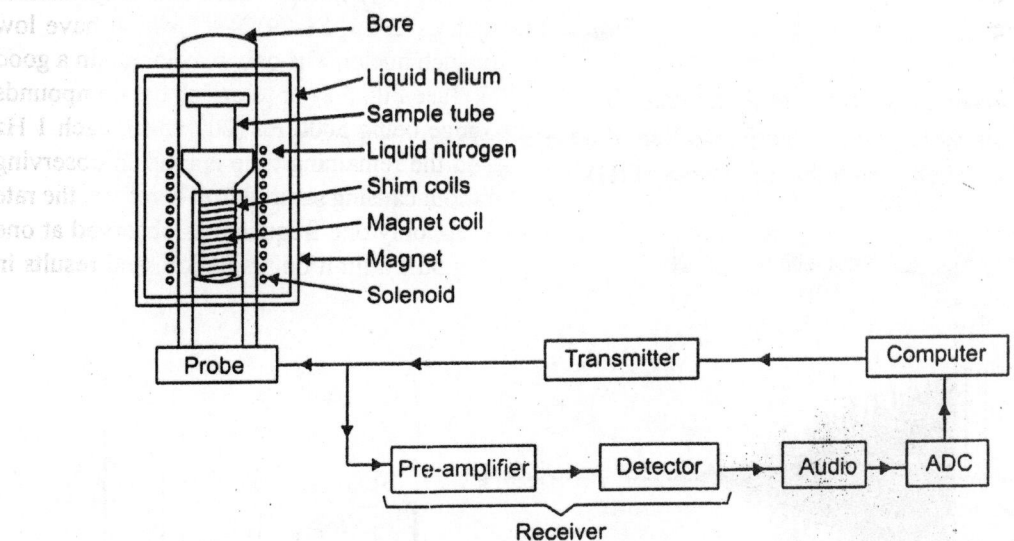

Fig. 5.3a. A schematic FT NMR spectrometer.

All resonances are observed at the same time by effectively applying all the frequencies at once. The signal due to all M_y's decaying away to zero over a second or two is recorded.

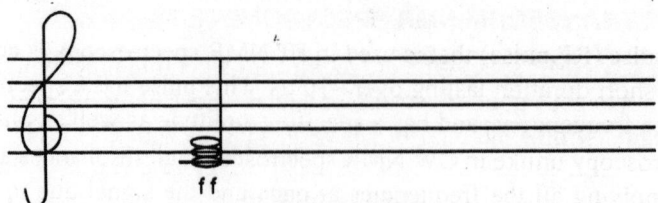

Fig. 5.3b.

A short pulse (duration t sec.) at v_o that is equivalent to supplying all frequencies in range $v_o \pm 1/t$ (Fig. 5.4a).

$25 \ \mu s \equiv 40 \ KHz$

v_o is called the "carrier frequency".

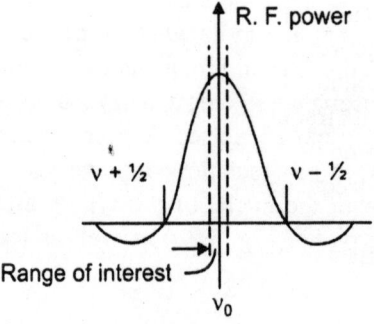

Fig. 5.4a.

Each M_y decay looks different to the detector
and total signal is sum or superimposition of decays from all resonances
And this is called Free Induction Decay (FID)

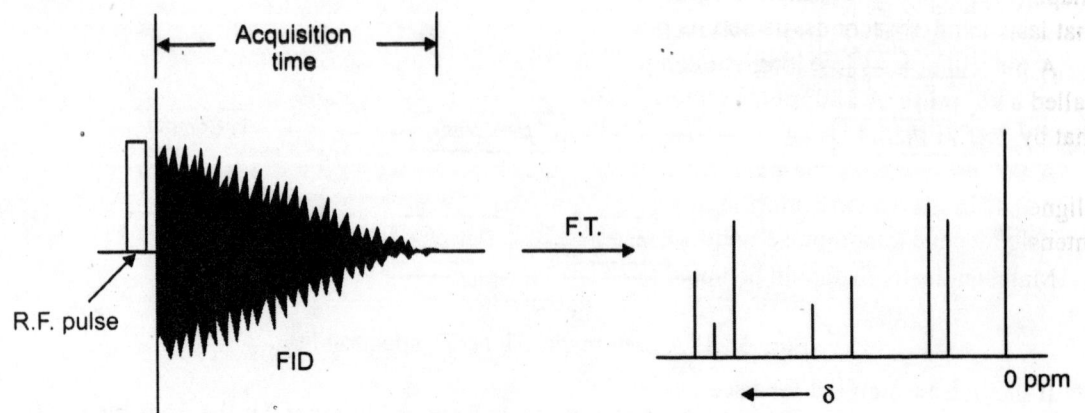

Fig. 5.4b.

Pulse

The radiofrequency pulse (RF pulse) that is used in FT NMR spectroscopy is actually a very powerful pulse (50–300 W) of short duration lasting over ~10 μs. This pulse has a specific frequency, identical to that of the reference frequency v_0 and has a specific amplitude as well as phase.

In FT NMR spectroscopy unlike in CW NMR spectroscopy, all resonances are detected at the same time by effectively applying all the frequencies at once and the signal due to all the My's decaying away to zero is recorded. Consequently, this complicated signal is transformed to a conventional NMR spectrum exhibiting absorptions plotted in the customary manner. **Now, a question arises as to how do we apply so many frequencies all at once?**

When a discrete fundamental frequency signal is turned on and off very rapidly so as to have a pulse lasting over t second, the result is the creation of a range of frequencies centred about that frequency whose bandwidth is about $1/t$ seconds. This can be inferred from a variation of the Heisenberg uncertainty principle: Although the frequency of the oscillator was fixed, but because its duration was short, so its frequency content was not certain as the oscillator could not get sufficient time to generate the solid discrete frequency. A short pulse can be represented as shown in the Fig. 5.4c as a plot of intensity versus time. So, a short powerful pulse behaves like a spread of frequencies. In other words, a pulse ts long would enable us to irradiate the nuclei in the sample all at once with every frequency in the range equal to:

$$F \pm 1/t.$$

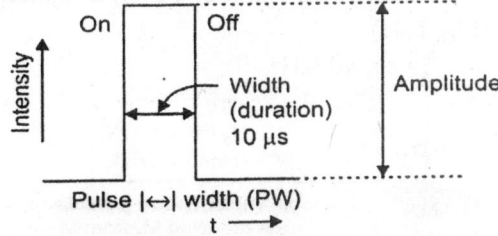

Fig. 5.4c. An RF pulse (rectangular).

Therefore, it seems possible to achieve simultaneous irradiation of the sample by selecting a suitably small value of time, t as shown in Fig. 5.4a.

An ideal pulse has constant amplitude and turns on and off instantly and show looks rectangular in shape (Fig. 5.4b). Its duration is called pulse width

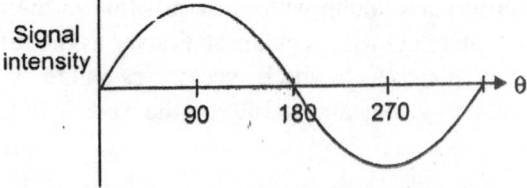

Fig. 5.4d. The varying phase with θ.

that lasts in microseconds, μs and its phase is determined by its starting point in the sine function.

A pulse that lasts just long enough to rotate the net magnetization vector M_z by an angle of 90° is called a 90° pulse. A 180° pulse rotates M_z by 180°, a 270° pulse rotates M_z by 270°, a 360° pulse does that by 360° (Fig. 5.4d).

A 90° pulse means the pulse width that is needed to precisely tip the sample magnetization, M_0 aligned with the +z axis into the x–y plane. This gives the maximum intensity FID signal. The peak intensity depends upon pulse width (PW) as shown in Fig. 5.4e.

Mathematically, it should be noted that the frequency of rotation of M_0 about the x'-axis is given by:

$$v_1 = \gamma \cdot \frac{B_1}{2\pi}$$

If the pulse is applied for t sec., M_0 will rotate through an angle θ rad, called pulse angle.

$$\theta = \gamma \cdot B_1 t \frac{360}{2\pi} \text{ deg.}$$

As already indicated the detecting coil is so designed in the NMR spectrometers that it detects the signals generated along the axis. To conclude, the M_o is tipped through an angle θ and the resultant component given by $M_o \sin \theta$ along the y′-axis is detected as an FID (Fig. 5.4f).

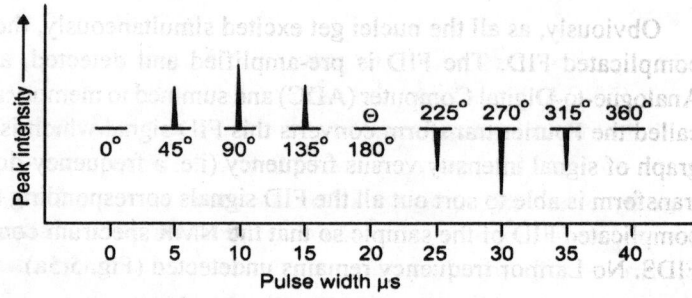

Fig. 5.4e. Variation of peak intensity with pulse width.

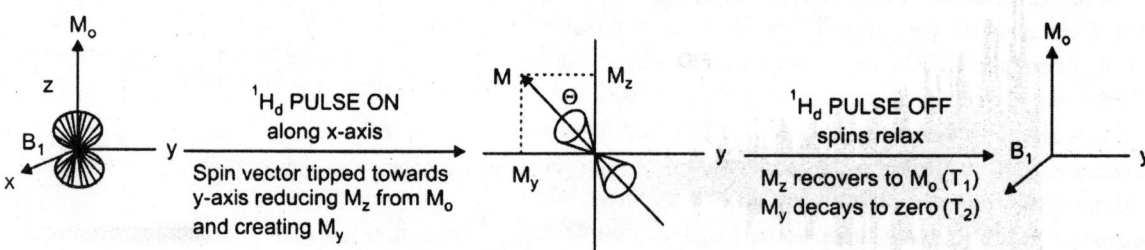

Fig. 5.4f. Application of pulse and detection of FID.

The phase of the pulse is determined by its starting point in the sine function.

As we use a rotating frame of reference instead of laboratory frame, it is therefore essential to know pulse phase along with pulse position in the rotating frame of reference. B_1 field vector that rotates counterclockwise remains stationary as the reference frequency is equal to the pulse frequency in the x′–y′ plane. At 0°, the B_1 vector lies on the +y′-axis; at 90° on +y′ axis; at 180° on the –x′ axis; at 270° on the –y′-axis and at 360° on the +z-axis (Fig. 5.4g).

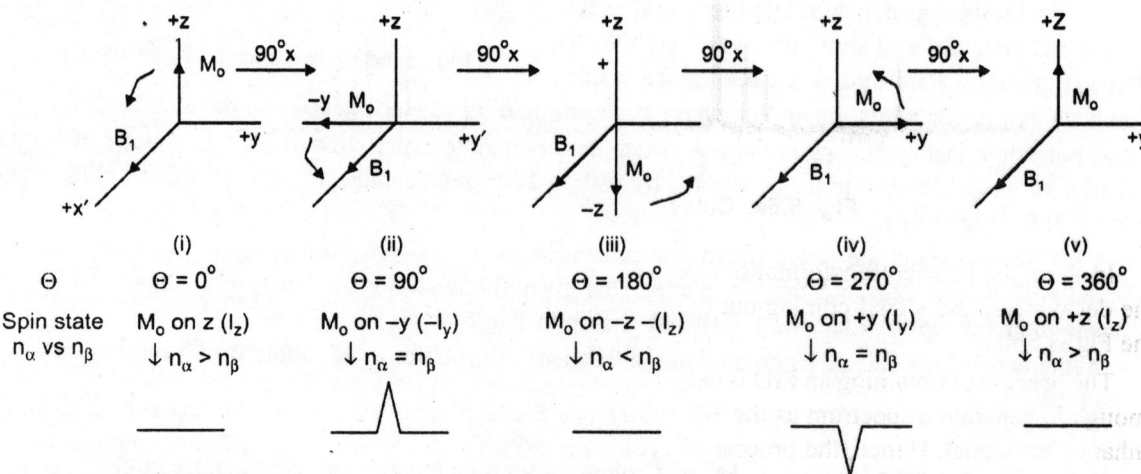

Fig. 5.4g. Phase of pulse and position of M_o w.r. to θ when B_1 lies along the +x′-axis. All pulse rotations are counterclockwise as we see them with B_1 pointing towards us.

Obviously, as all the nuclei get excited simultaneously, the FIDs of all the nuclei add together as a complicated FID. The FID is pre-amplified and detected, audio-filtered and then digitized by the Analogue-to-Digital Computer (ADC) and summed to memory and recorded. A mathematical calculation called the Fourier transform converts this FID signal which is a function of time (time-domain) into a graph of signal intensity versus frequency (i.e. a frequency-domain), the NMR spectrum. The Fourier transform is able to sort out all the FID signals corresponding to different Larmor frequencies from the complicated FID of the sample so that the NMR spectrum contains so many signals arising from these FIDS. No Larmor frequency remains undetected (Fig. 5.5a).

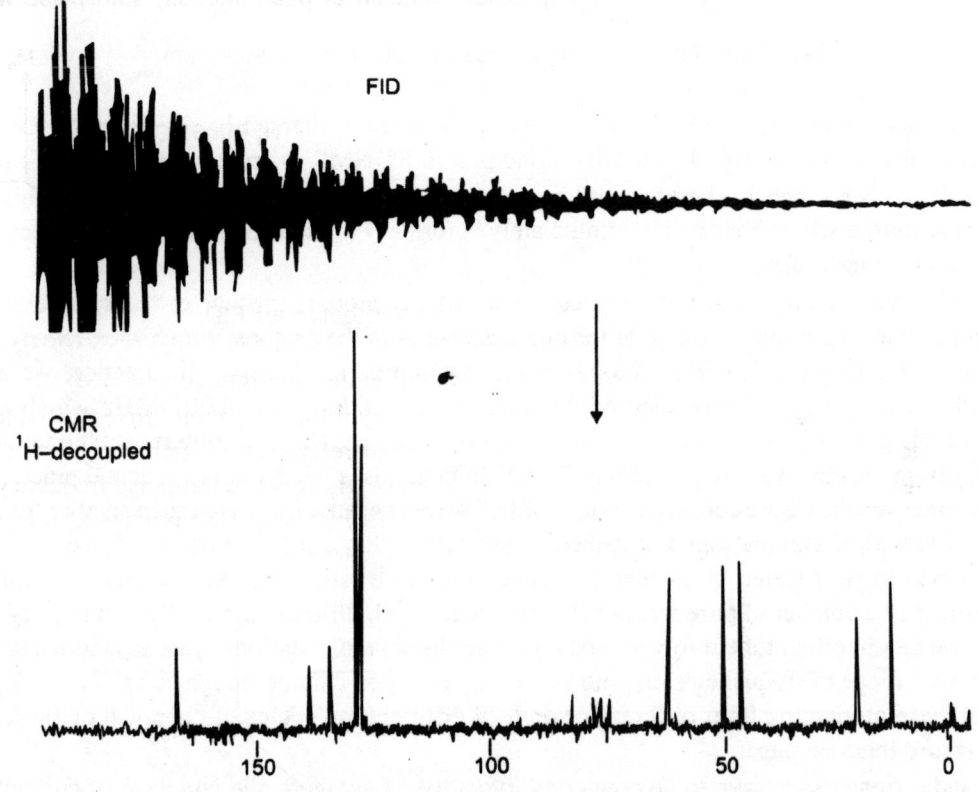

Fig. 5.5a. Obtaining a FT C–13 NMR spectrum.

In short, the Fourier transformation is analogous to playing a chord on the piano as well as recording the decaying sound signal coming out of a microphone. The complete process can be represented by the Fig. 5.5b.

The process of obtaining an FID is called **acquisition.** It needs to be noted that one single FID is not enough to generate a spectrum as the S/N ratio is in favour of noise. We need to cancel out noise and enhance the signal. Hence, the process of acquisition of FID is carried out many times. The obtained individual FIDs hundreds or even more are added up such that while noise goes down, the signal rises up. Furthermore, before the acquisition is repeated to get a FID, a small time interval usually of the order of a second or so (in case of protons) is allowed as a delay, called relaxation delay ("pulse delay")

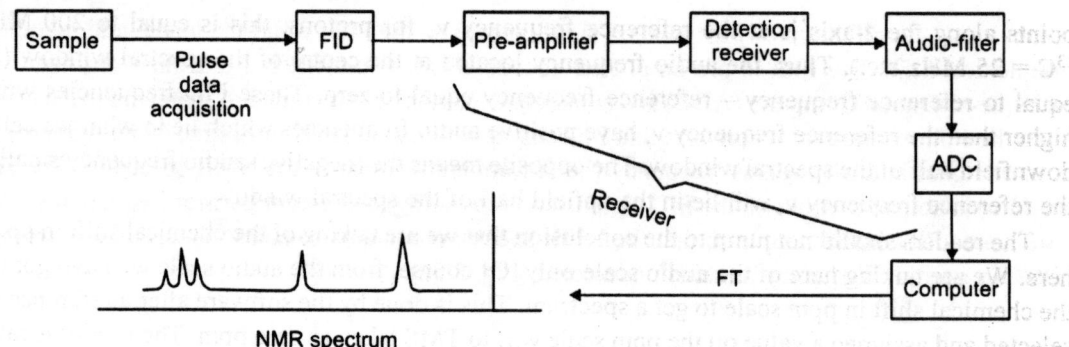

Fig. 5.5b. The FT NMR process of obtaining a spectrum.

between any two successive FIDs. This is necessary to allow Boltzman Excess to get re-established otherwise no signal is obtained. The details of the pulsed FT NMR instrumentation are as follows :

The FID is a weak signal. Therefore, it has to be pre-amplified before being detected. This is done by the pre-amplifier which does its job immediately before any thermal electric noise gets accumulated from the connecting cables.

The FID contains all of the Larmor frequencies of the protons present in the sample molecule. These frequencies represent the range of the chemical shifts of the protons, which is extremely narrow. For protons, this range is 199.999–200.001 MHz that represents 10 ppm. In practice, we are only interested in measuring this tiny slice of frequencies i.e. $- 0.001$ to $+ 0.001$ MHz which means $- 0.001 \times 10^6$ Hz to $+ 0.001 \times 10^6$ Hz $= - 1000$ Hz to $+ 1000$ Hz. So, why not subtract out the fundamental frequency from the observed frequencies $(v_o - v_r)$? In fact, this is what is done in actual practice by the sector. In other words, we are concerned with "audio" waves because these are much smaller frequencies $(- 1000$ Hz to $+ 1000$ Hz) that can be detected by our ears as they are sound waves. You can even listen to such waves in your stereo by connecting these to a pair of speakers! As the FID is nothing but a superposition of a number of pure frequencies associated with different kinds of protons present in the sample, you can in effect tune into very accurately to these "radio stations" just as stations come into time in a very range of frequencies on your FM radio. But, you cannot recognise each molecule, what to talk of these originating from different protons in different molecules of chemical classes. So, you need to record them on paper.

The audio frequencies have to be converted into a list of numbers, the language of computers. An Analogue-to-Digital Convertor (ADC) is used for this purpose. What the ADC does is that the voltage of each audio signal is sampled at regular time intervals. This is followed by converting each analog voltage level into an integer number.

This process of converting a FID into a long list of numbers followed by storage into memory is called **"sum of memory"**. As the FID signal is weak, therefore, several FID scans are acquired and stored into memory, obviously this sum leads to an improvement in the S/N ratio.

The resultant audio signal consists of frequencies that are equivalent to the difference between the real Larmor frequencies of the protons in the test sample and the reference frequency (i.e. $v_o - v_r$). In fact this subtraction of the observed frequencies from the reference frequencies is achieved by using the rotating frame of reference instead of the laboratory frame of reference wherein the net magnetization points along the z-axis is at the reference frequency v_r for protons, this is equal to 200 MHz, for ^{13}C = 25 MHz etc.). Thus, the audio frequency located at the centre of the spectral window (SW) is equal to reference frequency − reference frequency equal to zero. Those FID frequencies which are higher than the reference frequency v_r have positive audio frequencies which lie in what we call as the downfield half of the spectral window. The opposite means the (negative) audio frequency smaller than the reference frequency v_r will lie in the upfield half of the spectral window.

The readers should not jump to the conclusion that we are talking of the chemical shift in ppm scale here. We are talking here of the audio scale only. Of course, from the audio scale we have got to go to the chemical shift in ppm scale to get a spectrum. This is done by the software after a reference peak is selected and assigned a value on the ppm scale w.r. to TMS taken as zero ppm. The task of locating the audio frequency at the centre of the spectral window (i.e. at O), is achieved by what is called as **Quadrature Detection** which detects the audio frequencies in the range + SW/2 to − SW/2 through zero at the centre.

5.5 OVERSAMPLING

After the FID has been audiofiltered, the analogue-to-digital convertor or digitizer samples the FID voltage at regular time intervals, assigning a positive or negative value to the intensity at each sample time, thus converting the analog FID into a digital FID. That is necessary to do as computer only knows the language of numbers. The rate at which the ADC samples the raw analog FID into a digital FID is called the sampling rate. There occurs a delay between sampled successive data points in the FID. This is called Dwell time, DW. Thus, the rate of sampling is equal to 1/DW Hz. How fast can sampling be done? That is determined by the highest frequency signal to be digitized i.e. it depends upon what peak in the NMR spectrum is farthest from the reference or the centre frequency.

$$\text{Rate} = \frac{1}{DW} = DW = \text{Dwell time}$$

Now
$$DW = \frac{1}{2 \times SW}$$

$$\therefore \text{Rate} = \frac{1 \times 2 \times SW}{1} = 2 \times SW$$

Thus, dwell time (DW) is inversely proportional to the spectral width (SW).

On the 800 MHz, spectrometer, for a CMR spectrum (200 ppm) rate of sampling is equal to 2 × SW = 2 × 200 × 20 = 80,000 samples per second. For a proton NMR spectrum (10 ppm) on 800 MHz spectrum, the rate is equal to 2 × SW = 2 × 10 × 800 = 16,000 samples per second.

Older type ADC can operate at that sample rate. Modern generation ADCs can even sample at 400,000 samples per second. In other words, their ability at this rate is 32 times greater than that required for the proton spectrum. Such a rapid rate is called oversampling. Oversampling not only creates a larger spectral or sweep width and generates too much data to be conveniently stored. You might wonder about the use of oversampling. This helps in giving higher resolution. The net effect is that this increases the dynamic range of detecting even very weak signals in the presence of very strong signals.

5.6 NMR DATA PROCESSING

The NMR data processing can be conveniently investigated in three sub-processes:

1. Data manipulation before Fourier transformation.
2. Fourier transformation.
3. Data manipulation after Fourier transformation.

5.6.1 Data manipulation before fourier transformation

This involves the following two steps :

- Zero-filling
- Weighting (window functions)

5.6.1.1 *Zero-filling*

This is actually an optional operation whose purpose is to add to the quality of the NMR spectrum. That is to say it increase

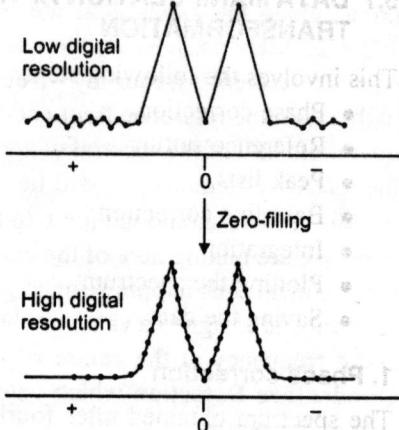

Fig. 5.6. Increase in digital resolution due to zero-filling.

the digital resolution as well as gives better shapes to sharp peaks. The graininess of the spectrum disappears and inaccuracies are eliminated. What is done is that zeros are added to the end of the list of the FID data. This way, you increase the number of points in the FID, which leads to greater digital resolution (see Fig. 5.6).

5.6.1.2 *Weighting (window functions)*

Weighting means laying "weight" on certain portions compared to other portions of a FID. The idea is to enhance the peak height by reducing the noise-contributing part. For example, suppose the FID of the last sample was acquired upto 1.2 seconds but the FID signal is useful just upto 0.3 seconds as after this time it just almost mixes up and disappears into noise. So, it is clear that the FID part from 0.3 to 1.2 seconds does not contribute to the signal height rather it only adds to the noise. Therefore, would it not be wise to lay emphasis on the FID part upto 0.3 seconds? One way could be eliminate all the FID data to zero after the desired 0.3 s time interval? This can be done but the result is the observation of a sharp discontinuity at 0.3 s in the FID under consideration. This leads to appearance of artifacts in the NMR spectrum. Fortunately, a more suitable method was found wherein the FID is multiplied by a suitable exponential decay function such that it achieves the desired target of emphasising The FID upto 0.3 s compared to the part upto 1.2 s (see Fig. 5.7 and 5.8).

Consequently, S/N ratio is improved. This technique is particularly useful in CMR spectra. Even though:

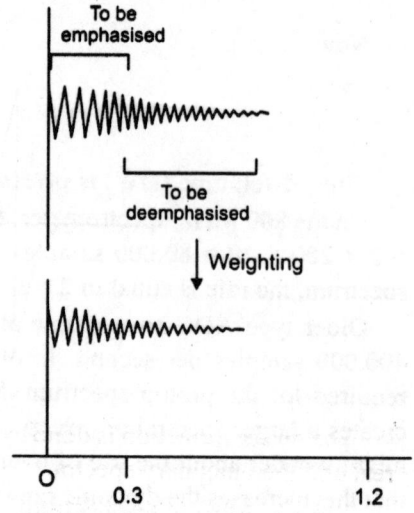

Fig. 5.7. Weighting of FID.

$$\text{Exponential multiplier} = e^{-LB \times t}$$

LB = line broadening, t = acquisition time

Although the peak height decreases and line broadening occurs, the improved *S/N* ratio is still worth achieving.

5.7 DATA MANIPULATION AFTER FOURIER TRANSFORMATION

This involves the following steps:

- Phase correction
- Reference setting
- Peak lists
- Base line correction
- Integration
- Plotting the spectrum
- Saving the data

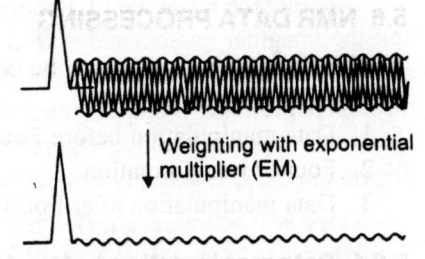

Fig. 5.8. Weighting leads to considerable improvement in S/N, although it leads to a decrease in peak height and line broadening.

1. Phase correction

The spectrum obtained after fourier transformation is now changed from the time domain into the desired frequency-domain spectrum. However, the spectrum may not contain the peaks with the right phase; it may have phase errors. The peak may be half-up-half down (dispersive) or upside down (inverted). Like we read earlier in the section on pulse, the shape of the peaks is dependent upon the starting point of the sine function i.e. 0° or 180° or + 90° or – 90° in the time-domain FID. Hence, it becomes necessary to phase the spectrum to get a zero-error phase to get what we call as absorptive peaks.

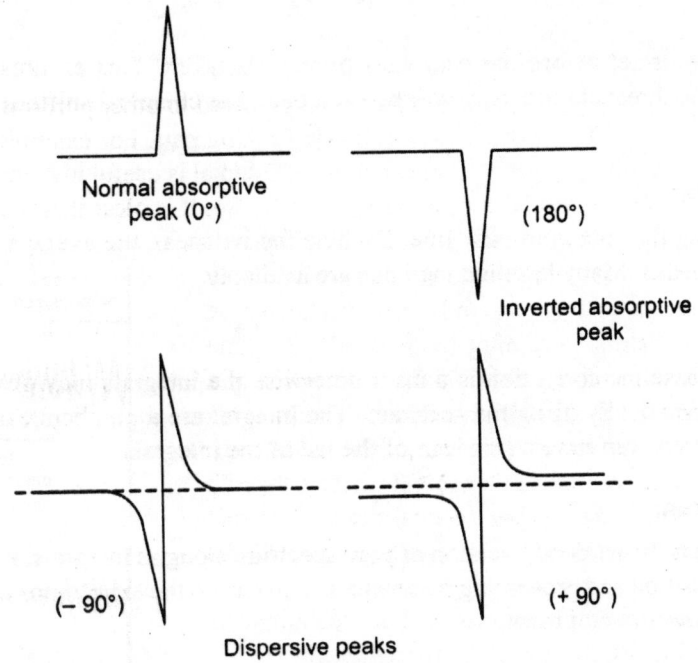

Normal absorptive peak (0°)

(180°)

Inverted absorptive peak

(– 90°)

(+ 90°)

Dispersive peaks

The phase correction is done by using the mathematical relation called the linear combination of the real and the imaginary spectra :

$$\text{Absorptive spectrum} = \text{Real spectrum} \times \text{Cos } \theta + \text{Imaginary spectrum} \times \text{Sin } \theta$$

As before the FT of the FID, there are two numbers - the real and the imaginary associated with a frequency point. In fact, a spectrum consists of absorptive co-error peaks as well as dispersive modes in linear combination. The angle θ is the angle between the two mutually perpendicular vectors – the real and the imaginary. Q is actually a linear function of chemical shift δ:

$\theta = $ (slope $m \times$ chemical shift) + zero-order phase correction, b

Slope M is also called the first-order phase correction. So, the phase correction is done by optimising the slope (first-order) phase correction m and the zero-order phase correction, b. Phase correction is represented by Fig. 5.9.

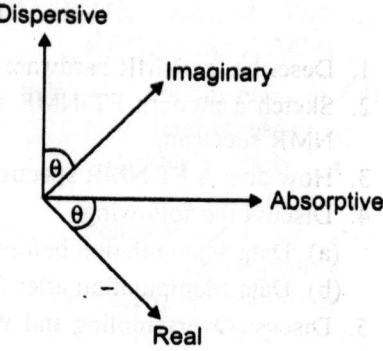

Fig. 5.9. Phase correction.

Reference setting

Like we have learnt before, routine NMR spectra are obtained by using TMS as a reference. So in setting the reference, the TMS peak is selected and assigned a 0.0 ppm chemical shift. As TMS contributes a very weak signal in CMR spectra, so the peak due to the solvent being used in the sample solution is selected instead. For example, in case of $CDCl_3$, the "triplet" is selected and assigned a value of 77.0 ppm.

Peak list printout

A threshold intensity is set before the peak lists printout is taken. This ensures that the peaks with intensity less than the threshold intensity will be excluded. The chemical shifts are printed out in ppm as well as Hertz.

Base line correction

This means flattening the spectrum base line. By baseline we mean the average of the noise regions where there are no peaks. Many baseline methods are available.

Integration

Before integration, baseline correction is a must otherwise the integrals may give inaccurate results. This is done by automatically using the software. The integral are a numbers can be printed directly next to each peak or you can have a print out of the list of the integrals.

Plotting the spectrum

The recorder print outs the hardcopy version of your spectrum along as integrals, integral areas, scale x, peak positions, acquisition and processing parameters. You can do the expansions of the smaller regions of the spectral window and plot them.

Saving the NMR data

The NMR data should be saved. In fact, this is saved as the raw FID for later flexible processing. It can be saved on a CD-ROM or DVD. For those researches who use NMR for qualitative and quantitative research works or thesis, this is absolutely essential to do that.

PROBLEMS

1. Describe the NMR hardware and software.
2. Sketch a modern FT NMR spectrometer. Describe its working leading to the recording of a NMR spectrum.
3. How does a FT NMR spectrometer differ from a Continuous Wave (CW) Spectrometer?
4. Discuss the following:
   (a) Data Manipulation before Fourier Transformation.
   (b) Data Manipulation after Fourier Transformation.
5. Discuss Oversampling and Weighting.

6

NOE and Applications

6.1 NUCLEAR OVERHAUSER EFFECT (NOE)

6.1.1 Introduction

When two nuclei such as protons in a molecule that are separated by 5Å or less in distance irrespective of whether they are bonded or not, irradiation and saturation of one nucleus at its resonant frequency, increases the signal intensity of the other nucleus. This effect is called Nuclear Overhauser Effect. The NOE depends upon the distance between the two interacting nuclei, that is to say, it is a through-space effect and occurs even if they are far apart in the bonding network of the molecule. The NOE varies in intensity as the inverse sixth power of the distance.

$$\text{NOE } \alpha \frac{1}{r^6} \quad \text{for H} \overset{r}{\rule{1cm}{0.4pt}} \text{H}$$

6.1.2 Significance of NOE

The NOE effect is a very useful effect of great significance. As mentioned earlier, it depends upon the distance between the interacting nuclei and varies in intensity of r^{-6}, the distance between the nuclei. Thus, the NOE is detected between the protons which are situated at a distance of 5Å or less. In other words, we get a useful information from the NOE experiments regarding the distance, r. In fact, it is these measured distances between the interacting the 3D-structures of proteins and nucleic acids.

Examples

1. The syn and anti-carbons in N,N–dimethylformamide resonate at 36.2 and 31.1 ppm respectively. When the aldehydic proton is irradiated at its resonant frequency, there occurs enhancement in the signal of the syn methyl carbon which is closer to the proton compared to the anti one. No NOE enhancement is observed for the anti-carbon as it is far away from the aldehydic proton.

174

Similarly, when the syn methyl carbon is irradiated while the proton magnetic resonance is being determined, NOE enhancement is observed for the aldehydic proton as expected. Irradiation of the trans methyl carbon does not, as anticipated, lead to an enhancement in the aldehydic proton's signal intensity.

2. When of the two methyl groups at 4–position the axial one was irradiated at its carbon's resonant frequency, about 12% enhancement in signal intensity was observed for deuterium at 2 position:

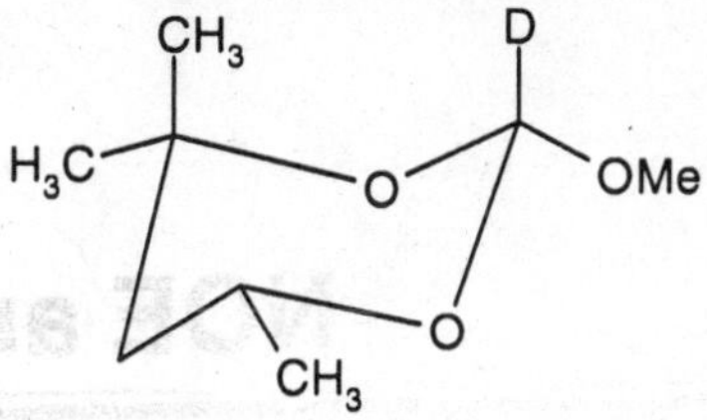

3. In the following pyrrole, when CH_2 protons signals at 3.8 ppm was irradiated, then an increase in signal intensities of the 3–methyl signal and ortho aromatic protons was observed by the author of this book.

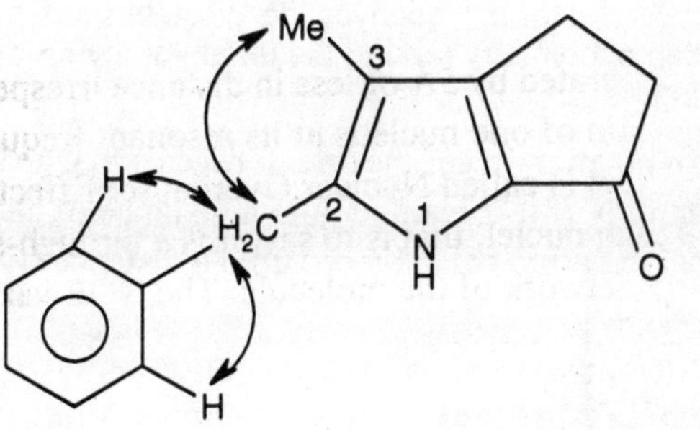

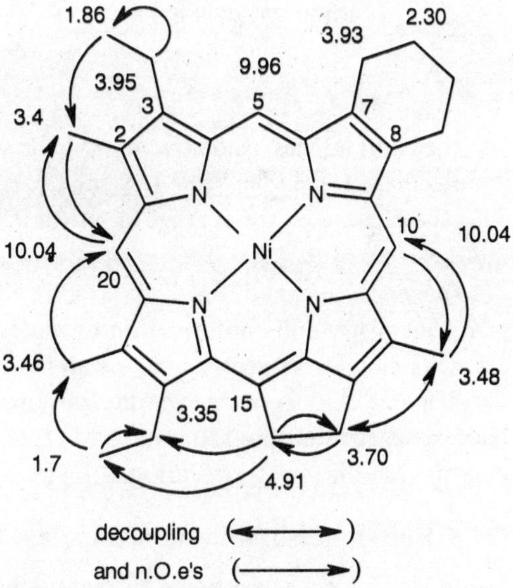

4. When C–3 CH_3 protons (δ 1.62 ppm) are irradiated, then considerable NOE enhancement is observed for 2–H proton (δ 5.49 ppm) in Nerol.

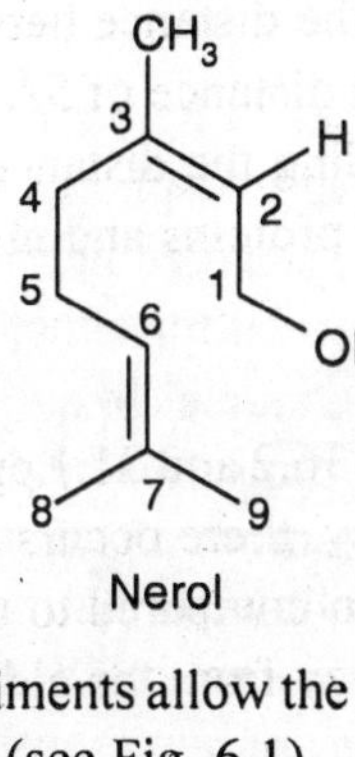

Nerol

decoupling ($\longleftrightarrow$)

and n.O.e's ($\longrightarrow$)

Fig. 6.1. ^{1}H NMR chemical shifts for a petroporphyrin nickel complex. δ 9.96 (2H) and 10.04 (1H) (5–, 10–, 20–H), 3.44 (2–Me), 3.48 (12–Me), 3.46 (18–Me), 3.95 (q, 3–Et) and 1.86 (t, 3–Et), 3.85 (q, 17–Et) and 1.70 (t, 17–Et), 4.91 and 3.70 (both m, 5–membered ring), and 3.93 and 2.30 (both m, 6–membered ring).

5. NOE experiments allow the follow of substitution pattern of the nickel complex of petroporphyrins completely (see Fig. 6.1).

6. The stereochemistry around the recently isolated tetrahydropyran ring in bromophycolide P (a potential anti-malarial compound) was established by NOE correlations as 10R, 11R, 14S. NOEs observed between H–14 (δ 5.08) and both H–13 (δ 1.88, 2.30), Me–26 (δ 1.36), and Me–27 (δ 1.09) suggested an equatorial position for H–14 within the tetrahydropyran ring of 7. Furthermore, 1,3–diaxial NOE correlations were observed between H–13b and Me–26. NOEs were also seen between equatorial Me–25 (δ 1.47) and both H–12 protons (δ 1.72, 2.35). Collectively, these data supported a configuration of 11R, 14S for 7.

Bromophycolide P

Key NOE correlations (double-headed arrows) observed for bromophycolide P established the stereochemistry around the tetrahydropyran ring as 10R, 11R, 14S

The NOE tells us as to how myopic the world is for an atom in a molecule. It reveals that an atom in a molecule can only feel the presence of another atom only if it is located upto a distance of about 5Å. As a C—H bond on the average is 1Å (or 0.1 nm) long, the atom can only see upto a distance five times the C—H bond length.

The measurement of the distance r via NOE experiments enables us to extract information regarding stereochemistry and conformation of molecules and 3–D structures of bigger molecules like proteins etc. wherein certain protons in one amino acid residue are constrained by the peptide bond such that they become close in space to certain protons in the next amino acid residue. In fact, the NOE experiments have given accurate 3–D structures of proteins and nucleic acids. That is why NMR technique is said to be a rival to the X-ray crystallography in this regard.

6.1.3 Homonuclear and Heteronuclear NOEs

When NOE is observed between two nuclei of the same type, it is called homonuclear. For example, the NOE correlation between say two protons, two carbon nuclei, two phosphorus nuclei etc.

The NOE that is observed between two different types of nuclei, is called heteronuclear NOE, for example, between ^1H and ^{13}C, ^1H and ^{31}P etc. The NOE can be observed for either atom.

It should be noted that if between the two interacting ^1H and ^{13}C nuclei in a C—H bond, the ^{13}C nucleus is irradiated at its resonant frequency while the NMR of the protons is being determined, very little increase in the proton signal is noticed. This is because the number of ^{13}C nuclei in the given molecule are very few. On the other hand, if, reverse method is followed, that is the ^1H nucleus is irradiated, while the spectrum of the carbons is being observed, considerable NOE enhancement in the signal of ^{13}C nuclei is observed. The reason is that while the protons are numerous, the ^{13}C nuclei are few because of their low natural abundance as already discussed. As the ^{13}C nuclei give weak signals in general, therefore, the NOE technique is used to enhance the sensitivity of the signals in CMR spectra because a much-needed enhancement in the S/N ratio is observed. So, NOE/ becomes further significant in that it can also be used for the purpose of peak enhancements. However, it should be noted that unlike the NOE observed between H—H interacting nuclei, the NOE observed for the ^{13}C nucleus between H and ^{13}C interacting nuclei is not used for measuring the distance r. This is because the major part of the NOE enhancement arises from the protons directly bonded to the carbon rather than from non-bonded protons and the bond distance in a covalent ^{13}C—H bond is already known to us. Further, unlike for the ^1H—^1H interacting nuclei, the NOE for ^{13}C varies with inverse third power of the distance r :

$$H \overset{r}{\text{——}} H \qquad NOE = f \frac{1}{r^6}$$

$$^{13}C \overset{r}{\text{——}} H \qquad NOE = f \frac{1}{r^3}$$

will NOE enhancement for all the carbons be identical in the CMR spectrum of a molecule?

It needs to be noted that the NOE enhancement for the ^{13}C nuclei will be different. That will depend upon the number of protons attached to a particular carbon. Greater the number of protons attached to a carbon, greater will be the NOE enhancement of that carbon. Thus, we would expect the following decreasing order for various types of carbons.

$$CH_3 > CH_2 > CH$$

As a quaternary carbon C_p does not possess a ^1H, so the NOE enhancement for this carbon will be the least.

6.1.4 Magnitude of NOE

The maximum NOE is given by :

$$(\eta_I S)_{max} = \frac{1}{2} \frac{\gamma_S}{\gamma_I}$$

where I is the spin observed and S is the nucleus that is irradiated and Y_S and Y_I are their magnetogyro ratios respectively. For homonuclear NOE, $\eta_{max} = 0.56$. So, maximum intensity observable is $1 + \frac{1}{2} \phi$ normal. Thus, the effect is small. For heteronuclear NOE, Y_S will naturally be different from Y_H. Under these circumstances, the NOE effect will be high. Furthermore, the η_{max} can be either positive or negative, depending upon the sign of Y.

Thus η_{max} for some nuclei is as follows with respect to proton :

Nucleus observe H	η_{max}	
H	0.5	(50% enhancement)
^{13}C	1.99	(200% enhancement)
^{19}F	0.53	
^{31}P	1.24	
^{15}N	-4.93	
^{29}Si	-2.52	

Increase in signal intensity due to NOE is given by :

$$1 + \eta$$

So, for $^1H^1H$ i.e. homonuclear NOE

$$\text{Increase in signal intensity} = I + \frac{1}{2}$$

For ^{13}C, ^1H heteronuclear NOE :

$$I = 1 + \eta$$
$$= 1 + 1.99 = 2.987$$

This amounts to about three-fold increase in signal intensity.

For ^{15}N, as γ_N is negative, therefore, the signal is reversed and is about ($I + h = 1 - 4.93 = -3.93$), $3.93 \approx 4$ times as large.

It should be noted that in case a nucleus has negative gyromagneto ratio γ (as in ^{15}N and ^{29}Si), η_{obs} may have a magnitude of -1. If that happens, the total intensity can be near zero. Therefore, in ^{15}N and ^{29}Si. NMR spectroscopy, this creates problem when the suppression of NOE has to be achieved.

Further, η depends upon the nature of the relaxation mechanism.

Maximum NOE is observed when the nuclei relax exclusively via dipolar relaxation . As C-13 relaxes via this mechanism mostly, therefore, the increase in line intensity I,

$$NOE_{max} (I) = 1 + \eta \text{ becomes}$$

$$= 1 + 2 \frac{T_1}{T_1 CH}$$

where T_{1CH} is the dipolar relaxation time of $^{13}C-^1H$ and T_1 is the overall spin-lattice relaxation time. T_1 is related to T_{1i} as follows :

$$\frac{1}{T_1} = \frac{1}{\sum T_1 i} \qquad \text{....(A)}$$

where $T_1 i$ is the relaxation time due to the i-th mechanism.

In case the $^{13}C-^1H$ interaction is dipolar in nature and is the only effective mechanism, then T_1 is equal to T_{1CH}. So, the increase in intensity I,

$$NOE_{max} (I) = 1 + 2 \frac{T_1}{T_{1CH}}$$
$$= 1 + 3$$
$$I = 3$$

becomes three-times more than the intensity observed without NOE enhancement. When T_1 is much smaller than T_{1CH} as happens when mechanisms other than the dipolar mechanisms operate, then no NOE enhancement occurs, so that the C-13 nuclei appear in the CMR spectrum with characteristically low intensity peaks. However, the low signal intensity of a C-13 nucleus can occur due to mechanisms other than discussed above and therefore, it does not indicate the absence of dominant dipolar relaxation mechanism necessarily. The probability of the other mechanisms becomes smaller if the $^{13}C-^1H$ dipolar relaxation time is smaller.

As already indicated NOE is a through-space effect, the interacting nuclei may or may not be directly bonded. So, even if the interacting nuclei are directly bonded, the rate of relaxation T_1 may arise by mechanisms other than via direct through space interaction. These may be the result of interactions with the dissolved paramagnetic species or interactions with the nuclei of the solvent. Under such situations, it may well be that only a fraction of the possible η_{max} is observed because of dipole-dipole relaxation mechanism. We can therefore, determine the proportion of the relaxation occurring as a result of dipole-dipole mechanism :

$$\frac{T_{1\,obs}}{T_{1\,DD}} = \frac{\eta_{obs}}{\eta_{max}}$$

Further, the percentage contribution by dipole-dipole mechanism, P_{DD} can be determined by the following relation :

$$P_{DD} = \frac{\eta \times 100}{1.987}$$

Therefore NOE investigations allow us to calculate the nature of the relaxation mechanism. Further, in general, no NOE is observed when quadrupolar relaxation occurs. Furthermore η may get reduced in case the interacting nuclei are not bonded directly and are further apart from each other in space.

It needs to be noted that when full NOE occurs for all nuclei, the relative line intensities are not influenced and that the equation (A) is valid only when the molecular rotational mobilities are high compared to the reciprocal of the resonance frequencies when the extreme narrow conditions are met. In practice, this is always true for small or medium-sized molecules in commonly used solvents at room temperature when the applied magnetic field strengths are low or medium. The equation becomes invalid at high magnetic field strengths (5–50 k gauss or higher) as the extreme narrowing condition does not apply even for medium-sized molecules. Under these conditions, therefore the observed NOE.

6.1.5 Quantitative Derivation of NOE

Let us consider a two-spin system. The possible energy states and transition probabilities are shown in Fig. 6.2.

We have to take into account the total magnetization vector M_z of each spin in the two spin system. Obviously, M_z will be equal to the population difference between $n\alpha$ and $n\beta$ spin-states at a point, other then equilibrium state.

$$Mz = n\alpha - n\beta$$

The M_z^o at equilibrium state will be:

$$M_Z^o = n_\alpha^o - n_\beta^o$$

$$= \frac{N}{2} \frac{Yh\,Bo}{2\pi\,kT} \quad \text{where k is Boltzman constant}$$

Y is the magnetogyro ratio of the molecules.

This can be shown on the basis of Boltzman distribution law:

$$\frac{n_\beta^o}{n_\alpha^o} = e^{-\Delta E/kT} = 1 - \Delta E/kT = 1 - \frac{Yh\,Bo}{2\pi kT}$$

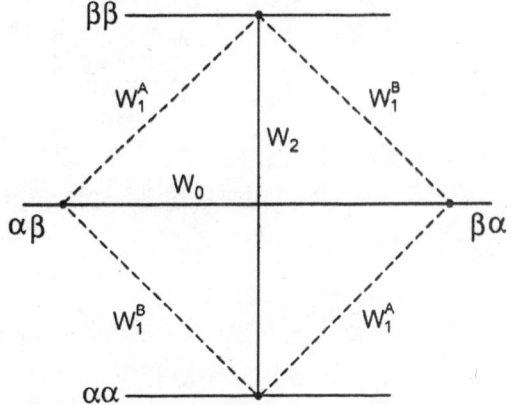

Fig. 6.2. The four energy states and the transition probabilities for a two spin system.

So, if we have a two-spin system (AB), then:

$$M_Z^A = \frac{N}{2} \cdot \frac{Y^A.h\,Bo}{2\pi kT}$$

and

$$M_Z^B = YB = \frac{N}{2} \cdot \frac{Y^B.h\,Bo}{2\pi kT}$$

or

$$\frac{M_Z^A}{M_2^{oB}} = \frac{YA}{YB}$$

Now, the nucleus A can relax from B spin state to a-spin state by transition $W_1^A + W_1^A + W_2 + W_0$. Therefore, rate of change of M_Z^A will be equal to:

$$\frac{dM_Z^A}{dt} = -(2W_1^A + W_2 + W_0)(M_Z^A - M_2^{oA}) - (W_2 - W_0)(M_Z^B - M_Z^{oB})$$

or

$$\frac{dM_Z^A}{dt} = -P.(M_Z^A - M_Z^{oA}) - \sigma(M_Z^B - M_Z^{oB})$$

If β-spin is totally decoupled, it gets saturated so that nb = na which means $M_Z^B = 0$. Under these equilibrium conditions, M_Z^{oA} will have new value. So,

$$\frac{dM_Z^A}{dt} = O = -P(M_Z^A - M_Z^{oA}) = \sigma M_Z^{oB}$$

or,

$$P(M_Z^A - M_Z^{oA}) = \sigma M_Z^{oB} = \sigma \frac{Y^B}{Y^A} \cdot M_Z^{oA}$$

or,

$$\frac{M^A}{M_Z^{oA}} = 1 + \frac{\sigma}{P} \frac{\gamma^B}{\gamma^A}$$

$$= 1 + \eta$$

η is called quantitative NOE.

As σ/P = 0.5 for majority of the spin system, so

$$\eta = 0.5 \frac{\gamma^B}{\gamma^A}$$

When we are dealing with the homonuclear NOE, $Y^B = Y^A$.

$$\eta = 0.5$$

That is to say NOE enhancement will be only 58%.

As Y^C is 1/4th of Y^H, therefore,

$$\eta = 1.987$$

and the enhancement in peak intensity will be $= 1 + \eta = 1 + 1.987 = 2.987$.η for $^{15}N = -4.93$. As ^{15}N has a negative γ, so $1 + \gamma = 1 - 4.93 = -3.93$. For ^{29}Si γ is also negative, so

$$1 + \eta = 1 - 2.52 = -1.52$$

So, you can see that an enhanced difference in the population of one nucleus after saturation of the second nucleus gives rise to an enhanced net magnetization vector M_Z compared to M_O (i.e. $M_Z > M_O$). That is why peak intensity is enhanced. Even as we talk of this effect in terms of enhanced M_Z, it also needs to be noted that the magnitude of the NOE effect diminishes with increasing internuclear distance r, $A \overset{\eta}{\text{———}} B$ between the interacting nuclei:

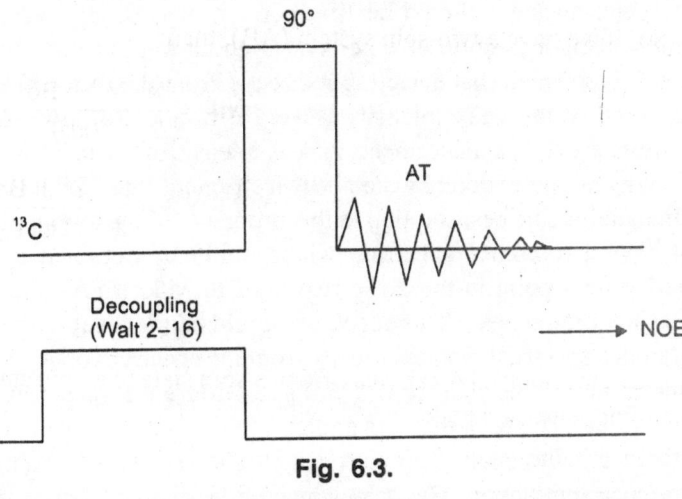

Fig. 6.3.

$$NOE \propto \frac{1}{r^6}$$

Therefore, if we know the magnitude of NOE, we can calculate the value of r between the interacting nuclei. This value of r is very important in case of protons as this helps us to determine the three-dimensional structure of bigger molecules like proteins etc. However, it is emphasised here that the NOE effect is not employed in CMR spectroscopy for determining the internuclear distance between the interacting nuclei such as C–13 and H because the distance between the chemically bound C and H (C–H) is well known as the NOE observed is actually contributed mainly by C–13 rather than by the carbon and hydrogen nuclei that are interacting.

We can say that in an NOE experiment, NOE builds up during the pulse delay as well as before the 90° pulse is applied. The NOE reaches a steady-state during the spin-lattice relaxation time, T_1.

It is possible to see NOE effect not only in a proton-decoupled CMR spectrum but also in a coupled CMR spectrum. In other words, it is possible to retain the signal enhancement due to NOE even in a coupled spectrum. This is done in Gated coupling.

$^{13}C \overset{1}{\text{———}} H$ $^{13}C \quad {}^{1}H$

Through | Bond   Through | Space

Major contribution to NOE   Minor contribution to NOE

Further, it needs to be noted that unlike in Homonuclear H—H NOE, all the hydrogens are irradiated rather than a selected one. This is achieved by $Walt_Z$–16 decoupling. Technique-wise, in order to observe NOE on ^{13}C signals, nothing special is to be done to irradiate all the protons. As the $Walt_Z$–16 decoupling is done anyway to obtain a proton noise (broad-band) decoupled spectrum during the process of acquisition of C–13 peaks, this decoupling is allowed to continue during the pulse delay as well rather than being turned off.

6.2 NOE DIFFERENCE SPECTRA

In the previous section of NOE, we learnt that saturation of one proton, A situated at a distance $< 5Å$ to another B in a molecule causes an enhancement in the peak intensity of B proton. Although theoretical peak enhancement should be fifty percent, it is usually very small (being a fraction of a percent to about ten percent). In fact, it is so small that detecting it directly from the difference observed in the peak intensity is very difficult. So, how to measure accurate enhancements in peak intensities due to NOE?

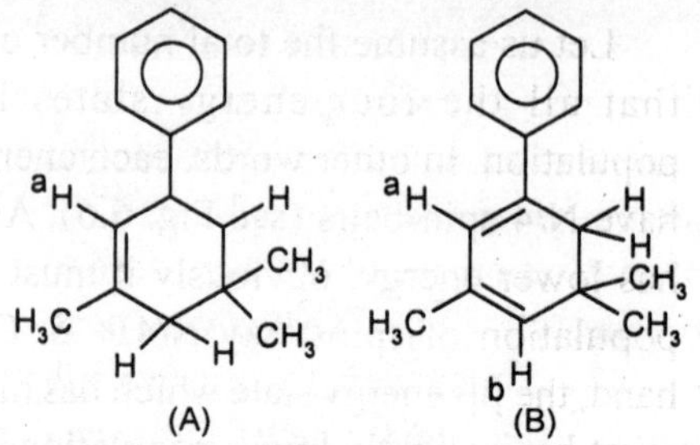

Why not get it done by the NMR instrument itself, why do it manually? The best solution to this problem will be to first of all have a reference spectrum which could be obtained by irradiating a point in the noise region of the spectrum rather than any proton peak. This spectrum would be identical to the normal 1D spectrum. Now subtract this reference spectrum mathematically from the spectrum obtained after NOE enhancement at every point. The result will be what we will call as a Difference Spectrum or NOE Difference Spectrum. How will it look like? The peak that was enhanced in signal intensity appears as a positive peak due to enhanced-reference subtraction. The peak which showed no NOE enhancement disappears due to reference-reference subtraction. The peak which underwent irradiation during the NOE experiment now appears inverted due to zero-reference peak. Fig. 6.4 illustrates the normal NOE and difference NOE spectra.

NOE difference spectra very closely enable us to distinguish between the two possible isomeric structures of a compound. For example the two isomeric substituted biphenyl compounds.

The compound B was synthesised in such a way that it could have two possible structures A and B (Fig. 6.4) as shown by its proton NMR spectrum (i). Now which is the right structure can be confirmed through NOE difference spectra readily.

Irradiation of $=C(CH_3)$ methyl proton should clarify this all. As per structure A, irradiation of this methyl group should lead to an NOE on H^a as well as CH_2. On the other hand, we would expect to see NOE on H_a and H^b rather than on CH_2 in structure B. When NOE difference spectra were run, it was found that the peak due to H^a and H^b underwent enhancement while the peaks due to all other protons disappeared as they did not experience any NOE, of course, the peak due to $=C—CH_3$ protons became upside down.

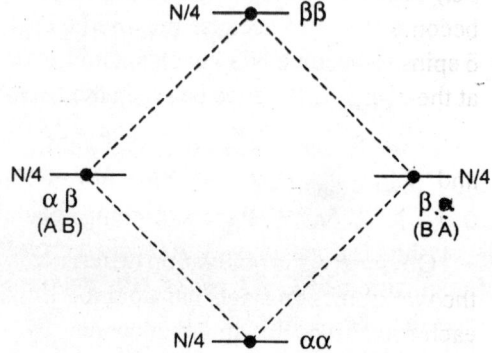

Fig. 6.4.

Cross-Relaxation (Cross Polarization)

The NOE is based on the fact that the difference between populations of nuclei in the higher-energy state and the lower-energy state is affected by the difference between the populations of (these two) energy states of the nuclei that are situated nearby in space within 5Å. Irradiation and saturation of one nucleus leads to equalization of its two spin states. That causes an enhancement in the population difference between the different energy states of the other interacting nuclei. This enhancement, therefore, leads to an enhancement in the peak intensity of this second nucleus. How does this enhancement occur, can be demonstrated as follows. Let us consider the A–B system. For this two spin system, four spin states are possible – αα, αβ, βα and ββ as shown in Fig. 6.5.

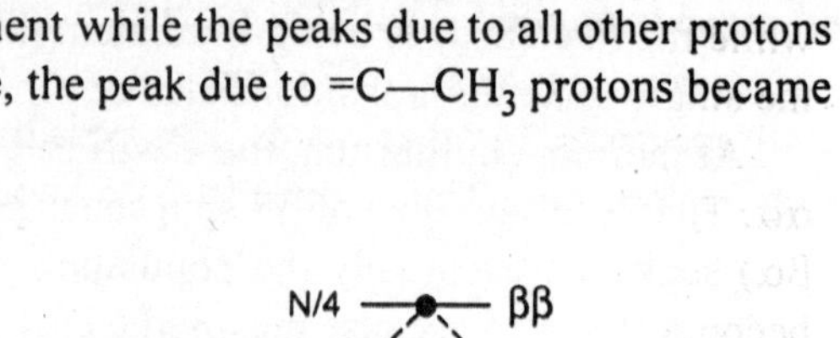

Fig. 6.5. Spin states and possible transitions and their populations. If N is the number of total spins, then each energy state should have N/4 population.

Let us assume the total number of spins as N that all the four energy states have equal population. In other words, each energy state will have N/4 spin-pairs (see Fig. 6.6). As αα energy has lower energy, obviously it must have higher population of spins, say N/4 + δ. On the other hand, the ββ energy state which has higher energy, must have slightly lower population say N/4–δ at Boltzman thermal equilibrium (Fig. 9.34). The αβ and βα energy states have equal energy i.e. N/4 each. The two allowed transitions will be αα → βα and αβ to αβ and the intensity of these allowed transitions will be proportional to the population

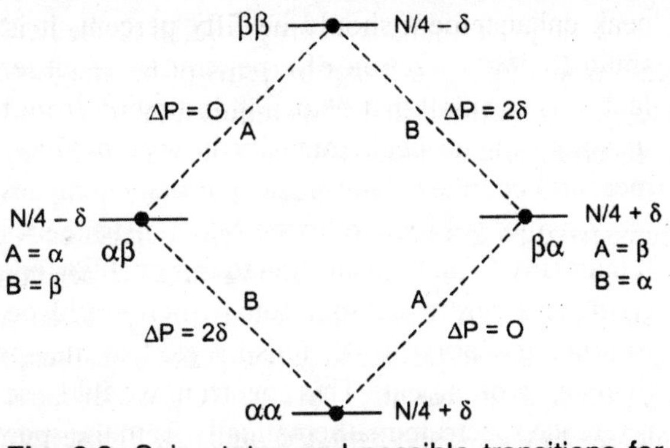

Fig. 6.6. Spin states and possible transitions for a two-spin system and population at Boltzman equilibrium.

difference between the involved spin states, $(P_{αα}-P_{βα})$ and $(P_{αβ}-P_{ββ})$ respec-tively. Let us consider the difference in the population of these two states at this point:

$$P_{αα}-P_{βα} = N/4 + δ - N/4 = δ$$
$$P_{αβ}-P_{ββ} = N/4 - δ - N/4 = δ$$

That is to say DP = d in each tran-sition. After the spin states are perturbed, they try to restore the equilibrium Boltzman population. They can relax by following the reverse path of the transitions shown. That is to say by "single-quantum" transitions in which one nucleus remains the same, the other undergoes transition. There is the other possibility, in which both the ββ spins relax directly back to αα spin states. This is called a "double-quantum" transition, a non-radiative pathway. This is also called **Cross-relaxation (cross-polarization) (simultaneous relaxation)**. When the nucleus A is being observed while the nucleus B is being irradiated, the "double-quantum" relaxation occurs efficiently. Although the single-quantum transitions also occur, we can forget about them as they do not cause NOE effect.

At thermal equilibrium, there will be a slight Boltzman excess of nuclei in the lower energy state, αα. That is to say some of ββ spin states have dropped down to the middle equal energy states (αβ and βα) such that eventually the population of the ββ state becomes N/2–2δ. The lower spin state will become N/4 + 2δ because the middle energy level spin states which initially become N/4 + δ each, lose δ spins to become N/34 each again. Let us now look at the energy difference between the two spin states:

$$P_{αα} - P_{βα} = N/4 + 2δ - N/4 = 2δ$$
and $P_{αβ} - P_{ββ} = N/4 - (N/4 - 2δ)$
$$= N/4 - N/4 + 2δ = 2δ$$

Obviously, the population difference ΔP between the two transition states has doubled from δ to 2δ in each transition. So, an enhancement by two fold is expected to occur. This process of pumping up the population of nucleus A by irradiating nucleus B is called **"spin pumping"**. The net change in the NMR spectrum starting from Fig. is shown in Fig. 6.7.

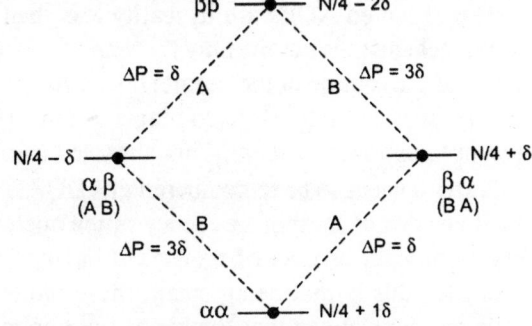

Fig. 6.7. Spin states and possible transitions for a two-spin system and populations after "double quantum" transitions.

As the peak intensity is proportional to the net Mz magnetization vector for each nuclear spin, it is clear from the Fig. 6.8 that in terms of net magnetization, the $M_Z^B = 3/2$ Mo (150%) while $M_Z^A = 1/2$ Mo, it is also clear that M_Z^A is reduced to 1/2 (50%) of M_Z^o (100%). So, while M_Z^B is increased by 50% of its equilibrium value (100%). This means the increase (50%) in M_Z^B is exactly equal to the decrease (50%) in M_Z^A. That also means that the Z-magnetization (Mz) lost by the proton A has actually been transferred on to proton B. Therefore, what does NOE mean in terms of magnetization vector, Mz point of view? This simply means that in NOE experiments, when two nuclei are close enough in space at a distance of < 5°A, irradiation and saturation of one nucleus leads to a transfer of a part of magnetization vector Mz of one nucleus to the other nucleus, thereby increasing the value of its Mz, the Z-magnetization vector. In short, we infer that an NOE experiment leads to a **transfer of Z-magnetization** from one nucleus to the closely situated nucleus. Please remember this conclusion as you are going to use this concept in the more advanced part of the spectroscopy called 2D NMR spectroscopy.

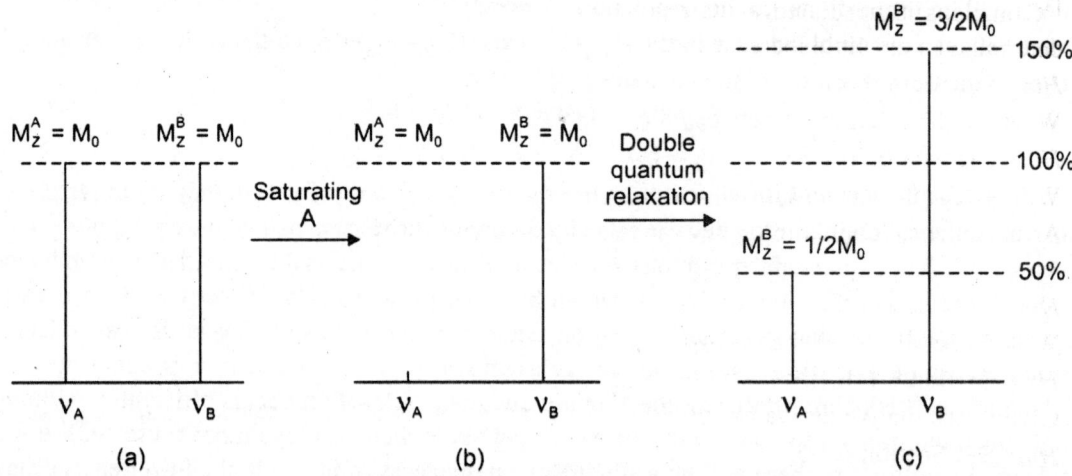

Fig. 6.8. Change in appearance of NMR spectrum of nuclei A and B (say proton), (a) at equilibrium, (b) after saturation of A by continuous irradiation, (c) after double quantum relaxation (DQR) in which the intensity of proton B has enhanced by two times.

The observed NOEs are in reality less than fifty percent. The reason is that the double-quantum (DQ) mechanism is not the only mechanism. There are other mechanisms in operation as well. The DQ as well as the routine or the normal relaxation processes go on together. In fact, a steady state is reached with the population levels becoming constant. The observable NOE is anything between a fraction of a percent to up to ten percent. This observed NOE is, therefore, also known as steady state NOE.

Note: It needs to be remembered that DQR is effected by magnetic fields that oscillate at a frequency two times that of Larmor frequency of the nucleus. Further, it needed to be noted that DQ relaxation is very significant in case of molecules having low molecular mass, say less than one thousand. The reason for this is that being small, these molecules have very rapid rate of tumbling and they have sufficient populations that tumble at Larmor as well as twice the Larmor frequency. Molecules with MW > 1000, it is the zero-quantum (ZQ) rather than the double-quantum (DQ) relaxation mechanism that is significant. A ZQ transition means one spin droping down and the other spin droping up i.e. $\alpha\beta$

→ βα. The large molecules have almost insignificant populations that tumble at single-quantum frequency or at the double quantum frequency. This gives rise to positive NOE, i.e. reduction of peak intensity. For small molecules, the NOE is negative, that is to say the peak intensity is decreased. In fact, molecules having MW 2000–4000 Da exhibit either little or no NOE at all, of course that depends upon the shape of the molecule, rigidity as well as viscosity of the solvent in use. Such molecules show what is called Rotating-Frame Overhauser Effect (ROESY).

PROBLEMS

1. What is Nuclear Overhauser Effect? What is its significance? Give some examples of NOE effect.

   Hint: See Section 6.1.1.

2. Comment on the statement "if between the two interacting ^1H and ^{13}C nuclei in a C–H bond, the ^{13}C nucleus is irradiated at its resonant frequency while the NMR of the protons is being determined, very little increase in the proton signal is noticed."

   Hint: See Section 6.1.3.

3. What are the differences between the NOE observed for ^1H–^1H and ^{13}C–^1H?

   Hint: See Section 6.1.3.

4. Will NOE enhancement for all the carbons be identical in th CMR spectrum of a molecule?

5. Arrange the following in the decreasing order of observed NOE enhancements:

   $$CH_3, \ CH_2, \ CH$$

   Hint: See Section.

6. Write in details about the magnitude of NOE.

   Hint: Section 6.1.4.

7. Give a quantitative derivation of NOE.

   Hint: See Section 6.1.5.

8. What is meant by NOE Difference Spectra?

7

Applications of ¹H NMR Spectroscopy Including Dynamic Processes

7.1 INTRODUCTION

Infrared and UV spectroscopies that employ higher frequency radiation are of limited use when we talk of dynamic processes. Evidently this is because the time-scale of the processes that can be studied by these spectroscopies is slow in comparison of the frequency employed so that rather than dynamic, it is actually the static picture that is observed. We can say that these two spectroscopic techniques work faster such that the averages of spectral parameters are hardly observed. The individual bands in these two spectroscopic techniques represent distinct energies; for instance a difference of 10 cm⁻¹ means an energy difference of about 120 J mol⁻¹. On the other hand, a difference of 100 Hz at a NMR instrument operating at 60 MHz amounts to an energy difference of a mere 4.2×10^{-7} J mol⁻¹. Little wonder then about the inability of IR and UV spectroscopic techniques that give us the static picture compared to the ability of NMR spectroscopic technique that provides us the dynamic picture of time dependant dynamic processes of such as those occurring in equilibrium or even those involving simple intramolecular motion, bond rotation etc.

It is not only the case of lower radio frequencies but also the smaller-line separations and the small natural-line widths in the spectra that enable NMR spectroscopy to capture many time-dependent phenomena as they occur. Of course, it does not mean that the NMR spectrometer can capture any motion at any speed it occurs. NMR spectroscopy does not compare to optical spectroscopies which work on a nanosecond or a picosecond or even faster time scales. NMR spectroscopy works on its own time scale called the NMR time scale that is of the order of milliseconds magnitude. Although the dynamic processes like those involving simple intramolecular motion or bond rotation occurs at a much faster rate compared to the NMR time scale, nevertheless NMR spectroscopy enables us to capture these events to the best of its abilities worth useful interpretation, not only from qualitative point of view but also from the point of view of quantitative analysis, that is to say from the reaction rates relationships as well.

When a process occurs on a time scale faster than the NMR time scale, the NMR instrument sees only an average picture of the change that is to say that it sees or catches a chemical shift that is the time average of the chemical shifts of the nucleus in two different environments. This inability, is actually an ability of the technique that gives us the ability to study these fast phenomena!

Let us consider two nuclei of the same element in a molecule in two different chemical environments.

$$H_a \underset{1/K^1}{\overset{K^1}{\rightleftharpoons}} H_b$$

Obviously, these will resonate in NMR at their own resonant frequencies at their own chemical shifts. Now, let us consider that the two atoms interchange their position only occasionally such that their lifetime τ, in any one environment is long, then we hardly observe a change in the NMR spectrum, we get two different resonance lines (Fig. 7.1a). Now suppose they interchange their position at a fast rate such that their residence time or lifetime τ is shorter than NMR time scale, then only one singlet is observed (Fig. 7.1c). If the life times are of intermediate values, a broadened line (Fig. 7.1b) is seen in the spectrum such that its shape is governed by the relation $\tau \, \nu_0 \, \delta$, ν_0 being the resonant frequency, δ its chemical shift in ppm.

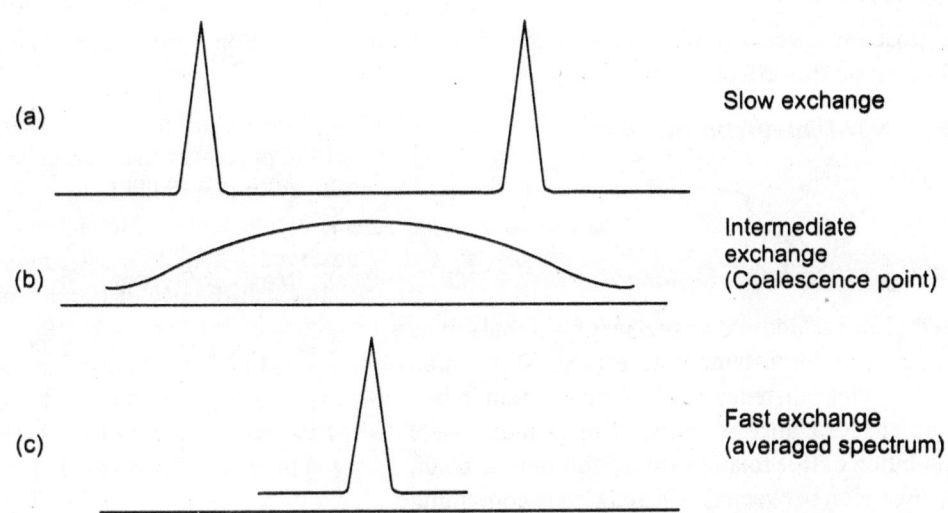

Fig. 7.1. NMR spectra of slow, intermediate and fast exchanges.

The temperature at which the two signals coalesce is called coalescence point, τ_C. The coalescence point τ_C is equal to :

$$\tau_C = \frac{2}{\pi \, (\nu_0 \delta)}$$

and

$$\frac{2}{\tau_C} = \frac{1}{\tau_A} + \frac{1}{\tau_B}$$

From these equations, we get very precise relation between the exchange rate and temperature.

The exchange broadening is used to measure the rate constants K^1 and $1/K^1$ as well as the energy of activation E_{act} for such processes.

Rate constant K^1 is given by the equation:

$$K^1 = \left(\frac{\pi}{2}\right) \cdot \Delta v \text{ where } \Delta v = (v_A - v_B)$$

or
$$K^1 = 2.22 \, \Delta v$$

ΔG, the free molar activation energy is related to K like this:

$$K^1 = \frac{kT_c}{h} \cdot e^{-\Delta G / R\tau_c}$$

where k is Boltzman constant, h is Planck constant, and R is gas constant. ΔG for a first-order exchange process will be given by the Eyring equation:

$$\Delta G = 1.91 \, \tau_c \, [10.32 + \log \tau_c / K^1] \times 10^{-3} \text{ kJ/mol}$$

Thus, for N,N-dimethyl acetamide having K^1 is calculated to be 17.8 s^{-1} at $\tau_c = 353$ K. ΔG_{353} is calculated to be 78.5 kJ mol^{-1}.

We shall now show how NMR helps us in investigating the following dynamic processes.

7.2 HINDERED ROTATION

NMR spectroscopy is very useful in studying the effect of hindered rotation in molecules. The following examples illustrate this effect.

Example 1 : N,N-Dimethylformamide

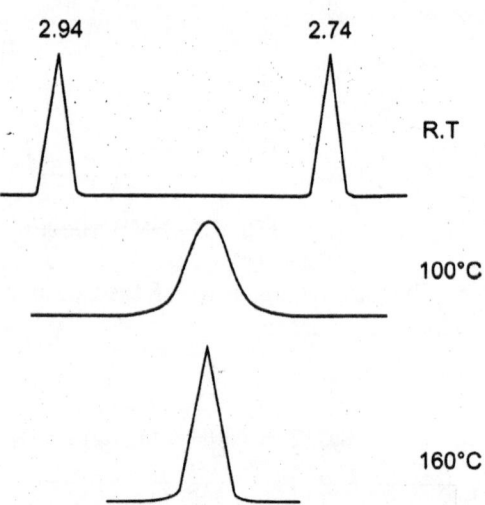

N,N-Dimethylformamide shows two methyl signals in its NMR spectrum at room temperature (Fig. 7.2) which clearly indicates the existence of hindered rotation in this molecule due to resonance as shown. Creation of C=N leads to inhibition of free rotation around this double bond. The interconversion between C—N and C=N containing resonating structures is slow as the energy barrier is high (88 kJ mol^{-1}) at room temperature. However, when this barrier is overcome by providing energy by raising the temperature, the interconversion becomes faster, as indicated by broadening of the two methyl singlets. Eventually the two singlets coalesce into one signal.

The methyl protons closer (or cis) to oxygen absorb at δ 2.94 ppm while the protons of the other (trans) methyl resonate at δ 2.79.

The resonance hybrid structure of this amide is therefore, like this in which the C—O and C—N bonds are partial double bonds and therefore, it is better to represent the interconversion around the C—N bond like this.

Fig. 7.2. NMR spectrum of N,N-Dimethyl-formamide as a function of temperature. The aldehydic proton is unaffected and therefore not shown.

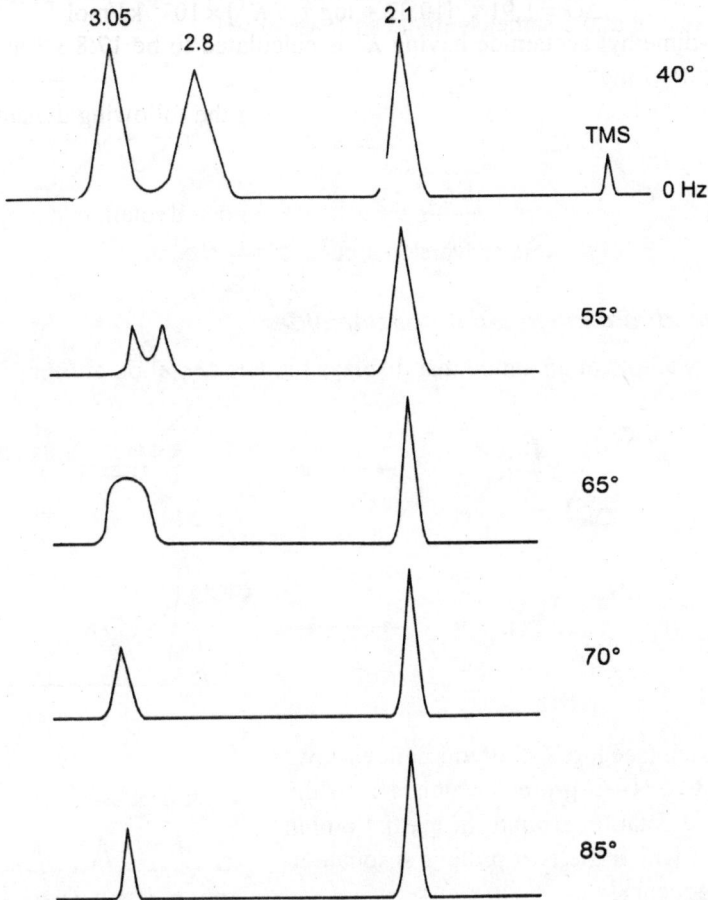

Example 2 : N,N-Dimethyl Acetamide

Like N,N-Dimethyl formamide this compound also shows hindered rotation around the amide bond, that is to say slow exchange of methyl protons attached to nitrogen occurs. The NMR spectrum of this molecule at room temperature shows two N—Me singlets as shown in Fig. 7.3.

Fig. 7.3. NMR spectrum of N,N–dimethyl acetamide as a function of temperature.

Intext Exercise

Q. Why does N,N–dimethylacetamide, $(CH_3)_2NCOCH_3$ show two N-methyl singlets at room temperature whereas it only shows one sharp peak due to these N-methyl groups at higher temperature at 110°C?

Evidently, the free rotation around the C—N bond is inhibited at r.t. due to resonance.

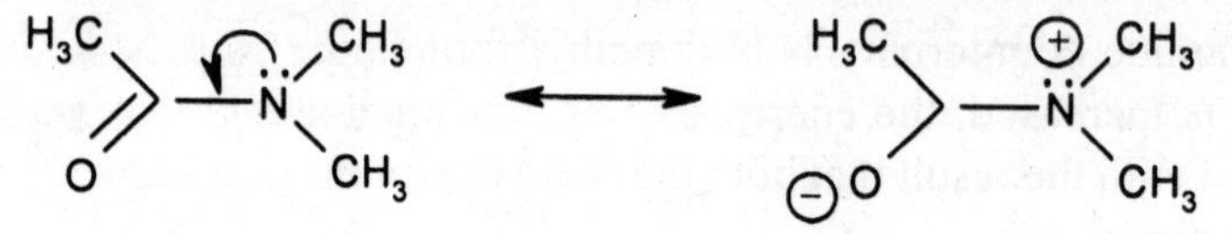

The formation of the C—$\overset{+}{N}$ bond does not allow free rotation to occur. Consequently, the Larmor frequencies of the two N—Me groups now become different. As the temperature is raised, the C—$\overset{+}{N}$ due to fast rotation, the Larmor frequencies of the two N—Me groups now become identical with the result that the two absorb at the same chemical shift as shown :

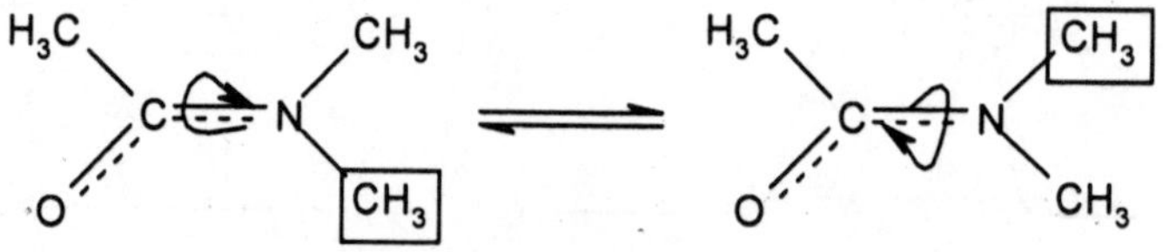

Interconversion around C --- N bond

Example 3: Hindered rotation in α-chloroacetamide

This is yet another example of an amide that displays hindered rotation at room temperature :

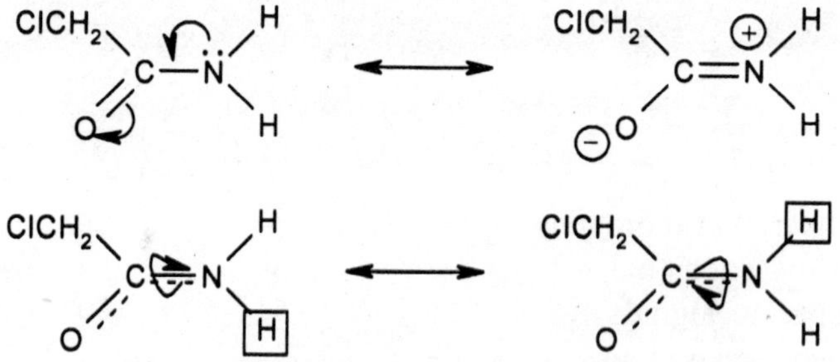

The NMR spectrum (see Fig. 7.4) of this amide shows two singlets for the two N—H protons which reflects the presence of hindered rotation around the partial amide bond, consequent to which the two protons resonate at different Larmor frequencies.

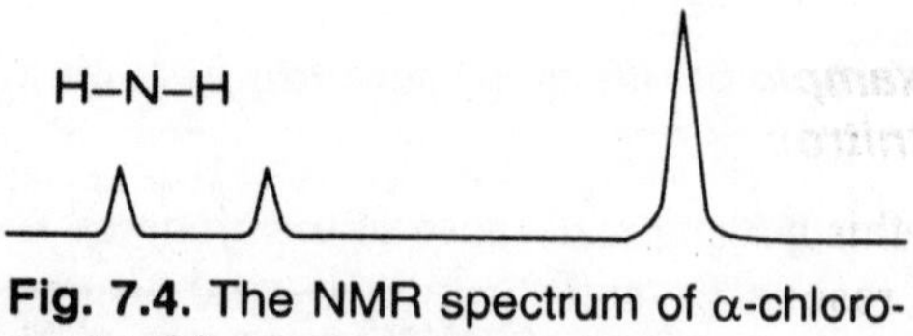

Fig. 7.4. The NMR spectrum of α-chloro-acetamide at room temperature.

Intext Exercise

The following compound shows two N—Me singlets in its PMR spectra at room temperature but only one at higher temperature. Explain why.

$$(CH_3)_2N—COOC_2H_5$$

Example 4: N,N-Dimethyl methane thiamide

This molecule like its amide counterpart, N,N-dimethyl formamide shows two methyl singlets at r.t. but as the temperature is increased, the energy barrier is overcome and internal rotation around N—C—S bond becomes fast with the result that both the N—Me protons now resonate at the same chemical shift and give only one signal.

Example 5: N,N-Dimethyl carbamate

Like amides and thioamides, carbamates also show hindered rotation :

The rotation being hindered at room temperature, the interconversion is slow such that the r.t. nmr spectrum shows two separate signals for the two N—CH₃ protons but the two signals merge as temperature is increased (see Fig. 7.5).

Example 6: Hindered rotation in N-Methyl-2,4,6-trinitroaniline

In this molecule, because of the hindered rotation due to resonance stabilisation by the N-methyl amino group, the two meta aromatic protons are non-equivalent as observed at –60°C analysis of its NMR spectrum shown in Fig. 7.6.

The rotation is very fast at room temperature in this molecule such that both the meta aromatic protons have identical Larmor frequencies. When the lower temperature slows down the rotation around the

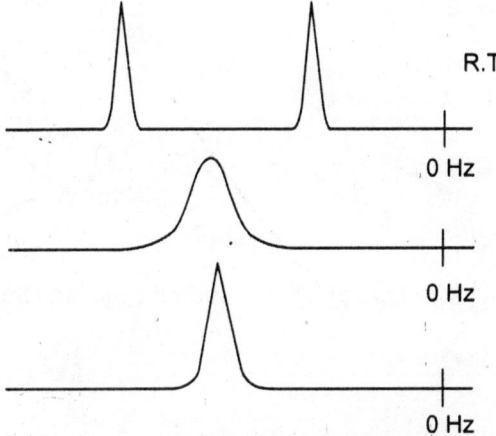

Fig. 7.5. NMR spectra of N,N-dimethyl-carbamate as a function of temperature. The CH₂CH₃ multiplets are not shown as they remain unaffected.

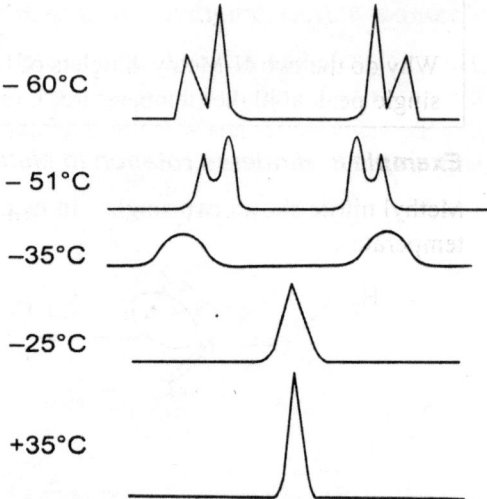

- 60°C

- 51°C

-35°C

-25°C

+35°C

Fig. 7.6. NMR spectrum of N-Methyl-2,4,6-trinitroaniline as a function of temperature with regards to aromatic protons.

C—N bond, then the two protons become non-equivalent and appear as a doublet each. In other words, the AB spin system degenerates into an A_2 spin system.

Why does the NMR spectrum of N-Methyl-2,4,6-trinitroniline change from an A_2 spin system to an AB spin system as temperature is decreased from 35°C–60°C. Explain.

Example 7: Hindered rotation in p-Nitroso N,N-dimethylamine

In this molecule, the two N-methyl groups protons have different resonant frequencies at room temperature. These appear as two separate signals. But with the rise in temperature, they coalesce into one signal as the interconversion around the partial double bound, C—N bond becomes rapid (Fig. 7.6).

The energy of activation for the hindered rotation has been calculated to be ~ 96 kJ mol⁻¹.

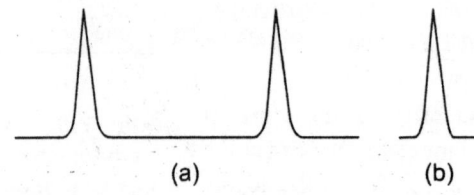

(a)   (b)

Fig. 7.7. NMR spectrum of p-nitroso N,N-dimethylaniline at (a) r.t. (b) at higher temperature.

Intext Exercise

Why do the two N-Methyl singlets of N-nitroso N,N-dimethylaniline observed at r.t. change into a single peak at higher temperature. Explain.

Example 8: Hindered rotation in Methyl nitrite

Methyl nitrite shows two singlets in its proton NMR spectrum at room temperature.

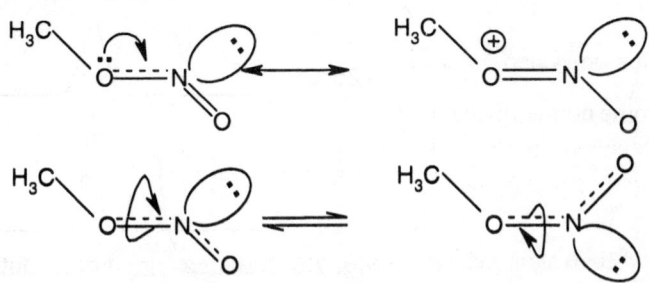

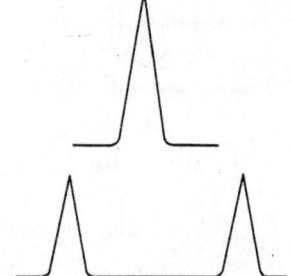

Fig. 7.8. NMR spectrum of methyl nitrite at (a) r.t., (b) higher temperature.

This is due to hindered rotation around O—N—O bond but which becomes rapid at higher temperature with the result that both the methyl groups protons now become equivalent and resonate at identical Larmor frequencies (Fig. 7.8).

7.3 ROTATION ABOUT SINGLE BONDS

NMR also helps us in the investigation of conformational equilibria in a cyclic as well as a cyclic systems.

7.3.1 Substituted Ethanes

NMR spectra of 2,2,3,3-tetrachloro butane shows one signal for the two methyl group protons at r.t. due to staggered conformation (a) (Fig. 7.9). Obviously the rotation around C—C single bond is rapid at room temperature. If the rate of rotation is lowered down by decreasing temperature, we should expect to see two signals for the methyl groups, of course, the intensity of the signals wil be proportional to the population of the conformational isomers b and c.

Intext Exercise

Q. How many signals should t-butyl cycloheptane show for its three methyl groups in its NMR spectrum?

Ans. If you write the most stable conformation of the molecule, which is obviously the staggered conformation, then it becomes clear that we should expect two signals for the three methyl groups in the ratio 2:1.

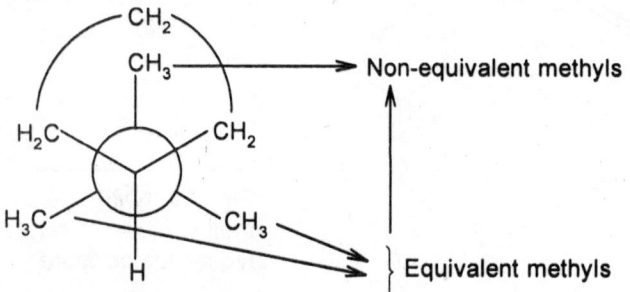

Staggered conformation

Indeed, the signals are obtained for the three methyl groups in the ratio expected. However, as the temperature is decreased to –126°, the two signals coalesce and eventually one signal is obtained.

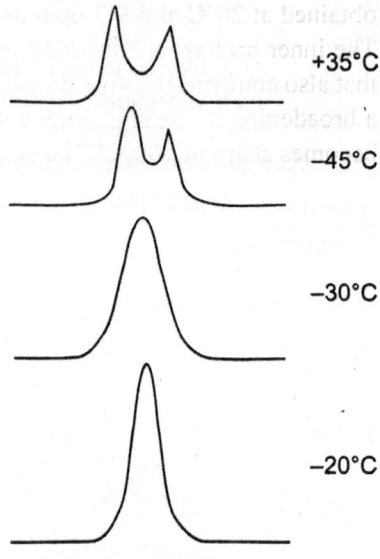

Fig. 7.9. The NMR spectrum of 2,2,3,3-tetrachlorobutane as a function of temperature.

7.3.2 Ring Inversion in Cyclohexanes

The cyclohexane chair conformations undergo interconversion at room temperature with the result that the axial and equatorial hydrogen interchange their positions accordingly. If we take the NMR of cyclohexane d_{11}, C_6HD_{11}, then variable NMR spectroscopy confirms this deuteration is necessary to prevent spin-spin splitting.

When the NMR is taken at room temperature then only one sharp peak is observed at S 1.84 ppm. However, when the ring inversion is frozen at –60°C, the signal becomes broad and eventually two signals are obtained at –68°C as shown in Fig. 7.10. From the coalescence point, the energy barrier was found to be about 45 kJ mol^{-1}.

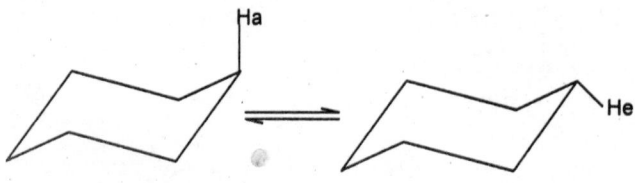

7.3.3 [18]-Annulene

Variable temperature NMR spectroscopy shows that occurs the exchange of 6 internal protons with the outer hydrogens by rotation around C—C single bonds. Two broad signals are

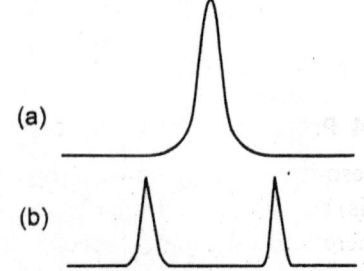

Fig. 7.10. The NMR spectrum of cyclohexane derivative C_6HD_{11} (a) at r.t. (b) –60°C.

obtained at 20°C at δ 9.3 ppm and at δ 3.0 ppm for the external and the internal protons respectively. The inner protons are shielded, while the outer 12 protons are deshielded due to magnetic anisotropy that also confirms the $4n + 2\pi$ electron aromatic character of the molecule. As the temperature is raised, a broadening of the signal occurs and an average weighted signal at δ 5.4 ppm is seen at 70°C which becomes sharp at 100°C. The spectra are recorded in Fig. 7.11.

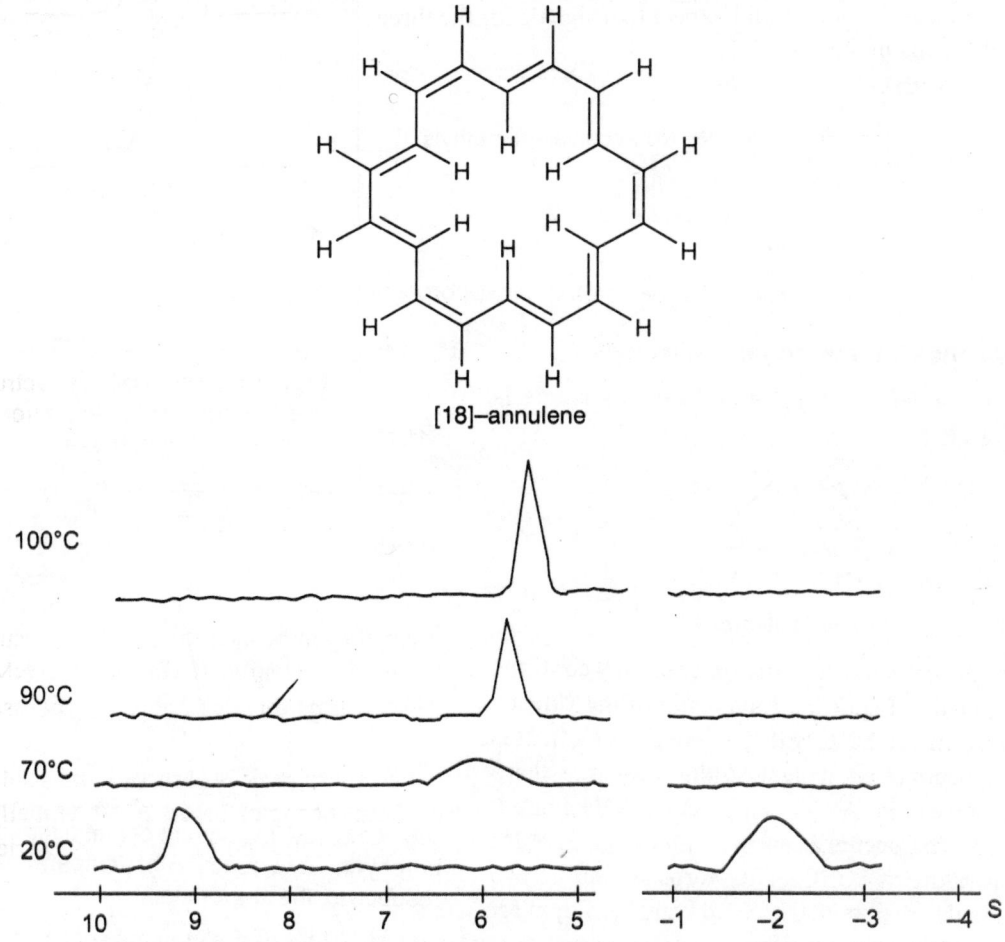

[18]–annulene

Fig. 7.11. The NMR spectrum of [18] annulene as a function of temperature.

7.4 Proton-exchange in Porphyrins

Meso-tetraphenyl porphyrin (Fig. 7.12) undergoes N—H protons exchange (in fact any porphyrin shows this) between the pyrrole rings as shown. As a result, the β-protons form two sets of equivalent protons. Therefore, we should expect two peaks from these protons. However, the NMR spectrum taken at room temperature at δ 8.75 shows only one signal. Obviously, this shows that the exchange process is very rapid at room temperature compared to NMR time scale. If that is so then we should expect to see two signals at lower temperature. Indeed, this was the case as shown in Fig. 7.12. The peak at δ 8.75

broadens at – 46° and then separates δ 8.95 and δ 8.75 apart into two peaks at – 60°C. The energy of activation was calculated to be 48.30 kJ/mol.

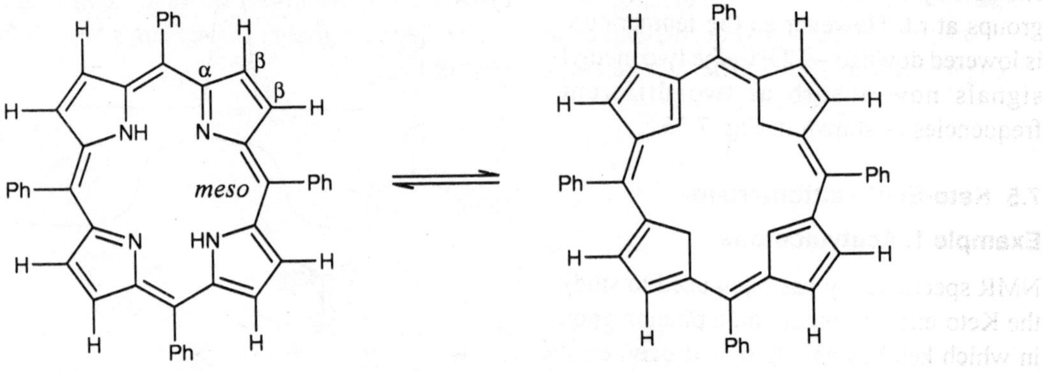

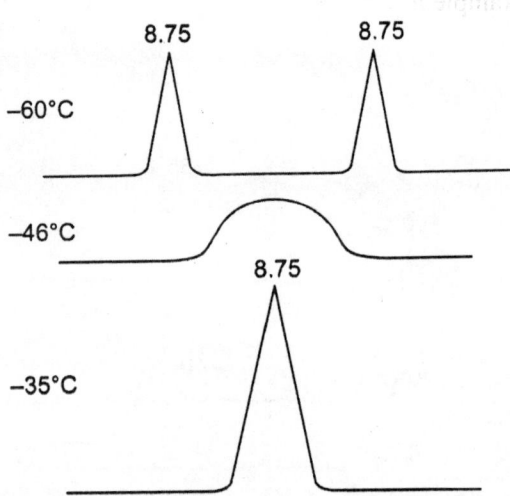

Fig. 7.12. Mesotetraphenyl porphyrin molecule.

7.4.1. Valence Tautomerism: Bullvalene

Bullvalene undergoes a series of valence isomerizations of the type of cope rearrangements.

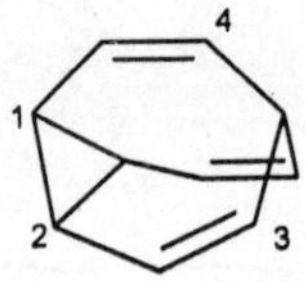

Frozen bullvalene

Variable temperature NMR spectroscopy confirms this as shown in Fig. 7.14. As a result of the valence isomerizations at 80°C, all the ten protons in this molecule become equivalent so that only one sharp singlet is observed. As the temperature is decreased, line broadening occurs as shown in the Fig. 7.14 for the temperature of 150°C. Afterwards at – 80°C, two broad signals are obtained at S 5.64 and 2.15 ppm for

8.75   8.75

–60°C

–46°C

8.75

–35°C

Fig. 7.13. NMR spectrum of meso tetraphenyl porphyrin as a function of temperature with respect to the β-protons.

the[6] and [4] protons respectively as expected for the frozen structure of the molecule. The energy of activation was calculated to be 49 kJ mol⁻¹.

7.4.2 Valence Isomerization of 2–methyloxepine and 2–methylbenzene oxide

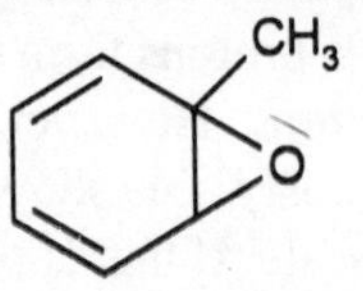

2-methylbenzene oxide 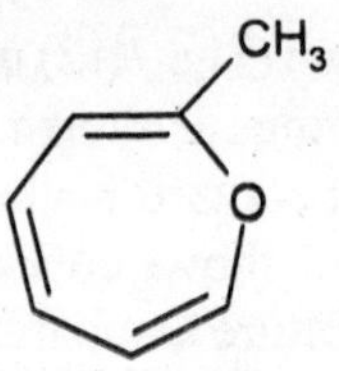   2-methyl oxepine

This interconversion is rapid at room temperature. Hence, the NMR spectrum shows only one singlet due to both the CH_3 groups at r.t. However as the temperature is lowered down to $-125°C$, the two methyl signals now absorb at two different frequencies as shown in Fig. 7.15.

7.5 Keto-Enol Tautomerism

Example 1. Acetylacetone

NMR spectroscopy has been used to study the Keto-enol tautomerism, a phenomenon in which ketones having α-hydrogen exist in equilibrium with its enolic form. An example is acetylacetone.

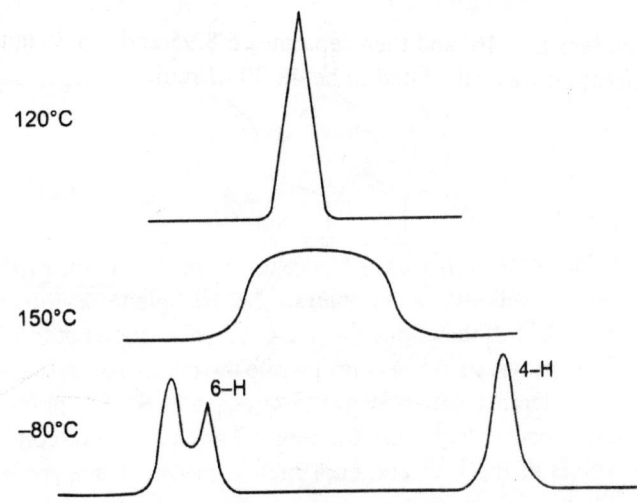

Fig. 7.14. NMR spectrum of bullvalene as a function of temperature.

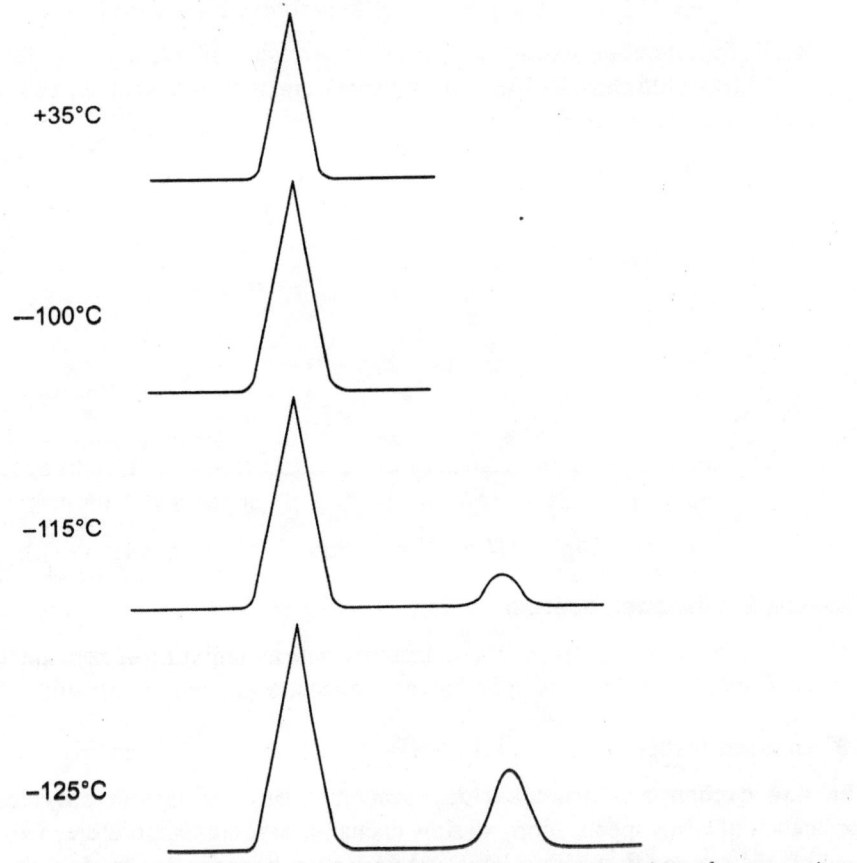

Fig. 7.15. NMR spectrum of α-methyloxepine w.r. to methyl protons as a function of temperature.

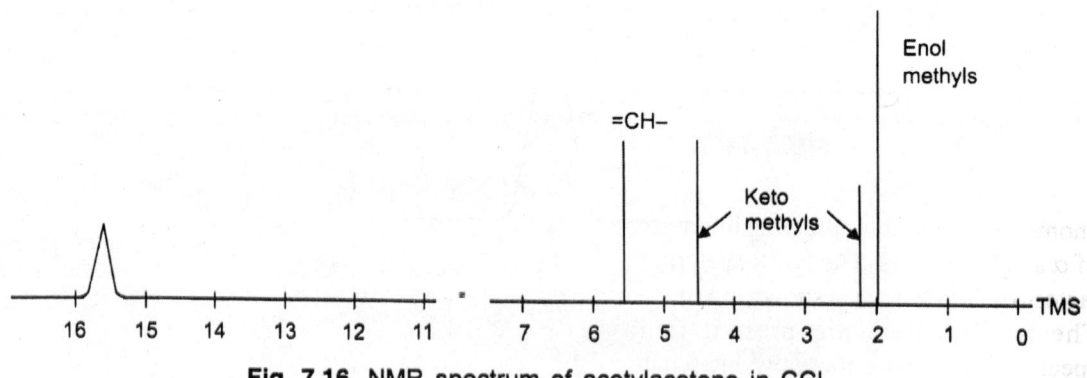

Keto   Enol

The NMR spectrum of acetylacetone is shown in Fig. 7.16. A careful interpretation shows the presence of both the tautomers. The methylene protons resonate as a singlet at δ 3.7 plan, while the olefinic CH of the enolic form appears as a singlet at S 5.7 ppm. The singlet at 2.2 ppm corresponds to methyl groups of th keto form, while the enolic methyls appear at 2.0 ppm. The enolic O—H as expected is considerably deshielded and appears at S 15.5 ppm. The enolic form is stabilised as a result of intramolecular hydrogen bonding. The equilibrium constant K can be determined by the ratio of the integrals of the keto and enol methyl peaks. While the enolic content is found to be 85%, keto term exists in 15% amounts.

$$K = \frac{\text{Integral area of Enol form } CH_3 \text{ group } 85}{\text{Integral area of keto form } CH_3 \text{ groups } 15} = 5.66$$

Clearly, the rate of the equilibrium or interconversion of keto and enol forms is slow. If it were fast then the NMR would show a time averaged spectrum, which is what happens as the temperature of this interconversion is increased.

Fig. 7.16. NMR spectrum of acetylacetone in CCl_4.

Example 2. Ethylacetoacetate

Fig. 7.16(b) shows the spectrum of ethylacetoacetate as a mixture of keto and enol forms in 78:22 ratio, of course, exact ratio depends upon solvent concentration and temperature.

7.6 Annomerization

The slow exchange in disaccharides: Annomerization in lactose provides an elegant example of application of NMR spectroscopy to slow exchange at room temperature. This disaccharide occurs as a mixture of its α and β anomers. This anomerisation happens due to ring opening and reclosing at the

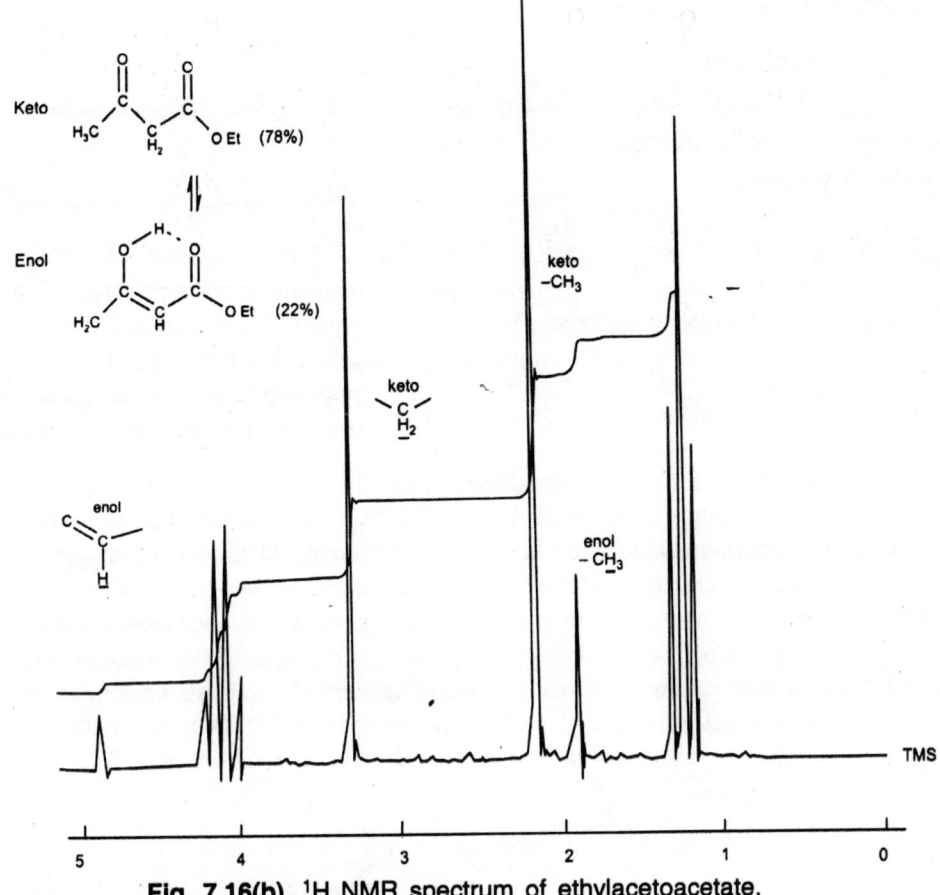

Fig. 7.16(b). ¹H NMR spectrum of ethylacetoacetate.

anomeric carbon, thus allowing interchange of α and β anomers. The NMR spectrum of lactose in $D_2O/NaOD$ is shown in Fig. 7.17. The two anomers are present in the spectrum, confining the slow interchange process. The doublet at 5.11 ppm (J = 3.8 Hz) is due to glucose + proton of the α-anomeric lactose. The doublet at S 4.45 ppm (J = 7.5 Hz) is due to the glucose–1–proton of the β-anomer.

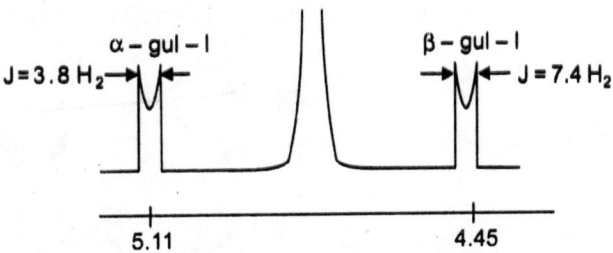

Fig. 7.17. The NMR spectrum of lactose in $D_2O/NaOD$, only the α-glu–1 and β-glu–1 part is shown.

The equilibrium constant K can be found out for the equilibrium α lactose $\rightleftharpoons$ β lactose.

$$K_{eq} = \frac{\text{Integral area of β-anomer}}{\text{Integral area of α-anomer}} = 1.81$$

Obviously, the β-anomer is present in larger amount over the α-anomer.

7.7 ORGANOMETALLIC CHEMISTRY

7.7.1 Trimethylaluminium

An elegant example of the application of NMR technique is the exchange in trimethyl aluminium. This occurs as a dimeric spcies as shows :

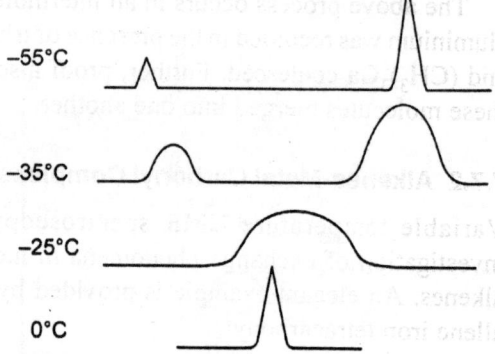

Fig. 7.18. Proton NMR spectra of aluminium trimethyl at a function of temperature.

The two methyls act as bridging methyls and the remaining four are the terminal methyl groups. The NMR spectrum of this compound in toluene or in cyclohexane shows only one sharp singlet (Fig. 7.18). This shows that all the six methyl groups protons are equivalent. However, when the temperature is lowered down to –50°C, its spectral behaviour changes. Thus, at 0°C, the line starts broadening that goes on till –25°C and then at –35°C two broad signals are obtained which eventually stand out clearly at –50°C. The two separated signals have the integral ratio of 1:2, corresponding to the two bridged and four terminal methyl groups. How does that happen? Clearly, the two Al(CH₃)₃ groups break off and then re-link together, such that the inner bridging methyls become terminal and the two terminal methyls become bridging methyls and this continues till all become equal. The exchanges are fast enough on the NMR time scale such that all the six methyl groups behave magnetically equivalent. The energy of activation was calculated to be about 65.3 kJ mol⁻¹.

The above process occurs in an intermolecular fashion. When the NMR spectrum of the trimethyl aluminium was recorded in the presence of trimethylgallium $(CH_3)_3Ga$, the signals arising from $(CH_3)_3Al$ and $(CH_3)_3Ga$ coalesced. Further, proof also comes from the fact that the averaged peaks from both these molecules merged into one another.

7.7.2 Alkenes-Metal Carbonyl Complexes

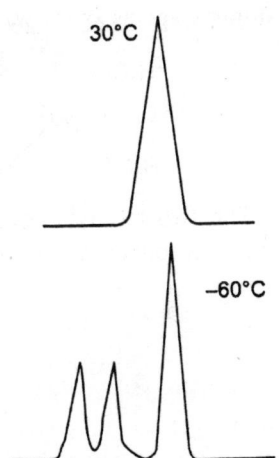

Variable temperature NMR spectroscopy is again helpful in the investigation of exchange phenomena in metal carbonyl complexes of alkenes. An elegant example is provided by the complex, tetramethyl-allene iron tetracarbonyl.

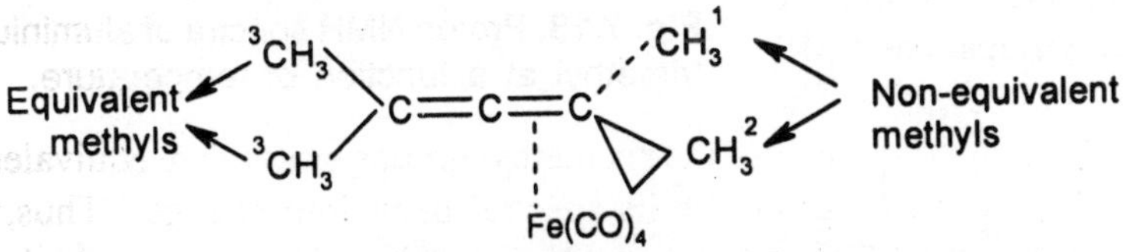

Fig. 7.19. NMR spectrum of tetramethyl allene iron tetracarbonyl complex as a function of temperature.

The NMR spectrum observed at room temperature (30°C) shows only one sharp signal for the for methyl groups as shown in Fig. 7.19. However, when the NMR spectrum recorded at –60°C shows that the exchange of $Fe(CO)_4$ group is slowed down so that complex shows three signals for the methyl groups in the integral ratio of 1:1:2, corresponding to CH_3^1, CH_3^2 and two $^3CH_3$ respectively as expected.

Further proof for the fast-exchange tautomerism in this molecule comes from the fact that the spectrum also shows the presence of uncomplexed excess tetramethyl allene molecule in the region of fast-exchange.

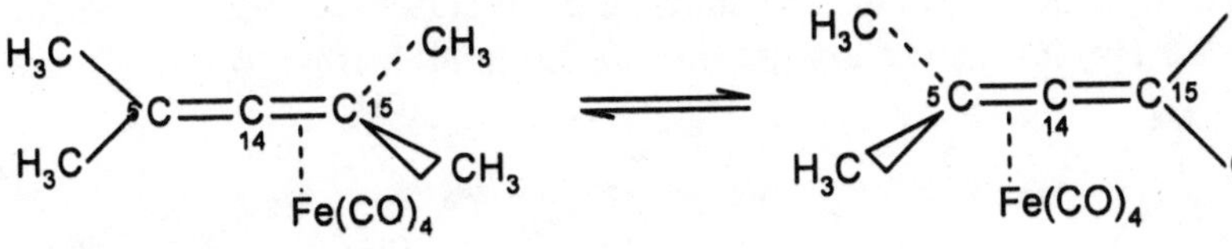

7.7.3 Exchange in Grignard Reagent

NMR spectroscopy is very useful in revealing the exact structure of Grignard reagent. An example is provided by the investigation of allyl magnesium bromide.

$$BrMg-\overset{3}{C}H_2-\overset{2}{C}H=\overset{1}{C}H_2 \rightleftharpoons \overset{1}{C}H_2=\overset{2}{C}H-\overset{3}{C}H_2-MgBr$$

The NMR spectrum of this compound shows a quintet δ 6.2 and a doublet at δ 2.5 in the integral ratio of 1:4 which is consistent with an AX_4 spin system. This is due to rapid equilibration of the two structures which arises due to attachment of the MgBr moiety at C–1 or at C–3 (Fig. 7.20).

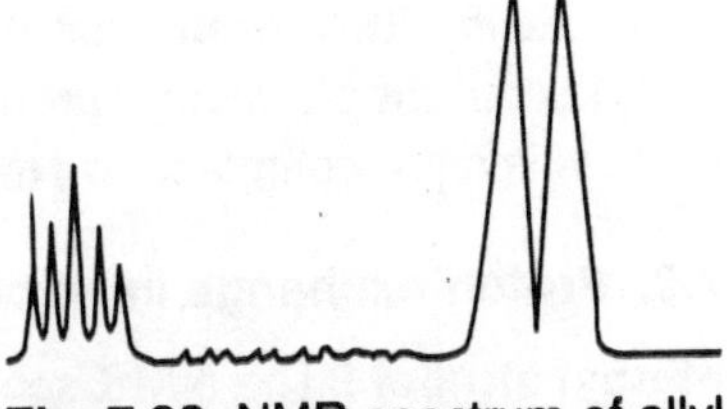

Fig. 7.20. NMR spectrum of allyl magnesium bromide.

7.8 STRUCTURE DETERMINATION AND PROTON EXCHANGE OF CARBOCATIONS

7.8.1 Structure Determination

NMR spectroscopy serves as an effective technique in confirming the structure of allylic-type carbocations such as A. When to this molecule, H_2SO_4 is added, it is converted into a allylic-type cation.

The PMR of the salt D formed, which is a resonance hybrid of the resonating structures (B–C) shows only three peaks in the ratio 6:4:1 corresponding to the six protons of the two equivalent methyls, four methylene protons and one C–H proton. Thus, nmr directly confirms the resonance hybrid structure of the salt formed.

7.8.2 Proton Shifts in Carbocations

The analysis by NMR spectroscopy of the σ-complexed carbocation obtained upon addition of hydrofluoric acid, Hf to hexamethyl benzene shows a doublet (J = 2.1 Hz) for the six methyl groups and a multiplet (J = 2.1 Hz) for the tertiary proton coupled to all methyl (6 × CH_3) protons.

Evidently, this means that the proton is shifting (probably 1,2-shift) from one carbon to another such that all the six methyl groups become equivalent. And that this can only happen if the exchange process is rapid compared to NMR time scale. The spectrum is shown in the Fig. 7.20.

7.9. Proton-exchange in alcohols

Methyl alcohol : The NMR spectrum of methanol at room temperature shows only two singlets, one due to OH protons and one due to CH_3 protons (Fig. 7.21). Clearly, here the expected spin–spin splitting from this AX_3 spin system is not seen. That means that the O—H protons are undergoing rapid exchange at room temperature at a rate faster than the NMR-time scale. If we can lower down this rate of exchange to lesser than the NMR-time scale we can hope to see the two signals being split into expected multiplicities. When the temperature was lowered down to –15°C, the two signals showed signs of splitting and at –60°C, the quartets (OH) and the doublets become distinct.

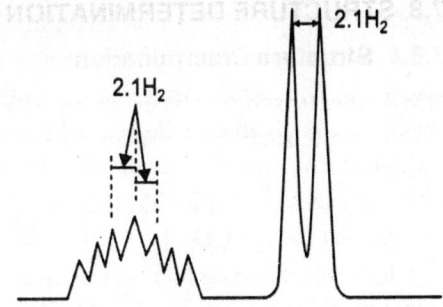

Fig. 7.21. NMR spectrum of σ-comple-xed carbocation of hexamethyl benzene in Hf at room temperature.

$$CH_3OH_A + CH_3OH_B \rightleftharpoons CH_3OH_B + CH_3OH_A$$

7.10 Chemical Exchange

Unlike methanol, ethanol shows spin–spin splitting at room temperature.

$$\underset{q}{CH_3}—\underset{m}{CH_2}—\underset{t}{OH}$$

We see a quartet due to methyl protons, the CH_2 protons couple with both OH and methyl protons appearing as an octet (Fig. 7.22). Obviously, in this case the OH exchange between the ethanol molecules is very slow compared to NMR-time scale. In order to prove this, we can either follow the variable temperature NMR technique i.e. we can increase the temperature or we can increase the rate of the exchange by addition of acid into it i.e. by chemical exchange.

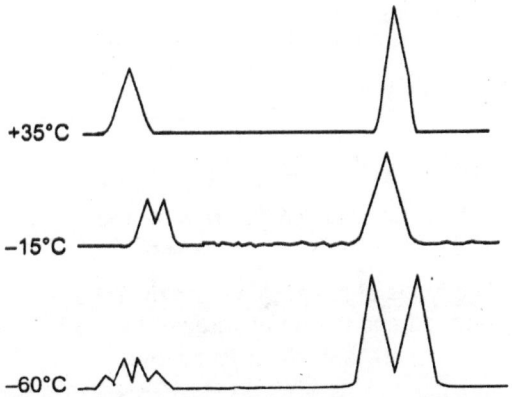

Fig. 7.22. NMR spectrum of methanol CH_3OH as a function of temperature.

$$CH_3CH_2OH_A + CH_3CH_2OH_B \rightleftharpoons CH_3CH_2OH_B + CH_3CH_2OH_A$$

Because of the following equilibrium, the OH-proton undergoes fast chemical exchange with the $H^{\oplus}$ added.

$$CH_3CH_2OH_A + H_B^{\oplus} \rightleftharpoons CH_3CH_2OH_B + H_A^{\oplus}$$

The net result is that the exchange rate being faster than the NMR time scale, the spin–spin splitting between CH_2 and OH is not seen by the NMR camera. So, the CH_2 octet is reduced to a mere quartet due to coupling with CH_3 protons alone. Similarly, the OH proton's multiplicity is reduced from a triplet to a singlet. Chemical change has therefore been prevented because of interchange of H_A and H_B. This interchange becomes faster with each addition of acid such that only 10^{-5} mol of acid is enough to decouple the OH completely from the $-CH_2-$ protons.

The OH_A proton remains attached to oxygen for a period (10^{-6} s) that is much less than the time period during which it remains unattached to oxygen. So, the OH proton cannot couple with the $-CH_2-$ proton during that small time period. What happens is that supposing an OH proton in one molecule was in the α spin state, it gets fast exchanged with a proton of OH of another molecule in the β spin state. Thus, the CH_2 spin sees a rapid blur of α and β spin states of the proton on oxygen. The NMR time scale for this exchange is given by 1/2. 22 J where J is equal to Δν, the difference in resonant frequencies of the α and β spin states of the proton for the CH_2.

It should be noted that we talk of ethyl alcohol being intermolecularly hydrogen bonded that:.

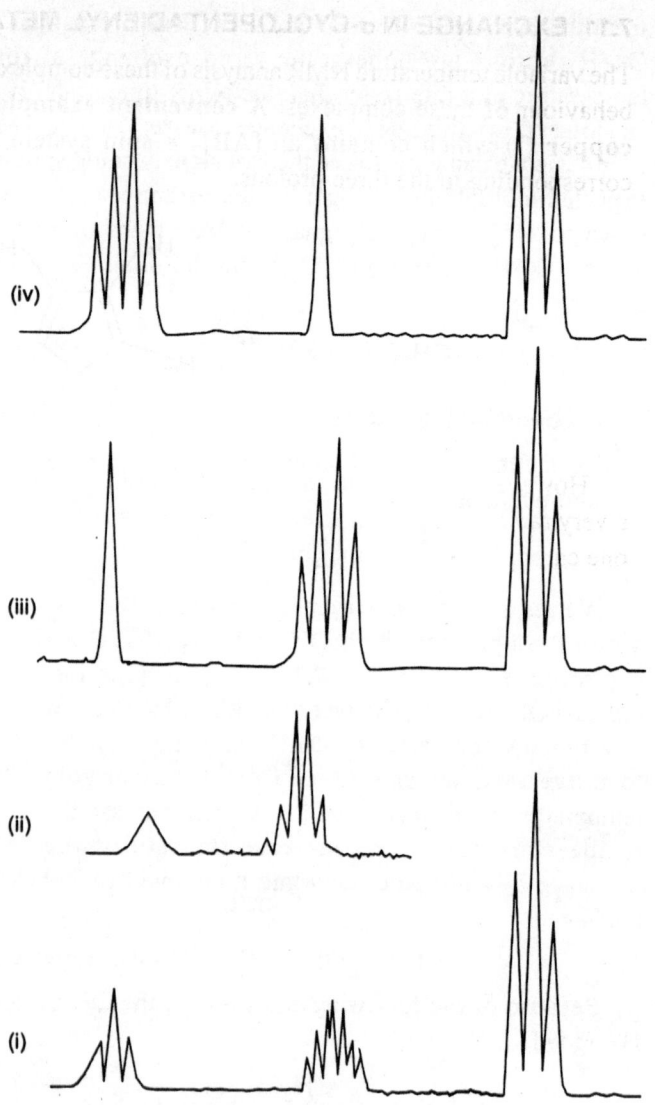

Hydrogen-bonded   Non-hydrogen bonded

Two types of molecules – the hydrogen-bonded and the non-hydrogen bonded in any sample of an alcohol

That does not mean all the molecules of ethyl alcohol in a sample are hydrogen-bonded. In fact, the degree of this special bonding is always found to be lesser than one hundred percent. What implication does that have for us from the point of view of its NMR spectrum? It simply means that there are two typs of ethyl alcohol molecules in a given sample of it – one, which are hydrogen-bonded and the

Fig. 7.23. NMR spectrum of ethyl alcohol (1) ultra pure, (2) and (3) with acid added, (4) 70% solution in $CDCl_3$.

other that are non-hydrogen-bonded as shown in Fig. 7.24. That means, two types of OH protons will have different Larmor frequencies but we only get one resonance in the spectrum. This is probably because the interchange or the exchange of protons between/within the two types of molecules is such that the signal observed is the concentration-weighted average of the expected two chemical shifts. This answers the question as to why upon addition of a *non-protonated* solvent into the alcohol, the chemical shift of the OH proton shifts to low field. This is because the extent of hydrogen-bonding is lowered.

7.11 EXCHANGE IN σ-CYCLOPENTADIENYL METAL COMPLEXES

The variable temperature NMR analysis of these complexes quite clearly sheds new light on the structural behaviour of these complexes. **A convenient example is σ-cyclopentadienyl (triethyl phosphine) copper** (I) which contains an $[AB]_2 \times$ spin system and therefore should give three resonances corresponding to the three protons.

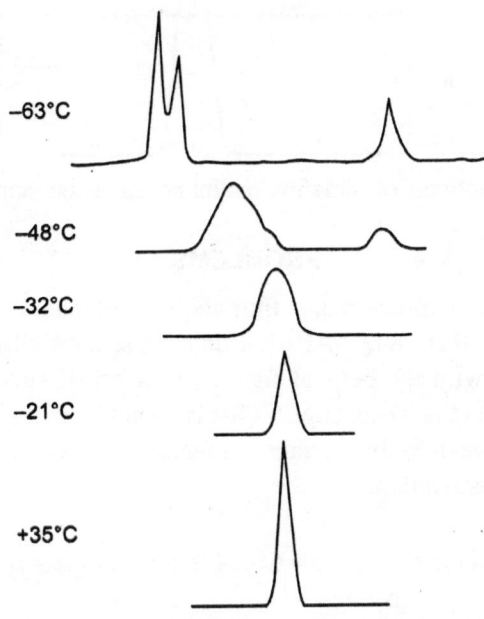

However, it shows only one peak in its PMR spectrum. In other words, it means that there is occurring a very rapid exchange at a rate faster than the NMR time scale and copper exchanges its position with one carbon to after another in a manner such that all the five protons become equivalent.

Fig. 7.24. The NMR spectrum of σ-cyclopentadienyl (triethylphosphine) copper (I) as a function of temperature.

7.12 Exchange in Dimethyl Cadmum, Cd(CH₃)₂

When the NMR of dimethyl cadmium, is recorded at room temperature, then besides the single peak due to equivalent protons, two satellites are obtained around this peak due to spin-spin splitting with the isotopic ¹¹³Cd and ¹¹¹Cd nuclei, the naturally occurring isotopes of Cd which have a natural abundance of 12% and 13% respectively. However, when the temperature is increased, the satellites broaden and then disappear under the major methyl peak. These changes are recorded in Fig. 7.25.

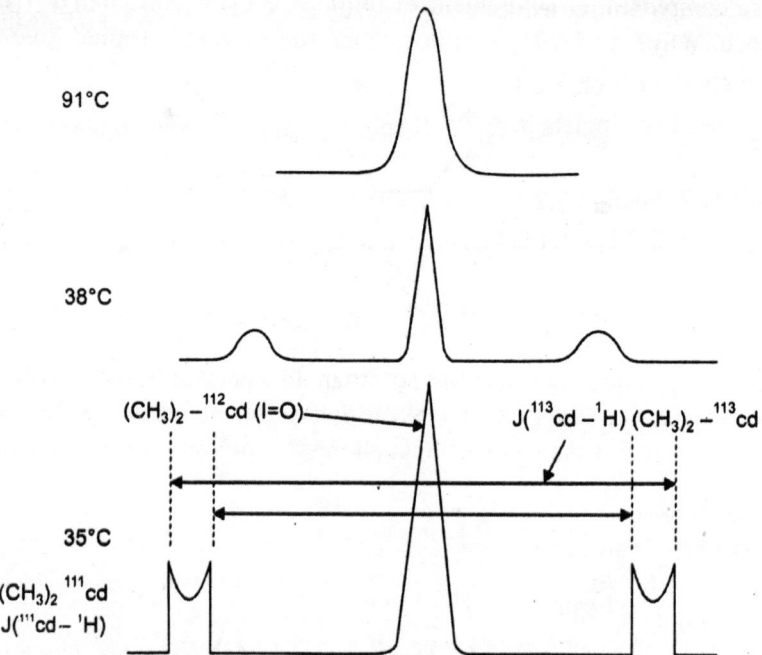

91°C

38°C

$(CH_3)_2 - {}^{112}cd \ (I=O)$ ────────→ $J({}^{113}cd - {}^1H) \ (CH_3)_2 - {}^{113}cd$

35°C

$(CH_3)_2 \ {}^{111}cd$
$J({}^{111}cd - {}^1H)$

Fig. 7.25. NMR spectra of dimethyl cadmium as a function of temperature.

PROBLEMS

1. NMR spectroscopy can capture many time-dependent phenomena as they occur but i.r.-spectroscopy cannot do that. Why? At what time scale does NMR work compared to optical spectroscopies? Show with the help of figures, how NMR spectra differ at slow exchange, intermediate exchange and fast exchange? What is meant by coalescence point? How can we get the precise relation between exchange rate and temperature as well as the rate constants K^1 and $1/K^1$ and the energy of activation.

   Hint: See Section 7.1.

2. Why does N,N-Dimethylacetamide show two N-methyl singlets at r.t. whereas it only shows one sharp peak at higher temperature.

   Hint: See Example 2, Section 7.1.

3. N,N-Dimethylmethane thiamide shows two methyl singlets at r.t. but only one at higher temperature. Why?

   Hint: See Example 4, Section 7.1.

4. N,N-Dimethylcarbamate exhibits two methyl singlets at r.t. but only one at higher temperature. Why?

   Hint: See Example 4, Section 7.1.

5. N-Methyl–2,4,6–trinitroaniline shows only one peak for the meta protons at 35°C but at lower temperature, we see two doublets for these proton. Why?

6. p-Nitroso N,N-dimethylaniline exhibits two singlets at r.t. but only one at higher temperature for the methyl group. Why?

   Hint: See Example 6, Section 7.2.1.

7. Methylnitrite shows two singlets in its PMR spectrum at r.t. but only one at higher temperature. Why?

   Hint: See Example 7, Section 7.2.1.

8. ^{1}H NMR spectrum of 2,2,3,3–tetrachlorobutane shows only one signal at r.t. but two signals at – 45°C. Why?

   Hint: See Example 7, Section 7.2.1.

9. t-Butylcycloheptane shows three methyl singlets at r.t. but only one at – 126°C. Why?

   Hint: See Intext Exercise 7.1.

10. The NMR spectrum of cyclohexane derivative, C_6HD_{11} shows one peak at r.t. but two at – 60°C. Why?

    Hint: See Section 7.3.2.

11. Two broad signals are obtained in the ^{1}H NMR spectrum of [18]–Annulene at r.t. but only one at 100°C. Why?

    Hint: See Section 7.3.3.

12. The N–H protons in meso-tetraphenylporphyrins appear as a single peak at 8.75 ppm at r.t. but as two separate peaks at – 60°C. Why?

    Hint: See Section 7.4.

13. Bullvalene exhibits only one peak at 80°C but two broad signals at " 80°C. Why

    Hint: See Section 7.4.1.

14. The ^{1}H NMR spectrum of 2–methyloxepine shows one singlet due to both methyl groups at r.t. but two different signals at – 125°C. Why?

    Hint: See Section 7.4.2.

15. Show the existence of keto-enol tautomerism in ethylacetoacetate.

    Hint: See Example 2, Section 7.5

16. How can you study annomerization in carbohydrates like lactose?

    Hint: See Section 7.6.

17. (a) Trimethylaluminium shows one peak at 0°C but two peaks at – 55°C. Why?

    (b) Show the application of NMR technique in studying exchange in organometallic chemistry by taking the example of trimethyl aluminium.

    Hint: See section 7.1.

18. The ^{1}H NMR spectrum of tetramethylallene iron tetracarbonyl complex shows only one signal at r.t. but three signals at – 60°C. Why?

    Hint: See Section 7.2.

19. The NMR spectrum of allyl magnesium bromide shows a quintet at 6.2 ppm and a doublet at 2.5 ppm in the relative ratio (1:4). What information does this reveal regarding the spectrum of this reagent?

    Hint: See Section 7.3.

20. Give an example to show the application of NMR spectroscopy to structure determination of carbocations.

    Hint: See Section 7.8.1.

21. Give an example to show the application of NMR spectroscopy to investigate proton shifts in carbocations.

    Hint: See Section 7.8.2.

22. The NMR spectrum of methanol at r.t. shows only two singlets but a quartet and a doublet at − 60°C. Why?

    Hint: See Section 7.

23. The NMR spectrum of an ultra pure sample of ethylalcohol shows a triplet, a doublet quartet (octet) and a triplet at r.t. but a singlet, a quartet and a triplet in presence of a small amount of acid added into the sample. Explain.

    Hint: See Section 7.10.

24. Two types of molecules - the hydrogen-bonded and the non-hydrogen bonded exist in ethyl alcohol, so we should see two different OH peaks. However, we only see one resonance for these in the NMR spectrum. Why?

    Hint: See Section 7.10.

25. The NMR spectrum of σ-cyclopentadienyl (triethyl phosphine) copper (I) shows only one peak although it contains three non-equivalent sets of protons. Explain.

    Hint: See Section 7.11.

26. The NMR spectrum of dimethylcadmium shows satellites around a single peak due to protons. Why?

    Hint: See Section 7.12.

27. Explain the use of NMR spectroscopy in the fluxional inorganic molecules.

    Hint: Discuss the following:
    (i) Trimethyl aluminium (see Section 7.7.1).
    (ii) Alkenes-metal carbonyl complexes like tetramethyl allene iron carbonyl (see Section 7.7.2).
    (iii) Exchange in Grignard Reagent like allyl magnesium bromide (see Section 7.7.3).
    (iv) Exchange in σ-Cyclopentadienyl metal complexes (see Section 7.11).
    (v) Exchange in Dimethyl cadmium (see Section 7.12).

8

Pharmaceutical Applications of ¹H NMR Spectroscopy

Although, we have seen the power of ¹H NMR for structure elucidation of organic compounds, we would learn here some special applications of this technique.

8.1 DETECTION OF IMPURITY IN DRUGS

If in the ¹H NMR spectrum of the known drug compound, we discover extra peaks, clearly the test sample is impure and therefore one can go for purification of the compound. For example, if an extra peak is seen in the spectrum of antipyretic drug paracetamol (crocin - trade name), the drug needs to be purified further before being distributed for sale as there are dangers that the impure drug might increase the fever of the patient instead of lowering it down to normal body temperature.

8.2 INVESTIGATION OF RELATIVE AMOUNTS OF COMPONENTS IN A MIXTURE SUCH AS ASPIRIN AND PARACETAMOL

The relative amounts as a molar ratio of aspirin and phenacetin in a mixture is determined by measuring the integration of the two sharp singlets at 2.1 and 2.3 δ, ppm due to the acetyl methyl groups in phenacetin and aspirin respectively. Aspirin and phenacetin are present in equimolar amounts in the spectrum (Fig. 8.1).

8.3 MOLECULAR MASS OF AN UNKNOWN COMPOUND

This can be determined by dissolving in the sample solution a standard compound containing a common proton group (such as methyl etc.). What is done next is to that the intensities of the recognisable peaks

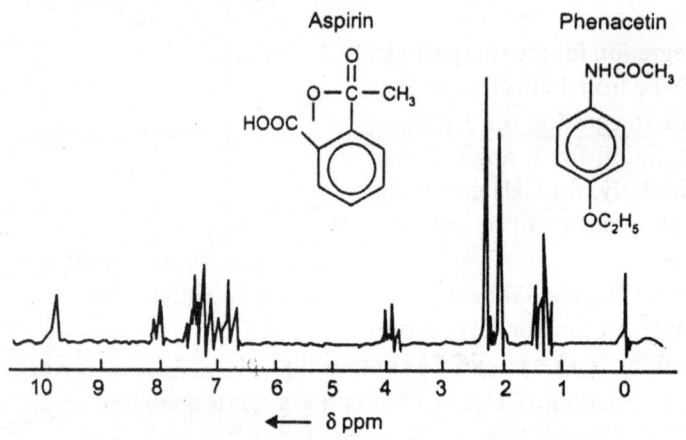

Fig. 8.1. ^{1}H NMR spectrum of a mixture of Aspirin and Phenacetin.

of the test sample I_t as well as the standard I_s are noted in the spectrum obtained. Then by using the following equation, the molecular mass is readily obtained:

$$\frac{M_t}{M_s} = \frac{I_t \times n_s \times W_t}{I_s \times n_t \times W_s}$$

wherein n_s and n_t are respectively the number of protons contributing to the recognizible peak in the test sample as well as the standard. W_t and W_s represent weights in mg of the test and standard respectively.

Hexamethylcyclotrisiloxane is the standard normally used as its resonance at 9 Hz is distinctly removed from other usual absorptions.

Note: It can rightly be concluded that this formula presupposes that the unknown compound exists in the monomer state.

8.4 DETERMINATION OF THE PERCENTAGE OF HYDROGEN

This is done by mixing the unknown compound with a weighed quantity of a standard compound with a known hydrogen percentage. Integration of the spectrum then enables one to determine the percentage of hydrogen straight away.

8.5 DETERMINATION OF ETHANOL CONTENT IN ALCOHOLIC LIQUOR

In many countries the alcoholic liquors must contain at least 40% alcohol. In order to verify this the analysis of liquors being sold in the market is done via NMR analysis.

First of all, the PMR spectrum is recorded. It shows three sets of peaks; one a triplet at 1.2 ppm due to methyl protons of the ethyl group, another a quartet at 3.8 ppm due to the methyl group. The third sharp singlet appears at δ 5.00 ppm, due to both OH and H_2O protons. So, if we can calculate the integration for OH proton, then subtraction of this value from the total integration at 5 ppm gives us the real integration due to water protons (Fig. 8.2).

Suppose the integration for the triplet due to CH_3 protons at δ 1.2 ppm is x mm, and that for quartet due to CH_2 group at δ 3.8 ppm is y mm.

Let z mm be the integration for the sharp singlet centres at δ 5.0 ppm arising from both OH and H_2O protons. As x mm is the integration for 3 protons in CH_3 group, the integration for 1 single proton will be equal to $x/3$. Similarly, for CH_2 group, the integration for one single proton will be half of y mm $= y/2$ mm $= x/3$ mm.

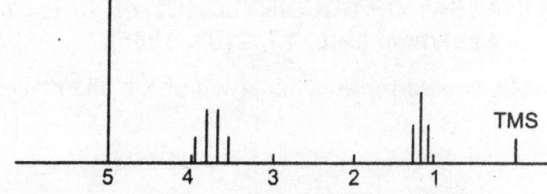

Fig. 8.2. Proton NMR spectrum of Ethanol in alcoholic liquid.

Now, as integration for OH should be equal to integration for one single proton for CH_2 group $= y/2$. Hence, integration for $H_2O = z - y/2$ % composition.

Ratio of water (H_2O): Alcohol (CH_3CH_2OH) based upon the number of protons present in H_2O (i.e. 2H) and ethyl alcohol (2H, due to CH_2 group $= y$ mm) $= (z - y/2) : y$.

However, the % composition cannot be correct as the relative molar masses (RMMs) and densities of water and the alcohol are different. While density of water $= 1.00$ g mL^{-1} that of alcohol is 0.968 mL^{-1}.

So, $\dfrac{\text{Mass of water}}{\text{mass of alcohol}} = \dfrac{(z - y/2) \times 18/I}{(y \times 46)/0.0.96}$ $\quad \therefore \% \dfrac{46y/0.96}{46y/0.96 \times 18\,(z - y/2)} \times 100$

where 46 is the RMM of alcohol while 18 is the RMM of water.

8.6 INVESTIGATION OF INTERACTIONS BETWEEN DRUG MOLECULES AND PROTEINS

NMR spectroscopy has been utilized to investigate the interactions between drug molecules and proteins like enzymes, proteolipids etc. Binding of physo-stigmine enzyme to acetylcholine-esterase has also been studied. Similarly, binding of atropine analogues to acetyl choline-esterase has been studied. Interactions between cholinergic ligands and housefly brain have also been explored with the aid of NMR spectroscopy.

8.7 COMPLEXATION OF CAFFEINE WITH L-TRYPTOPHAN (Kato G, Mol. Pharmacol. 8; 575, 1972; ibid. 582, 1972; ibid. 7, 33, 1971)

^{1}H NMR spectroscopy has been exploited to study the complexation of caffeine with L-tryptophan wherein it was shown that caffeine interacts with L-tryptophan at a molar ratio of 1:1 by parallel stacking. Complexation was shown to be a consequence of polarisation and π-π interactions of the aromatic rings. Stacking involved benzene ring of the tryptophan getting located above the pyrimidine ring (Nishijo, J., Yonetani, I., Uvamoto, E., J. Pharm. Sci. 79, 18, 1990) of caffeine, while the pyrrole ring of L-tryptophan above the imidazole ring of caffeine:

8.8 ASSAY OF SUCCINYLCHOLINE INJECTIONS (Hanna, G.M. and Lau-Cam C.A.; Analytical Lett., 18, 2183, 1985))

NMR is used for direct analysis of the pharmaceutically important succinylcholine injections.

$$\begin{bmatrix} CH_2COOCH_2CH_2\overset{\oplus}{N}Me_3 \\ | \\ CH_2COOCH_2CH_2\overset{\oplus}{N}Me_4 \end{bmatrix} 2Cl^{\ominus}$$

In the assay of this compound (which is a nondepolarizing neuromuscular blocking agent), a known amount of acetamide is added as an internal standard to a freeze-dried sample of succinylcholine chloride injection. A solution of the mixture is obtained in D_2O and subjected to analysis by NMR. The relative integral intensities of the singlet at 3.27 ppm due to 18 methyl protons in succinylcholine and that at 2.01 ppm arising from 3 methyl protons of acetamide (CH_3CONH_2) are the peaks of concern to us. Thus, the amount of succinylcholine chloride present in the sample can be obtained by using the equation:

$$C = \frac{W}{V} \times \frac{I_s}{I_a} \times \frac{EW_s}{EW_a}$$

wherein W is the weight in mg of the standard acetamide, V is the volume in mL containing succinylcholine chloride. EW_s is the molecular mass of succinylcholine chloride divided by 18 (the number of 18 protons due to 6 methyl protons) while EW_a represents the molecular mass of acetamide divided by 3 (the number of protons in the methyl group).

Note: In this method, acetamide is used as a standard as it does not react with succinylcholine chloride. It was primarily selected as the standard as it contains a methyl group (whose CH_3 singlet absorbs at a distinct position at 2.01 ppm from those of the six methyl protons of succinylcholine chloride that resonate at 3.27 ppm). The methyl group is common to both the test sample as well as acetamide. That is why this compound was chosen as the standard. Although there are 18 protons in the test sample due to 6 methyls and only 3 protons (due to $1CH_3$) in acetamide, still one can easily equalise the intensity per proton by dividing the intensity of the signal of the methyl protons in the test sample by 18 and that in acetamide by 3.

8.9 ASSAY OF DIPHENYLHYDRAMINE (Benadryl) HYDROCHLORIDE CONTENT IN CAPSULE FORMULATION, $Ph_2COCH_2CH_2NMe_2.HCl$

This is done in a manner similar to that described for succinylchloline injection. Here t-butyl alcohol is used as an internal standard. By using the equation, concentration of the test sample in the capsule can be determined easily.

$$C = W \times \frac{I_d}{I_{BuOH}} \times \frac{EW_d}{EW_{BuOH}}$$

I_d stands for the integral intensity of the 6 N-methyl protons of diphenyl-hydramine peak at 2.85 ppm. BuOH stands for the integral intensity of the 9 methyl protons of test butanol. EW_d stands for the molecular mass (291.9) of the sample divided by 6 and EW_{BuOH} represents the molecular mass (74.1) of test. BuOH divided by 9. It should be noted that Diphenyl hydramine or Benadryl hydrochloride is an ethanolamine antihistamine with significant anticholinergic activity.

Intext Exercise

1. What will be the amount of diphenyl hydramine hydrochloride in a capsule if its solution containing tert butylalcohol as an internal standard) as analyzed by NMR shows peaks at 2.85 and 1.27 ppm in the average relative integral ratio of 1 : 5.88. Formula mass of diphenylhydramine hydrochloride is 291.9 g mol^{-1} and that of tert butyl alcohol is 74.1 g mol^{-1}. Weight of tert butyl alcohol used is 25 mg.

   Solution:

$$C = W \times \frac{I_d}{I_{BuOH}} \times \frac{EW_d}{EW_{BuOH}} = \frac{25 \times 1}{5.88} \times \frac{291.9 \times 9}{74.1 \times 6} = 25 \text{ mg}$$

PROBLEMS

1. Describe some pharmaceutical applications of ^{1}H NMR spectroscopy.
2. How can you do the assay of succinylcholine injections with the aid of ^{1}H NMR spectroscopy?
   Hint: See Section 8.
3. How can you do assay of diphenylhydramine hydrochloride content in capsule formulation by ^{1}H NMR spectroscopy?
   Hint: See Section 9.
4. How can you determine the relative quantities of aspirin and phenacetin using ^{1}H NMR spectroscopy?
   Hint: See Section 2.

9

NMR Relaxation, T_1 and T_2 Measurement

9.1 SPINS AS VECTORS

Each nuclear spin can be represented by a magnetic vector and its strength is determined by γ. This is called vector model. In fact, this model is a very simple model that helps us to understand the NMR phenomenon, which is a quantum phenomenon, by application of laws of classical physics before we can understand the true meaning and mechanistic picture of NMR phenomenon.

9.2 ALIGNMENT WITH B_0 AND NET MAGNETIZATION

When a sample is immersed in an applied field B_0, then according to statistical mechanics, the spin of the assemblage of protons orient themselves with respect to the applied field in two possible ways. Some align themselves into a precessing cone at an angle of 45° from +Z axis in the directions of and around the field. We call that the α-state precession. Similarly, other spins orient themselves in a cone precessing around the field but in the opposite direction at an angle of 45° from –Z axis what we call as the β-spin state. These two spin states occur in thermal equilibrium, of course, with a slight Boltzman excess in the lower energy α-spin state.

There is **one thing in common** within both the α- and the β-spin cones. That is all the spins are rotating with **random phase.** That is to say they are pointing in different direction at any point in time such that some are in $+x$, some in $-x$, others are in $+y$, still others in $-y$ axis and so on in any possible direction (Fig. 9.1). In other words, the spins are randomly oriented or that spins are **not in phase coherence** in both the cones.

Now, as per statistical mechanics, all vectors, let us say $N/2$ except δ out of a force of $N/2 + \delta$ vectors in the upper α-cone along +Z axis will have vectors numbering $(N/2 – S)$ in the δ-cone pointing in exactly the opposite direction in the –Z direction. Therefore, these will cancel out each other. However, as we have a slight population excess in the α-cone, we would still be left with the spins numbering 2δ, which of course, as already discussed is equal to 1 is 10^6 nuclei.

214

Let us now concentrate upon the population excess vectors as it is these which lead to a signal in NMR phenomenon. It needs to be emphasised again that these excess vectors are pointing in all possible directions in the cone as explained above. There is equal distribution as per statistical mechanics and there is no preferred direction or phase. We can say that the vectors or the spins are **non-coherent** or are in random phase.

Spins point in all possible directions $+z, -z, +x, -x, +y, -y$ within both the precessing cones.

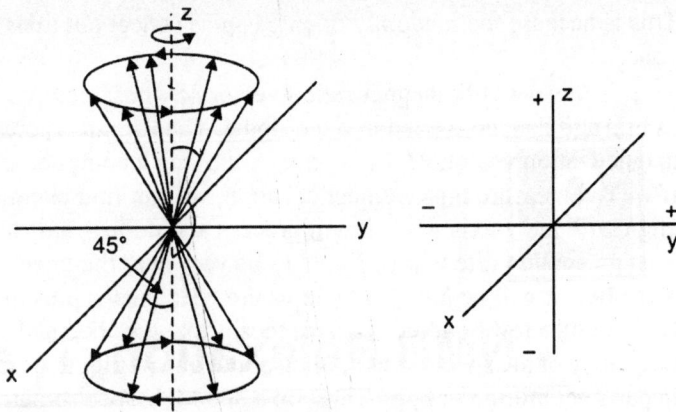

Fig. 9.1. Incoherence (no phase coherence) or random phases on application of a magnetic field B_0.

9.3 RF PULSE CREATES COHERENCE AMONG SPIN VECTORS

The effect of RF pulse is to create a team work among these spin vectors. In other words, when a suitable RF pulse is applied, then all these spin vectors show what we can call as a team-work in that they are forced to point in the same direction at any particular point in time. That is to say instead of being randomly oriented, they are now oriented in the same direction, in the same phase (Fig. 9.2). Or that the **phase incoherence** (randomness in phase) has been converted into **phase coherence** (order in phase). This team work of the spins has the effect that their individual vectors now add up. The result is the net magnetization also called **bulk magnetization, M,** rotates in the same direction that is counterclockwise direction with same Larmor frequency in the cone. In the absence of the pulse, the bulk magnetization is not detectable. The reason is clear that the spins are incoherent that there is phase randomness among the spins in the cone. That is why there is no (bulk) magnetization worth detection.

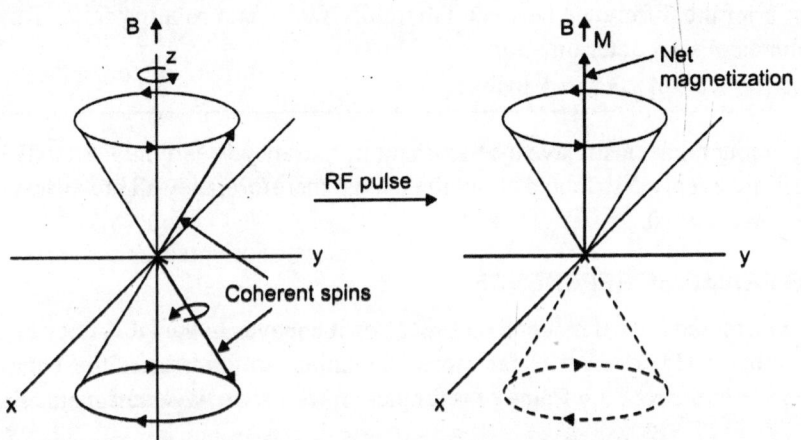

Fig. 9.2. Coherent spins : all spins pointing in the same direction (phase) at any particular point in time during application of Rf pulse.

This is because the randomly oriented spins cancel out their motions due to random distribution in the cone.

It is this net bulk magnetization vector M whose component along the $+z$-axis, Mz that is detected as FID and then converted into the signal. The RF pulse actually measures the z component of the bulk magnetization vector, M by creating a moving z component out of this stationary bulk magnetization. If we can measure this net magnetization, we can find chemical shift. This can be done by forcing it to align with the y-axis when it will precess about the Z axis and the precession rate will be determined. This precession rate will be found to be very near the operating frequency of the spectrometer, says at 800 MHz, it will be $800 \pm x$ MHz where x Hz means plus or minus a few hundred Hz. This distance x Hz is about a few hundred Hz. This means that the chemical shifts are very small compared to operating frequency of the spectrometer, often about one millionth of the total rate. That is why, they are reported in parts per million or ppm. Thus, on a 800 MHz spectrometer, 1 ppm is equal to a mere 800 Hz, 2 ppm being 2×800 Hz = 1600 Hz and so on.

The question now is how to force the net magnetization Mz align with the y-axis so that the chemical shift could be measured. Of course, it also needs to be noted that it would certainly be very difficult to follow such a fast precession of Mz with our eyes. The net magnetization Mz precesses about the fixed Z axis at nearly the operational frequency of the spectrometer say about 800 MHz at 800 MHz. Here the fixed Z axis is actually represents the Z axis of the fixed frame or also called "Laboratory frame". So, you see, it will be difficult to detect the Mz along the y-axis in the "laboratory frame". Therefore, what can we do to detect Mz easily. We would like to detect the chemical shift i.e. x Hz out of $(800 \pm x)$ *MHz straight away. Can that be done? Yes. How? By using a "rotating frame" of reference.* In the rotating frame, the precession rate is determined in terms of chemical shift itself in Hz straightaway (which is of course, is converted into ppm). This is what is plotted in one-dimensional NMR spectrum against intensity. Evidently, when a sample contains more than one kind of proton, there will be more than one precessional rate and we will have to measure all these precessional rates or chemical shifts, giving us the corresponding number of peaks in the spectrum.

Intext Question

1. Explain in brief the difference between laboratory frame and rotating frame from the point of view of chemical shift determination.

   Hint: Describe section 9.3 as an answer.

Individual spinning nuclei also have a component $\mu_{x, y}$, transverse to the field axis in the horizontal xy plane. As these are evenly distributed about the z-axis, therefore, they all are average to zero. That is to say $Mx = My = Mx - y = 0$.

9.4 ROTATING FRAME OF REFERENCE

So far, we have considered the net magnetization M_0, as it behaves in the laboratory or stationary frame of cartesian references. However, it is far more convenient to investigate the behaviour of the net magnetization vector in the rotating frame of reference in which we have designated the x and y axis as x' and y' axes.

The rotating frame of reference as per its name is rotating around the z-axis, it is not stationary. The x' and y' axes in this frame precess about the Z-axis at a rate of the operating frequency of the NMR instrument (say 800 MHz). **The precession in this frame is not nearly as fast as that in the laboratory frame. In fact, the precessional rate is just the chemical shift rate.** A magnetic vector that rotates around the z-axis with the velocity of the rotating frame, would appear stationary in this rotating frame of reference (Fig. 9.3). A magnetic vector that travels at a velocity faster than that of the rotating frame would rotate clockwise about the z-axis (Fig. 9.4). A transverse magnetic vector that rotates around z-axis with a velocity lesser than that of the rotating frame would appear counter-clockwise about the z-axis (Fig. 9.5).

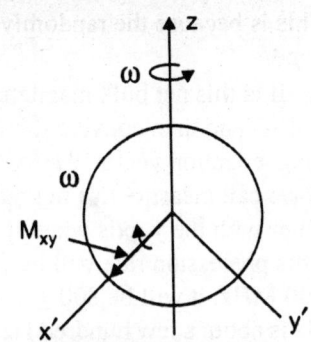

Fig. 9.3. A stationary transverse vector M_{xy} as ω of $M_{xy} = \omega$ of rotating frame of reference.

If a coil that passes an alternating current having the same Larmor frequency as that of the rotating frame is moved about the rotating coordinates system, then it induces a pulsed magnetic field B_1, around the x'-axis when the alternating current is turned on and off (Fig. 9.6a).

What is the effect of the pulsed magnetic field B_1 around the x'-axis on magnetic vector M_z in rotating frame versus laboratory frame?

The effect of the pulsed magnetic field B_1 around the x'-axis is that the nuclear spin vector behave in a manner such that the net magnetization vector M_0, is forced to rotate (precess) about the direction of this field B_1. At what angle, does the M_0 now rotate about B_1? This is governed by the equation:

$$\theta = 2\pi y \tau B_1$$

where τ is the duration of the pulse and Y is the gyromagneto ratio.

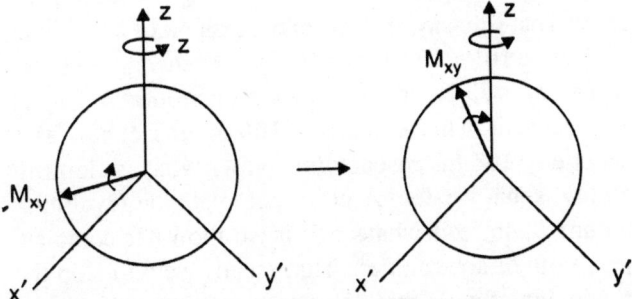

Fig. 9.4. A clockwise rotating transverse vector M_{xy}. The M_{xy} rotates clockwise as its velocity is higher than that of the rotating frame of reference.

Let us understand this effect in more details. In the rotating frame of reference, when a pulsed magnetic field is applied along the x'-axis, this field will have a tendency to force the bulk magnetization M_0 into the x'-direction. However, M_0 just does not get turn around into the x'-direction. Rather, like a gyroscope, M_0 starts precessing about the x'-axis (see Fig. 9.7).

Supposing the strength of B_1, pulsed magnetic field was 2.5×10^{-4} T, and B_0

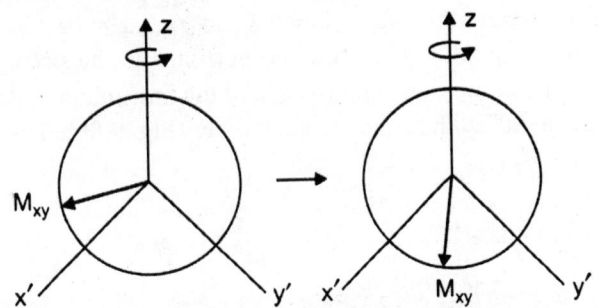

Fig. 9.5. A counter-clockwise rotating transverse vector M_{xy}. The Mxy rotates counter-clockwise as its velocity is smaller than that of the rotating frame of reference.

was 100 MHz, then, the rate of the precession of B_1 around x'-axis will be :

$$\frac{\text{Strength of } B_1}{\text{Strength of } B_0} = \frac{2.5 \times 10^{-4}}{2.5} = 10^{-4}$$

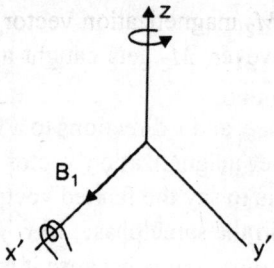

Fig. 9.6a. Generation of pulsed magnetic field B_1 along x'-axis in the rotating frame of reference.

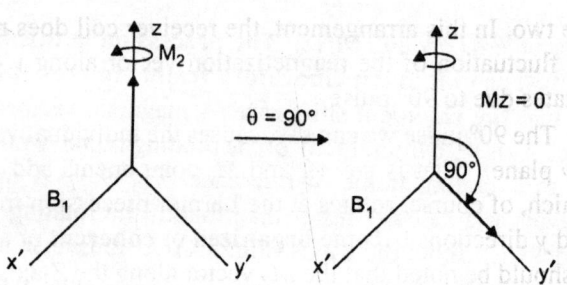

Fig. 9.6b. Rotation of M_z down to y' axis upon application of a 90° pulse in the rotating frame of reference.

So, the M_0 will precess at 10^{-4} times the precessional frequency caused by the main field B_0 (pointed at Z-axis). That is to say, the rate of precession of M_0 around B_1 will be $10^8 \times 10^{-4}$ Hz or 10^4 Hz per second. In other words, M_0 will complete a revolution around B_1 in just 10^{-4} seconds. This amounts to 100 microseconds (as 1 second = 10^6 microseconds). Now, what is done in reality is that we do not let M_0 complete the revolution around B_1. Instead, what we do is we allow it to complete just 1/4th of a revolution. That means we will stop the revolution after 25 microseconds i.e. a 90° pulse.

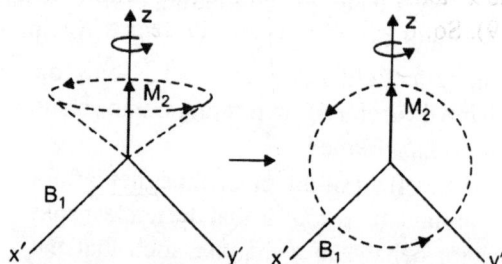

Fig. 9.7a. M_0 along z-direction. (b) When B_1 is applied, M_0 is forced to precess around B_1 along x'- direction.

The effect of a 90° pulse is shown in Fig. 9.8a in which we see that M_0 has moved by an angle of 90°. It needs to be emphasised here that the duration in microseconds (μs) of a 90° pulse will depend upon the strength of the pulsed magnetic field B_1 applied along the x'-direction. It was just for the sake of discussion that we assumed B_1 to be 2.5×10^{-4} T. Further, the rate of precession of M_0 aroud B_1 along x'-direction is directly proportional to the strength of the applied field.

The geometrical arrangement of the transmitter coil (x'-direction) and the receiver coil (y'-direction) is set at 90° with respect to each other (Fig. 9.8b). This is done to prevent any direct coupling between

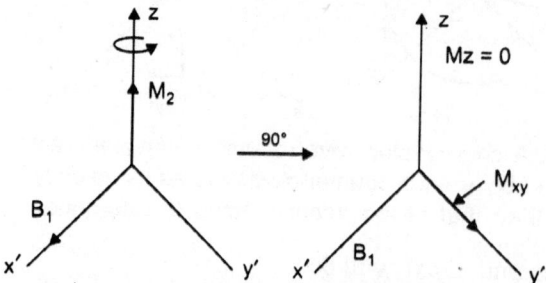

Fig. 9.8a. Effect of 90° pulse on M_z in rotating frame.

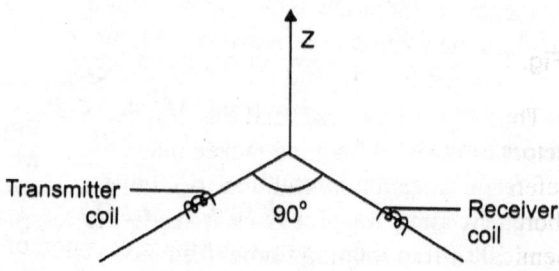

Fig. 9.8b. Geometrical arrangement of transmitter and receiver coils at 90°.

the two. In this arrangement, the receiver coil does not record the M_Z magnetization vector as there is no fluctuation of the magnetization vector along y'-direction. However, M_Z gets caught as M_{xy} as it rotates due to 90° pulse.

The 90° pulse we can say, causes the individual vector spins in the x and y directions to add up in the x-y plane. That is the M_x and M_y components add up to form a net magnetization vector in the M_{xy} which, of course, rotates at the Larmor precession frequency. That is to say the fanned vectors in the x and y directions become **organized** or **coherent** or are distributed in the same phase, in x–y direction. It should be noted that the M_Z vector along the Z-axis is not directly measurable because it is stationary and does not rotate. Therefore, it has to be detected by tipping it around.

So, in the rotating frame, when a 90° pulse is applied along the x'-axis, it rotates M_Z, the net magnetization vector by 90° about x' axis such that the net magnetization rotates down to y'-axis.

However, in the laboratory or the stationary frame of reference, when a 90° pulse is applied along the x'-axis, it forces net magnetization vector, M_Z to **spiral down** around the z-axis to xy-plane (Fig. 9.9). So, it will be difficult to detect M_Z along y-axis in the laboratory frame.

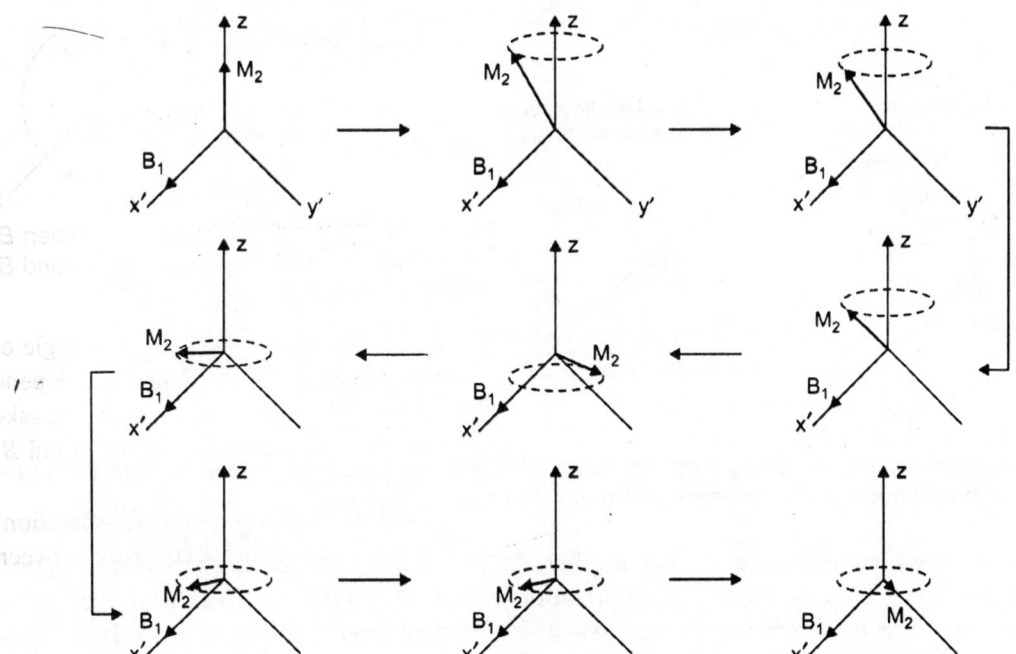

Fig. 9.9. Spiralling down of M_Z net magnetization vector to check direction on application of B_1.

Thus, It can be concluded that it is much more convenient to investigate the behaviour of nuclear vectors towards the applied pulsed magnetic field. That is why, a rotating frame of reference is used in preference to stationary (laboratory) frame of reference in FT NMR spectroscopy. Further, while in the laboratory frame, M_Z precesses at nearly the operating frequency, say $(800 \pm x)$ MHz where XHz is the chemical shift in rotating frame, the precession rate is the chemical shift value rather than the operating frequency i.e. x Hz and not $800 \pm x$ Hz. It is the chemical shift x in Hz which after conversion into ppm is plotted against intensity in the NMR spectrum.

9.5 EFFECT OF THE RF PULSE: DETECTING THE SIGNAL

The net or the bulk magnetization vector M that is acting along B_0 is very small, and undetectable. In order to detect it, we have to perturb the system as already mentioned.

A RF pulse is applied with the larmor frequency ν_0, along the x'-axis in the rotating frame of reference for a short period and then removed abruptly (Fig. 9.10). This pulse is a pulse magnetic field B_1 rotating in the xy plane at the same Larmor frequency. As B_1 is rotating with the same angular velocity or the frequency ($w_0 = \gamma B_0$), as the nuclei, therefore, it would no longer appear to precess and become stationary and coincident with the applied field (see Fig. 9.11). The magnetic behaviour can now be completely described by a stationary M_0, the bulk magnetization vector.

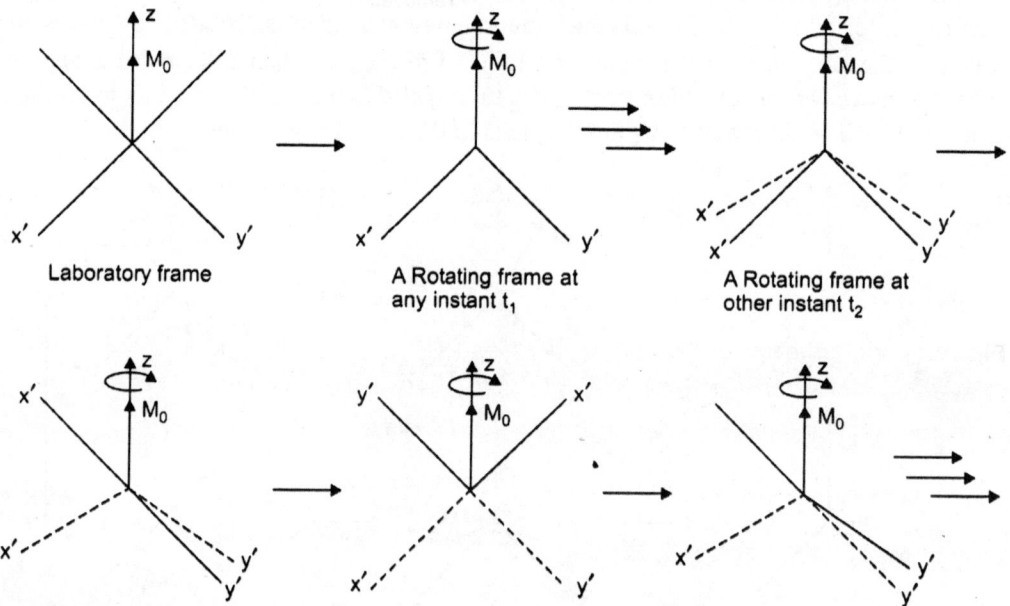

Fig. 9.10. Laboratory frame versus rotating frame of reference about the z-axis. In both the frames M_0 is along the z-direction. M_0 appears stationary in rotating frame.

The nuclei now precess around B_1 also. Further, the precession cone axis gets displaced from the main field axis. The bulk or the net magnetization vector M, rotates around the B_1 vector in a counterclockwise direction from the $+Z$ axis to $-y$, $-z$, $+y$ and finally returns to $+z$ axis. When the pulse is removed abruptly at a time when it ends on the $-y$ axis, it is called a 90° pulse (Fig. 9.12 and 9.13). At this point, there is no difference in the population between α and β spin states such that $M_z = 0$.

As at this point in time i.e. after a 90 pulse, spinning nuclei or vectors do not now all have the identical component in the x–y plane, this gives a resultant magnetization M_{xy} transverse to the main field rotating at the Larmor precession frequency. M_{xy} now induces a radiofrequency current or a FID signal in the coil (Fig. 9.14) that is placed around the sample to detect it. The FID gradually decays to zero as the spin coherence is lost. It should be noted that in case B_1 is not allowed to precess at the same frequency as the nuclei, then under these conditions, the nuclear precession about B_1 is always changing

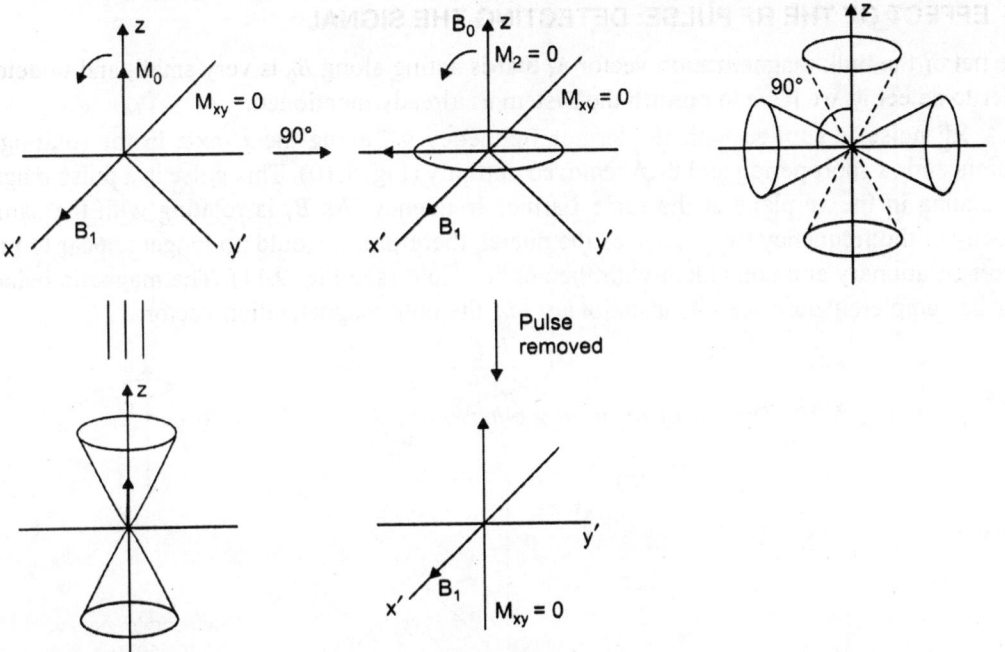

Fig. 9.11. Perturbation of the spin orientation from z-direction on application of a 90° pulse.

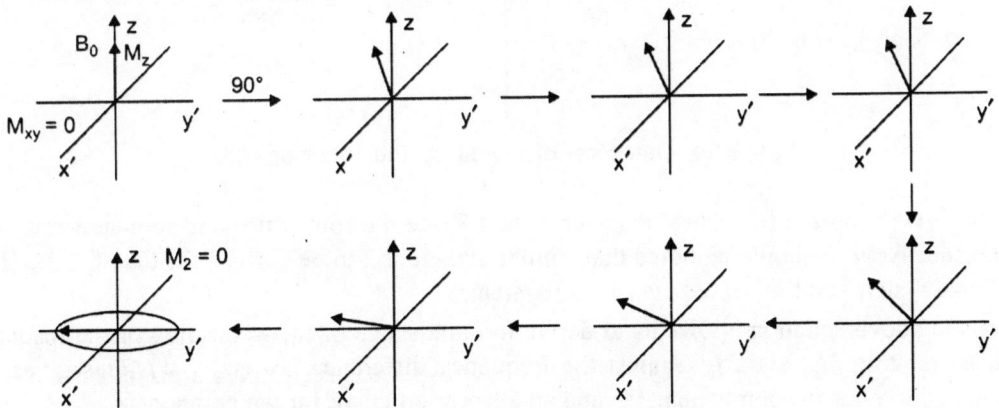

Fig. 9.12. Effect of a 90° pulse : gradual tipping of M_z at 90° w.r. to z-axis.

directions such that M_{xy} can never become significant. Thus, it is necessary to set B_1 such that it precesses at the same frequency as the nuclei, otherwise, the signal cannot be obtained.

Bloch showed that the magnitude of the transverse magnetization My' is given by the following equation :

$$My^1 = \frac{-M_0\, Y\, B_1\, T_2}{1 + T_2^2\, (w_0 - w)^2 + Y^2\, B_1^2\, T_1\, T_2}$$

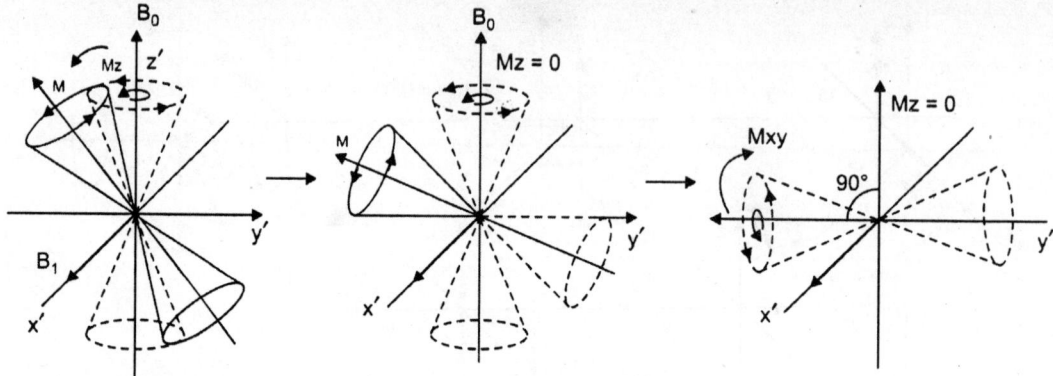

Fig. 9.13. Tipping of M_0 from z-direction to xy direction with cones.

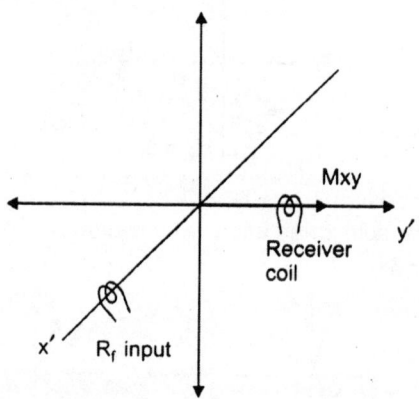

Fig. 9.14. Detection of signal by the receiver coil.

where $w_0 - w$ means the frequency, distance T_1 and T_2 are the spin lattice and spin-spin-relaxation times respectively. It should be noted that similar equations can be derived for the $M_x{}^1$, M_y (fixed coordinate system) and M_x (fixed coordinate systems).

In fact, the above equation allows us to derive the line space of the absorption or the resonance signal on plotting $M_x{}^1$ and $M_y{}^1$ against the frequency difference Dw $(w_0 - w)$. This gives us a dispersion curve for the component M_x. and an absorption curve for the component M_y.

Thus, the effect of a 90° pulse of the B_1 field vector is to swing the precession cone axis into the xy plane out of the z-direction so that the bulk magnetization vector becomes detectable as magnetization vector M_{xy} (see. Fig. 9.14).

It should be noted that if enough energy is put into the system, then M_z goes on decreasing and in fact, it can be reduced to zero i.e. $M_Z = 0$. This is shown in Fig. 9.16. At this stage population of α-spin states N_α, becomes equal to population of β-spin states N_β i.e. $N_\alpha = N_\beta$. So, there will be no signal in NMR. This is called "Saturation". Therefore, this phenomenon is undesirable and has to be avoided (see also Fig. 1.15a and 1.15b).

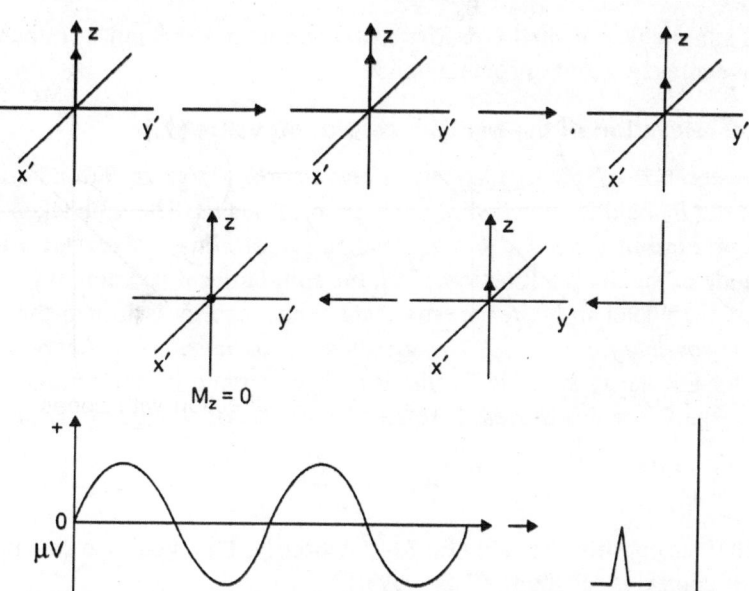

Fig. 9.15. The undesirable saturation state in NMR ($M_z \to 0$).

9.6 RELAXATION AND MECHANISM

After the pulse has been removed, the perturbed spin system relaxes back to the equilibrium in two separate processes. This is called Relaxation.

In one process, the Boltzman population excess is restored due to nuclei relaxing from the β-spin state to the α-spin state. In other words, the magnetization along the z-direction grows from zero and becomes equal to the original equilibrium value, M_0. This is called **spin-lattice relaxation.**

The second process involves decay of M_{xy} to zero magnitude. This is called **spin-spin relaxation.** When these two processes are complete, we once again have $M_{xy} = 0$ and

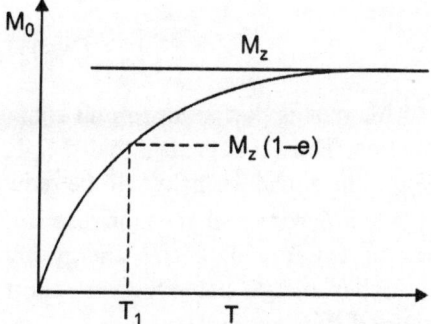

Fig. 9.16. A decaying FID that gives rise to a spectrum.

bulk magnetization M equal to M_0 magnitude. The NMR repeats the process to get FIDS. Successive FIDs are added up by the computer to cancel out the noise thereby increasing the S/N ratio to give us the usual spectrum (Fig. 9.16).

9.6.1 Mechanism of Spin-lattice Relaxation

As already mentioned, after the removal of the B_1 pulse you need to wait till the perturbed system has returned to its original position. This process is called relaxation. Evidently, relaxation consists of two processes :

1. Longitudinal relaxation of the M_z from zero to M_0 value (spin-lattice relaxation).
2. Transverse relaxation of the M_{xy} to zero value ($M_{xy} = 0$) (spin-spin relaxation).

For the sake of simplicity, we shall consider relaxation after a 90° pulse (rather than 180° pulse) about which we have already learnt in some details :

9.6.2 Longitudinal relaxation of the M_z from zero to M_0 value (T_1)

This involves the restoration of the net magnetization vector M_z from zero to its original equilibrium value of M_0. When the B_1 field is switched off, this process begins. The time taken by this process is called **spin-lattice relaxation time, T_1.** It is also called **longitudinal relaxation time.** Thus, we can say that the magnitude of the M_z is a function of T_1, the spin-lattice relaxation. It is also defined as the average life time of the nuclei in higher energy state. Thus, energy is lost to the surroundings (the lattice). *The simplest possible form for this energy release is assumed to be that of a first order decay.* The time constant for this decay is called T_1 that is a characteristic for the efficiency of this process. According to Bloch, the T_1 for this process is related to the rate of change of M_z like this :

$$\frac{dM_z}{dt} = \frac{M_0 - M_z}{T_1}$$

where M_0 is the Boltzman equilibrium value for M_z. Obviously, $1/T_1$ would be the rate constant for this process, K which, of course, is related to $t^{\frac{1}{2}}$ as $0.693/t^{\frac{1}{2}}$.

Further, it is the value of T_1 which is one of the factors that determines the form of the NMR signal.

It can be deduced from the equation that :

$$I(w_0) = \frac{\text{constant}}{B_1 T_1} \quad \text{where } I = \text{intensity}$$

This means that at maximum signal ($w = w_0$) the intensity of the signal would be given by this equation. Thus, it is evident that if T_1 is high and the amplitude of the oscillating field B_1 is also high, then, I, the signal intensity will be reduced. This is called **saturation of the resonance line.**

When T_1 are small, then the resonance lines get broadened. Under these conditions the nuclei return very quickly from the higher energy spin states to the lower energy spin states. That means they stay in the higher energy states for very short time intervals. This leads to uncertainty in determining the energy difference.

We know that as per Heisenberg principle,

$$\Delta E \cdot \Delta t \approx h/2\pi$$

Also
$$\Delta E = h \, \Delta v$$

Putting the value of ΔE from first equation into second equation, gives us the relationship :

$$h \, \Delta v \cdot \Delta t \approx h$$

or
$$\Delta v \cdot \Delta t = \frac{I}{2\pi}$$

or
$$\Delta v = \frac{I}{2\pi \cdot \Delta \pi}$$

$$\Delta v = \frac{I}{2\pi \cdot \Delta t}$$

As is evident from from this equation, the uncertainty in the determination of the resonance frequency Δv is inversely proportional to T_1. As T_1 for organic protons is equal to few seconds or even lesser, in general, the contribution to line width is not more than 0.1 H_z by the spin-lattice relaxation time. The Bloch equation can also be written in the form :

$$M_z = M_0 \left(1 - e - \frac{t}{\pi}\right)$$

for a 90° pulse so that T_1 is then the time required to change the M_z, the z component of the net magnetization by a factor of e. Or **we can also say that T_1 is the time that reduces the difference between the longitudinal magnetization M_z and its equilibrium value, M_0 by a factor of e.** A plot of M_z versus tune looks like as shown in Fig. 9.16.

9.6.3 Transverse Relaxation, T_2

After the pulse is turned-off, the net magnetization vector in the x'-y' plane starts to dephase as each of the spin packets which make it up now start experiencing a slightly different magnetic field and so rotates at its own Larmor frequency. The process of dephasing increases with time. In other words, the transverse magnetization M_{xy} starts decaying with time to equilibrium value. The time taken by this process is constant and is called T_2.

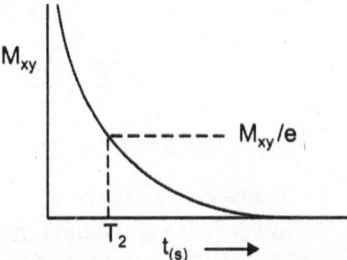

Fig. 9.17. Variation of M_{xy} with time.

$$M_{xy} = M_{xy} \cdot e^{-t/T_2}$$

Variation of M_{xy} with t is shown in Fig. 9.17.

So, we can say that T_2 is the time required to reduce the transverse magnetization by a factor of e.

It should be noted that the magnitude of the x-y magnetization as well as the peak height are actually determined by T_2. That is to say the magnitude of T_2 determines the decay rate of the FID. Thus, larger value of T_2 means rapid decay of FID. Conversely, smaller value of T_2 means decay or a ringing FID and a broader peak after FT. T_2 yields sharp or narrow peak after FT. Narrow peak in the spectrum means better interpretation whereas broader peak means poor resolution and hence poor interpretation.

Intext Exercise

Which one would you prefer and why?

a. $T_1 > T_2$ b. $T_1 < T_2$

Hint: As many working hundreds of scans have to be taken for a spectrum, therefore, we would like that T_1 be shorter then T_2. In fact, this is what a person on an NMR spectrometer would like. But the real situation is the other way around. T_2s are always shorter than T_1s. In fact, this much is quite thinkable that magnetization cannot reestablish along z-direction faster than it decays from xy-direction as otherwise, it would mean that at some point in time the total net magnetization taking a vector sum along z-direction and in xy-direction could become more than we began with, M_{zo}. That would mean we are getting something from nothing. Actually, we cannot get something from nothing. So, it is quite clear that magnetization will decay faster from xy-direction than it reestablishes along the z-directions that there would be less total magnetization than M_z at equilibrium (M_{zo}). That means we are getting nothing from something.

In a field that is perfectly homogeneous, the FID decays to zero exponentially, the time having characteristic value of T_2. As there always is present inhomogeneity in the field, it is observed that the FID decays faster than it would do otherwise. This is characterized with a time constant called T_2^* such that T_2^* is always less than T_2. The line width of the peak after FT, that is to say the full width of the peak at half of the peak height ($\Delta V\frac{1}{2}$) is given by the equation :

$$\Delta V\frac{1}{2} = \frac{1}{\pi T_2^*}$$

Thus, T_2^* can be easily founded out by measuring the width of the peak (Fig. 9.18). Now, T_2^* is related to T_2 and T_2^i, the inhomogeneity decay constant like :

$$\frac{1}{T_2^*} = \frac{1}{T_2} + \frac{1}{T_2^i}$$

Hence, T_2 can be easily found out.

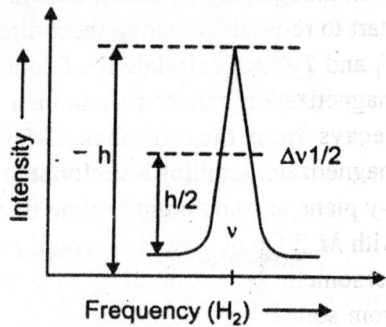

Fig. 9.18. Relationship between line width ($\Delta v\frac{1}{2}$) and T_2^*.

9.7 FACTORS AFFECTING T_2

1. Transverse relaxation time T_2 is affected by the number of molecules tumbling at the frequencies lower (zero quantum) than the Larmor frequencies (single quantum) as in case of molecules having higher MW for small molecules. On the other hand, T_1 is determined by the number of molecules tumbling at the Larmor frequencies (single quantum). In case of molecules with higher MW as the number of molecules tumbling at the Larmor frequencies is higher than those at lower frequencies, so $T_2 < T_1$. Proof for this comes from the fact that for molecules with smaller MW since the number of molecules tumbling at Larmor frequencies and at lower frequencies is almost equal, so $T_2 \approx T_1$.

2. Although spin-exchange does not affect T_1, it does affect T_2. The reason is that phase coherence of the transverse magnetization is lost during the spin-exchange. The reason as to why T_1 does not get affected is that the distribution of spin between upper and lower states is not altered.

$$A\uparrow + B\downarrow \longrightarrow A\downarrow + B\uparrow$$
Spin-exchange

3. Chemical exchange destroys phase coherence of the transverse magnetization. So T_2 gets affected. It should be noted that T_1 is also affected as energy is transferred from one nucleus to another.

$$EtOH_A + H_BO \rightleftharpoons EtOH_B + H_AOH$$

9.8 T_1 vs. T_2

Experiments have shown that T_1 is always longer than T_2. The decay of x-y magnetization compared to re-establishment of magnetization is much faster. What is the relation between the two? If we look at the equations for M_z, M_x and M_y, they are independent of each other :

$$M_y = -Mo \cos (2\pi v_o t)e^{-t/T_2}$$
$$M_x = -Mo \sin (2\pi v_o t)e^{-t/T_2}$$
$$M_z = -Mo \cos (1 - e^{-t/T_i})$$

What does that imply? That means that there is no relationship between them. However, T_1 and T_2 relaxation are not completely independent of each other. The loss of xy magnetization is measured in the T_2 experiment. However, even though magnetization decays from x-y plane it may also start to re-establish along the z-direction. Therefore, how are T_1 and T_2 rates correlated? of course, it is very clear that the magnetization cannot re-establish itself z-axis faster than it decays from the x-y phase. If it were not so, the total magnetization, taking a vector sum along the z-axis or and in x-y plane at some point in time be more than what we began with M_{zo}! Obviously, that would be incongruent; you cannot get something from nothing. You can conceive getting nothing from something. That is to say x-y magnetization decay can occur at a faster rate compared to recovery of magnetization along $+ z$ direction so that at some point, you can have less total magnetization compared to M_{zo}.

Hence, $$T_2 \leq T_1$$

As it is the recovery of the M_o that enables us to get the NMR spectrum, clearly T_1 determines the rate of obtaining an NMR spectrum; longer T_1 will mean longer relaxation delay. On the other hand, as the magnitude of T_2 determines the rate of decay of the FID, it is clear that shorter the time duration of the FID i.e. shorter T_2, the resultant peak in the spectrum will be broader. If the T_2 is long, the rate of decay of FID will be longer and so the peak in the spectrum will be sharper. **Hence, any one working with an NMR spectrometer would always like a world in which all T_1 are very short and all T_2 are very long so that the rate of acquisition is fast and the signal obtained is sharp. However, this does not happen that way. T_1 is always larger than T_2.** This is because, while T_1 is basically determined by the number of molecules tumbling at the Larmor frequency, T_2 is basically determined by the number of molecules that tumble at the low frequencies. T_1 is almost equal to T_2 for small molecules. For large molecules, $T_1 \gg T_2$ as the number of molecules tumbling at the low (zero-quantum) frequencies is much greater than those tumbling at the Larmor or single-quantum frequency (Fig. 9.19 and 9.20).

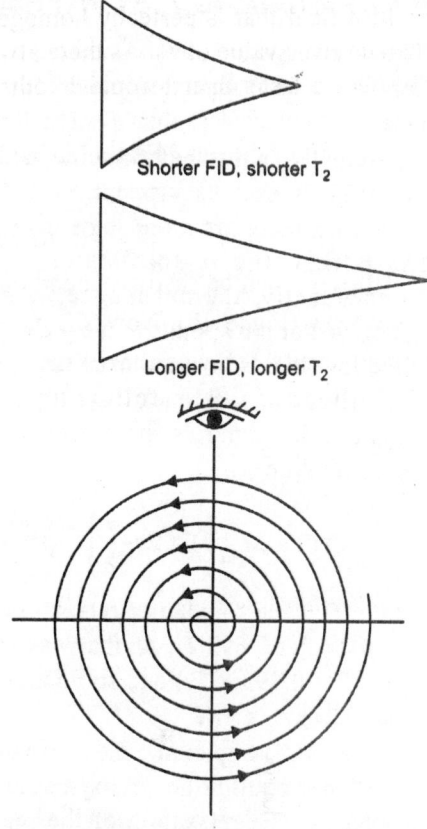

Shorter FID, shorter T_2

Longer FID, longer T_2

Fig. 9.19. Spiraling of the T_2 coherence as seen from the top (Z) direction.

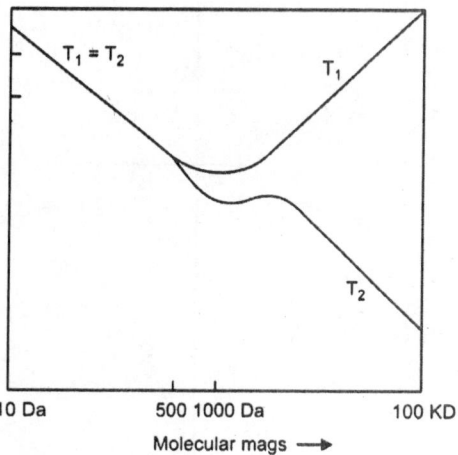

$T_1 = T_2$

T_1

T_2

10 Da   500 1000 Da   100 KD

Molecular mags ⟶

Fig. 9.20. T_1 and T_2 as a function of molecular mass.

9.9 DETERMINING T_1 BY INVERSION-RECOVERY METHOD

The is inversion recovery method is so called as the net magnetization of the nuclei is inverted by applying a 180° inversion pulse followed by recovery or relaxation of this magnetization along the z axis.

Actually, in this method some half a dozen of 180°–τ–90–τ experiments are carried out as shown in Fig. 9.21. In each experiment, first of all a 180° pulse is applied that inverts the Boltzman population excess i.e. there are more spins in the β than the α spin-states. Consequently, the net magnetization vector now points in the $- Z$ direction (it gets inverted from the $+ Z$ direction). The following equation that controls the relaxation with time (t).

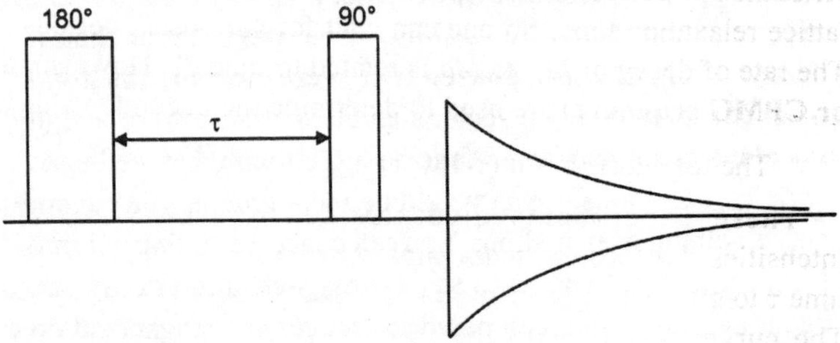

$$M_z(T) = M_{z_o}\left(1 - 2e\frac{-t}{T_1}\right)$$

Fig. 9.21. A 180°-τ-90° experiment for T_1 measurement.

where T_1 is the spin lattice relaxation time and M_{zo} is the magnetization vector at the end of 180° pulse ($t = 0$). After 0.693 T_1, M_z that was equal to $-M_o$ now becomes zero. M_z becomes ½Mo after two half-lives (2 × 0.693 × T_1) and so on and after a long time, t_α it becomes equal to Mo in the $+ Z$ direction (Fig. 9.21).

Now M_z is tipped into the x-y plane so that it could be detected by applying a 90° pulse when it will spiral up to equilibrium giving a decaying signal, of course the spectrum obtained will be negative (out-of-phase). The relaxation of the magnetization vector into its final equilibrium continues after the

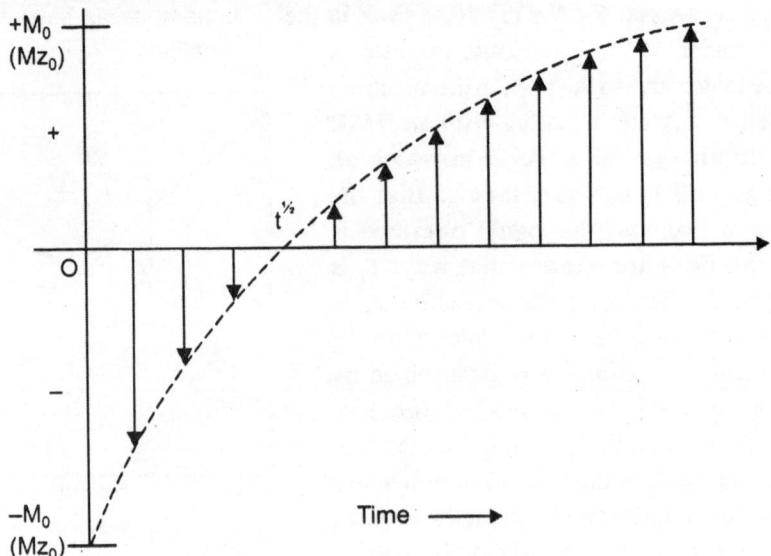

Fig. 9.22. Exponential curve for variation of M_z with time after 180° pulse.

initial signal is observed. Now as the subsequent relaxation is dependent upon field inhomogeneities as well as spin-spin relaxation time T_2, so we do not go that further.

The data obtained is fitted into the above equation which gives us the value of T_1. All this is done by the computer. The spectra appear in the form of stacks as shown in Fig. 9.23.

9.10 SPIN-SPIN LATTICE TIME (T_2) MEASUREMENT

After the 90° pulse, the M_z tipps into x-y plane. The M_{x-y} now decays to zero with time T_2, the spin-spin lattice relaxation time. So one can wait for various T_2 periods and measure the spectrum (Fig. 9.23). The rate of decay of M_{xy} to Mo is related to time T_2. However, a series of τ-180-τ (**spin echo element or CPMG sequence**) are used to determine the accurate value of T_2 (Fig. 9.24–9.26).

The total time τ = n (τ-180-τ)

These experiments give rise to intensities that are plotted against total time τ to give a curve shown in Fig. 9.26. The curve is fitted into the following equation :

$$M_{xy}(T_2) = M_{zo}\, e\frac{-\tau}{T_2}$$

It is clear from this equation that at time τ equal to zero which means immediately after the 90° pulse,

$$M_{xy(o)} = M_{zo}$$

As T approaches infinity (∞) M_{xy} approaches zero (see Fig. 9.23).

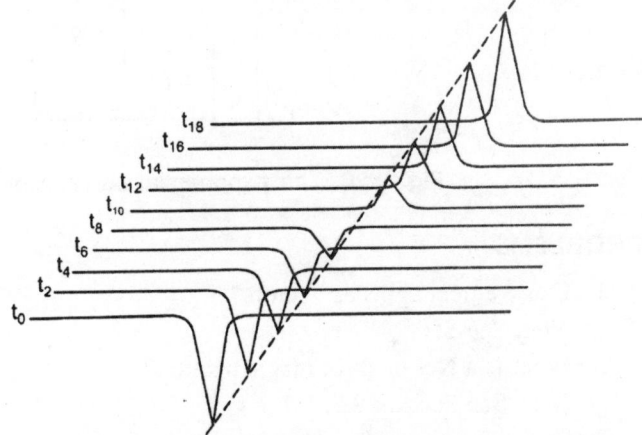

Fig. 9.23. 180°-τ-90° generated stacked spectra.

Note : The purpose of spin-echo element or CPMG sequence is to prevent dephasing due to non-uniform field i.e. the dephasing that occurs during the first τ period is rephased during the second τ period.

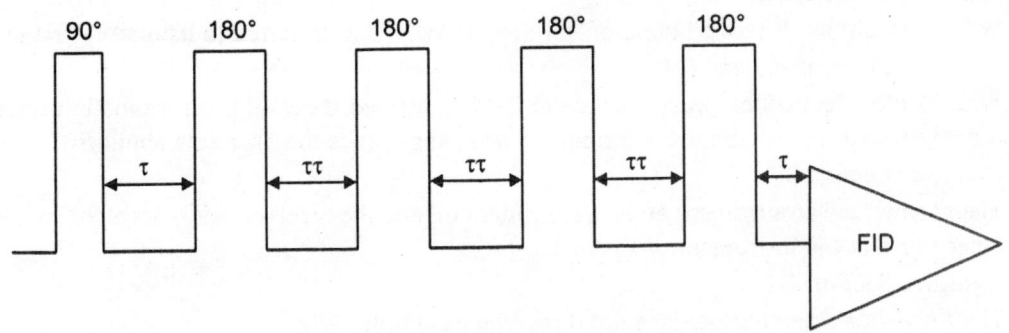

Fig. 9.24. An initial 90° pulse followed by variable pulse delay τ.

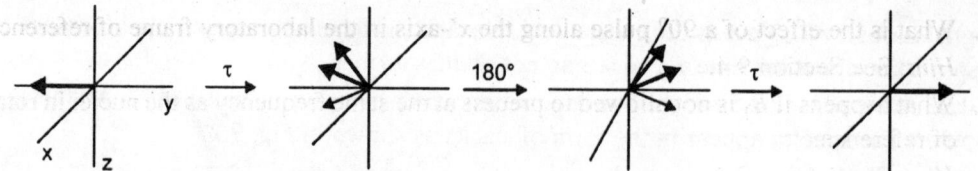

Fig. 9.25. τ–180°–τ spin echo experiment.

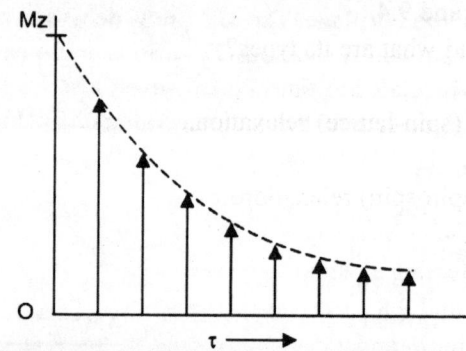

Fig. 9.26. The exponential curve depicting variation of M_z with τ.

PROBLEMS

1. Can we treat spins as vectors?
   Hint: See Section 9.1.

2. What is a Net or Bulk magnetization?
   Hint: See Section 9.2.

3. Define incoherence and coherence.
   Hint: See Section 9.2.

4. Can we detect Net magnetization in the absence of the *rf* pulse?
   Hint: See Section 9.3.

5. What is the difference between laboratory frame and rotating frame from the point of view of chemical shift determination?
   Hint: See Section 9.3.

6. What is meant by Rotating Frame of Reference? Why is it preferred to laboratory frame?
   Hint: See Sections 9.3 and 9.4.

7. What is the effect of the pulsed magnetic field B, around the x'-axis on magnetic vector M_z in rotating frame versus laboratory frame? At what angle does the M_0 rotate about B_1.
   Hint: See Section 9.4.

8. The geometrical arrangement of the transmitter coil and the receiver coil is set at 90° w.r. to each other in FT NMR instrument. Why?
   Hint: See Section 9.4.

9. The M_z vector along the z-axis is not directly measurable. Why?
   Hint: See Section 9.4.

10. What is the effect of a 90° pulse along the x'-axis in the laboratory frame of reference?

    Hint: See Section 9.4.

11. What happens if B_1 is not allowed to precess at the same frequency as the nuclei in rotating frame of reference.

    Hint: See Section 9.4.

12. Explain in details the rotating frame of reference.

    Hint: See Section 9.3 and 9.4.

13. What is Relaxation and what are its types?

    Hint: See Section 4.6.

14. Explain Longitudinal (spin-lattice) relaxation.

    Hint: See Section 4.6.

15. Discuss Transverse (spin-spin) relaxation.

    Hint: See Section 4.6.

16. Discuss (a) factors affecting T_2 and (b) T_1 versus T_2.

    Hint: See Section 9.7 and 9.8.

17. How can you determine T_1 and T_2?

    Hint: See Sections 9.9 and 9.10.

10

Carbon-13 Nuclear Magnetic Resonance

10.1 SENSITIVITY OF C-13 VERSUS ^{1}H

Carbon-12 has an equal number of protons and neutrons, so that its nuclear spins are paired. Consequently, it has spin I = O. Therefore, it is NMR inactive. This seems surprising even though it is the most abundant isotope of carbon and all organic compounds are made up of carbon. As we will see later on, it is good that C-12 is NMR-inactive, otherwise the carbon magnetic resonance spectra could have been very complicated, difficult to interpret. Carbon-13 which has an extra neutron has I = ½ and hence it is NMR-active. However, the problem with C-13 nucleus is its low natural abundance which is 1.11%. Further, the nuclear magnet strength of C-13 is about one-fourth of that proton. Hence, due to the dual factors of low natural abundance combined with low gyromagnetoratio, the sensitivity of carbon-13 nuclear magnetic resonance experiment is significantly lower than that of proton. Its sensitivity, γ^3 compared to proton is 1/64 as its γ is 1/4 of γ for proton. The overall sensitivity of C-13 compared to proton would, therefore, be equal to:

$$\text{Overall sensitivity} = \text{sensitivity} \times \% \text{ natural abundance} = \frac{1}{64} \times 1.11\% = 1.72 \times 10^{-4}$$

Now as S/N ratio is proportional to the square root of number of scans, therefore, in order to get an identical S/N ratio for C-13 relative to a single scan hydrogen, we will have to take some 33,850,000 scans! That is why, there were difficulties in getting C-13 spectra worth interpretation in the beginning. As a result, the time required for obtaining a C-13 spectrum would be very large using a CW spectrometer as it requires about 100–500 s to take a spectrum even for protons. Obviously, as several thousands of scans are required for C-13 observation, therefore, difficulties were encountered using CW spectrometers. Furthermore, large amount of sample is required as well compared to that required routinely for observing proton signals.

But modern Fourier transform NMR spectroscopy makes it possible for us to obtain CMR spectra worth interpretation in a very small period of time. Even as we complain of low natural abundance of C-13 nucleus, it is worth noting that this low figure is of great use to us as well. If C-13 had 100% natural abundance like proton, then spin-spin interactions could have enormously complicated the proton NMR spectra of organic compounds and indeed it would not have been possible to develop proton

NMR spectroscopy if the technique of heteronuclear double resonance were not known. It is this low natural abundance of 1.11% which means that most of the carbon nuclei are not involved in NMR resonance phenomenon. In other words, a majority of the molecules of the given compound sample do not contain C–13 nuclei. Consequently, there is very little chance that for a particular C–13 nucleus present in the molecule, any neighbouring carbon is also C–13. As probability of seeing a C–13 nucleus in a molecule is just its natural abundance i.e. 0.01, therefore, the chance of seeing two C–13 nuclei in fixed positions is equal to its (natural abundance)^2 : $0.01 \times 0.01 = 1 \times 10^{-4}$. Hence, for all practical practical purposes, the chances for finding two coupled C–13 nuclei in the same molecule is negligible. That is why $^{13}C–^{13}C$ splitting is not seen in CMR of samples containing only the natural abundance of carbon–13 nucleus.

Fourier transform NMR spectrometry requires little amounts of the sample. Thus, while 1 mg quantity of the organic compound is enough for obtaining one single scan, about 30 mg of the sample is required in order to obtain one thousand scans of the C–13 nmr spectrum.

10.2 EQUIVALENT AND NON-EQUIVALENT CARBONS

Those carbons in a molecule which have the identical chemical environment, that is to say which are equialent by symmetry within the molecule are called equivalent carbons.

The carbons in a molecule which have different chemical environments are called non-equivalent carbons.

Examples of equivalent carbons

Some examples of all carbons being equivalent carbons in a molecule are ethane, dimethyl ether, cyclopropane, cyclobutane, cyclopentane, cyclohexane, benzene, acetylene, ethene etc.:

CH_3CH_3
Ethane

CH_3OCH_3
Dimethyl ether

Cyclopropane

Cyclobutane

Cyclopentane

Cyclohexane

Benzene

$CH_2{=}CH_2$
Ethene

$CH{\equiv}CH$
Acetylene

All equivalent carbons in a molecule

Non-equivalent carbons

The carbons in a molecule that have different chemical environments are called non-equivalent carbons.
Examples of molecules in which all C are non-equivalent:

CH_3CH_2Cl
Chloroethane

CH_3CH_2OH
Ethanol

$CH_3CH_2OCH_2CH_3$
Diethyl ether

$CH_3CH_2CH_2Cl$
Chloropropane

$CH_3CH_2CH_2OH$
Propanol

$CH_3CH_2CH_2OCH_2CH_2CH_3$
D-n-propyl ether

13·6 22·1 29·2 32·7 44·3
$CH_3\ CH_2\ CH_2\ CH_2\ CH_2Cl$
1-chloropentane

14·1   22·9   32·1   29·3   29·1   34·1   139·1   114·2
$CH_3-CH_2-CH_2-CH_2-CH_2-CH_2-CH=CH_2$
Oct–1–ene

68·4   84·5   18·3   30·9   22·1   13·7
$HC\equiv C-CH_2-CH_2-CH_2-CH_3$
Hexyne–1

113   140   23·8   9·3
$CH_2=CH-CH_2-CH_3$
But–1–ene

70·9   39   32   9·5
$CH_2-CH_2-CH-CH_3$
|
Br

CH_3 9·5
1–Bromo–3–methyl butane

18·7   136   115
$CH_3-CH=CH_2$
Propylene

$CH_3-CH-CH_2$
Propyne

Molecules containing all non-equivalent carbons

Examples of molecules containing both equivalent and non-equivalent carbons

Molecule

Mesitylene

Sets of non-equivalent carbons

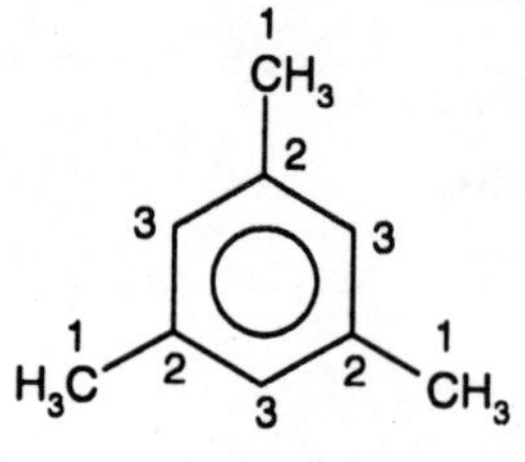

Contains 3 sets of equivalent carbons shown as 1, 2 and 3
Three carbons marked as 1 are all equivalent
Three carbons marked as 2 are all equivalent
Three carbons marked as 3 are all equivalent

$$\overset{1}{C}H_3 \ \overset{2}{C}H_2 \ \overset{1}{C}H_3$$

Propane

Contains two sets of equivalent carbons shown as 1 and 2
Two terminal carbons (1) are both equivalent
The middle carbon (2) is different from the terminal carbons

$$\overset{1}{C}H_3 - \overset{2}{C}H - \overset{3}{C}H - \overset{4}{C}H_3$$

$$\overset{1}{C}H_3 \qquad Cl$$

2–chlorobutane

Contains only four different kinds (non-equivalent) carbons
1, 2, 3 and 4 as two CH_3 carbons marked as 1 are equivalent
between themselves

$$\overset{1}{C}H_3$$

$$\overset{1}{C}H_3 - \overset{2}{C} - \overset{3}{C}H_2 - \overset{4}{C}H_3$$

$$Cl$$

2-chloro–2–methylbutane

Contains only four different kinds of carbons as two CH_3
carbons marked as 1 are equivalent between themselves

$$\overset{1}{C}H_2 - \overset{2}{C}H_2 - \overset{3}{C}H - \overset{4}{C}H_3$$

$$Cl \qquad \overset{4}{C}H_3$$

1-chloro–3–methylbutane

Contains only four types of carbons as carbons marked as 4
are equivalent

$$\overset{1}{C}H_3 - \overset{2}{C}H_2 - \overset{3}{C}H_2 - \overset{3}{C}H_2 - \overset{2}{C}H_2 - \overset{1}{C}H_3$$ Contains only three sets of equivalent carbons

n-hexane

$$\overset{1}{C}H_3$$

$$\overset{1}{C}H_3 - \overset{2}{C}H - \overset{3}{C}H_2 - \overset{4}{C}H_2 - \overset{5}{C}H_3$$

2–Methylpentane

Contains only four different kinds of carbons as two carbons
marked as 1 and 1 are equivalent

$$\overset{1}{C}H_3 - \overset{2}{C}H_2 - \overset{3}{C}H = \overset{3}{C}H - \overset{2}{C}H_2 - \overset{1}{C}H_3$$ Contains only three non-equivalent sets of carbons

But–3–ene

$$\overset{1}{H_3C} \diagdown \qquad \diagup \overset{1}{C}H_3$$
$$\overset{2}{C} = \overset{2}{C}$$
$$H \diagup \qquad \diagdown H$$

cis–2–butene

Contains only two non-equivalent sets of carbons marked 1,
1 and 2,2

$$\overset{1}{H_3C} \diagdown \qquad \diagup H$$
$$\overset{2}{C} = \overset{2}{C}$$
$$H \diagup \qquad \diagdown \underset{1}{C}H_3$$

trans–2–butene

Contains only two non-equivalent sets of carbons marked
1,1 and 2,2

$$\overset{1}{H_3C}-\overset{2}{CH}-\overset{1}{CH_3}$$

Contains only eight sets of non-equivalent carbons as carbons marked 3 and 3 are equivalent. Similarly, carbons marked 4 and 4 are equivalent

$$CH_3-\underset{\underset{O}{\|}}{C}-CH_3$$

Contains two sets of non-equivalent carbons.

Intext Exercise

1. How will you distinguish between 2–bromopropane and 1–bromopropane on the basis of number of peaks alone in their CMR spectra?

Answer

Structural formula of 2–bromopropane and 1–bromopropane are as follows :

$$\overset{a}{CH_3}-\underset{\underset{Br}{|}}{\overset{b}{CH}}-\overset{a}{CH_3} \qquad CH_3-CH_2-CH_2Br$$

2–bromopropane   1–bromopropane

We would expect only two peaks in case of 2–bromopropane as it contains only two different kinds of carbons instead of three. On the other hand, we would expect three peaks in the CMR of 1–bromo-propane as all the three carbons in it are non-equivalent.

10.3 TYPICAL CMR SPECTRUM

A typical CMR looks ^{13}C NMR spectrum of Oesterone acetate is shown in Fig. 10.1. As with PMR spectra, the following information becomes available from CMR spectra as after all, the basic principle of NMR spectroscopy remains the same, whatever the nuclei being observed in the NMR experiment.

1. Number of signals.
2. The position or the chemical shift of a signal.
3. Spin-spin splitting from a CMR spectrum which is not hydrogen-decoupled.

1. Number of signals

The number of signals in a CMR spectrum gives us the message as to how many different carbons or different sets of equivalent carbons are present in the molecule. If one signal is obtained, despite the presence of more than one carbon as indicated by the molecular formula, it means all the carbons are alike or equivalent. If number of signals obtained is less than the actual number of carbons present in the molecular formula, it shows the presence of some equivalent carbons that absorb at the same position, thereby reducing the number of signals. For example, only one signal is obtained for all the six carbons of benzene. Similar is the situation for ethane, CH_3-CH_3. Fig. 10.1 shows all the 20 carbons present in the molecule of Oesterone acetate as all of them are non-equivalent.

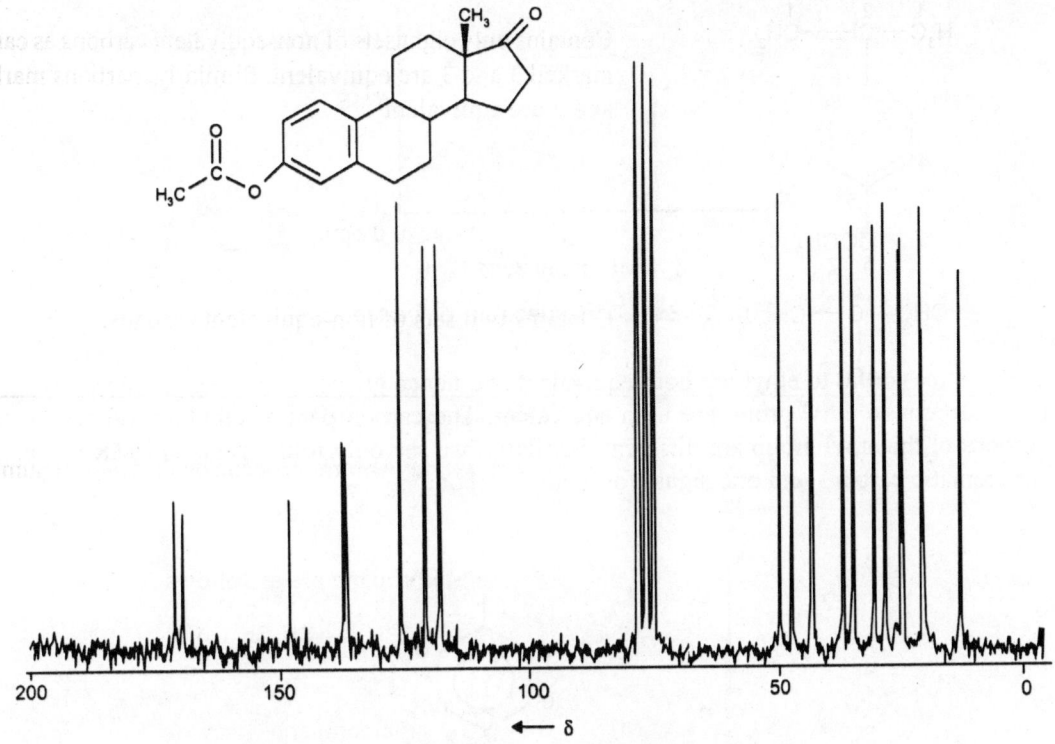

Fig. 10.1. CMR spectrum of Oesterone acetate.

Examples

1. **Benzene :** All carbons are equivalent so only one signal is obtained in CMR spectrum as shown in Fig. 10.2a.

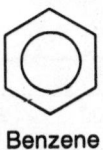

Benzene

2. **Ethyl benzene :** Ethyl benzene shows five signals only in its CMR spectrum (Fig. 10.2a) despite the presence of eight carbons in it. This is because, there are two sets of two carbons each, cc and dd that are equivalent in nature i.e. :

$$
\begin{array}{c}
\text{b} \quad \text{a} \\
29\ CH_2 \!\!-\!\! CH_3\ \ 15.6 \\
\end{array}
$$

144.2   c   c (127.9)

d   d (128.4)

e (125.7)

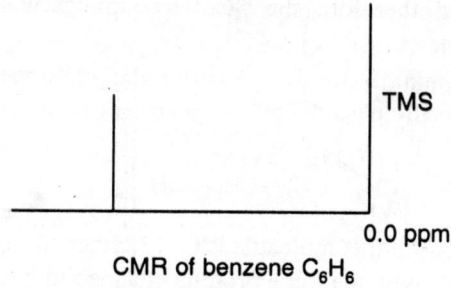

CMR of benzene C_6H_6

Fig. 10.2a. CMR spectrum of benzene.

Carbons (cc) ortho to ethyl are both equivalent and hence give only one signal. Similarly, meta (d,d) carbons to ethyl group are both equivalent. The carbon para to ethyl as well as the two carbons of the ethyl group are different. Similarly, we see only four signals in CMR of toluene for aromatic carbons and one signal for methyl carbon.

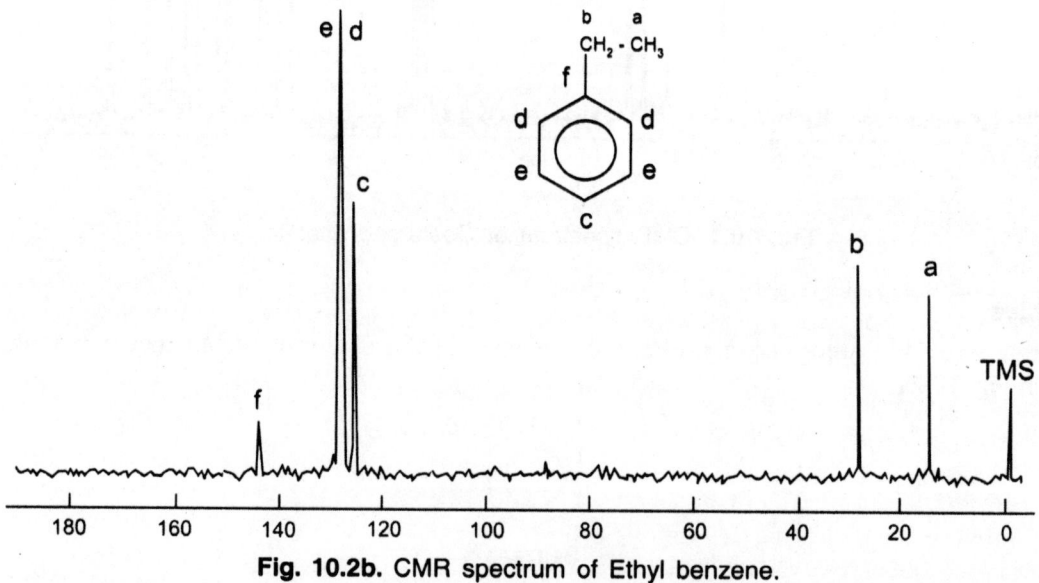

Fig. 10.2b. CMR spectrum of Ethyl benzene.

10.4 BROAD-BAND OR PROTON-NOISE DECOUPLING (PROTON-DECOUPLED SPECTRA)

We have already talked of the differences between C–13 and H–1 spectroscopy. Although the low natural abundance of C–13 (1.11%) is an advantage that $^{13}C-^{13}C$ couplings do not occur, however $^{13}C-H$ coupling occurs extensively. The $^1J_{CH}$ coupling is very large to the extent of about 150 Hz. This means that all methine carbons (CH) will show wide doublets, all methylene carbons (CH$_2$) will give triplets and all methyl carbons (CH$_3$) will give quartets. Of course, the quaternary carbon which is not attached to a proton will not show any coupling. A very complicated C–13 spectrum will be obtained that will not be worth interpretation. There is a further complication as well which arises from long-range $^{13}C-H$ coupling such as $^1J_{CH}$ ($^{13}C-H$), $^2J_{CH}$ ($^{13}C-C-H$) etc. Now, as the H-1 nucleus has one hundred per cent natural abundance, therefore, the ^{13}C–^{1}H couplings will appear completely in the form of peaks rather as small satellites.

Consequently, the spectra will contain extensively overlapping multiplets that will be very difficult to analyse. This can be understood easily from the C–13 spectrum of the simple molecule, 1–propanol:

$$\overset{13}{\underset{3}{CH_3}}-\overset{12}{\underset{2}{CH_2}}-\overset{12}{\underset{1}{CH_2}}-OH$$

Let us first of all consider that C–3 of this molecule is C–13, other two carbons being C–12. As per the n + 1 rule, this carbon will couple with the three protons attached to it to give a quartet ($^1J_{CH}$ ~ 125 Hz). Each line within this quartet will be split apart into a triplet owing to coupling with the adjacent CH_2 protons ($^2J_{CH}$ ~ 15 Hz) thus giving a total of twelve lines. Each of these twelve lines will in turn be split apart into a triplet. This is shown in Fig. 10.2c. The net result is the appearance of small thirty six peaks.

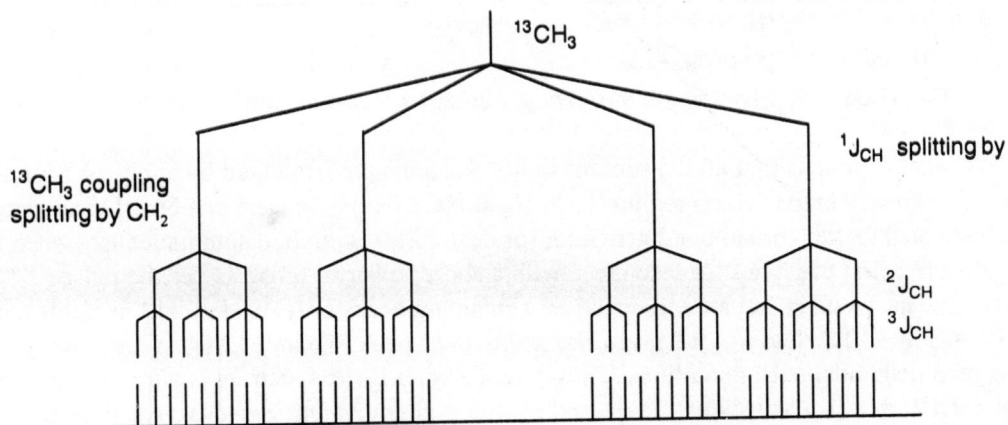

Fig. 10.2c. 36 lines arising from the coupling of CH_3 in propanol–1 due to $^1J_{CH}$, $^2J_{CH}$ and $^3J_{CH}$ coupling in the molecule, CH_3–CH_2–CH_2OH in which only CH_3 carbon is C–13.

If we consider C–2 being C–13 in some other molecules and the remaining two carbons being C–12, and similarly the C–1 being C–13 in some other molecules and the remaining two carbons being C–12, we can see extensive overlapping peaks intermingled with noise in the CMR spectrum.

The overall result of such ^{1}H–^{13}C couplings is a very complicated spectrum with the overall sensitivity being cut down further in terms of time as well if we have to get a good signal-to-noise ratio of 2^{2n} times that requires a single uncoupled line.

So, what should we do in order to get only C–13 signals? Obviously, it is essential to remove all ^{13}C–^{1}H couplings if we want to get a meaningful CMR spectrum worth structural elucidation. Although we can aim at decoupling **selective** ^{13}C–^{1}H couplings in the spectrum, it will be more time-saving and more simplified a spectrum if all the ^{13}C–^{1}H couplings are eliminated in the spectrum together. The difference between these two modes is shown in Fig. 10.3.

Therefore what should we do? We have already learnt of double resonance technique. Why not apply that technique to all the protons instead of choosing only one additional larmor frequency of a

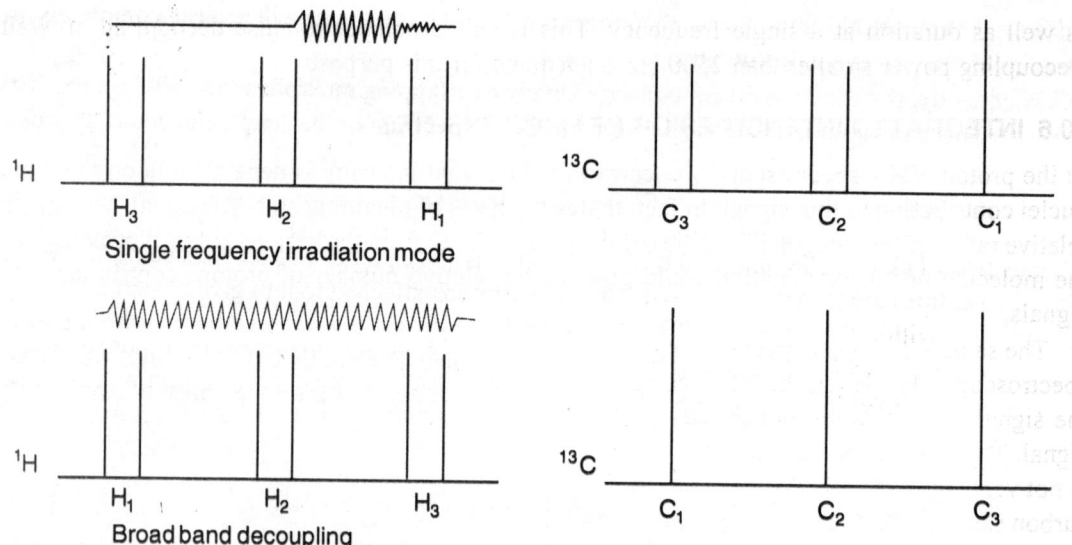

Fig. 10.3. Proton decoupling via single frequency irradiation mode as well as broadband decoupling.

proton. So, what is done is that all the protons in the molecule are irradiated by applying **broad band** decoupling frequency in the proton region (1000 Hz at 100 MHz) by means of a broad band generator. It should be noted that the broad bond generator (or decoupler) is applied simultaneously when all the C-13 nuclei are being observed for resonance with a short powerful pulse as per the pulsed FT NMR technique. The net result is that a CMR spectrum containing peaks only due to C–13 nuclei is obtained as shown in Fig. 10.2. Each C–13 gives rise to its own peak. Today, CMR spectra are generally speaking recorded under such conditions. Thus, a broad band CMR spectrum is very simple, chemical shift for each carbon is easily identifiable and all the non-equivalent carbons give their own peaks irrespective of their numbers – twenty or even thirty or more. Fig. 10.1 shows 20 peaks arising from all the twenty non-equivalent carbons present in oesterone acetate.

All multiplets arising due to 13C–H couplings ($^{1}J_{CH}, ^{2}J_{CH}, ^{3}J_{CH}$) collapse under these conditions thereby improving S/N ratio. In fact, the broad-band decoupling not only decouples all $^{13}C....^{1}H$ couplings but also leads to a considerable, almost threefold increase in S/N in addition to that resulting from the elimination of the complex cascade of multiplets. This phenomenon is called Nuclear Overhauser Enhancement (NOE). Consequence of NOE effect is a substantial decrease in the time required for recording of CMR spectrum as now lesser number of FIDs are required than would be needed in the absence of such an effect.

Further the hydrogen-decoupled spectrum is very simple in its appearance all single peak. It becomes quite convenient to identify the chemical shift at which a particular carbon resonates, despite the large number of carbons being present in a molecule, may be upto 30 even!

10.5 COMPOSITE-PULSE DECOUPLING OR WALT$_{Z}$–16

The broad band decoupling of protons has to be done by as low as possible decoupling power. This is achieved by applying repeated train of a phase-cycled pulses that is by pulses that have different phase as well as duration at a single frequency. This is called composite-pulse decoupling or $Walt_Z$–16. Decoupling power smaller than 2500 Hz is adequate for this purpose.

10.6 INTEGRATED INTENSITIES OR PEAK INTENSITIES

In the proton NMR spectroscopy we learnt that the signal intensity is dependent upon the number of nuclei contributing to that signal. In fact, that is the basis of obtaining an NMR signal. We saw that the relative ratios of the integral intensities of the peaks arising from the various kinds of protons present in the molecule under examination could give us the relative number of protons contributing to those signals.

The same feature is expected to be observed in CMR spectroscopy as well (or indeed in any other spectroscopy). However, the ^{13}C spectra are not integrated as is done in proton spectra! This is because the signal intensities are not exactly proportional to the number of C–13 nuclei contributing to the signal. That is to say the integral intensities do not turn out to be reliable. In any case, this disadvantage is not very significant as this does not lead to loss of structural information that is needed to reveal the carbon skeleton i.e. the number of carbons present in the given molecule. That is why we do not bother to get relative intensities of the C–13 signals.

From the above observations, it must not be concluded that as the basic principle of an NMR signal being proportional to the number of nuclei contributing to the signal is not being followed, therefore, the principle of C–13 NMR spectroscopy is different from the proton or any other type of NMR spectroscopy.

Therefore, what are the reasons behind the unreliable relative integral intensities in CMR spectroscopy? There are two reasons. One, the relaxation times of ^{13}C nuclei are longer than the relaxation times of various kinds of protons. After the FIDs of various nuclei are collected and then the pulse is repeated, there is allowed a short time decay called relaxation (pulse) delay during which the excited nuclei relax back to their α-spin state. In case of protons, their relaxation times are very short so that they relax quickly within seconds before the pulse sequence is repeated. However, it is not so for C-13 nuclei whose relaxation times (the spin lattice relaxation times T_1) are quite variable. What happens is that while some C-13 nuclei relax quickly within seconds, others may require longer times ranging over minutes. In other words, all the C-13 nuclei do not relax back to ground state equally between the pulses applied. In case of those C-13 nuclei having longer relaxation times, the FID is already ceased so that not all such nuclei have relaxed back to α-spin state. Evidently, the FIDs of such nuclei will give weaker signals compared to those C-13 nuclei which relax completely during the relaxation delay and hence contribute completely and give strong signals. Complete relaxation yields strong signals. Incomplete relaxation yields weaker signals (see Fig. 10.4). Consequently, the relative peak intensities are not satisfactory reliable. What could be the solution? Simple, increase the delay time between the pulses till all the C-13 nuclei have relaxed completely. That can be done but that is usually not done as it will require lot of time. So, the principle of C-13 NMR spectroscopy is still the same as that of proton nmr spectroscopy but the differences between the two are due to the differences in the techniques being followed for duration of the relaxation delay periods between the pulses.

Secondly, under conditions of protons decoupling, as we have already seen, there occurs a peak enhancement due to Nuclear Overhauser Enhancement (NOE) to different extents for different C-13 nuclei. In general, it is found that the peak due to methyl, CH_3 carbon is stronger than that due to a

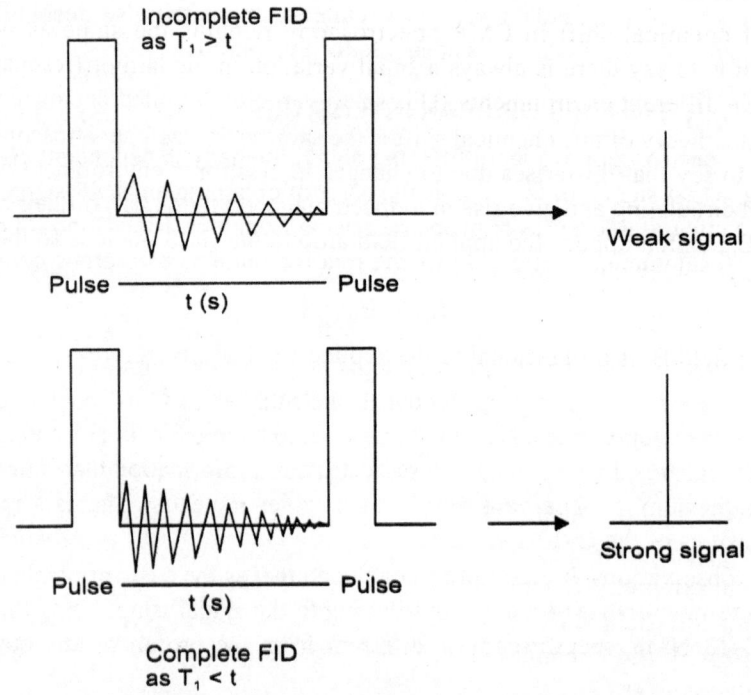

Fig. 10.4. Illustration of FIDS during relaxation (pulse) delay period t (a) incomplete FID giving a weak signal, (b) complete FID giving a strong signal. Note the relaxation (pulse) delay period t (s) is the same in both cases for these carbons present in the same sample being investigated.

methylene, CH_2 carbon which is of course, stronger than that due to a methine, –CH– carbon. As the spin-lattice relaxation for C–13 nuclei is based upon the dipole-dipole interaction with protons attached directly to the carbons, therefore, the quaternary carbons which do not have protons, have very long spin-lattice relaxation times. The result is that the quaternary carbons show either little or none of any NOE enhancement. That is why, it is rather advantageous in recognizing a quaternary carbon due to their small peaks.

Thus, it is clear now as to why, peak intensities in CMR spectra are not reliable under the routine NMR conditions.

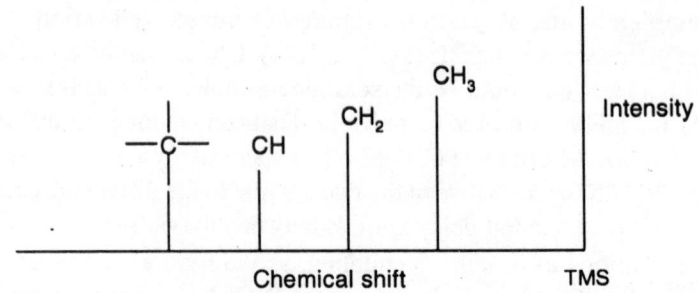

Fig. 10.5. A schematic relative signal intensity due to CH_3, CH_2, CH and quaternary carbons in a molecule in a proton decoupled CMR spectrum.

10.7(a) CHEMICAL SHIFT

The definition of chemical shift in CMR spectroscopy remains the same as we learnt in PMR spectroscopy. That is to say there is always a small variation in the larmor (resonant) frequencies of different carbons in different environments. This small variation is called chemical shift.

The origin or the theory of this chemical shift is the same as in PMR spectroscopy, we discussed in Chapter 2. Again to say that this arises due to changes in electronic environment of the 13-C nuclei. The electrons start circulating and give rise to induced magnetic fields (B') of their own in presence of the applied field B_0, which oppose the applied field around the C-13 nucleus so that the B_{eff} is never equal to B_0 i.e. :

$$B_{eff} = B_0 - B'$$

As the induced field B' is proportional to the applied field, B_0, therefore :

$$\begin{aligned} B_{eff} &= B_0 - B' \\ &= B_0 (1 - \sigma) \end{aligned}$$

where σ is the screening constant in units of parts per million (ppm). The value of σ is proportional to the electron density of the p-orbitals. The value of σ in protons is proportional only to the electron density in 1s orbital as the protons do not contain p-orbitals. The p electrons in non-spherical molecules which lack spherical symmetry generate large magnetic fields at the nucleus and cause low-field shift or deshielding. **This low-field shift or the deshielding is known as paramagnetic shift. This is the basic reason as to why the chemical shift range for C-13 nuclei is large compared to that for protons. While the shift for C-13 nuclei is 0-200 ppm, that for protons is 0-10 ppm (see Fig. 10.6).** There is only diamagnetic and not paramagnetic shift in protons unlike in C-13 nuclei. It should be

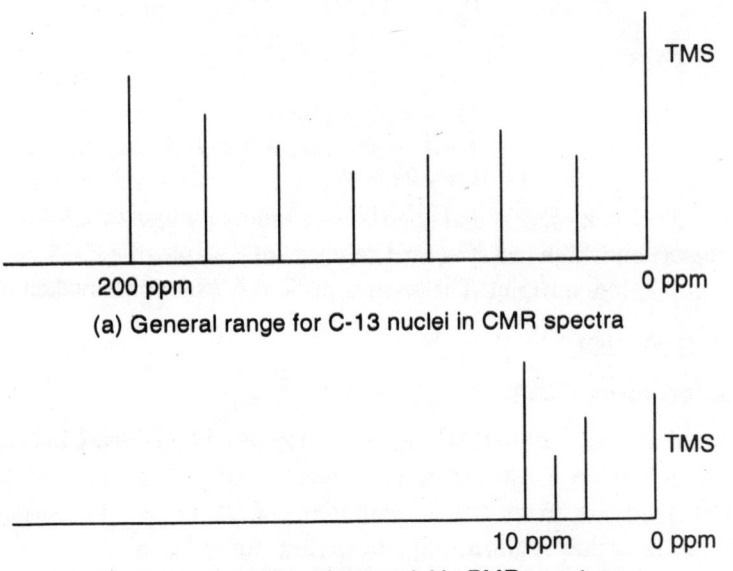

(a) General range for C-13 nuclei in CMR spectra

(b) General range for H-1 nuclei in PMR spectra

Fig. 10.6. (a) The large general range for C-13 nuclei (0–200 ppm) due to paramagnetic shift. (b) The small general range for H–1 nuclei (0–10 ppm) due to diamagnetic shift.

noted that as the range C-13 nuclei is very large, so almost each non-equivalent carbon atoms in the given molecule give a distinct peak at a different chemical shift in the spectrum. The kinds of overlappings seen in PMR spectra are rarely seen in CMR spectra.

As in case of protons, the resonance frequencies of the C-13 nuclei, are measured with reference to a standard or reference compound whose carbon-13 nuclei resonate at the extreme right or most up-field end of the spectrum and so are assigned a value of 0 ppm ($\sigma = 0$). The frequency difference (in Hz) between the C-13 nucleus in the sample and that of the reference is divided by the operational frequency (in Hz) as in PMR or any other spectroscopy so as to make it independent of the operational frequency of the NMR spectrometer and also multiplied by 10^6 to express it in a convenient manner i.e. in ppm, easy to remember :

$$\delta = \frac{V_{sample} - V_{reference} \ (Hz) \times 10^6}{V_0 \times 10^6 \ Hz}$$

$$= 0 - 200 \ ppm$$

Fortunately for us the reference compound chosen for recording CMR spectra is the same as used in PMR spectra i.e. tetramethylsilane, which is a good thing as you can record both PMR as well as CMR spectra with the same sample in the nmr tube. These days for obtaining CMR spectra TMS is not actually added into the sample. Rather the peak due to ^{13}C of the deuterated solvent (such as $CDCl_3$) is used as an internal reference. Of course, the spectrum is still presented with reference to TMS at 0.0 ppm at the extreme right. When

Tetra methyl silane
Most upfield ^{13}C (and ^1H)
$\delta = 0.0$ ppm

$CDCl_3$ is commonly used as a solvent that appears as a relatively weak triplet centred at 76.9 ppm due to coupling with deuterium which has spin I = 1. As per 2nI + 1 rule, the C-13 nucleus in $CDCl_3$ is split apart into (2 × 1 × 1 + 1) into a triplet. The control peak at δ 76.9 ppm is taken as the reference peak.

10.7(b) SOLVENTS IN CMR

1. Deuterated Chloroform, $CDCl_3$

$CDCl_3$ is usually used as a solvent in CMR spectroscopy. As an FT-NMR instrument requires a lock-signal of heteronucleus as an additional control mechanism to provide the required stability that electromagnets can not provide, so the deuterium present in $CDCl_3$ serves the purpose. This is particularly necessary for ^{13}C spectra as they require long time periods for accumulation of a large number of scans. This way, it becomes possible to make corrective adjustments between the electromagnetic and the electronics. That is to say, the rf and the magnetic fields are always locked, in keeping with the relation:

$$v_0 = \gamma B_0/2\pi$$

Deuterium, ^2H is an NMR active nucleus $I = I$. As its γ is different from that of the C–13, therefore, it does not absorb in the CMR spectrum. However, spin of the carbon of $CDCl_3$ gets split due to coupling with the spin of deuterium as per the $(2nI + 1)$ rule. That is, it gives a $(2 \times 1 \times 1 + 1)$ "Triplet". This triplet is different from a routine triplet in the sense that the ratio of component peaks is 1:1:1 rather than 1:2:1.

The three peaks are, of course, equally spaced.

The triplet is observed at 77.0 ppm. The three peaks are seen because of three possible spin-states, +1, 0 and –1. The relative ratio of peaks in the triplet is 1:1:1 as these three spin states have equal populations statistically speaking.

It needs to be noted that J_{CD} in $CDCl_3$ is ~ 20 Hz. This is about 1/7 of the J_{CH} value in $CHCl_3$. Why so? The answer is not far to seek. A comparison of Y_H and Y_D shows that Y_H/Y_D is equal to about 7 Hz. Further, the triplet at 77.0 ppm serves as a chemical-shift reference particularly when you forget to add the TMS as the primary reference. Even when TMS is used, it is used in very small amount of ~ 0.02% so that the TMS peak is often lost in the noise. **These days TMS is actually not added.**

2. d₂–Dichloromethane, CD₂Cl₂

This solvent gives a quintet centred at 54.0 ppm. Their relative ratios are 1:2:3:2:1, again different from that in a quintet in a PMR spectrum. The coupling constant, J is equal to 27 Hz. The quintet can be predicted on the basis of the formula:

$$2nI + I$$

In CD_2Cl_2, n, the number of D atoms = 2. $I = I$.

$$\therefore \qquad \text{multiplicity} = 2 \times 2 \times 1 + 1 = 5$$

How can we explain the multiplicity? First of all, the C–13 peak is split into three equally spaced peaks by one deuterium. Then each line is further split by the second deuterium giving a five-line pattern as shown in Fig. 10.7a.

3. Deuterated Acetone (Acetone-ds), CD₃COCD₃

This solvent shows a septet at 29.9 ppm as well as a carbonyl carbon peak at 206.7 ppm as expected.

The "septed" contains seven lines in the relative ratio of 1:3:6:7:6:3:1 with coupling constant J = 18 Hz. The septet is to be expected on the basis of the multiplicity formula $2nI + 1$. As n = 3, therefore $2 \times 3 \times 1 + 1 = 7$. Now, you try yourself to show the origin of the septet and their relative integral ratios.

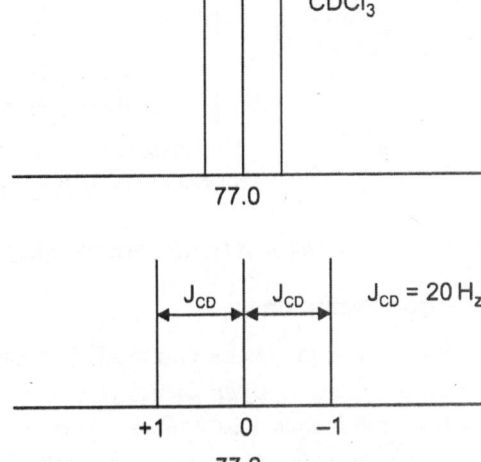

Fig. 10.7a. Origin and intensities of lines in quintet of CD_2Cl_2. A↑ means an +I spin state, A↓ means a –1 spin state and o means spin = 0.

4. Dimethyl sulfoxide–d₆ (DMSO–d₆), CD₃SOCD₃

This is used when $CDCl_3$ is not very suitable on grounds of solubility mainly. This is commonly used for carboxylic acids. As expected on the basis of the multiplicity formula $2nI + I$, DMSO–d₆ shows a septet centred at 39.5 ppm with J ~ 40 Hz.

5. Dioxane–d₈ appears as a quintet at 66.5 ppm

This is less frequently used as is Methanol–d_4 which appears as a septet at 49.0 ppm. Finally, it should be noted just like spin–1/2 Pascal triangle, it is possible to write one (Spin–I Pascal triangle) for as well:

					1							$D = 0$
				1	1	1						$D = 1$
			1	2	3	2	1					$D = 2$
		1	3	6	7	6	3	I				$D = 3$
	1	4	10	16	19	16	10	4	1			$D = 4$
1	5	15	30	45	51	45	30	15	5	I		$D = 5$

Hint: How to remember the relative ratios? Easy. Each number is actually the sum of the number placed directly on top of it as well as the number on the left and right of this top number. For example:

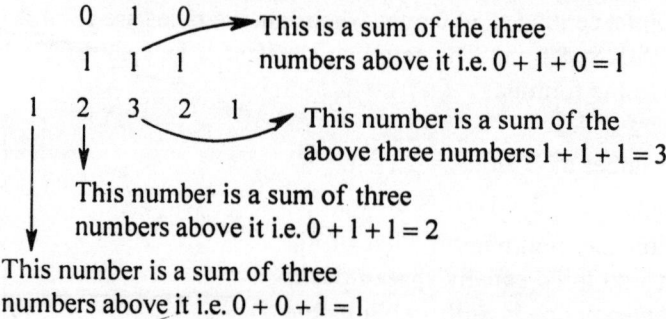

$$0 \quad 1 \quad 0 \rightarrow \text{This is a sum of the three}$$
$$1 \quad 1 \quad 1 \qquad \text{numbers above it i.e. } 0 + 1 + 0 = 1$$

$$1 \quad 2 \quad 3 \quad 2 \quad 1 \quad \text{This number is a sum of the}$$
$$\text{above three numbers } 1 + 1 + 1 = 3$$

This number is a sum of three
numbers above it i.e. $0 + 1 + 1 = 2$

This number is a sum of three
numbers above it i.e. $0 + 0 + 1 = 1$

10.8 THE CORRELATION CHART AND CHEMICAL SHIFT CORRELATIONS

The correlation chart

Chemical shift ranges for common functional groups are shown in the correlation chart in Fig. 10.7b.

As a student is often asked questions regarding the range of some selected functional groups' carbon both in theory as well as in practical class work including viva-voce, this author has arranged the selected functional groups carbon chemical shift in some approximate range that is easy to remember. This is shown in Table 10.1. For alkanes, the range is 8–30 ppm and for C-halogen, it is 30–65 ppm. Next range starts from 65 to 100 ppm for acetylenic carbons. For C = C and aromatics, the range is 100–175 ppm. The next range that begins at 150 ppm and ends at 185 ppm is that for carbonyl C in acids, esters and amides. The next range that begins with 185 ppm and ends upto 220 ppm is for the aldehydic and ketonic carbons. *This, I feel, is necessary to ward off pressure from the minds of the students to memorize the finer details of the real range. In fact, these five functional groups are of wide interest to students. Of course, if the students can remember the correlation chart (Table 8.7) that will be very helpful but why tax one's brain.* After examining the spectrum on the basis of Table 10.1, students should then go to Fig. 10.7b.

Types of Carbon

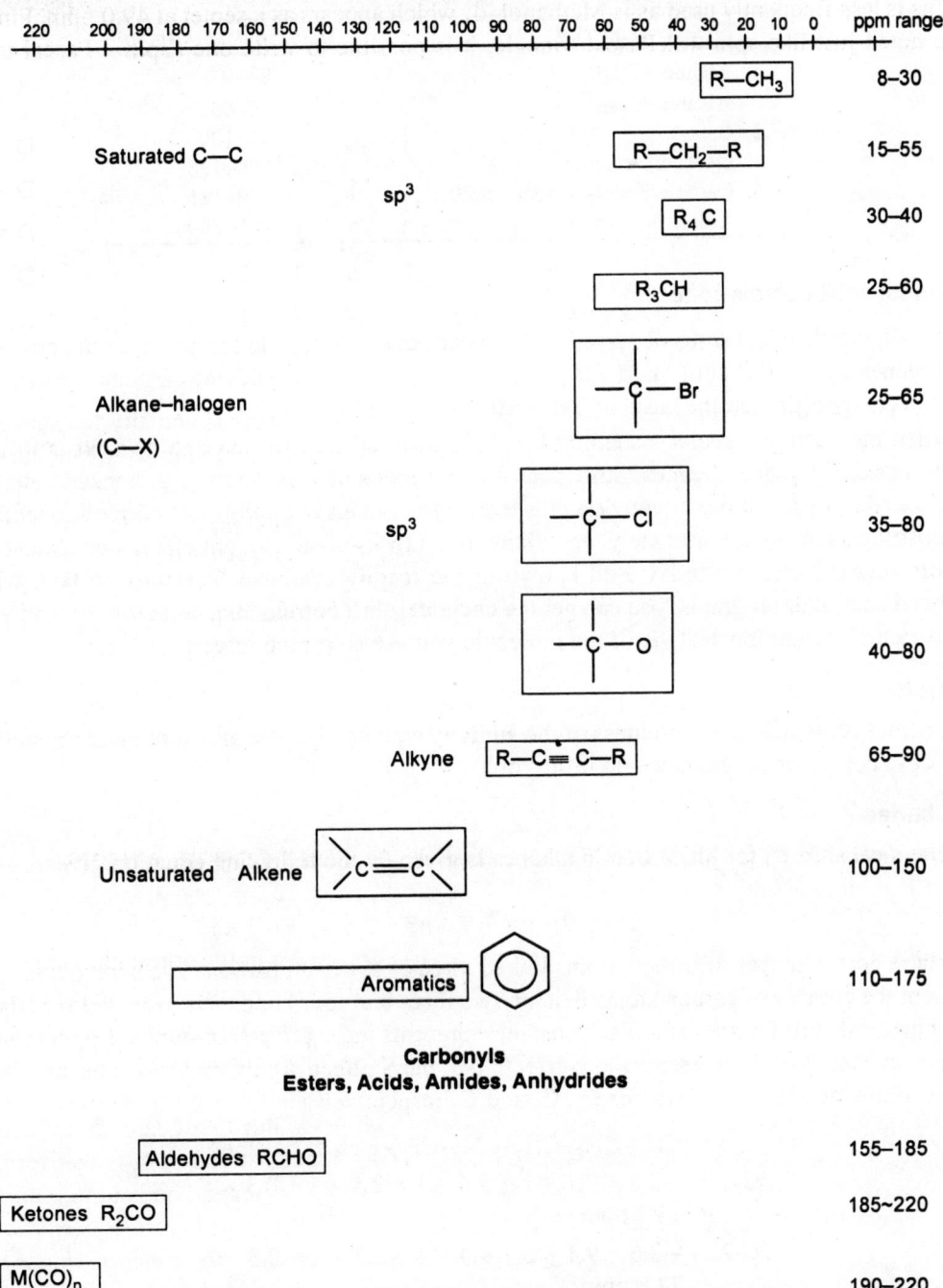

Saturated C—C

sp³

R—CH₃ 8–30

R—CH₂—R 15–55

R₄C 30–40

R₃CH 25–60

Alkane–halogen
(C—X)

sp³

25–65

35–80

40–80

Alkyne   R—C≡C—R   65–90

Unsaturated   Alkene   100–150

Aromatics   110–175

Carbonyls
Esters, Acids, Amides, Anhydrides

Aldehydes RCHO   155–185

Ketones R₂CO   185~220

M(CO)ₙ   190–220

Fig. 10.7b. Correlation chart for common functional groups.

Table 10.1. The chemical shift (approximate) for some selected functional groups

Structural carbon	Chemical shift (ppm)
1. Alkane–C (sp^3)	8–60
Alkane–X (sp^3)	30–65
2. C≡	65–100
3. C=C + aromatic	100–175
4. Carbonyl acids, esters, amides	150–185
5. Aldehydes, ketones	185–220

Chemical shift correlations

First of all, the chemical shifts observed in the spectrum of the sample are noted for their chemical class in the general chemical shift chart for good clues regarding the types of carbons present, molecular skeleton present (first on the basis of Table 10.1 and then Fig. 10.7).

When the basic molecular skeleton class is known, all that we have to do next is to look at the related basic, reference chemical shift data for that molecular skeleton (e.g. benzene etc.) and then using the additivity equations already established we have to make appropriate correction increments for the substituents present. Fortunately, equations for additivity of substituent effects for almost all classes of molecular skeleton are today well known in the readily available literature. In fact, with today's advanced computer programs, you can get the chemical shift correlations done for you and you can get a predicted spectrum for the type of the molecule you sketch on the screen.

Example

I will demonstrate here the usefulness of the additivity equation in case of alkanes and aromatics only as these days computer programmes do it for you!

(a) Alkanes

The chemical shift δ_i, for ith carbon in alkanes is given by the following equation given by Grant and Paul.

$$\delta_i = 2.6 + 9.1\ n\alpha + 9.4\ n\beta - 2.5\ n y + 0.3\ n\delta$$

Where $n\alpha$ = Number of carbon atoms linked directly to the ith carbon. The symbols $n\beta$, ny and $n\delta$ represent the number of carbon atoms that are two three and four bonds removed. – 2.6 S, the constant is the chemical shift for methane. The constant represents the α effect, constant 9.4 ppm represents the β-effect, constant – 2.5 represents the y-effect : 0.3, the S effect. Applying these rules to n-hexane, we get the following chemical shifts for C_1, C_2 and C_3 respectively.

$$\delta = CH_3–CH_2–CH_2–CH_2–CH_2–CH_3 \text{ n hexane}$$
$$\delta C\text{-}1 = -2.6 + 9.1 \times 1 + 9.4 \times 1 \times 2.5 \times 1 + 0.3 \times 1$$
$$= 13.7 \text{ ppm as}$$
$$\delta C\text{-}2 = -2.6 + 9.1 \times 2 + 9.4 \times 1 - 2.5 \times 1 + 0.3$$
$$= 22.8 \text{ ppm}$$
$$\delta C\text{-}3 = -2.6 + 9.1 \times 2 + 9.4 \times 2 - 2.5 \times 1$$
$$= 31.9 \text{ ppm}$$

The observed C-1, C-2 and C-3 chemical shifts are 13.7, 22.7 and 31.8 ppm respectively. The calculated values of 13.7, 22.8 and 31.9 ppm thus tally well with these observed values.

Observed   13.7 22.7 31.8

$$CH_3-CH_2-CH_2-CH_2-CH_2-CH_3$$

Calculated 13.7 22.8 31.9

(b) Aromatics

Thus, let us calculate the chemical shifts for p-nitro phenol. Base value for benzene is 128.5 ppm. We will take values from the Table 10.2 for the substituents :

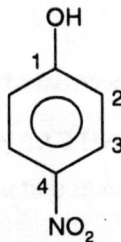

Table 10.2. Substituent chemical shifts (δ_c) in benzenes

Benzene $^\circ C = 128.5$, + to the left, the right

Substituent	C_1	C_2 ortho	C_3 meta	C_4 para
NO_2	19.6	5.3	0.9	6.0
$COOCH_3$	2.0	1.2	– 0.1	4.8
$COCH_3$	7.8	– 0.4	– 0.4	+ 2.8
CHO	8.2	1.2	0.6	5.8
CN	– 16.0	3.6	0.6	4.3
F	35.1	– 14.3	0.9	– 4.5
Cl	6.4	0.2	1.0	– 2.0
Br	– 5.4	3.4	2.2	– 1.0
I	– 32.2	9.9	2.8	– 7.3
OH	26.6	– 12.7	1.6	– 7.3
OCH_3	31.4	– 14.4	1.0	– 7.7
$OCOCH_3$	22.4	– 7.1	– 0.4	– 3.2
COOH	2.8	1.3	0.4	4.3
NH_2	19.2	– 12.4	1.3	– 9.5
NMe_2	22.4	– 15.7	0.8	– 11.8
CH_3	9.3	0.7	– 0.1	– 2.9
CH_2CH_3	15.3	– 0.5	0.0	– 2.6
$CH(CH_2)_2$	20.1	– 2.0	0.0	– 2.5
$- C(CH_3)_3$	22.9	– 3.4	– 0.4	– 3.1
$- C \equiv CH$	– 5.8	6.9	0.1	0.4
– Ph	12.1	– 1.8	– 0.1	– 1.6

Calculated chemical shifts for C_1, C_2, C_3 and C_4 taking base value for benzene as 128.5 ppm :

$\delta C_1 = 128.5 + 26.6 + 6.0 = 161.1$

$\delta C_2 = 128.5 - 12.7 + 0.9 = 116.7$

$\delta C_3 = 128.5 + 1.6 - 5.3 = 124.8$

$\delta C_4 = 128.5 + 19.6 + 7.3 = 140.8$

Comparison of calculated and observed data :

	Calculated (ppm)	Observed (ppm)
δC_1	161.1	161.5
δC_2	116.7	115.9
δC_3	124.8	126.4
δC_4	140.8	141.7

Thus, the utility of the corrective additions are demonstrated quite clearly.

10.9 CHEMICAL SHIFTS OF PROTONS AND CARBON-13: A COMPARISON

Although the range for C-13 is about twenty times that of proton : while C-13 range is 0–200 ppm, it is a mere 0–10 ppm for protons; the orders in C–13 chemical shifts are somewhat (roughly) similar to those observed in proton shifts. Moving downfield from the reference (TMS = 0 ppm), the order for C-13 as well as H is overall similar as shown in Table 10.3 and Fig. 10.8.

TMS $\longrightarrow$ Alkanes $\longrightarrow$ Olefins $\longrightarrow$ aromatics $\longrightarrow$ aldehydes

Table 10.3. Increasing chemical shifts order for ^{13}C and ^1H shifts in ppm

Chemical class	δC-13	δH
Alkanes	8–60	0.5–1.5
Alkones	100–150	4.5–6.5
Aromatics	110–175	6.0–8.5
Aldehyde	185–220	9–10.5

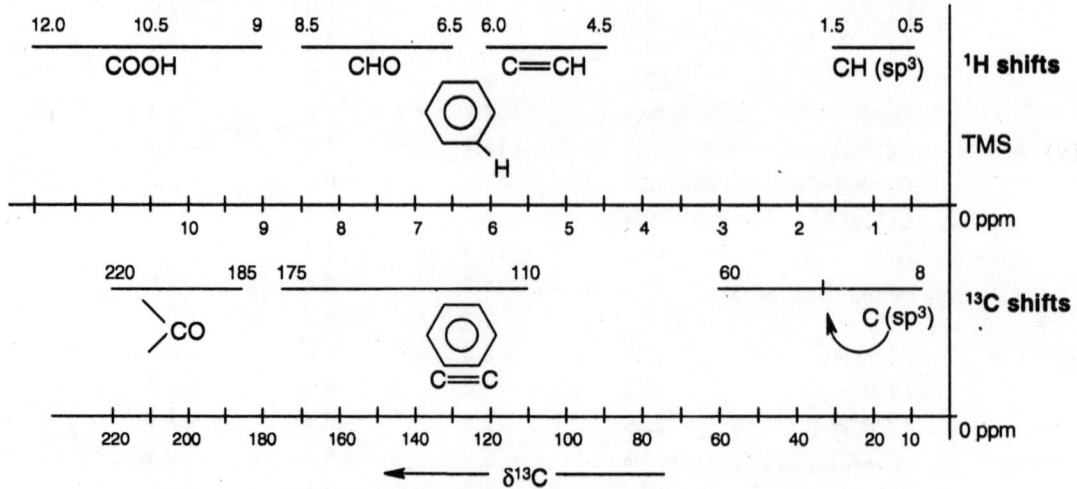

Fig. 10.8. Analogy between δH and δC on TMS scale

(a) Similarities

(i) The factors such as electronegativity and anisotropy and hybridisation which affect ^1H shifts as we saw in Chapter 2, also affect the C-13 shifts as well in about the same way. The downfield shift in ^{13}C shifts due to electronegativity is more in ^{13}C than in ^1H because the electronegative atom is directly attached to the ^{13}C atom whereas the ^1H is effected indirectly, through two bonds i.e. X–C–H.

(ii) When we look at hydrocarbon without any nearby electronegative or unsaturated groups, we find that the chemical shift of both ^{13}C and ^1H are at the right edge of the range i.e. 8–30 ppm for ^{13}C and 0.8–1.6 for ^1H. For each substitutions on the hydrocarbon part, there occurs a small downfield shift in both cases (^{13}C and ^1H) :

$$-\overset{|}{\underset{|}{C}}H \;>\; \overset{|}{\underset{|}{C}}H_2 \;>\; -CH_3$$

30	20	10	^{13}C shift
1.6	1.2	0.8	^1H shift

(iii) **Electronegativity** causes identical effect of deshielding in ^{13}C shifts as we see in ^1H shifts. The more electronegative between oxygen and nitrogen causes stronger downfield shift.

For CH–O–
^{13}C shifts	50–85 ppm
^1H shifts	3–4 ppm

(iv) Downfield shifts are observed for increasing substitution on C–O bonds :

$$-\overset{|}{\underset{|}{C}}-$$

	^{13}C ppm
	85
$-\overset{|}{C}H-O$	75
$-CH_2-O$	65
CH_3-O	55

40

(v) Anisotropy effect that is seen in ^1H spectra, also affects ^{13}C shifts.

Thus, when a substituent is near an unsaturated group as C == O, the effect is clearly discernible in ^{13}C as in ^1H shifts. The deshielding is observed.

Example :

(a) CH$_3$ being attached to C == O :

$$\begin{array}{c} H_3C \\ \diagdown \\ \diagup \, C == O \\ H_3C \end{array}$$

The ^{13}C of the CH$_3$ absorbs downfield at 30 ppm like ^1H of the CH$_3$ resonates downfield at 2.1 ppm. The CH$_3$ group in acetone is in the plane of the C == O group and is, therefore, affected by anisotropy.

(b) Anisotropic effect is also seen in alkenes both for ^{13}C and ^1H :

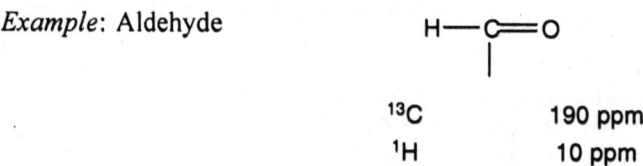

^{13}C	100–150 ppm
^1H	4–6 ppm

(vi) Combined effect of electronegativity and unsaturation or anisotropy is visible in both ^{13}C and ^1H.

   Example: Aldehyde   H—C=O

^{13}C	190 ppm
^1H	10 ppm

(vii) **Hydrogen bonding** with polar solvents leads to downfield shifts in both ^{13}C and ^1H.

(viii) The acetylenic carbons resonate in the range of 65–90 ppm that is in between the range for sp^3 (δ–30 ppm) and sp^2 carbons (100–175 ppm). This is similar to the situations in ^1H shifts while the sp^3 C–H protons absorbs at 0.5–1.5 ppm, and sp^2 at 4.5–6.5 ppm, the acetylenic protons resonate at 2.5–3.5 ppm :

	^{13}C ppm	^1H ppm
C–CH	8–30	0.5–1.5
C≡CH	65–90	2.5–3.5
C=CH	100–175	4.5–6.5

(b) Divergences

However, there are some divergences as well.

(i) While ^{13}C shifts for aromatic and olefinic carbons are almost the same (100–175), it is not so in ^1H spectroscopy. Further while th alkene protons absorb at 4.5–6.5 ppm, the aromatic protons resonate at 6–8.5 ppm. So **PMR spectroscopy is better in this respect for making distinction between C = CH and aromatic C = CH bonds compared to C–13 NMR spectroscopy.**

	^{13}C ppm	^1H ppm
Olefinic aromatic	100–175 ppm	6–8.5 ppm
		4.5–6.5 ppm

Intext Question

2. Which is better in making distinction between aliphatic and aromatic compounds — PMR or CMR?

   Hint: Answer as above in (i).

(ii) The electronegativity effect in ^{13}C and ^1H are dissimilar. While the electronegativity effect leads only to deshielding and gets reduced with distance, in ^{13}C the situation is different. Although the electronegativity effect leads to deshielding or downfield shift in the α and β carbons, it causes the opposite effect on γ carbon i.e. it causes a small upfield or shielding effect. That is to say while an electronegative substituent (iodine being an exception) at α or β-position, deshields the carbon, that in the γ-position shields it. This effect is called **γ-effect.** This γ-effect is of great importance in doing conformational analysis we will see later on.

Intext Question

3. What are the similarities and divergences between proton and C–13 chemical shifts?

   Hint: See answer as above.

10.10 FACTORS AFFECTING CHEMICAL SHIFTS OF C-13 NUCLEI–

1. π-Charge density effects
2. Resonance effects
3. Neighbour anisotropy effect and chemical shift anisotropy
4. Isotope effect
5. Hybridisation effects
6. Substituent effects (α, β and γ-effects)
7. Steric effect due to induced polarization of C–H
8. Hyperconjugation effects

10.11. π-CHARGE DENSITY EFFECTS

In ions containing π-bond, the C-13 shifts can be correlated with π-charge density. While negative charge density leads to shielding, positive charge causes deshielding. Greater the negative charge, greater the shielding. Greater the positive charge, higher the deshielding. That is to say as the π-charge density increases from positive to negative, chemical shift decreases. This is shown in Fig. 8.9.

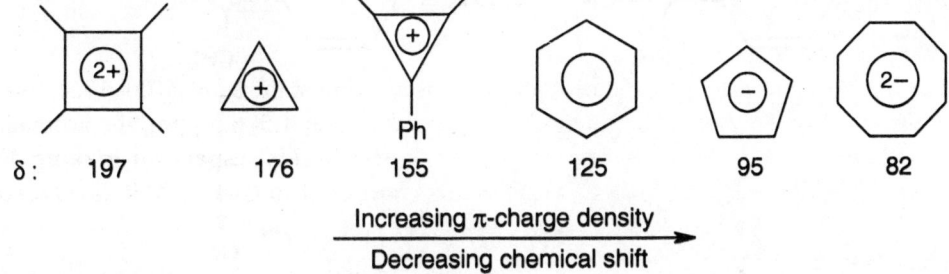

δ: 197   176   155   125   95   82

Increasing π-charge density
Decreasing chemical shift

Fig. 10.9. Correlation between π-electron densities and chemical shift in aromatic system based upon charge density of benzene carbons.

10.12 RESONANCE EFFECTS

Resonance leads to charge separation in the molecules making one carbon atom positive, and the other negative. The positively charged carbon thus gets deshielded and resonates at higher chemical shift compared to the carbon that develops negative charge and therefore gets shielded.

Examples

Ketene : In ketene, while the CH_2 carbon resonates at δ 2.5 ppm, the carbonyl carbon absorbs at δ 194.0 ppm.

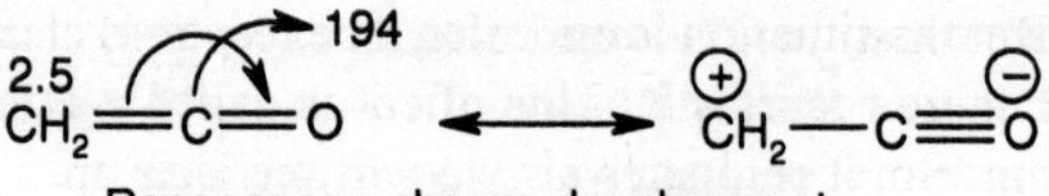

Resonance : charge development

2-cyclohexenone :

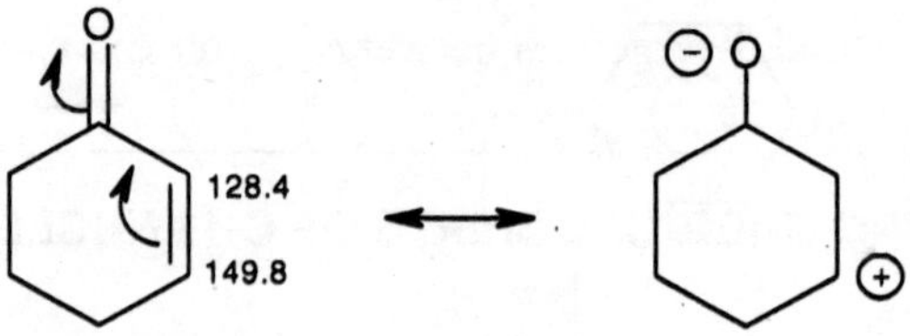

128.4

149.8

The carbocations having alkyl substituents are more deshielded compared to the carbocations having substituents which take up the positive charge on to themselves through resonance. Thus the central carbon in tert-butyl carbocation resonates at 328 ppm, while that in phenyl dimethyl methane carbocation absorbs at δ 254 ppm.

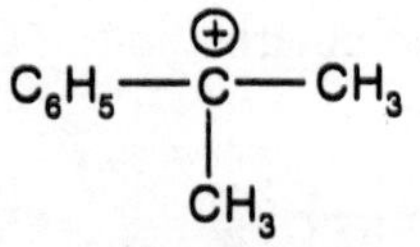

$(CH_3)_3\overset{\oplus}{C}$

328 ppm

$C_6H_5\overset{\oplus}{-}\overset{|}{C}-CH_3$

CH_3

254 ppm

The phenyl group stabilises the carbocation through resonance, thereby reducing the positive charge on the central carbon :

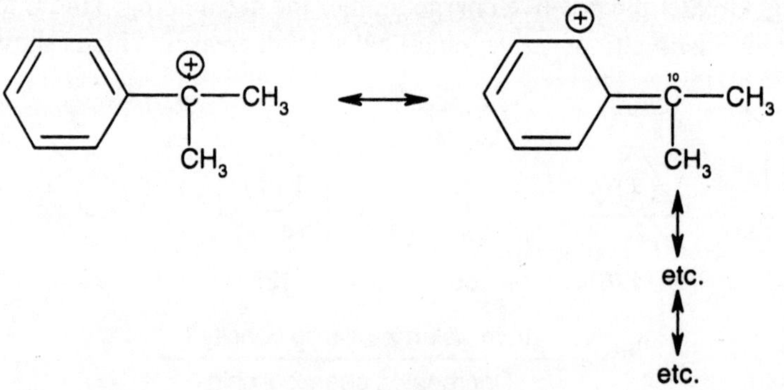

etc.

etc.

Similarly, while phenyl di-methyl carbocation resonates at 254 ppm, the diphenyl methyl carbocation absorbs at 198 ppm. This is because of greater reduction of positive charge by the greater resonating effect of the two phenyl groups in the latter.

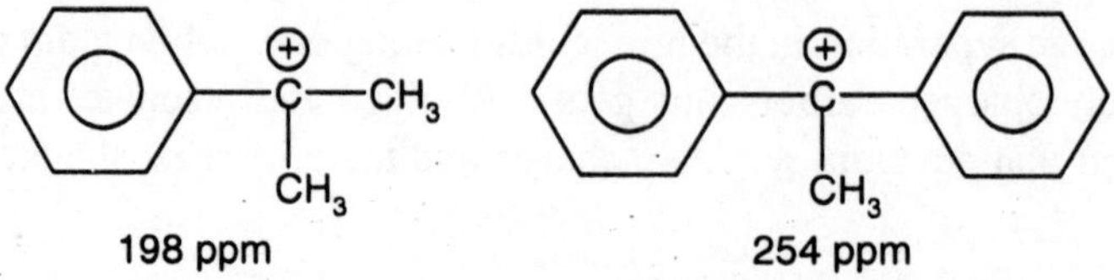

198 ppm

254 ppm

In triphenyl methane carbocation, the central carbon absorbs at 211 ppm, even though it has three phenyl groups that should reduce the positive charge even further at the central carbon compared to diphenyl methyl carbocation. But the situation is opposite. The reason is clear. With the introduction of the third phenyl group instead, there occurs inhibition of co-planarity in the molecule, a condition that is a must for resonance to occur. So, it resonates at a lower chemical shift compared to the diphenyl methyl carbocation.

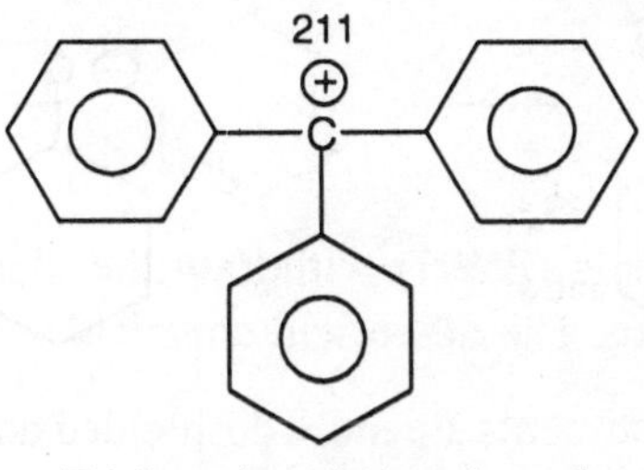

Triphenyl methyl carbocation

Steric factor prevents phenyl groups from assuming a co-planar arrangement.

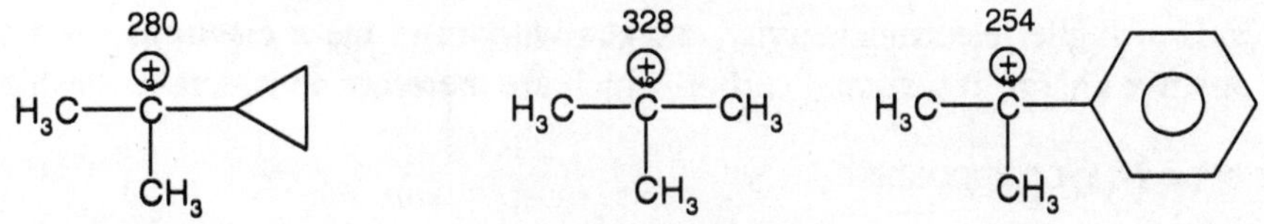

Cyclopropyl dimethyl carbocation   Trimethyl carbocation

The ^{13}C shift of cyclopropyl dimethyl carbocation (280 ppm) is in keeping with the reduced positive charge on the central carbon. In fact, this confirms the special stability of this carbocation, even more stability than the benzyl type carbocations. This extra stability is due to conjugation between the vacant pure p orbital of the central carbon with the bent orbitals of the cyclopropyl ring :

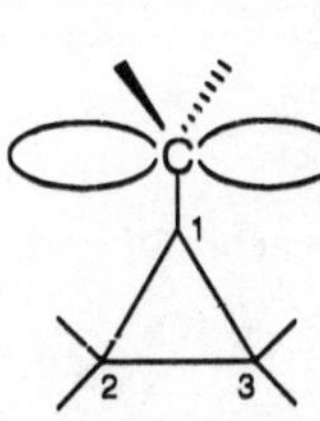

The conjugation is possible as the p orbital is oriented parallel to C_2–C_3 bond of the cyclopropane ring. If it were at right angle to it, the conjugation would not have been possible.

As the number of cyclopropyl groups increases, stability of the carbocation increases in that order, reducing the positive charge on the cationic carbon even further due to the same reason.

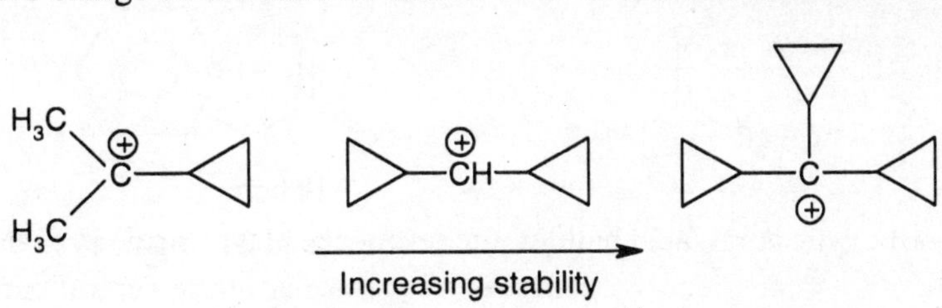

Increasing stability

Electron-donating substituents (EDG) activate the ortho and para carbons increasing charge density at such positions in benzene. This leads to paramagnetic shielding.

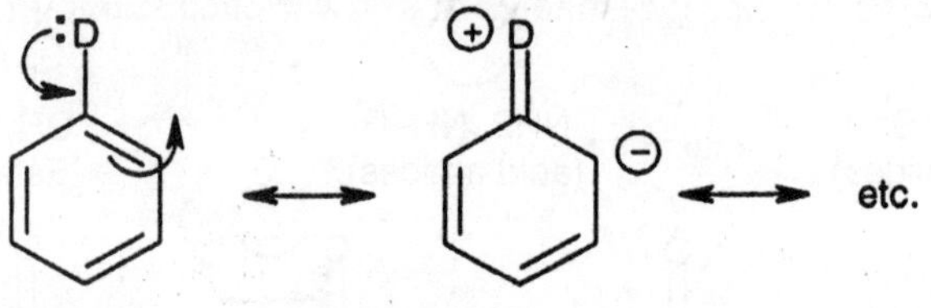

etc.

Electron withdrawing substituents (EWG) withdraw the electron density from ortho and para positions, thus leading to deshielding. The downfield chemical shifts of carbonyl carbons also occurs due to resonance :

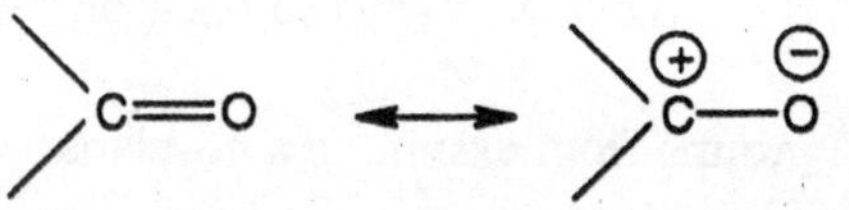

As a result of higher electronegativity, oxygen withdraws the π electrons towards itself, thereby leading to positive charge at carbonyl carbon which are therefore considerably deshielded.

Examples of carboxyl compounds

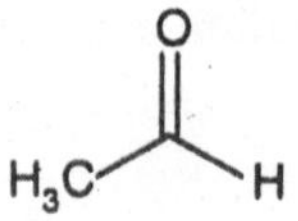

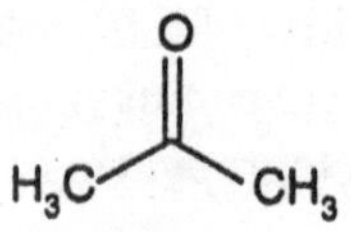

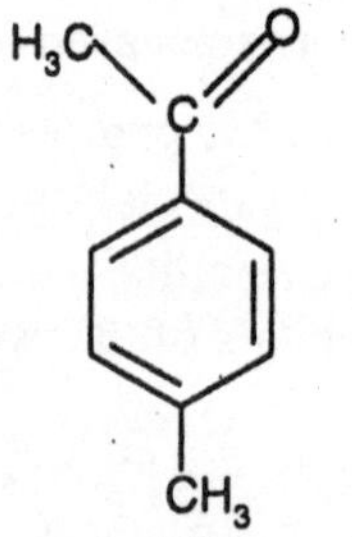

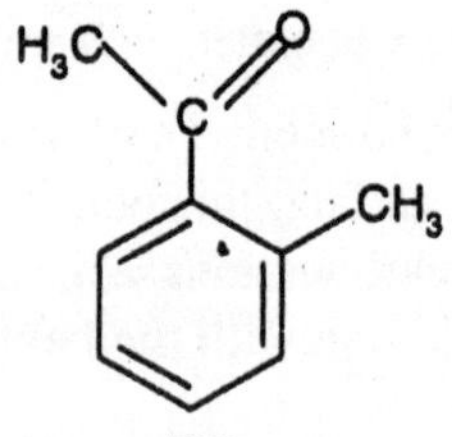

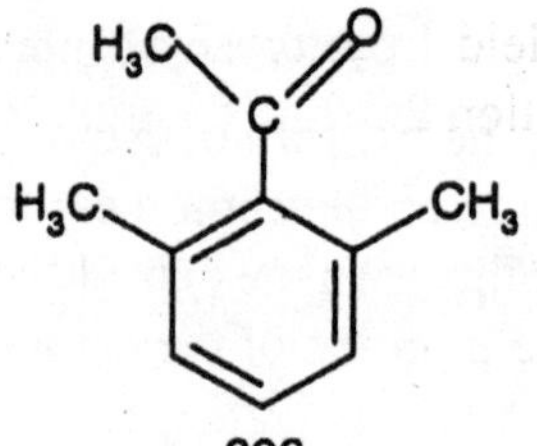

In unsaturated compounds, the effect on carbonyl carbon occurs as follows :

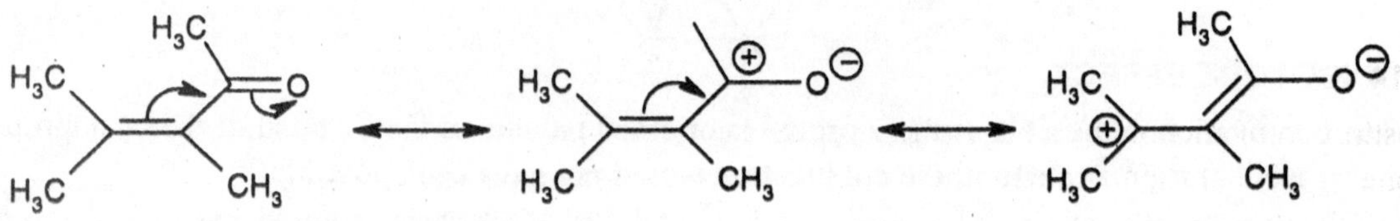

Examples

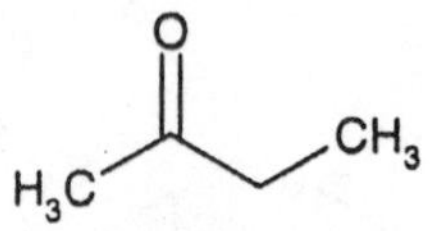

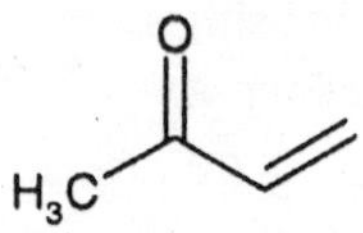

Amides, esters, carboxylic acids, acid halides, the resonance plays its role in deshielding the central carbon nuclei :

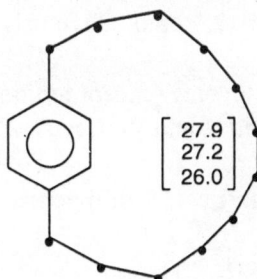

| X = Cl, Br, I | NH2, NH–R | OR, OH etc. |
| (acid halides) | (acid amides) | Ester, acids |

H_3C—OH 177 H_3C—OCH$_3$ 171 H_3C—NH$_2$ 172 H_3C—NH—CH$_3$ 172

H_3C—Cl 170 H_3C—Br 167 H_3C—I 160

10.13 NEIGHBOUR ANISOTROPY EFFECT AND CHEMICAL SHIFT ANISOTROPY

As in proton NMR spectroscopy, the neighbouring group anisotropy causes shielding of ring carbons. An example is [12]p–cyclophane in which the most shielded ring carbons appear at about 0.7 ppm upfield from those of cycloheptadecane. For a discussion of Chemical Shift Anisotropy (CSA), see Section 2.5.2.4 (Example 15).

$$\begin{bmatrix} 27.9 \\ 27.2 \\ 26.0 \end{bmatrix}$$

10.14 ISOTOPE EFFECT

Substitution of an atom by a heavier isotope causes an upfield shift of the carbons located at a distance of one or two bonds. Of course, there are examples that show downfield isotope effects.

10.15 HYBRIDISATION EFFECTS

As already stated the effect of hybridisation becomes clear as we find three different chemical shift regions for alkenes (sp^3), alkenes (sp^2) and acetylenes (sp) :

Alkanes (sp^3)	0–30 ppm
Alkynes (sp)	65–85 ppm
Alkenes (sp^2)	100–150 ppm

We will study the examples of these three classes later.

10.16 SUBSTITUENT EFFECTS IN ^{13}C CHEMICAL SHIFT: α, β AND γ EFFECTS

Alkanes

The effect of an electronegative element like chlorine is to withdraw the electron density away from the carbon atom to which it is covalently bonded towards itself. The net result of this removal of electron density from around the carbon will be to deshield it. *This is what we observe in PMR spectroscopy as well as in CMR spectroscopy but with a difference. The electronegativity effect diminishes with carbon chain in proton nmr spectroscopy. However, these effects are bigger in CMR spectroscopy and are felt farther away along the carbon chain and not only that, they also fall into different patterns as well.*

Let us consider the effect of chlorine on absorptions of carbons along a chain.

13.6   22.1   29.2   32.7   44.3   13.7   22.6   34.5   22.6   13.7

CH_3—CH_2—CH_2—CH_2—CH_2 CH_3—CH_2—CH_2—CH_2—CH_2

| |

Cl   H

1-Chloropentane   n-pentane

The C_1 resonates at δ 44.3 in 1–chloropentane compared to C_1 of pentane that resonates at δ 13.7 ppm. There is a downfield shift of δ 3.06 ppm. This shift is called the **α-effect.**

When we look at the chemical shift difference between C-2 (δ 22.6 ppm) of n-pentane and C-2 (δ 32.7 ppm) of 1–chloropentane, we find it is a downfield shift of + 10.1 ppm, although it is not as large as in α-effect. This is called **β-effect.**

But when we go to γ-carbon, we find the opposite situation! The carbon-3 is no longer deshielded! Rather it is shielded! It absorbs upfield unexpectedly! While C-3 of n-pentane absorbs at δ 34.5 ppm, the C-3 of 1–chloropentane absorbs at δ 22.1 ppm. Obviously the γ-carbon is upfield by – 5.3 ppm. This shift is called the γ-**effect.**

Not only chlorine, but all other substituents (except iodine) show the same substituent effects of absorption by sp^3 carbons : the downfield α and β-effects, of course the α-effect is bigger than the β-effect and the γ-effect that is upfield.

The α-effects of some other substituents at C-1 of n-pentane are as follows:

83.8

F + 70.1 ppm in F–CH_2–CH_2–CH_2–CH_2–CH_3

33.0

Br + 19.3 ppm in Br–CH_2–CH_2–CH_2–CH_2–CH_3

43.4

NH_2 + 29 ppm in H_2N–CH_2–CH_2–CH_2–CH_2–CH_3

62.0

OH + 48.3 ppm in HO–CH_2–CH_2–CH_2–CH_2–CH_3

78.2

NO_2 + 64.5 ppm in O_2N–CH_2–CH_2–CH_2–CH_2–CH_3

In fact, now it is possible to predict the chemical shift of any carbon having any substituent at any position in the linear or branched alkanes and cycloalkanes by adding shifts to the base value that can be calculated using a particular equation?

It should be noted that α, β and γ-effects are smaller for alkyl groups than for other substituents. In fact, the α- and β-effects are almost same for the methyl group, though the γ-effects are smaller and upfield.

For example, if we consider n-hexane to be n-pentane having been substituted at C-1 with a methyl group :

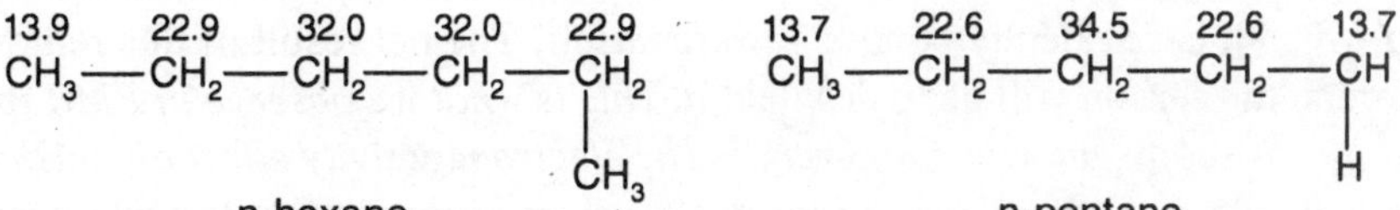

n-hexane

n-pentane

From the δC values indicated, it is clear that the substituent effect of methyl group is at : α-carbon $22.9 - 13.7 = + 9.2$ ppm; β-carbon $32.0 - 22.6 = + 9.4$ ppm; γ-carbon $(34.5 + 32.0) = -2.5$ ppm. The γ effect is illustrated as follows :

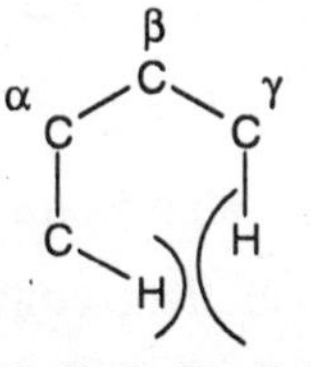

γ (C–C–C–C) effect

The γ-effect, the upfield shift at a γ-carbon due to a substituent has been interpreted as a result of a steric shift. This is suggested because most methyl and methylene carbons that experience a γ (C–C–C–C) gauche steric interactions appear upfield as compared to examples of molecules in which such interactions do not exist.

γ-effect in cyclohexanes

The γ-effect is also noted in cyclohexanes and that too to different extents for the axial and equatorial methyl substituents.

The equatorial methyl carbons absorb at about δ 22–23, while the axial methyl carbons appear at δ 18–19 ppm, there is a sizeable upfield shift of ~ 4–7 ppm for the axial γ-carbons, while there is a 0–3 ppm upfield shift for equational γ-carbon. It is therefore a matter of good news to us. How? Because it becomes possible to differentiate between axial and equatorial substituents. Hence, the γ-effect assumes great importance from the point of view of conformational analysis where the stereochemistry of different conformational isomers can be done with the aid of ^{13}C chemical shift data :

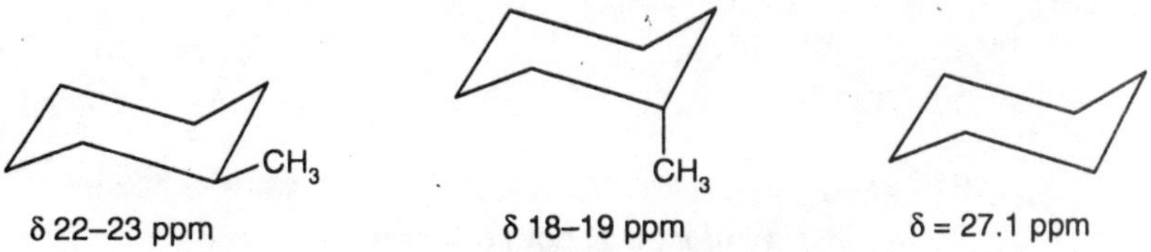

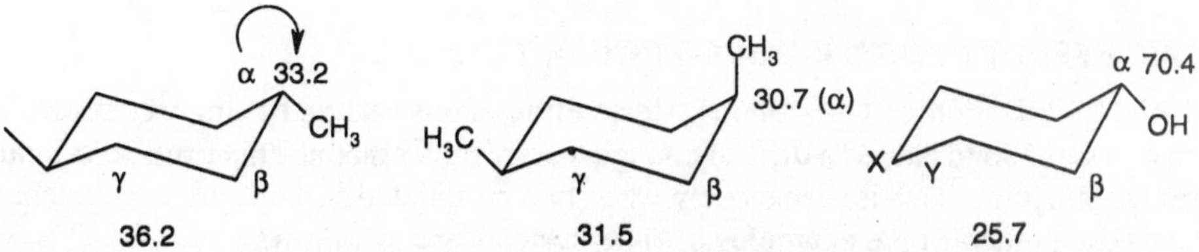

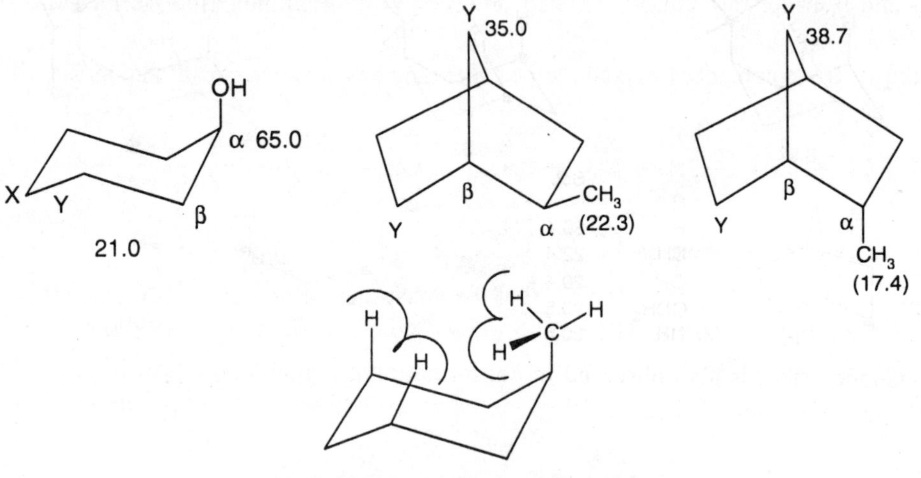

Y (C–C–C–C) interaction in cyclic systems

Further proof for such type of interactions is that as anticipated, the γ-effect in open chain molecules lies in between these values.

γ-effect in alkenes

Now, you must be wondering about the situation in cis (Z)– trans (E) isomeric carbons. Well, cis groups are usually shielded compared to the trans carbons by 4–6 ppm is due to γ-effect.

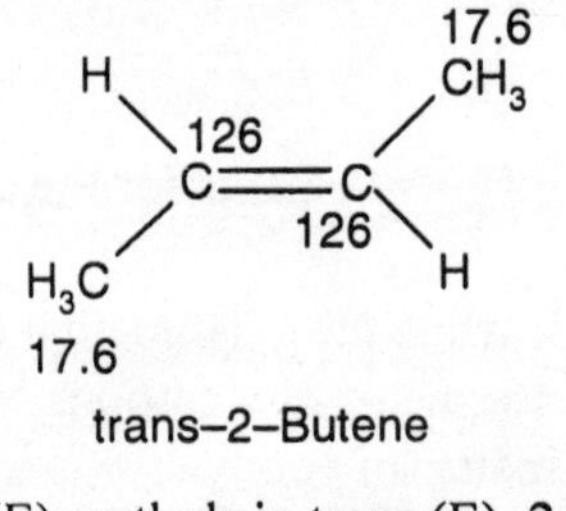

trans–2–Butene

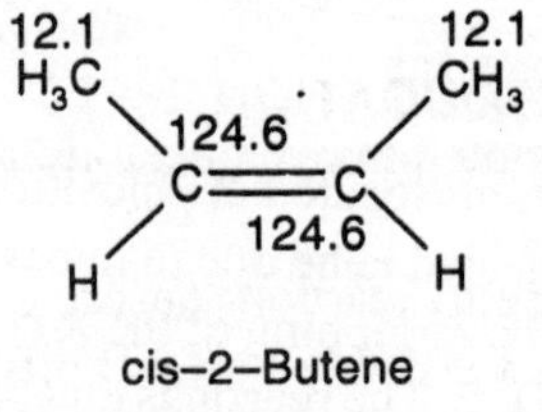

cis–2–Butene

Thus the trans (E) methyls in trans (E)–2–butene resonate at 16.8 ppm while the cis(Z)–methyls are shielded and absorbs at 11.4 ppm. This is illustrated by another example as well, the cis-trans 3-hexenes.

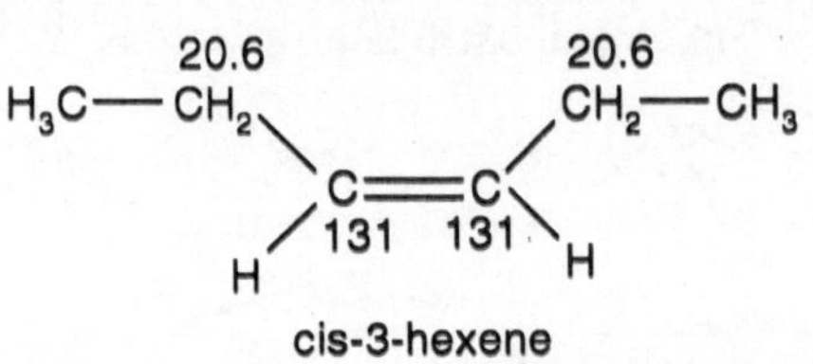

cis-3-hexene

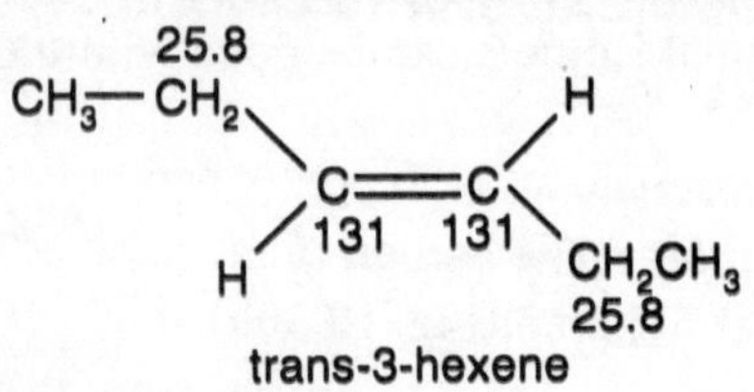

trans-3-hexene

Shift induced at dotted ● carbon

10.17 STERIC EFFECT DUE TO INDUCED POLARIZATION OF C–H

Due to induced polarization of C–H bonds, steric effect shows its effect on ^{13}C shifts. Thus, steric perturbation of a C–H bond causes a drift of change towards the carbon. This leads to orbital expansion and so increased shielding. This is seen closely when two protonated carbons are in γ-gauche orientation with respect to each other. Some examples of rigid systems are as follows :

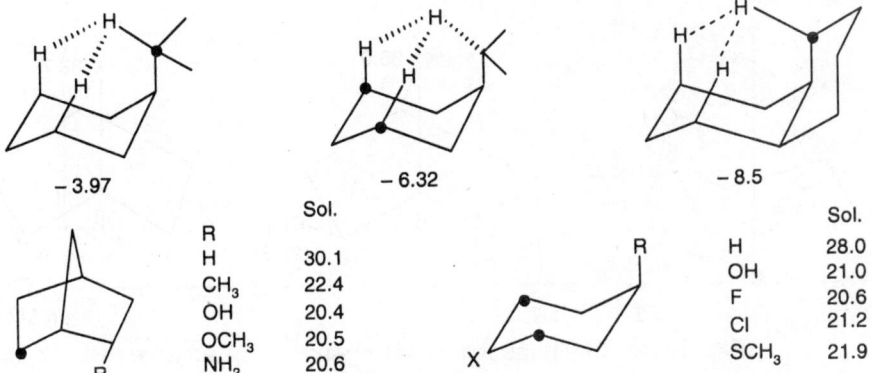

–3.97			–6.32		–8.5	

Sol.

R				R		Sol.
H	30.1			H		28.0
CH$_3$	22.4			OH		21.0
OH	20.4			F		20.6
OCH$_3$	20.5			Cl		21.2
NH$_2$	20.6			SCH$_3$		21.9

The γ-gauche effect is also observed in conformationally mobile systems. In open chain alkanes whereby the gauche rotamer exists in 30% population, upfield shifts of –2 ppm are noticed at γ-carbon.

$$\overset{\alpha}{X} - \overset{\beta}{CH_2} - \overset{\gamma}{CH_2} - CH_2 - CH_2 -$$

X	α	β	ψ
CH$_3$	+9	+10	–2
SH	+11	+12	–6
NH$_2$	+29	+11	–5
Cl	+31	+11	–4

Other substituents also cause similar upfield shifts of – 1 to – 5 ppm.

10.18 HYPERCONJUGATION EFFECTS

First row hetero-atoms located at γ-position and antiperiplanar to the C-13 nucleus cause upfield shifts. This has been suggested to be due to hyperconjugation. The effect leads to an increased electron density at γ-carbon. Partial overlapping of the lone pairs of the hetero-atom X with pπ orbitals of C_α is specially favourable for N, O, F. The reason is that the C–X bond is short while the pπ orbital radii are comparable to that of the carbon.

10.19 CHEMICAL SHIFTS OF CHEMICAL CLASSES

1. Alkanes

Alkanes resonate at 0–30 ppm when not substituted by hetero atoms.

Examples : The carbon in methane absorbs at – 2.3 ppm (Fig. 10.10a) while the carbon in ethane resonate at 5.7 ppm (Fig. 10.10b).

(CH$_3$)$_4$Si	CH$_4$	CH$_3$—CH$_3$	
0.0	–2.2	5.7	5.7

That is as the C gets substituted, its shift goes downfield.

In propane, the chemical shifts of terminal and middle carbons are respectively.

CH$_3$	CH$_2$	CH$_3$	n-propane
15.8	16.3	15.8	

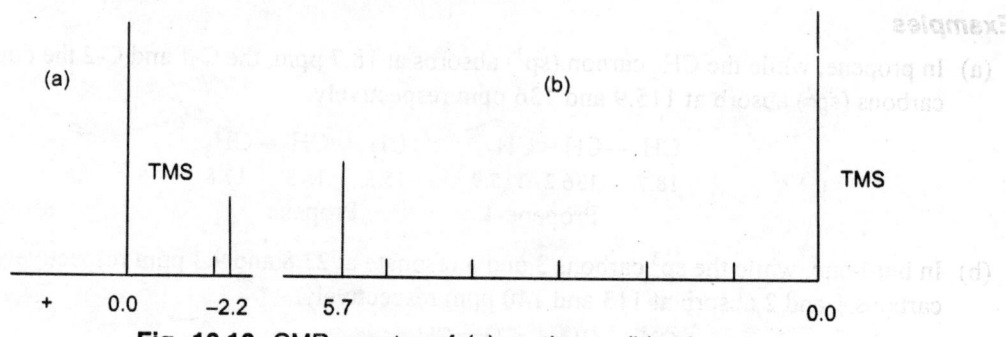

Fig. 10.10. CMR spectra of (a) methane, (b) ethane.

The trend continues in butane and pentane:

$$\underset{13.4}{CH_3} \quad \underset{25.2}{CH_2} \quad \underset{25.2}{CH_2} \quad \underset{13.4}{CH_3} \qquad \text{n-butane}$$

$$\underset{13.9}{CH_3} \quad \underset{22.8}{CH_2} \quad \underset{34.7}{CH_2} \quad \underset{22.8}{CH_2} \quad \underset{13.9}{CH_3} \quad \text{n-pentane}$$

Comparison of the alkenes C-shifts with those of the corresponding alkanes, shows that the olefinic double bond causes an upfield shift (though small) effect on the chemical shifts of the sp³ hybridised carbons in the molecule.

$$\underset{15.8 \quad 16.3 \quad 15.8}{CH_3-CH_2-CH_3} \qquad \underset{18.7 \quad 136.2 \quad 115.9}{CH_3-CH=CH_2}$$

That is to say that while the CH_3 carbon absorbs at 18.7 ppm in 1–propene, the CH_3 of n-propane absorbs at 15.8 ppm.

$$\underset{13.9 \quad 22.9 \quad 32.0 \quad 32.0 \quad 22.9 \quad 13.9}{CH_3-CH_2-CH_2-CH_2-CH_2-CH_3}$$
$$\text{n-hexane}$$

Below are some examples of cycloalkenes with shifts of sp³ carbons :

30.2 H₂C——CH 137.2

H₂C——CH

Cyclobutane

130.8
22.1
32.6
Cyclopentene

127.3
22.1
24.5
Cyclohexene

36.2   107.1
        CH₂
28.9
       149.7
26.9
Cyclohexylmethylene

113.3
–CH=CH₂
137.1
Styrene   cf

29.1   15.6
–CH₂—CH₃
Ethyl benzene

Alkenes

For alkenes, sp² carbons, the chemical shifts are in the range 100–150 ppm.

Examples

(a) In propene, while the CH_3 carbon (sp^3) absorbs at 18.7 ppm, the C-1 and C-2 the doubly bonded carbons (sp^2) absorb at 115.9 and 136 ppm respectively.

$$CH_3—CH=CH_2 \qquad CH_3—CH_2—CH_3$$

$$\text{18.7} \quad \text{136.2} \;\; \text{115.9} \qquad \text{15.8} \quad \text{16.3} \quad \text{15.8}$$

$$\text{Propene-1} \qquad\qquad \text{Propane}$$

(b) In but-l-ene, while the sp^3 carbons 3 and 4 resonate at 23.8 and 9.3 ppm respectively, the alkene carbons 1 and 2 absorb at 113 and 140 ppm respectively.

$$CH_3—CH_2—CH=CH_2$$

$$\text{9.3} \quad \text{23.8} \quad \text{140} \quad \text{113}$$

(c) The chemical shifts of some other olefinic carbons is depicted below.

$$CH_3—CH_2—CH_2—CH=CH_3$$

$$\text{138.5} \;\; \text{114.3}$$

$$\text{Pentene-1}$$

$$CH_3—CH_2—CH_3—CH_2—CH_3=CH_2$$

$$\text{138.7} \;\; \text{114.5}$$

Further, it needs to be noted that the terminal methylene group, $=CH_2$ is shielded while the internal $=CH-$ is deshielded as shown below :

$$\text{109.3 } H_2C \diagdown \qquad CH_2 \diagup$$
$$CH \qquad CH_3$$
$$\text{149.3} \;|$$
$$CH_3$$

$$H_3C \diagdown \qquad\qquad CH_3$$
$$\qquad\qquad \text{131.4} \diagup$$
$$C=CH$$
$$\qquad\qquad \text{118.7}$$
$$H_3C \diagup$$

Now, you must be wondering about the situation in cis (Z)– trans (E) isomeric carbons. Well, cis groups are usually shielded compared to the trans carbons by 4–6 ppm, due to γ-effect.

$$\text{17.6}$$
$$H \diagdown \qquad CH_3$$
$$\text{126} \diagup$$
$$C=C$$
$$\qquad \text{126} \diagdown H$$
$$H_3C \diagup$$
$$\text{17.6}$$
$$\text{trans–2–Butene}$$

$$\text{12.1}$$
$$H_3C \diagdown \qquad CH_3$$
$$\text{124.6} \diagup$$
$$C=C$$
$$\qquad \text{124.6} \diagdown H$$
$$H \diagup$$
$$\text{12.1}$$
$$\text{cis–2–Butene}$$

Thus the trans (E) methyls in trans (E)–2–butene resonate at 16.8 ppm while the cis(Z)–methyls are shielded and absorbs at 11.4 ppm. This is illustrated by another example as well, the cis-trans 3-hexenes.

$$\text{20.6} \qquad\qquad \text{20.6}$$
$$H_3C—CH_2 \diagdown \qquad CH_2—CH_3$$
$$C=C$$
$$\diagup \text{131} \;\; \text{131} \diagdown$$
$$H \qquad\qquad\qquad H$$
$$\text{cis-3-hexene}$$

$$\text{25.8}$$
$$CH_3—CH_2 \diagdown \qquad\qquad H$$
$$C=C$$
$$\diagup \text{131} \;\; \text{131} \diagdown CH_2CH_3$$
$$H \qquad\qquad\qquad \text{25.8}$$
$$\text{trans-3-hexene}$$

3. Alkynes

The alkyne carbons with alkyl substituents resonate in between the range for sp^3 and sp^2 carbons as is the case with protons i.e. at 65–90 ppm.

Further, in general $C \equiv C$ leads to shielding of the directly substituted sp^3 carbon by around 5–15 ppm when compared to its counterpart in alkanes.

Examples

$$\overset{22.1}{CH_3} - \overset{18.3}{CH_2} - CH_2 - CH_2 - \overset{84.5}{C} \equiv CH \qquad \overset{76.9}{CH_3 - CH_2 - CH_2 - C} \equiv C - CH_3$$
$$13.7 \qquad 30.9 \qquad 68.4 \qquad\qquad\qquad 73.7 \; 2.7$$

1–Hexyne   2–Hexyne

$$\overset{84.7 \quad 67.0}{CH_3 - CH_2 = C \equiv CH} \qquad \overset{73.6 \quad 73.6}{CH_3 - C \equiv C - CH_3}$$

But–1–yne   But–2–yne

$$-CH == CH- \qquad -HC \equiv C- \qquad -CH_2 - CH_2-$$
$$\delta \quad 150{-}100 \qquad\quad 90{-}65 \qquad\qquad 30{-}0 \text{ ppm}$$

4. Aromatic carbons

Unlike in PMR spectra, the aromatic and $C == C$ carbons absorb almost in the same range, 100–175 ppm. Therefore, PMR spectroscopy is more helpful when compared to CMR spectroscopy in distinguishing between the alkenes and aromatic molecules. However, as in general, few other carbons absorb in this region, the presence of peaks in this chemical shift range of 100–175 ppm indicates the presence of sp^2 and or aromatic carbons, without an iota of doubt.

Examples

Benzene carbons absorb at 128.5 ppm. Polynuclear aromatic hydrocarbon examples:

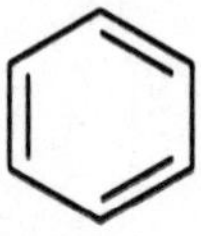

128.5 ppm 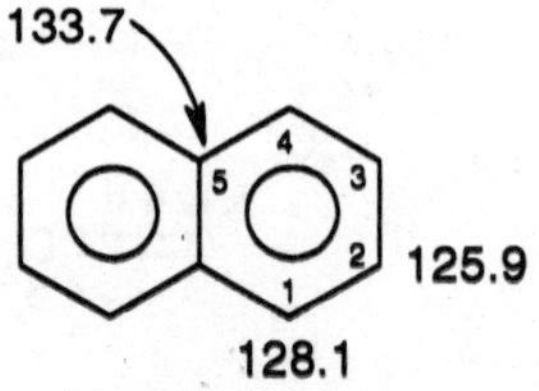   Naphthalene 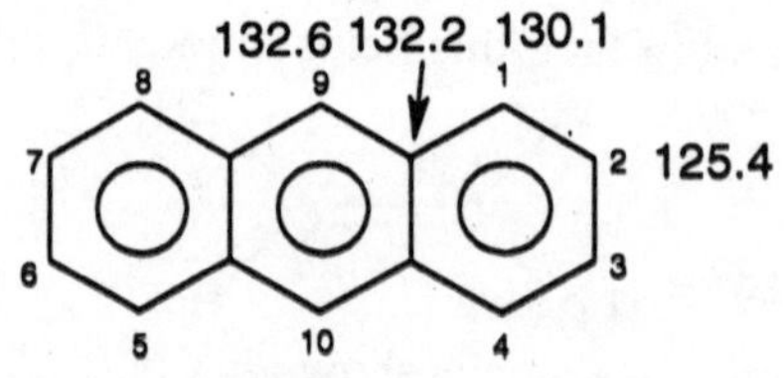   Anthracene

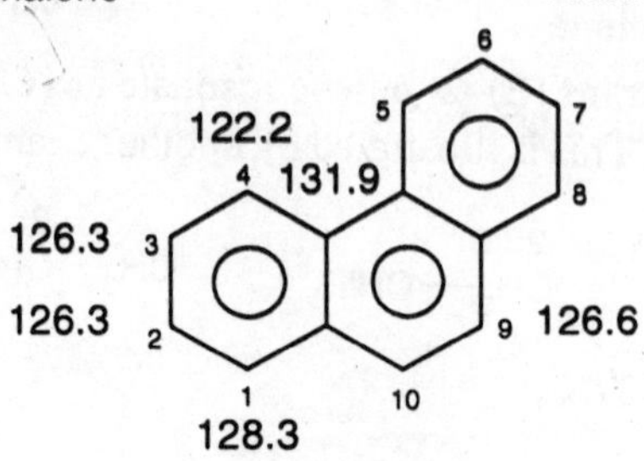

Phenanthrene

Substituted benzenes

All benzene carbons being equivalent resonate at 128.5 ppm. We will now consider mono-, di- and tri-substituted benzenes.

(i) Monosubstituted benzene

CMR of a monosubstituted benzene contains only four signals for the benzene nucleus, although, it possesses six carbons. As each signal in CMR recognizes a carbon atom in one particular chemical environment within the molecule, therefore, we can not expect six lines in its spectrum. We should expect only four lines because both the ortho as well as both the meta carbons are exactly equivalent i.e. each pair has exactly the same chemical environment. So, both the ortho carbons should have identical larmor frequencies and hence will contribute only one signal. Similarly, both the carbons will also contribute one signal instead of two.

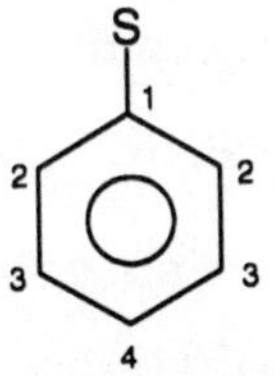

S = substituent

Four types of carbons in monosubstituted benzene ring

Further both the ortho and meta carbons contribute strong singlets in comparison to the para one. The ipso carbon to which the substituent is attached contributes a very weak signal. This is because this carbon is a quaternary carbon C_q which has no proton attached to it. As a quaternary carbon has a relatively long relaxation time T_1 and also as it has no protons to help in its relaxation, therefore, the enhancement in signal intensity that results for other types of carbons having protons, its signal is always weak and in fact, this helps in identifying its presence in the molecule.

Examples

1. Ethyl benzene

The CMR of ethylbenzene is shown in Fig. 10.11. The two ortho protons absorb at 127.9 ppm, in meta protons at 128.4 ppm, the para at 125.7 and the quaternary ipso carbon at 144.2 ppm. The CH_2 and CH_3 carbons of the ethyl group that are sp^3 appear in the region expected for sp^3 carbons, at 29.1 and 15.6 ppm respectively. Notice the weak intensity of the quaternary ipso carbon.

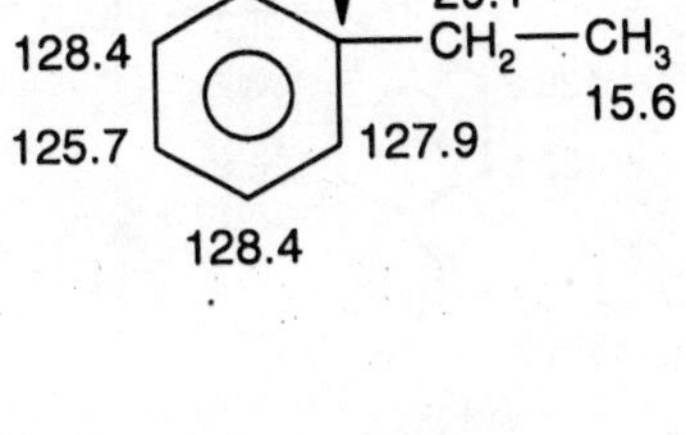

2. Acetophenone

As expected, the acetophenone molecule shows a total of six peaks in CMR spectrum shown in Fig. 10.11b. Two peaks are from the side chain i.e. the CO absorbing at the low field at 197.8 ppm and the CH_3 at 26.3 ppm.

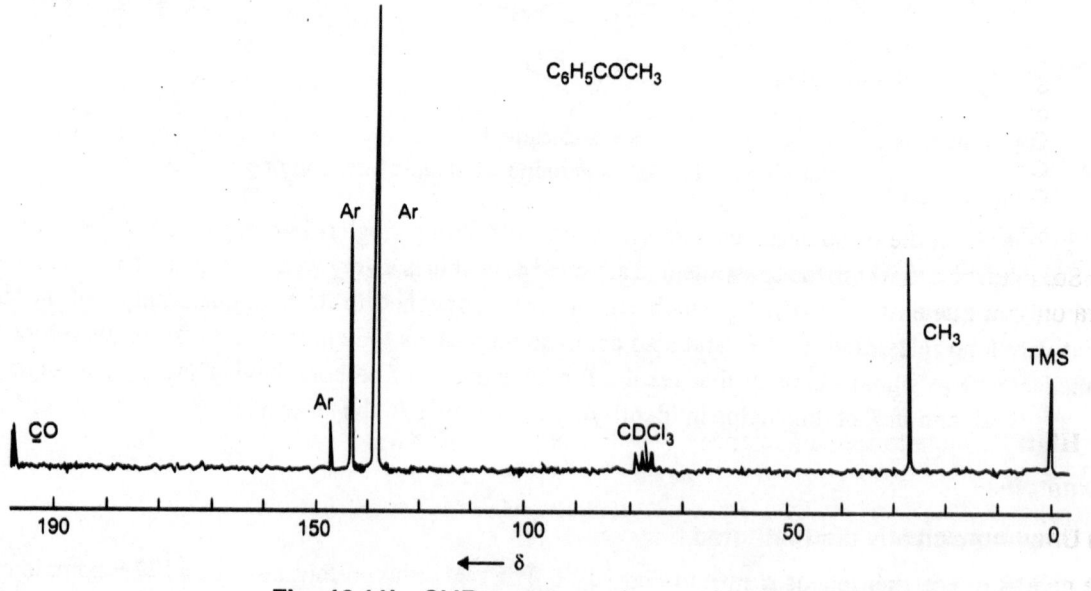

The remaining four peaks are due to the monosubstituted ring carbons.

The ipso carbon resonates at 137.1 ppm. As this is quaternary in nature, therefore, it contributes a weak signal (of course, the peak at 197.8 is also weak as the carbonyl carbon is also a quaternary carbon). The two ortho carbons give a strong peak at 132.9 ppm. Similarly, the two meta carbons also give rise to a strong peak at 128.2 ppm. The para contributes a peak at 128.4 ppm.

Fig. 10.11b. CMR spectrum of acetophenone.

3. Benzyl alcohol

The CMR spectrum of benzyl alcohol as expected contains five peaks.

The CH_2 carbon resonates at 64.5 ppm. The remaining four peaks (as expected) are due to the six carbons of the ring. Obviously the two ortho carbons are equivalent and contribute only one signal at 128.2 ppm. The two meta carbons resonate at δ 126.8 ppm. The signal at 127.2 is due to para carbon while the peak at 140.8 ppm is due to the quaternary ipso carbon. This is a weak signal as expected.

Disubstituted benzenes

(a) Symmetrically disubstituted benzenes

CMR can be used to distinguish very clearly between three isomeric disubstituted benzenes.

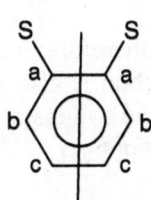 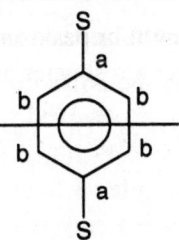

ortho	meta	para
3 peaks due to three sets of C	4 peakd due to four sets of carbon	2 peaks due to two sets of carbons
One simple axis	One simple axis	Two simple axis
One plane	One simple plane	Two planes
One symmetry plane in the plane ring	One symmetry plane in the plane of the ring	One symmetry plane in the plane of the ring

So, while the meta isomer gives four signals in broad-band spectrum, ortho gives three peaks and para only two peaks.

	m	o	P
	4	3	2

Hint: Formula for rememberance :

	m	o	P
	4	3	2

(b) Unsymmetrically disubstituted benzenes

We give here one example of p–nitrophenol.

Here obviously, benzene ring will give four peaks corresponding to carbons – a, b, c and d. This is observed indeed. The carbons a and d being quaternary give weaker signals.

The carbons a, b, c and d appear respectively at 161.5, 115.9, 126.4 and 141.7 ppm.

Intext Exercise

4. How will you distinguish the three disubstituted dibromobenzenes?

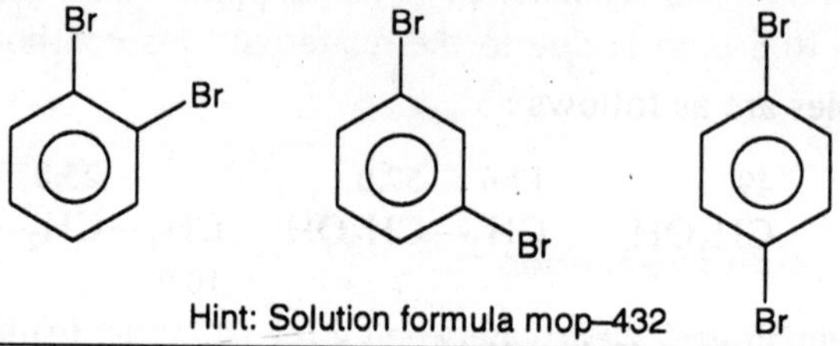

Br

Br

Br

Br

Br

Br

Hint: Solution formula mop–432

(iii) Trisubstituted benzenes

Depending upon the polysubstitution patterns as many as six peaks can be observed.

Symmetrically substituted benzenes show only two peaks. For example, 3,5–trimethyl benzene called mesitylene, contains only two sets of three equivalent carbons masked 1,3,5 and 2,4,6.

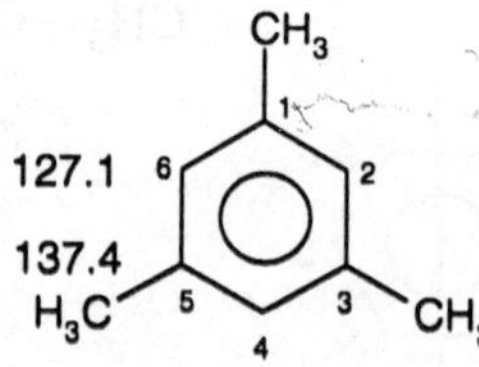

CH₃

127.1 6

137.4 5

H₃C   3 CH₃

4

2

C–1,3,5   137.4

C–2,4,6   127.1

Two sets of carbons: 1,3,5 and 2,4,6

5. Hetero aromatics

The ^{13}C shifts for some representative heteroaromatic compounds are given below.

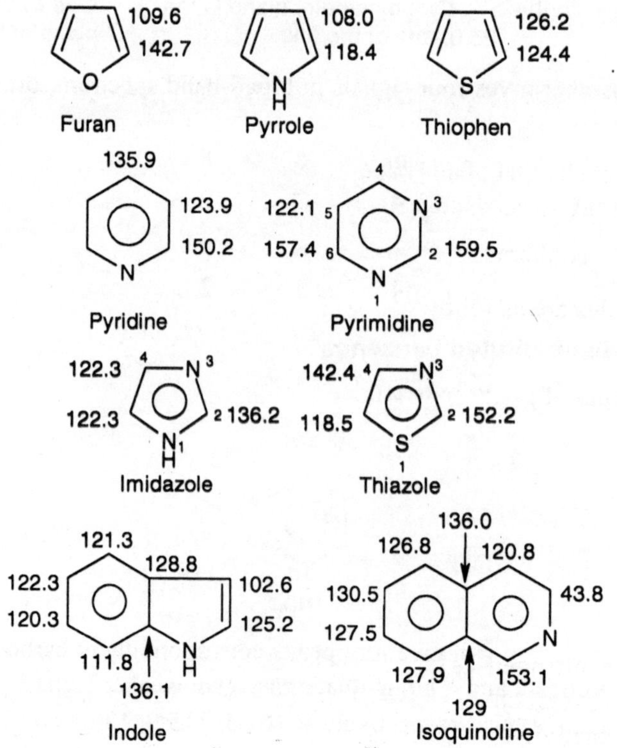

109.6
142.7

O

Furan

108.0
118.4

N
H

Pyrrole

126.2
124.4

S

Thiophen

135.9

123.9
150.2

N

Pyridine

122.1 5
157.4 6

4
N 3
2 159.5
N
1

Pyrimidine

122.3
122.3

4 N 3
2 136.2
N₁
H

Imidazole

142.4 4
118.5

N3
2 152.2
S
1

Thiazole

121.3
128.8

122.3
120.3

111.8
136.1

N
H

102.6
125.2

Indole

136.0
126.8   120.8

130.5
127.5

127.9   153.1
129

43.8

N

Isoquinoline

As we can seen from the above examples, carbon–2 of nitrogen and oxygen containing rings is shielded compared to carbon–3.

6. Alcohols

Some representative examples are as follows :

$$\underset{\text{49}}{CH_3OH} \qquad \underset{17.6 \quad 57.0}{CH_3-CH_2OH} \qquad \underset{\quad\quad 10.0 \quad\quad 63.6}{\overset{25.8}{CH_3-CH_2-CH_2OH}}$$

$$\underset{\substack{| \\ OH}}{\overset{63.4 \quad 25.1}{CH_3-CH_2-CH_3}} \qquad \underset{\quad\quad 19.1 \quad 35.0}{\overset{13.6 \qquad\qquad\qquad 61.4}{CH_3-CH_2-CH_2-CH_2OH}}$$

$$\underset{\substack{99 \\ \quad\quad\quad | \\ \quad\quad\quad OH}}{\overset{32.0 \quad 68.7 \quad 22.6}{CH_3-CH_2-CH-CH_3}} \qquad \underset{\substack{|68.4 \\ OH}}{\overset{CH_3 \\ | \quad 31.1}{CH_3-C-CH_3}}$$

Ipsenol

In general, replacement by OH of an H at C–1 leads to deshielding by 35–52 ppm, by 5–12 ppm for carbon–2. Replacement at C–3 leads to a shielding by 0–6 ppm.

7. Amines

Some illustrative examples are as follows :

$$\underset{\text{26.9}}{CH_3NH_2} \qquad \underset{17.7 \quad 35.9}{CH_3CH_2NH_2} \qquad \underset{\quad\quad 27.3}{\overset{11.2 \qquad\qquad 44.9}{CH_3-CH_2-CH_2NH_2}}$$

$$\underset{\substack{| \\ CH_3}}{\overset{47.5 \quad CH_3 \\ \quad\quad\quad | \\ CH_3-N}}{}$$

The electronegative nitrogen as expected leads to considerable deshielding by ~30 ppm at carbon–1 and by 11 ppm at carbon–2, which is slightly lower than that observed in alcohols, as expected on the basis of electronegativity.

8. Carboxylic acids, esters, amides, anhydrides

These absorb in the region 155-185 ppm.

10.20 THE OFF-RESONANCE DECOUPLED SPECTRUM

It is advantageous to have proton-noise decoupling for obtaining simple spectra for easy interpretation. However, it is equally important to know what kind of carbon is present in the molecule from the point of view of attached hydrogens. Is the carbon present as a CH_3, CH_2 or CH? This is done by means of off-resonance decoupling, a technique for obtaining partially decoupled spectrum in the sense that except $^1J_{CH}$ (one bond) coupling all other couplings will be removed i.e. the couplings between the carbon and more remote protons $^2J_{CH}$, $^3J_{CH}$ etc. What is done is that the sample is irradiated with a second radio frequency source whose major frequency is 1000 to 2000 Hz outside (off) the proton region. Remember, for broad band decoupling, the major frequency is set in the middle of the proton decoupling regions. A CH_3 carbon gives a quartet in which the ratio of the component peaks is 1:3:3:1 as per the N + 1 rule.

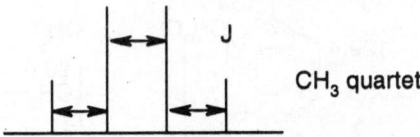

A CH_2 carbon appears as a triplet with the component peaks in the ratio of 1:2:1.

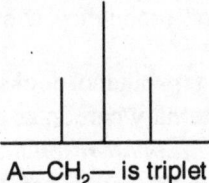

The methine carbon appears as a doublet.

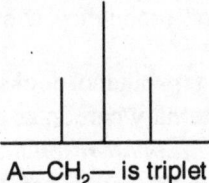

A quaternary carbon will appear only as a singlet. So, we can say that if a singlet peak due to ^{13}C observed in a broad-band spectrum remains a singlet under off resonance conditions, it is certainly due to a quaternary carbon.

A weak singlet due to —Ċ—

Example

An example of off-resonance spectrum is shown in Fig. 10.11c for butanone. This must have become clear to you by now as to the purpose of obtaining an off-resonance spectrum – it is of course, concerned with assigning peaks. For this purpose, both the broad-band and off-resonance spectra are, of course, required.

Another example is butanone.

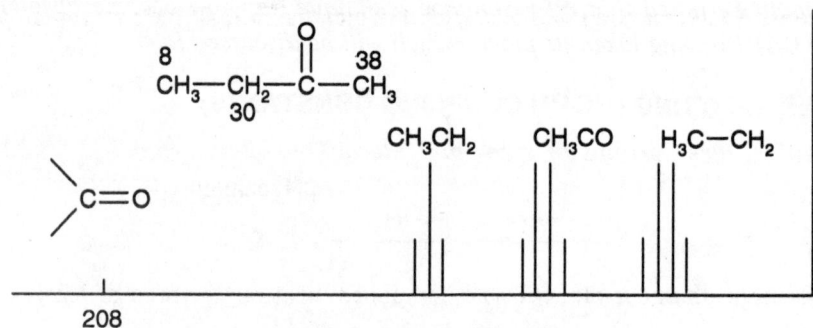

In its off-resonance spectrum, one singlet and three multiplets are observed as shown.

208

Fig. 10.11c. The off resonance spectrum of butanone.

Similarly, off-resonance spectrum of tert-butanol looks like as shown in Fig. 10.11d. The three methyl carbons and a quartet and the quaternary carbon as a weak signal.

It needs to be noted that under conditions of off-resonance, the apparent magnitude of the coupling constants gets reduced to about 30–50 Hz (although you have learnt in PMR spectroscopy that the value of coupling constant J is always constant).

The extent of the residual splitting (J_R) is proportional to the original $^1J_{CH}$ coupling, the irradiating power of the decoupler as well as its separation (in Hz) from the proton being decoupled :

$$J_O = J_R \left[1 + \left(\frac{\gamma B_2 / 2\pi}{\Delta v} \right)^2 \right]^{\frac{1}{2}} \qquad \qquad ...(1)$$

When $\gamma B_2 / 2\pi >> \frac{1}{2}(J_O - J_R)$

where J_O is the original C—H coupling, Δv is the proton resonance frequency in Hz, γB_2 (Hz) is the decoupler irradiating power and J_R is the observed residual splitting.

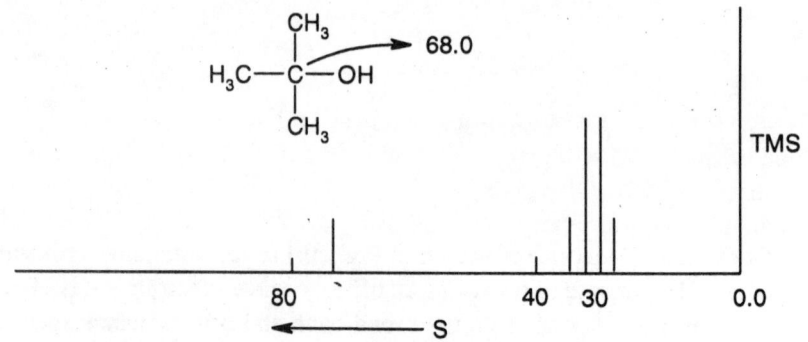

Fig. 10.11d. Off-resonance spectrum of t-butyl alcohol.

or
$$J_R/(J_O^2 - J_R^2)^{1/2} = \Delta v/(\gamma_H.B_2/2\pi)$$

So, greater J_R value means the proton resonance is farther away from the decoupler frequency i.e. Δn is larger. J_R value becomes smaller when more decoupler power (higher $\gamma_H B_2/2\gamma$) is used.

The importance of this equation (1) is that this is used both for calibrating the decoupler power as well for deducing the size of J_O and J_R and Δv. This helps in spectral assignment.

Finally, it should be noted that off resonance technique has now become obsolete with a new technique called DEPT having taken its place, which will be discussed later.

10.21 SPIN–SPIN SPLITTING ($^{13}C-^1H$ COUPLING CONSTANTS)

As discussed earlier, *three groups of spin-spin interactions* are observed in ^{13}CMR. These are $^{13}C-^1H$, $^{13}C-^{13}C$ and $^{13}C, X$ (X = an other NMR active nucleus) coupling constants.

$^{13}C-^1H$ coupling constants

These interactions are of three types :

   (a) $^{13}C-^1H$ ($^1J_{CH}$)
   (b) $^{13}C-C-H$ ($^2J_{CH}$)
   (c) $^{13}C-C-C-H$ ($^3J_{CH}$)

(a) $^{13}C-^1H$ ($^1J_{CH}$)

This is the coupling between ^{13}C and the hydrogen directly attached to this carbon. That is why, it is called one-bond coupling. The spin of ^{13}C is split into a doublet by the proton directly attached to it :

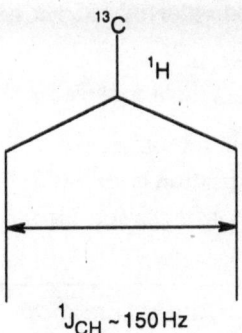

The size of $^1J_{CH}$ is very large compared to that observed in proton-proton couplings, (^2J, ^3J etc.) being about 100–150 Hz (^3J for proton-proton couplings being about 1–20 Hz).

Thus, a methine carbon (CH) will give only a doublet, a methylene (CH$_2$) will give a triplet and a methyl (CH$_3$) a quartet in CMR. Of course, a quaternary carbon signal will not be split. Further of course, if the methylene protons are non-equivalent, then we will get a pair of doublets.

C—H	$^1J_{CH} \approx 125$–150 Hz
C—C—H	$^2J_{CH} \approx 5$–10 Hz
C—C—C—H	$^3J_{CH} \approx 0$–1 Hz

$^1J_{CH}$ (125–150 Hz) is higher than $^2J_{CH}$ (5–10 Hz) which in turn is higher than $^3J_{CH}$ (0–1 Hz) as expected. The $^1J_{CH}$ couplings are observed as ^{13}C satellites of the ^1H spectrum as shown in Fig. The $^2J_{CH}$ and $^3J_{CH}$ are buried under the large ^{12}C—H resonances, and therefore, cannot be usually measured from the PMR spectra and are, therefore, determined from the CMR of enriched samples.

Obviously, the $^1J_{CH}$ are of considerable importance to chemists. So, they have tried to explore the structural dependence of $^1J_{CH}$. It has been found that the $^1J_{CH}$ is directly proportional to the fraction of s-character (ρ) of the C—H bond. The empirical relation is :

$$^1J_{CH} = 5000\ \rho$$

Further, as the s-character is related to the hybridization, parameter λ^2 of the carbon orbital sp^{λ^2}, therefore information concerning the hybridization of a particular carbon atom via $^1J_{CH}$ measurements can be obtained. Thus, by using the equation the $^1J_{CH}$ for methane (sp^3), ethane (sp^2) and acetylene (CH) has been determined to be 125, 167 and 250 Hz respectively and the calculated couplings are in line with the observed couplings.

	$^1J_{CH}$ calculated (Hz)	$^1J_{CH}$ observed (Hz)
Methane	125	125
Ethene	167	156
Acetylene	250	248

Therefore, the $^1J_{CH}$ values have been used to ascertain hybridization in molecules whose bondings are uncertain.

For instance, in cyclopropane, there are uncertainties regarding the exact bonding. However, J_{CH} value of 162 Hz is line with the predicted value of 167 Hz for sp^2 hybridisation :

△ ^1J observed = 161Hz

Based upon above empirical equation, therefore, we can say that about 32% s-character is present in C, H bond orbitals which means hybridisation is $sp^{2.1}$ (82% p-character is found for the C—C bonds). Further example, which prove the utility of equation for sp^2 hybridisation is illustrated by following rings are :

Intext Question

8. Can we use $^1J_{CH}$ couplings to predict hybridization of the carbon involved? If yes, give examples to demonstrate that what does the value of $^1J = 161$ Hz for cyclopropane tell us about the hybridisation state of its carbons?

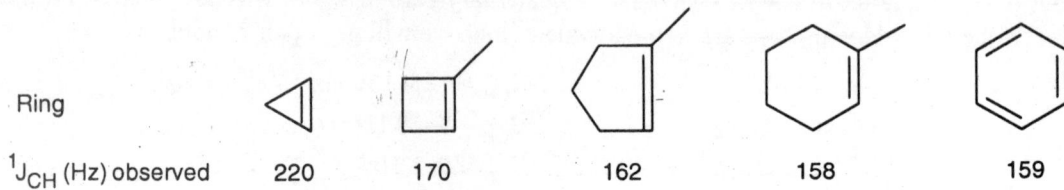

Ring					
$^1J_{CH}$ (Hz) observed	220	170	162	158	159

Effect of electronegative elements

The $^1J_{CH}$ of methanes substituted with electronegative elements changes although hybridization still remains the same (sp^3).

Table 10.3. Effect of electronegative elements on methanes

Methanes	J_{CH} observed
Methane	125
CH_3F	149
CH_3Cl	150
CH_3Br	152
CH_3I	151
CH_2Cl_2	178
$CHCl_3$	209
$CH_2(OC_2H_5)_2$	161

In general, these effects are additive, and therefore, they can be used to predict the $^1J_{CH}$ for multi-substituted molecules. Thus, the predicted value for 1,1,2,2–tetrabromoethane on the basis of values reported in Table 10.1 comes to be 179 Hz while the observed value is 181 Hz.

$$BrCH_2—CH_2Br \qquad ^1J_{CH} \text{ predicted} = 179 \text{ Hz}$$
$$^1J_{CH} \text{ observed} = 181 \text{ Hz}$$

Olefins

Here, the effects are more clear as shown in Table 10.4. While the α-effect of fluorine in vinyl fluoride is 44 Hz, it is 24 Hz in CH_3F. On the other hand, the β-effect is much less but about the same for cis as well as trans CH protons. The $^1J_{CH}$ for some other sp^2 systems are as follows :

CH_3CHO	173
$H—\underset{\underset{O}{\|\|}}{C}—NH_2$	188
$H—\underset{\underset{O}{\|\|}}{C}–N(CH_3)_2$	207
$H—\underset{\underset{O}{\|\|}}{C}—OH$	222

Table 10.4. Effects of electronegative substituents on $^1J_{CH}$ couplings in $CH_2 == CH—X$ vinyl halides

X	α	cis	trans
F	200	159	162
Cl	195	163	161
CN	177	163	165
CHO	162	157	162

Obviously, these systems show large α-substituent effects.

J_{CH} for some cycloalkanes, all of which have sp³ hybridization but different internal angles are :

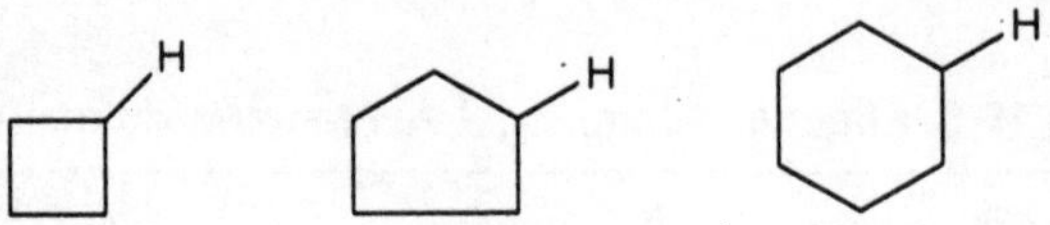

134.0   128.0   123.0

The $^1J_{CH}$ for some bicyclic systems are :

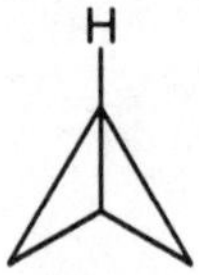

205.0

J_{CH} for pyridine are :

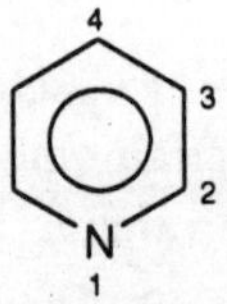

$^1J_{C_2H}$	$^1J_{C_3H}$	$^1J_{C_4H}$
170	163	152

For 5-membered heterocyclic systems, the $^1J_{CH}$ are as follows :

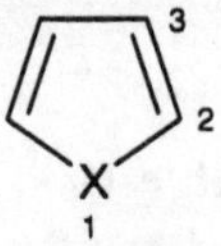

	$^1J_{C_2H}$	$^1J_{C_3H}$
X = 0	201	175
X = S	185	167
X = NH	184	170

$^2J_{CH}$ and $^3J_{CH}$ couplings

These coupling constants have smaller values than the corresponding H–H couplings. This is to be expected as the ratio of magnetic moments of carbon and hydrogen suggest : $J_{CH} \approx \frac{1}{4}J_{HH}$ for electronic transmission. However, the couplings are larger than this because the carbon nucleus has large electron density

Examples

We can obtain the values for CH couplings if we multiply the HH couplings by 0.65 (65%) in case of formaldehyde, ethylene and ethane. Thus, the calculated and observed $^2J_{CH}$ values are :

	Calculated	Observed
CH_3CHO	^2J + 26.7	26.7
$C—CH_2—CH_3$	^2J 1.6, ^3J 7.6, ^3J trans = 12.4	^2J 4.1, ^3J 7.6 cis, ^3J 14.1 trans
CCH_2CH_3	^2J − 8.1, ^3J = 5.2	^2J − 4.5, ^3J = 4.9

From this general rule, we can conclude that it is highly likely that both CH as well as HH couplings follow the same mechanism because the substituents on the coupling carbon affect the coupling only to a minor extent.

Examples

CH_3—*CR	^2J
*CR	
CH_3	– 4.5
CH_2I	– 5.0
CHO	– 6.6
CO_2Me	6.9
Ph	6.0

$(CH_3)_3C$—CR	^2J
*CR	
CH_3	4.65
CH_2I	5.99
CHO	– 6.6
CO_2Me	6.9
Ph	–

For benzene, the ^2J, ^3J, ^4J values are 1.0, 7.4 and – 1.1 respectively. So, $^2J_{CH}$ is less than $^3J_{CH}$ (while $^2J_{HH} < {}^3J_{HH}$)

$^2J = 1.0$
$^3J = 7.4$
$^4J = -1.1$

Indeed, this is so in aromatic compounds, $^3J_{CH}$ being often a trans-oriented coupling.

In alkenes, orientation affects the $^2J_{CH}$ size with the increasing electronegative substituents.

	OAc	Cl	CO_2H
$^2J_{cis}$ (C^1H^α)	– 7.9	– 8.3	– 4.55
$^2J_{trans}$ (C^1H^β)	+ 7.6	+ 7.1	+ 1.55
^3J (C^2H^γ)	– 9.7	– 6.8	– 0.6

$^3J_{cis}$ is always less than $^3J_{trans}$ in alkenes. So, it can be used to know which geometric isomer we are dealing as is the case with $^3J_{HH}$. $^3J_{HH}$ is dependant upon the dihedral angle just as we saw in $^3J_{HH}$. Thus $^3J_{gauche} < {}^3J_{trans}$ for example in amino acid fragments.

$$^3J_{gauche} = 0.5 \text{ Hz}$$
$$^3J_{grans} = 12 \text{ Hz}$$

Note that the $^3J_{CH}$ values are roughly comparable to $^3J_{HH}$ values. The long range couplings like ^4J, ^5J etc. are small.

Some representative $^2J_{CH}$ for sp^3 carbons are :

$CH_2 = CH_2$	$(CH_3)_2CO$
– 2.4 Hz	5.5 Hz

Few examples of some representative $^2J_{CH}$ for sp carbons are :

$$CH \equiv CH \qquad C_6H_5O-C \equiv OH$$
$$49.3 \qquad\qquad 61.0 \qquad :$$

J_{CC} coupling constants

These are observed in C labelled molecules.

$^1J_{CC}$ are smaller than $^1J_{CH}$ as per expectations due to smaller magnetic momnt of carbon versus hydrogen. The $^1J_{CC}$ can be used diagonistically for single, double and triply bonded couplings i.e. for knowing hybridisation of the coupled carbons.

$$C—C \qquad\qquad C = C \qquad\qquad C \equiv C$$
$$35\text{--}40 \qquad\qquad 65\text{--}75 \qquad\qquad 170\text{--}175$$
$$CH_3—CH_3 \qquad CH_2 = CH_2 \qquad CH \equiv CH$$
$$34.6 \qquad\qquad 67.6 \qquad\qquad 171.5$$

Some more examples are :

$$\triangledown \qquad\qquad CH_3COCH_3 \qquad\qquad \bigcirc$$
$$10\ Hz \qquad\qquad 56.7 \qquad\qquad\qquad 57.0$$

Further, **a** general approximation is applicable to $^1J_{C-CH_3}$ and $^1J_{C-H}$:

$$^1J_{C—CH_3} = 0.27\ ^1J_{C—H}$$

$^2J_{CC}$ coupling constants

Again these are observed in ^{13}C-enriched molecules. They are much smaller than $^1J_{CC}$ as anticipated. In saturated systems $^3J_{CC} < 3\ Hz$.

Examples

$$CH_3—^*CH_2—C(OH)CH_3.^*CH_3 \qquad 2.4\ Hz$$

$$\text{[cyclohexane structure with CH}_3\text{]} \qquad\qquad 1.7\ Hz$$

In propionnitrite, it is exceptionally large, 33 Hz :

$$^*CH_3CH_2{}^*CN \quad 33\ Hz \qquad\qquad CH_3—C \equiv CH \quad 12\ Hz$$

It is about 16 Hz in acetone and similar molecules :

$$^*CH_3CO^*CH_3 \quad 16\ Hz$$
$$^*CH_3—CO—^*CH_2—CH_3 \quad 15\ Hz$$

$^3J_{CC}$ coupling constants

A dihedral angle dependence of $^3J_{CC}$ as seen in $^3J_{CH}$ couplings is also operational.

Examples

Butane : $*CH_3-CH_2-CH_2-*CH_3$

ϕ	0	30	60	90	120	150	180
$^3J_{CC}$	5.8	4.0	1.9	0.6	1.5	3.3	4.6

It can be seen that $^3J_{CC}$ at 0° is > $^3J_{CC}$ at 180° which is reverse to that observed for $^3J_{HH}$ at 0° and $^3J_{HH}$ at 180°.

The Karplus curve for $^3J_{C-C}$ is shown in Fig. 10.10. It shows the dependence of $^3J_{CC}$ on dihedral angle ϕ. The $^3J_{CC}$ Karplus curve is however, somewhat different from its counterpart in $^3J_{HH}$. For sp³–sp³ couplings, $^3J_{CC}$ at 180° ϕ is < $^3J_{CC}$ at 0° ϕ.

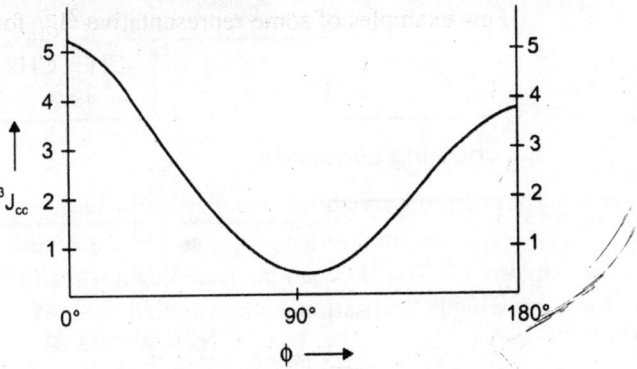

Fig. 10.11d. Karplus curve for dependence of $^3J_{CC}$ vs ϕ for sp³–sp³ systems.

10.22 GATED DECOUPLING

This is a decoupling technique that allows us to retain the increase in S/N ratio which occurs due to NOE effect.

The overlapping signals obtained in coupled CMR spectra are not only complex but also very weak due to poor S/N ratio. Would you not like to have a technique by which you get NOE enhancement for the coupled spectra as well? Obviously, you will. This is made possible by what is called Gated Decoupling, which actually means coupling with NOE enhancement.

In this technique advantage is taken of the fact that the appearance of coupling in CMR depends on presence or absence of proton noise decoupling during the acquisition period only and not upon decoupling conditions used before or after the acquisition period. So, the broadband proton decoupler is applied only during the relaxation (pulse) decay in order to get benefit of the heteronuclear NOE. The broad-band decoupler is "gated" off simultaneously with the ^{13}C pulse and acquisition period but "gated" on only throughout the relaxation delay. The NOE builds up before the ^{13}C pulse although it always starts decaying but that happens only partially. The result is that we have taken advantage of part of the NOE in our coupled spectrum. As the decoupler is turned off during the acquisition of the real signal, so that no decoupling occurs i.e. a coupled spectrum is obtained. This is how the technique affords the ^{13}C signals a much-needed enhancement in the S/N ratio. Gated technique is shown in Fig. 10.11f.

Undecoupled CMR spectrum of dioxan with gated decoupling versus without gated decoupling spectrum is shown in Fig. 10.12.

Example: The gated decoupled spectrum of dioxan is shown in Fig. 10.12.

10.23 INVERSE GATED DECOUPLING FOR QUANTITATIVE ANALYSIS

We have already discussed that the integral intensities in routine CMR spectra are not quantitative unlike in PMR spectra. Therefore, the routine CMR spectra cannot be used for quantitative analysis unlike PMR spectra which give us the relative integral intensities that are quite reliable.

You must be wondering whether we can get CMR spectra after all for obtaining relative ratios of

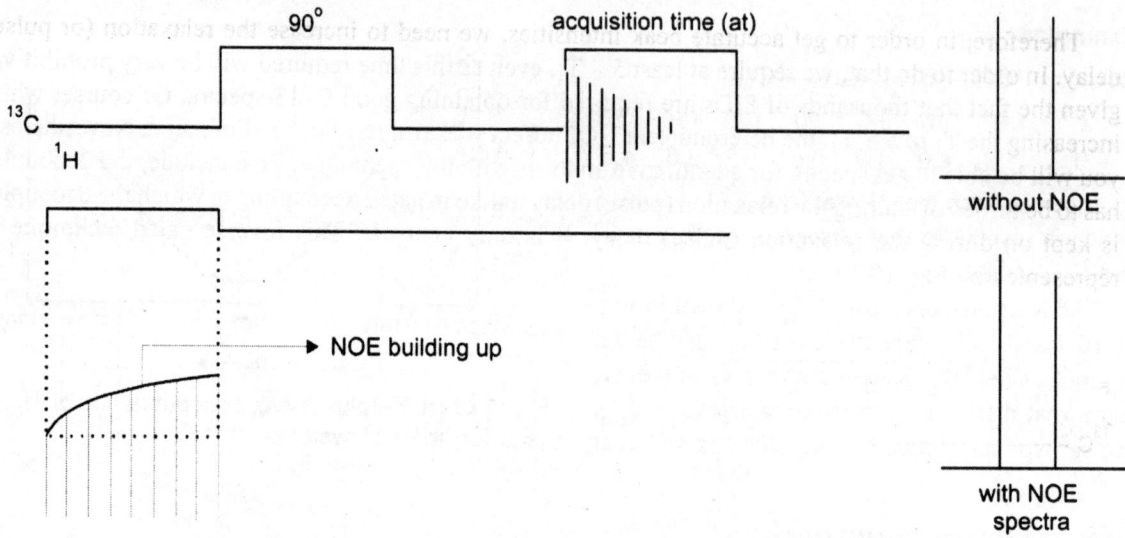

Fig. 10.12a. Gated decoupling (coupling with NOE effect).

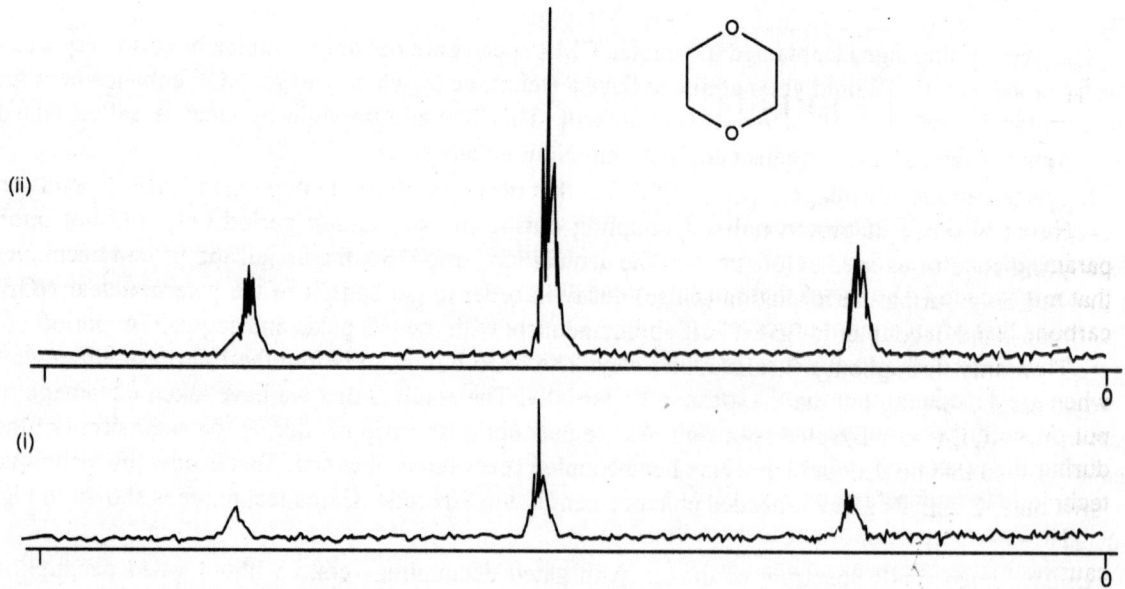

Fig. 10.12b. Undecoupled CMR spectrum of dioxan: (i) with gated decoupling to retain NOE; (ii) without gated decoupling.

the carbons present in the molecule. You can indeed get such spectra. You must also have wondered about discussing this point immediately after the Gated decoupling! Herein lies the solution. Why not do the reverse of gated decoupling? That is to say you get decoupled spectra which do not contain any increase in signal intensity due to NOE effect. As we discussed previously in details, NOE effect is different for different carbons, the reason for unreliable intensities of C–13 peaks.

Therefore, in order to get accurate peak intensities, we need to increase the relaxation (or pulse) delay. In order to do that, we require at least $5 \times T_1$, even as this time required will be very prohibitive, given the fact that thousands of FIDs are required for obtaining good C–13 spectra. Of course, while increasing the T_1 to $5 \times T_1$, the heteronuclear NOE effect will also have to be eliminated. Nevertheless, you will be able to get spectra for quantitative analysis with this technique. To conclude, the decoupler has to be turned off during the relaxation (pulse) delay unlike in gated decoupling in which the decoupler is kept on during the relaxation (pulse) delay. It is only kept off. This inverse gated technique is represented by Fig. 10.13.

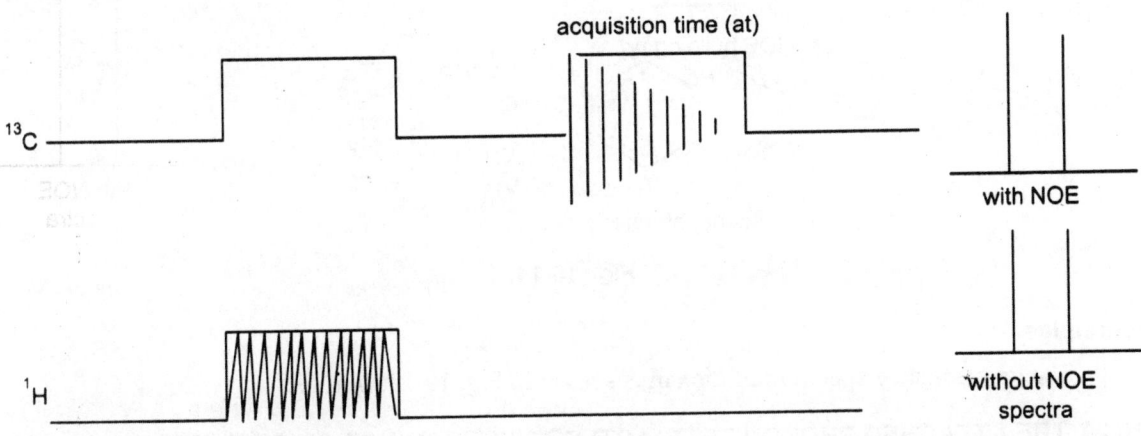

Fig. 10.13. Inverse Gated technique for obtaining decoupled spectra without NOE effect.

Note : As $5 \times T_1$ means a costlier loss of time, the time needed is cut down by using what are called paramagnetic relaxation agents like Cr (acac)$_3$ which further leads to loss of any NOE enhancement that might occur. The use of these metal complexes is particularly important for carboxyl or quaternary carbons that often are not observed in routine CMR spectra.

Thus, in order to ensure that the peaks heights are reliable, we need to do away with the NOE effect when the decoupled spectrum is being obtained. Therefore, we do the inverse gatting. The decoupler is put on with the simultaneous application of the pulse and during the acquisition time but gated off during the relaxation (pulse) delay. The decoupling is effective only during the acquisition time. The technique is represented by Fig. 10.13.

However, it is important to note that besides NOE, there is yet another factor that is at work in causing inaccurate peak intensities in CMR spectra. That is the rates of relaxation of different C–13 nuclei are different within a molecule. While some relax quickly, others relax very slowly. In case of C–13 nuclei that relax slowly, the FID is already ceased. Complete relaxation yields strong peaks while incomplete relaxation yields weak signals. Hence, in order to remove the inaccuracies due to difference in relaxation times, the relaxation delay (pulse delay) is increased to $5 \times T_1$, where T_1 is the relaxation (spin-lattice) time of the most slowly relaxing C–13 nuclei.

However, the price paid for quantitative analysis by using $5 \times T_1$ is very high as will be clear from the following example.

For example, the T_1 for C–9, C–11 and C–12 in acenapthene are 66, 112 and 72s respectively. Their peak heights are very small, particularly for C–11 and C–12 under the conditions : 25.2 MHz (1.5 g/2 ml), PW 3 μs (22°), AT 1.0s, no pulse delay, number of transients equal to 400. But if a pulse delay of 400 s is used, then under the conditions : 25.2 MHz (1.5 g/2 ml), PW 12 μs (90°), AT 1.0 s, pulse delay of 400 s, *then even after a mere 16 number of transients, the time increases from 7 min. to 1.8 h! And still the peak intensities are found to be unreliable! So, when inverse gated decoupling was used along with pulse delay of 400 s only then reliable peak intensities could be obtained after 150 number of transients. But you know how much time had it taken by then? The time had increased from 7 min to 18 h!* The spectra are shown in Fig. 10.14.

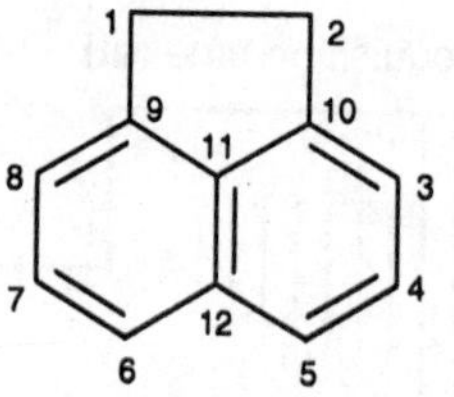

Carbon	T_1s
C_9	66
C_{11}	112
C_{12}	72

Acenaphthene

Fig. 10.14.

Examples

1. The inverse-gated spectrum of dioxan is shown in Fig. 10.12a and b.

10.24 THE ATTACHED PROTON TEST (APT) FOR DETERMINATION OF THE NUMBERS OF ATTACHED PROTONS

Would you like to have a method in your hand to know the number of protons attached to a carbon in the molecule so that you could distinguish between carbons that have different number of protons attached to them? With this test in your hand, you will be able to know whether a carbon is a CH_3 (methyl), CH_2 (methylene), CH (methine) or even a carbon having no proton (quaternary) attached to it. In other words, you can be in a position to say whether the number of attached protons is even as in CH_2 or quaternary or odd as in CH or CH_3.

Such a test exists and is called the Attached Proton Test (APT). When you take the ^{1}H-decoupled spectrum of a compound based upon APT technique, then the CH_3 and CH carbons give "up" (positive) peaks while CH_2 and quaternary carbon C_p give you the "down" (negative) peaks as is schematically shown in Fig. 10.15 for the compound 4–chloro–3–methyl–2–butanone, $CH_3COCH(CH_3)CH_2Cl$.

You would wonder as to why do we need the APT spectrum. Well, for a simple molecule such as 4–chloro–3–methyl–2–butanone, it may not be of great importance but it proves its worth for bigger complicated molecules like steroids etc. wherein we find that a peak often represents two overlapping carbons in the CMR spectrum. The APT test aids us in assigning these peaks to the appropriate carbons in the molecules.

For example, let us consider the CMR spectrum of cholesterol. The peak that appears at 32 ppm is actually contributed by two carbons–7 and 8. How do we say that? This is the message we get from the APT spectrum. In the APT spectrum, we get a "down" peak (due to $^7CH_2$) and an "up" peak (due to ^8CH) at about 32 ppm (Fig. 10.15b).

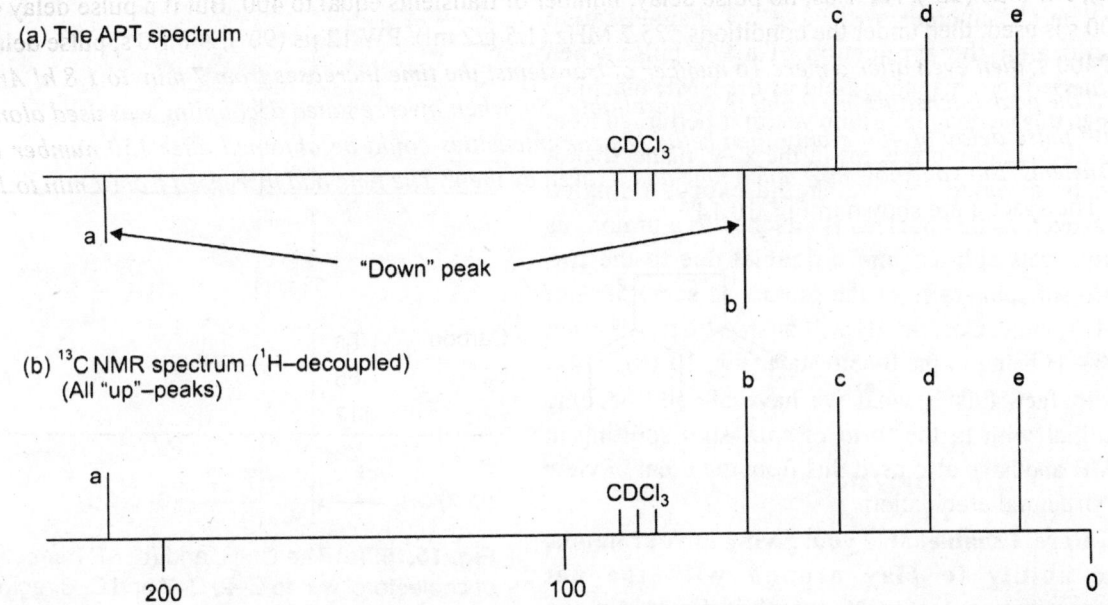

Fig. 10.15a. (a) The APT spectrum, (b) The [1]H-decoupled CMR spectrum for 4–chloro–3–methyl–2–butanone.

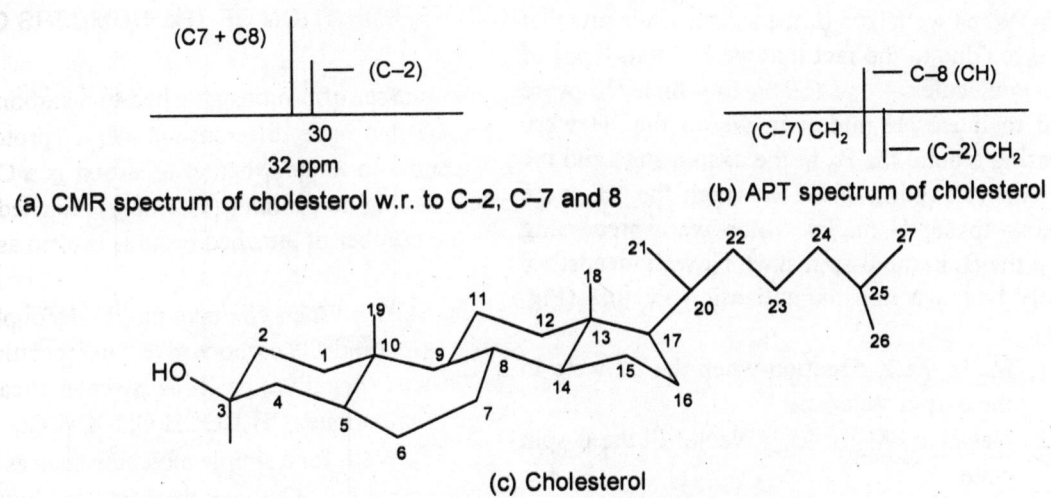

Fig. 10.15b. CMR (a), APT (b), spectra for cholesterol (c).

Theory of the APT

1. The Methine carbon

Let us consider a ^{1}H—^{13}C (CHCl$_3$) system, the simplest case of scalar (J) coupling.

$$^1H \xrightarrow{\ ^1J_{CH}\ } {}^{13}C$$

The ^{13}C nucleus will have net magnetization vector after the application of a 90° pulse when immersed in a magnetic field of the NMR machine. When this net magnetization vector is perturbed from the z'–direction to precess in the x'–y' plane, then it can be detected and we should expect a singlet. However, as this nucleus is attached to a proton, its signal gets splitted into a doublet due to the two different spin states of the proton. In some 50% of $CHCl_3$ molecules, the ^1H will be in α-state, the other 50% ^1H being in the β-spin state (Fig. 10.16).

In fact, this is what we have already become familiar with in the form of spin–spin splitting in CMR and have also used this from the point of view of structural elucidation.

Here, I shall enable you, giving in your hands, the ability to play around with the net magnetization vector, M_z which is directed along the z'–direction in the rotating frame of reference.

Let us re-consider the above simplest ^1H–^{13}C system. When we talked of the splitting, we saw that it occurred due to the fact that we had two types of $CHCl_3$ molecules – one (50%) in which ^{13}C were joined to those ^1H nuclei in which the ^1H were precessing around the B_0 in the α-spin state and the other (the remaining 50%) in which the ^{13}C were joined to those ^1H nuclei which were precessing around the B_0 in the β-spin state. Now, it means, we actually had two net magnetization vectors (Fig. 10.17):

1. M_Z in the Z direction when the ^1H were in the α-spin state.
2. Negative $-M_Z$ or $M_{(-Z)}$ vector in the β-spin state.

Although there will be an overall excess of M_Z, that does not mean that the two vector M_Z and $M_{(-Z)}$ will not exist independently. In fact, they do. How can we describe the motion of these magnetization vectors, M_Z and $M_{(-Z)}$? Let us select the rate of rotation of the rotating reference. The chemical shift position of the 13–C i.e. ν_o. This means we have placed the centre of the spectral window

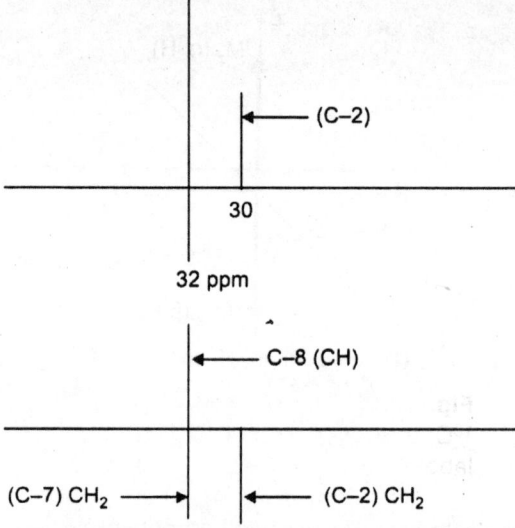

Fig. 10.15. (a) The CMR, and (b) APT spectra of cholesterol w.r. to C–2, C–7 and C–8 region at about 30–32 ppm, (c) the cholesterol molecule.

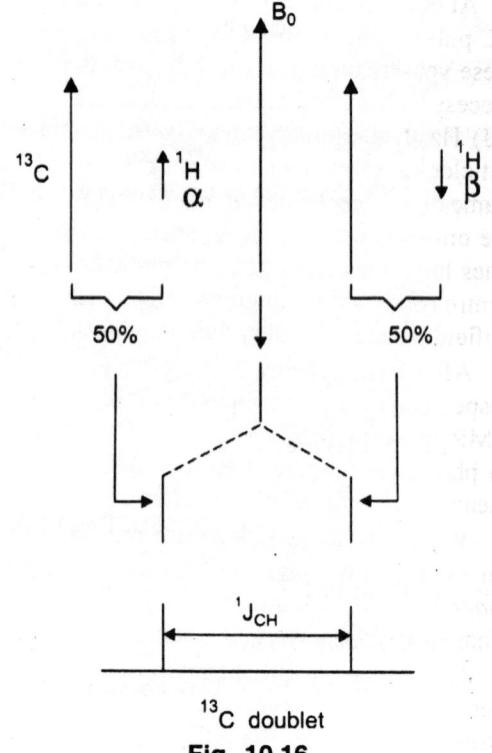

^{13}C doublet

Fig. 10.16.

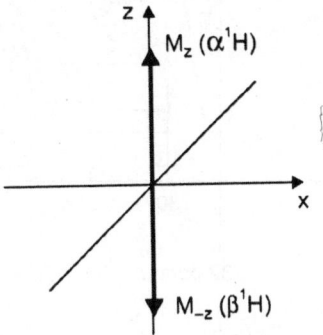

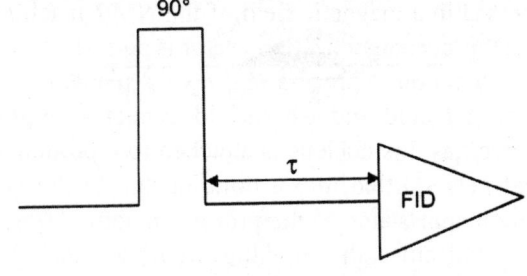

Fig. 10.17. The M_z and M_{-z} vectors of ^{13}C due to α^1H and β^1H protons in laboratory frame.

Fig. 10.18. A 90° pulse followed by a variable delay τ before FID.

precisely between the two component peaks of the ^{13}C doublet i.e. "on resonance" such that $\Delta v = 0$. Thus, the $+J/2$ and $-J/2$ will be the rotating-frame frequencies for the peaks due to α^1H and β^1H respectively. Here J means the one-bond ^1H—^{13}C coupling constant equal to about 150 Hz. So, the rate of precession (angular velocity) for the ^{13}C with α^1H will be in Hertz $\Delta v + J/2$ and $\Delta v = -J/2$ with β^1H nuclei attached.

At equilibrium, both the net magnetization vectors will be directed along the +Z axis. When a 90° ^{13}C pulse on the y' axis is applied along the –x' axis (not x axis), it will have the effect of rotating both these vectors on to the +y' (not y) axis (Fig. 10.18). Both of these net magnetization vectors will now precess for a period equal to 1/J (J ~ 150 Hz). The "–^1H" vector will rotate with a velocity equal to +1/(2J) Hz in a counter-clockwise manner towards the –X' axis. The "β-^1H" vector will rotate in an anticlockwise manner towards the +X' axis with a velocity to –1/(2J) Hz. Recapitulated the rotating frame of reference: the net magnetization vector stands still in the x'–y' plane if the resonance frequencies are on-resonance i.e. lie precisely at the centre of the spectral window whereas the "off-resonance" lines have magnetization vectors rotating in the x'→y' plane. Those peaks that are downfield of the centre rotate with + angular velocity i.e. counterclockwise from x' → y' – x' → –y' etc.; peaks that are upfield, rotate with negative angular velocity i.e. clockwise (Fig. 10.19).

After a short delay of period (τ) equal to 1/2J Hz, the two vectors will lie on the +y' and –y' axes respectively opposing each other. Now, if you collect the FID at this antiphase stage, you would get a CMR spectrum containing a doublet but in this doublet you will see one component peak being opposite in phase. (Remember that this spectrum would be obtained by doing a 90° phase correction which means changing the phase reference to –x' axis from y' axis).

When $\tau = 1/J$, then, it means that the α^1H and the β^1H vectors are 180° out of phase with each other on –x' axis. (We shall call this as the antiphase stage and the magnetization at this stage as *antiphase magnetization*. We shall show you later as to how to use this phenomenon for playing further games. That is why we have given some name to this stage for future reference).

If you take the CMR spectrum at this stage, you will get a doublet along +x' axis. If you did proton decoupling while you collect the FID, you will get a singlet that will be "upside-down" or "inverted". Now, as in general, the APT spectrum is phased with –x' axis, rather than +x' axis, it means the peak will be **positive** (Fig. 10.19).

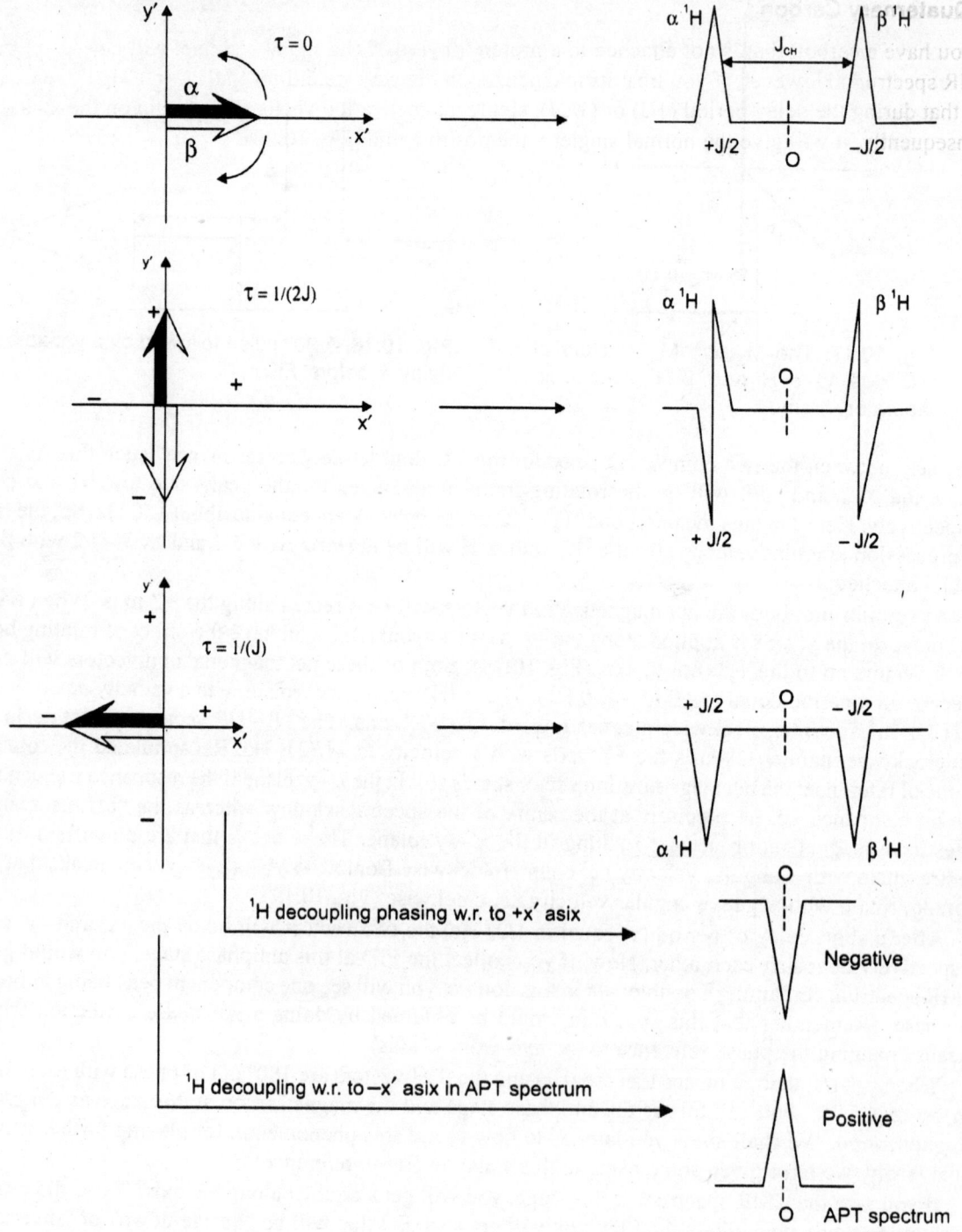

Fig. 10.19. The movement of magnetization vectors of carbon–13 in ^{13}CH during the APT test as seen from the z (top axis).

2. Quaternary Carbon

If you have a carbon that is not attached to a proton, obviously, its signal – singlet will not be split in CMR spectrum. However, if you treat its magnetization the way we did for the ^{13}C in $CHCl_3$, you will see that during the delay period (1/J) or (1/2J), single magnetization vector will remain on the x′–axis. Consequently, it will give the normal singlet – the positive one (Fig. 10.20).

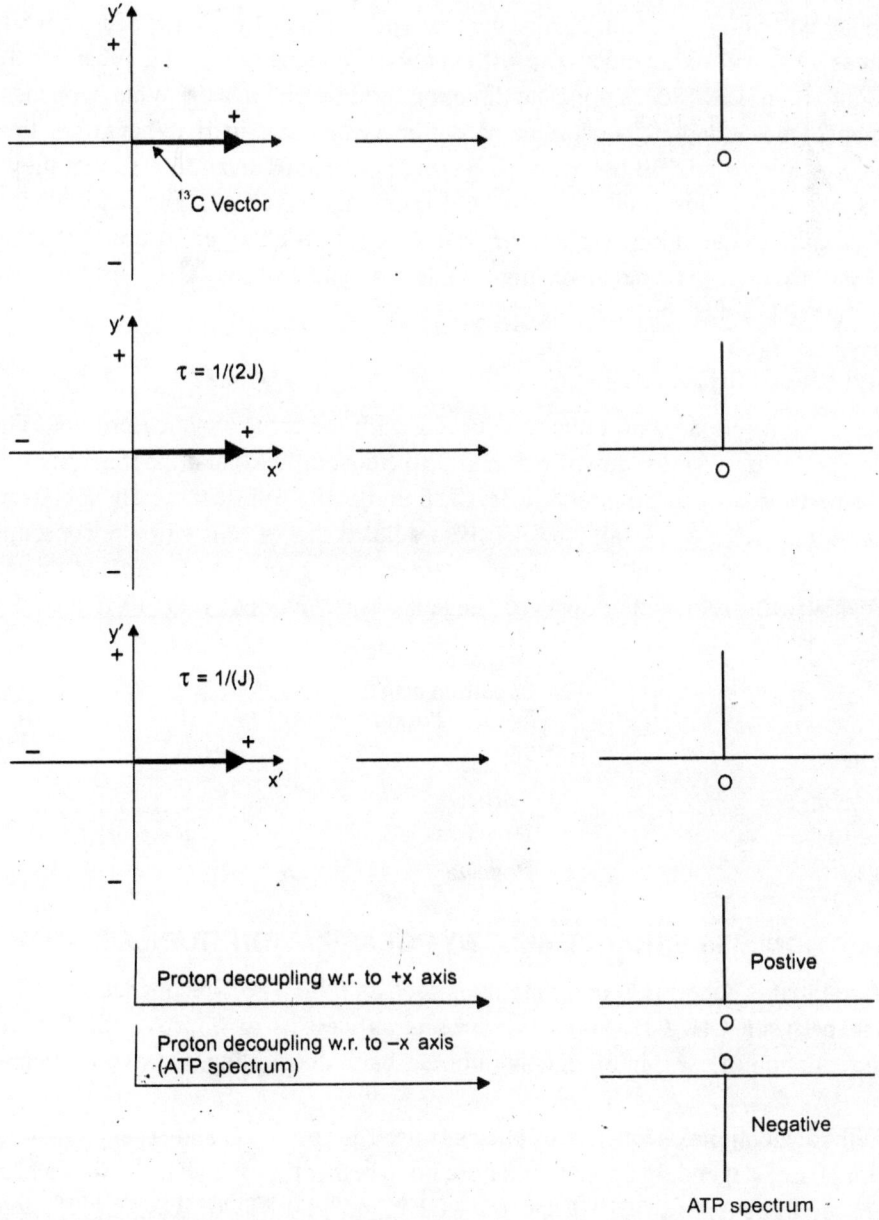

Fig. 10.20. The movement of ^{13}C magnetization vector in Cq in APT test.

But as we normally do the referencing in an APT spectrum with $-x'$ axis rather than $+x'$-axis, it means the peak for this quaternary carbon Cq, will be **negative** rather than positive.

3. Methylene, CH$_2$ group

The ^{13}C of CH$_2$ will give a triplet in the CMR spectrum such that the central peak ($\alpha\beta$ or $\beta\alpha$) of this triplet will lie exactly on $\nu = 0$ (i.e.) on "resonance" along the y'-axis. The downfield component peak (α, α) will rotate with in a counterclockwise manner with angular frequency of J Hz while the upfield component peak ($\beta\beta$) will rotate clockwise with angular frequency of $-J$ Hz. When $\tau = 1/(2J)$, the $\alpha\alpha$ and $\beta\beta$ vectors have moved 180° in opposite directions and lie on $-re$ axis. What happens to the central peak component? Does it budge? No, it remains stationary on the x'-axis. What after a total delay of 1/J? After this delay the $\alpha\alpha$ and $\beta\beta$ have moved respectively +360° and $-360°$ so that they lie along the x'-axis. If we take FID at this point with proton-decoupling, the obtained triplet will give us positive singlet. Now usually, as mentioned earlier, the APT spectrum is obtained by doing phasing using the $-x'$ (instead of $+x'$) axis, we get a negative singlet. The movement of the $-$CH$_2-$ magnetization vector as it happens in the APT test is shown in Fig. 10.21.

4. The Methyl group, CH$_3$

The ^{13}C signal is split into a quartet due to coupling with the three attached protons. The outer lines correspond to vectors $\alpha\alpha\alpha$ (most downfield) and $\beta\beta\beta$ (most upfield) and the inner ones correspond to vectors due to ($\alpha\alpha\beta$, $\alpha\beta\alpha$ and $\beta\alpha\alpha$) and ($\beta\beta\alpha$, $\beta\alpha\beta$ and $\alpha\beta\beta$). When these are subjected to the APT test, then after a total delay of 1/J, all the four vectors lie on the $-x'$ axis with the consequence that the quartet obtained is "upside-down". If we do the ^{1}H decoupling and take the FID at this stage, we will get a singlet which will be "upside-down" or "negative" or "inverted" (Fig. 10.22)

Conclusion	Phase in APT spectrum with ref. to **$-x'$ axis**
Methine CH	Positive
Quaternary Cq	Negative
Methylene CH$_2$	Negative
Methyl CH$_3$	Positive

10.25 DISTORTIONLESS ENHANCEMENT BY POLARIZATION TRANSFER (DEPT)

This is a method that is superior to other methods such as INEPT, off-resonance and APT and is used to distinguish between CH, CH$_2$ and CH$_3$ carbons as well as to improve the S/N ratio. Despite considerable reduction of overlap of signals in broad-band decoupling, the overlap remains a serious problem.

In this method, a complex sequence of pulses is used for both ^{13}C and ^{1}H such that the ^{13}C signals show different phases depending upon their nature i.e. whether they are CH, CH$_2$ or CH$_3$ or a quaternary carbon. There are three types of DEPT spectra – DEPT 45°, DEPT 90°, DEPT 135°, depending upon the pulse width (45°, 90° and 135° in that order) of the final ^{1}H pulse.

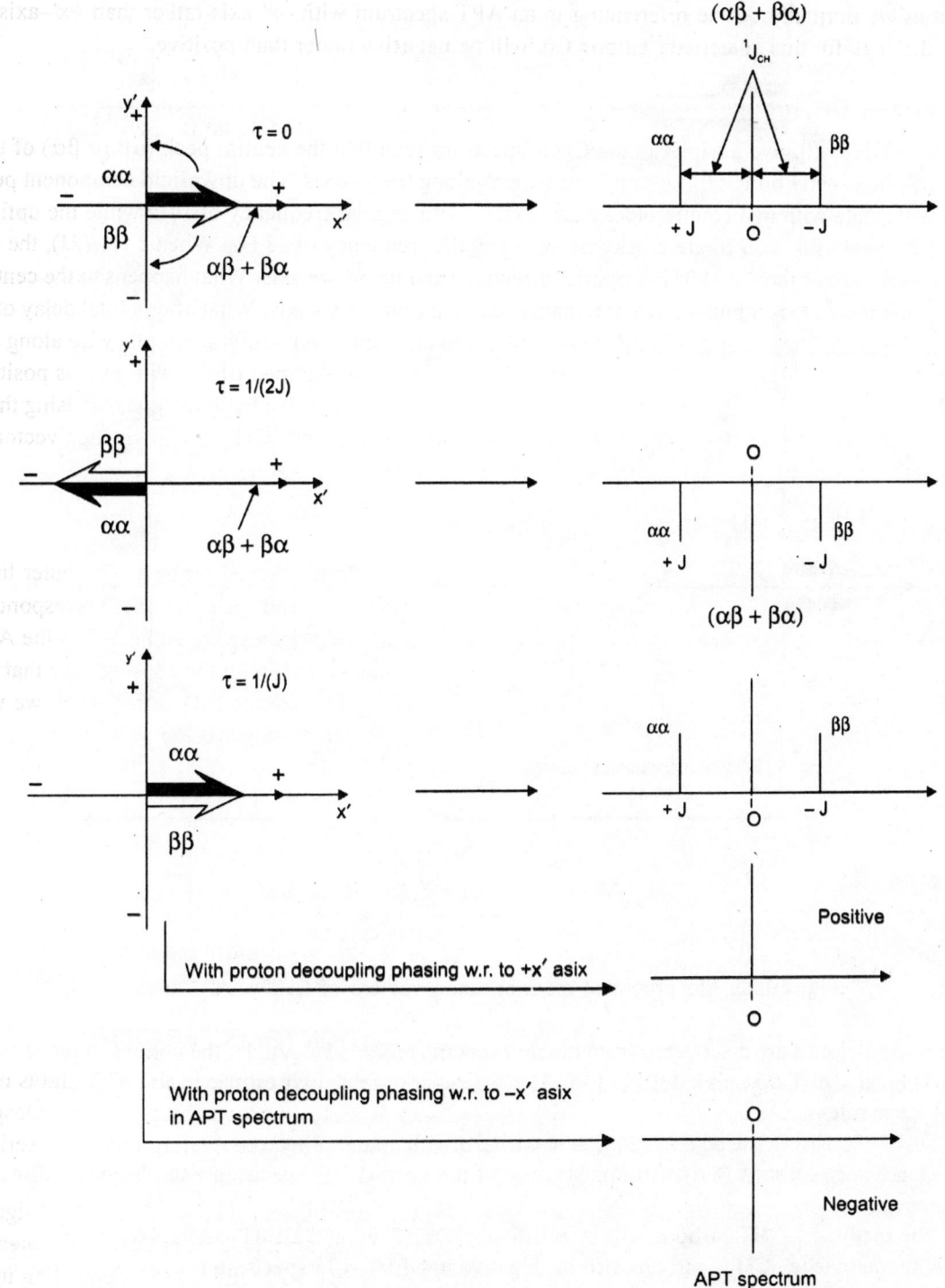

Fig. 10.21. Movement of ^{13}C magnetization vectors in CH_2 in APT test.

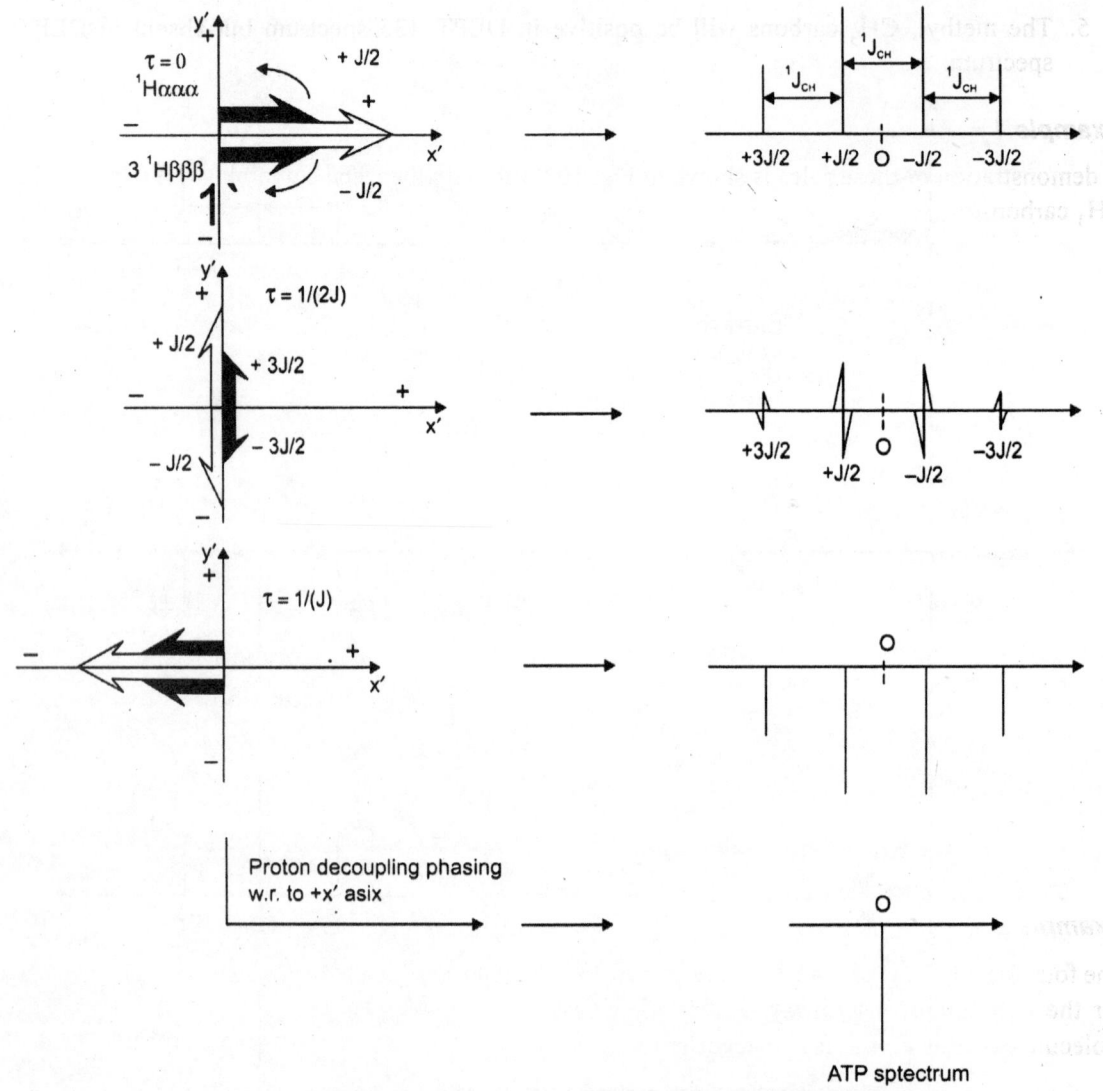

Fig. 10.22. Movement of magnetization vectors of CH_3 in APT test.

The DEPT results are discovered from the four spectra, recorded together : the normal ^{13}C spectrum, a DEPT-45, a DEPT-90 and a DEPT-135. The inferences are drawn on the basis of the following behaviour or rules :

1. DEPT–45 shows the peaks only due to carbons with attached protons.
2. Quaternary carbons (Cq) will appear only in the normal ^{13}C spectrum and absent in all other spectra.
3. The methine, –CH– carbons will be positive in DEPT–90 and DEPT–135 spectra.
4. The methylene –CH_2– carbons will be negative in DEPT–135 spectrum but absent in DEPT–90 spectrum.

5. The methyl, CH_3 carbons will be positive in DEPT–135 spectrum but absent in DEPT–90 spectrum.

Example 1

A demonstration of these rules is shown in Fig. 10.23 for ethylbenzene containing CH (ring), CH_2 and CH_3 carbons.

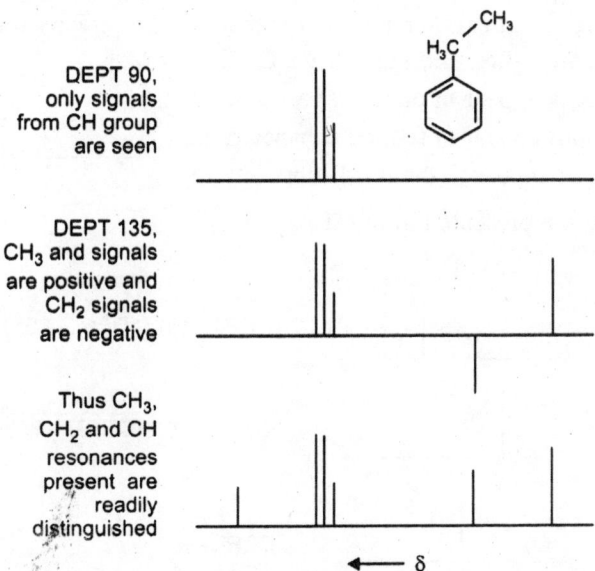

DEPT 90, only signals from CH group are seen

DEPT 135, CH_3 and signals are positive and CH_2 signals are negative

Thus CH_3, CH_2 and CH resonances present are readily distinguished

← δ

Fig. 10.23. The DEPT 90° and DEPT 135° spectra for ethyl benzene.

Example 2

The four spectra for DEPT analysis are presented in Fig. 10.24a for the compound, 4-hydroxy–3–methyl–2–butanone. This molecule contains all the four categories of carbons.

$$\overset{e}{CH_3}$$
$$\overset{d}{CH_3}-\overset{a}{\underset{\underset{O}{\parallel}}{C}}-\overset{}{\underset{c}{CH}}-\overset{b}{CH_2OH}$$

a is a quaternary carbon, d and e are two methyl carbons, b is a methylene carbon and c is a methine carbon. Normal ^{13}C spectrum shows five peaks at 213, 64, 50, 29, and 16.5 ppm.

As the peak at 213 ppm seen in normal ^{13}C spectrum disappears in all the DEPT spectra, it is clear that it must correspond to the quaternary carbon a.

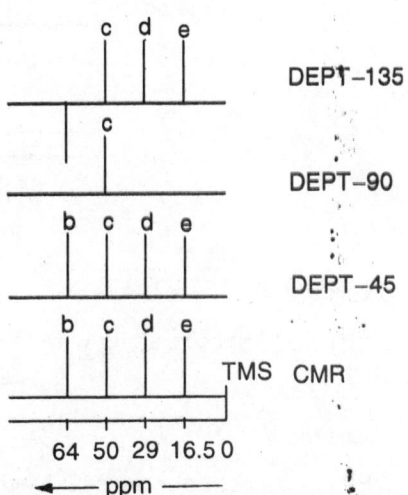

DEPT–135

DEPT–90

DEPT–45

TMS CMR

64 50 29 16.5 0

← ppm →

Fig. 10.24a. DEPT subspectra for 4–hydroxy–3–methyl–2–butanone.

The peak at 64 ppm seen in DEPT–135 because of its negative phase is obviously due to methylene carbon b. As the peak at 50 ppm is the single peak in the DEPT–90, it must be due to methine carbon CH, e.

So, we are left with only two peaks now at 29 and 16.5 ppm to be assigned. As these are present in DEPT–135 but absent in DEPT–90, these correspond to the two methyl peaks, d and e.

Further, it should be noted that it is also possible to further simplify the presentation of the DEPT experiment as four spectra by linear combinations of the four spectra recorded for the DEPT experiment. The net result of such mathematical manipulation is that we can directly read off the assignments in three ways. Such spectra are called "Edited" DEPT C–13 spectra:

1. Only the CH_3 carbons appear in one subspectrum.
2. Only the CH_2 carbons appear in second subspectrum.
3. Only the CH carbons appear in the third subspectrum.

The above subspectra are presented in Fig. 10.25.

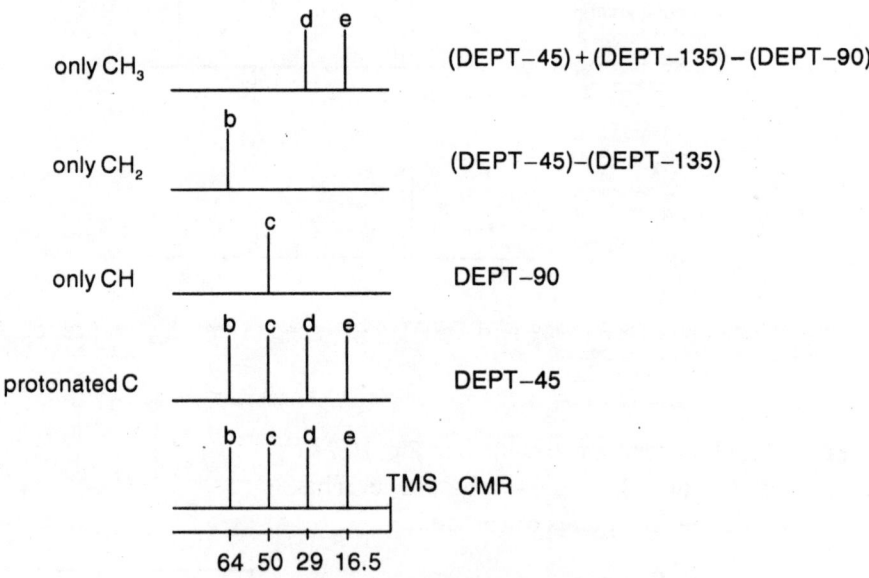

Fig. 10.24b. Edited DEPT spectra.

Example 3

DEPT C–13 spectra along with "Edited" DEPT spectra for a steroidal compound are recorded in Fig. 10.25.

Example 4

DEPT subspectra for trans–2–Methylcyclopentanol as shown in Fig. 10.26.

As can be seen the three CH_2 carbons (negative) peaks while CH (79.0) and CH_3 (17.9) carbons give positive peaks.

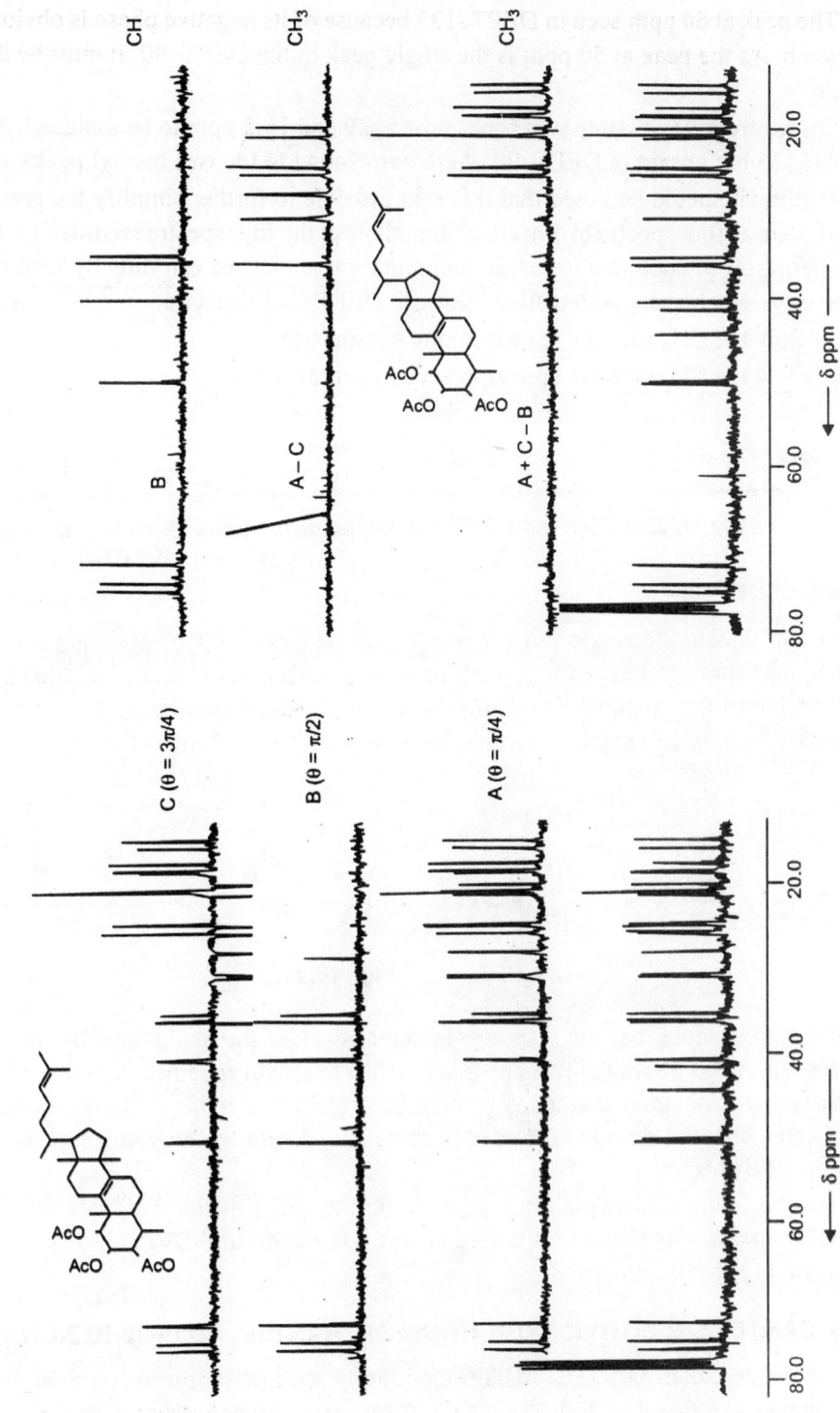

Fig. 10.25. DEPT Carbon–13 spectra and "Edited" DEPT Carbon–13 spectra.

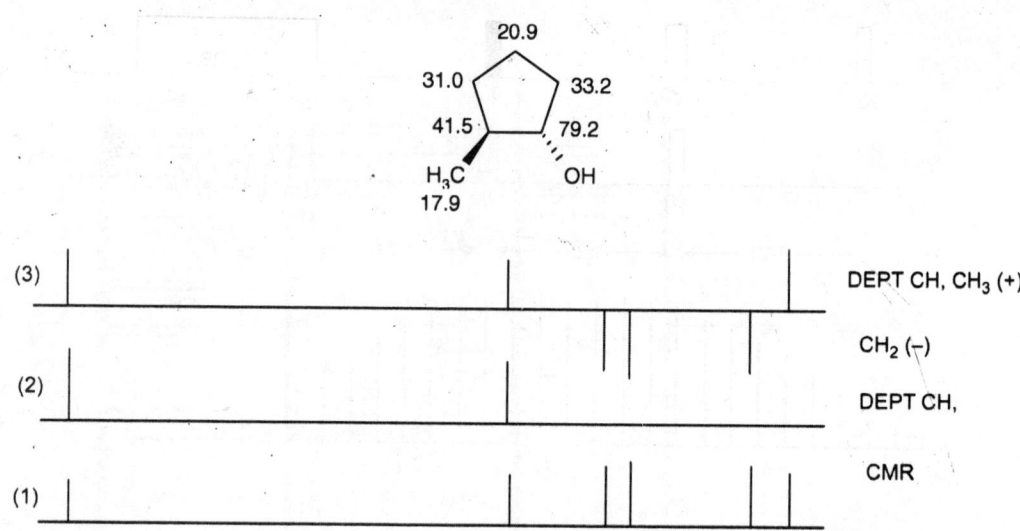

Fig. 10.26. CMR and DEPT subspectra for trans–2–methyl cyclopentanol.

Theory of DEPT

Recall that the simple single pulse n.m.r. experiment consists of applying a single radio frequency pulse to the sample to excite the spins followed by detection of the emitted free induction decay (FID) which is then Fourier transformed to yield a conventional spectrum. A standard broad band proton decoupled carbon–13 experiment could be represented as follows (Fig. 10.27):

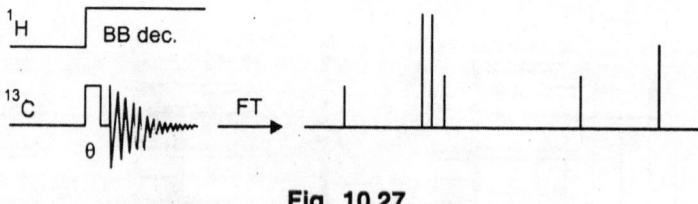

Fig. 10.27.

In particular note that the response is detected **after** the excitation. By using a carefully chosen sequence of pulses instead of just one it is possible to obtain spectra in which certain lines are absent or inverted depending upon how many protons each carbon atom bears. This is done in what looks rather complicated but all it does is to excite the spins in different ways by pulsing both protons and carbons to give useful spectra.

Thus the intensities of the lines depends on the value of the θ-pulse and how many protons the Carbon atom bears as shown in the Fig. 10.28a. DEPT 90° and DEPT 135° spectra for Ethyl benzene are shown in Fig. 10.28b.

10.26 DANTE : SELECTIVE EXCITATION OF ¹H-COUPLED C–13 RESONANCES

This technique called DANTE, 'delays alternating with mutation for tailored excitation' is used for separation of individual proton coupled C–13 resonances when strong overlap of individual multiplets

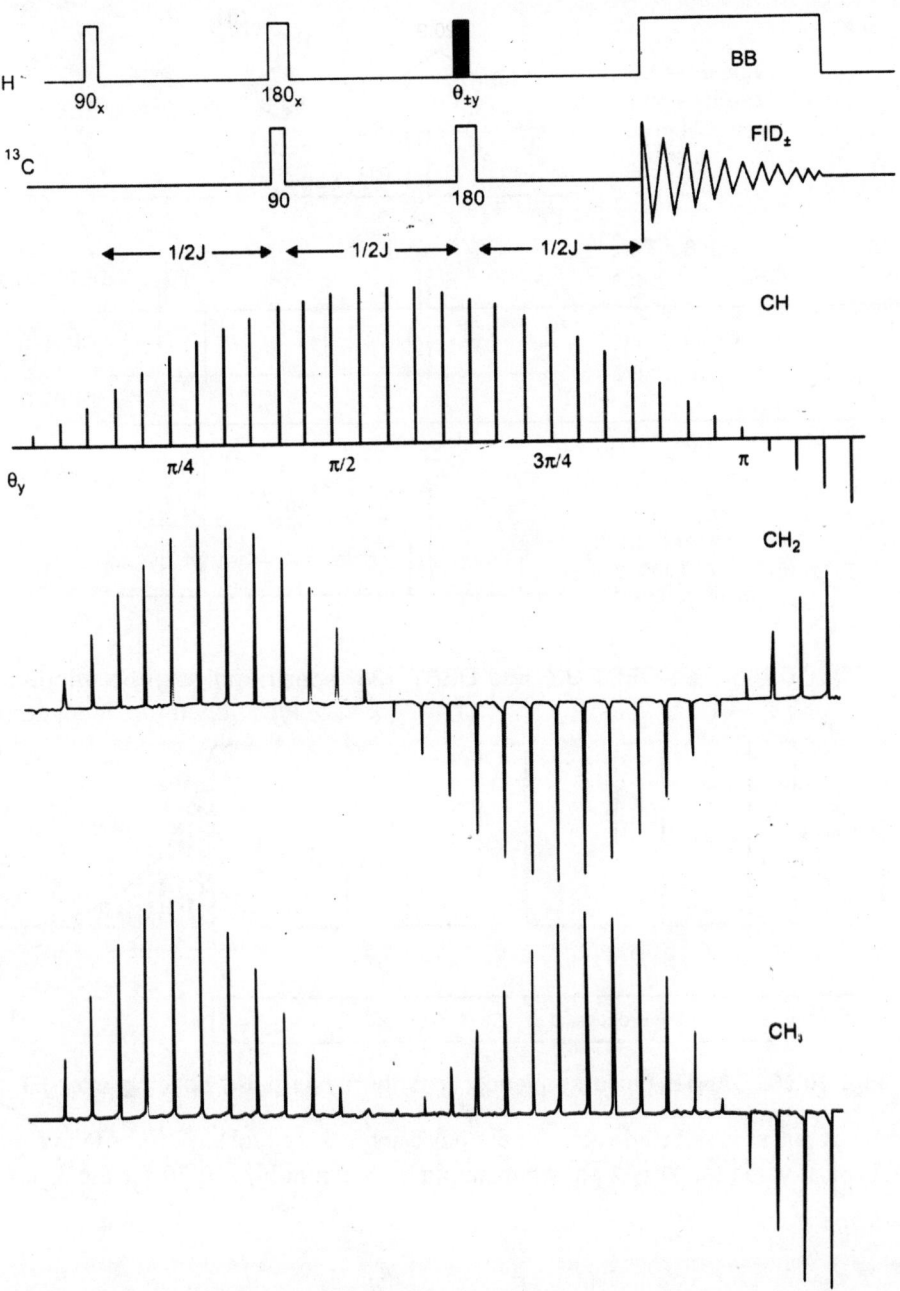

Fig. 10.28a. Distortionless Enhancement by Polarisation Transfer (DEPT).

occurs. What is done is that a single C–13 resonance whose frequency is determined in the ^{1}H-decoupled spectrum is selectively excited and ^{1}H-coupling is permitted during the FID detection with the result that the fully coupled multiplet of the selective C–13 is recorded without any overlap with other resonance. The DANTE pulse sequence is shown in Fig. 10.29.

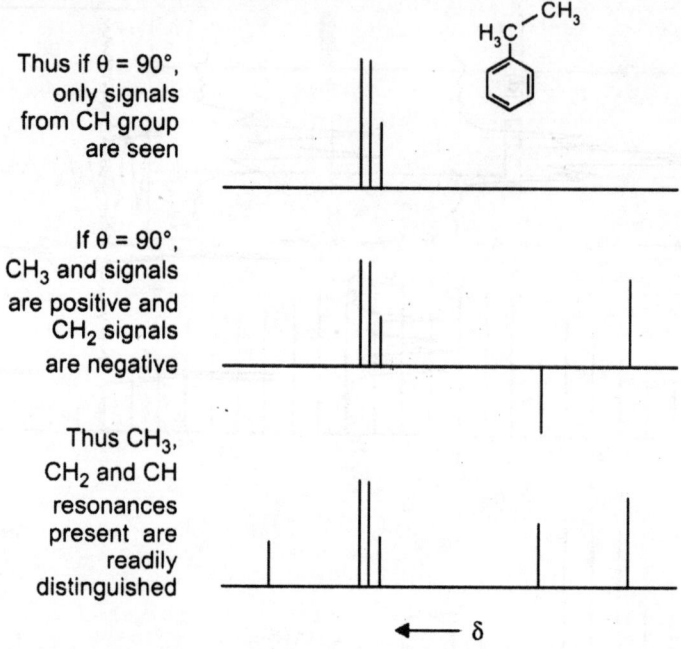

Thus if θ = 90°, only signals from CH group are seen

If θ = 90°, CH₃ and signals are positive and CH₂ signals are negative

Thus CH₃, CH₂ and CH resonances present are readily distinguished

⟵ δ

Fig. 10.28b. The DEPT 90° and DEPT 135° spectra for ethyl benzene.

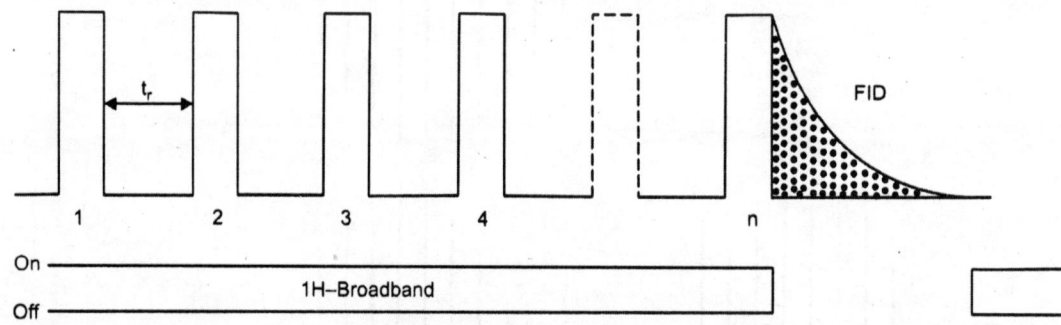

Fig. 10.29. DANTE pulse sequence, tr is the small pulse spacing after FT.

The number of pulses is selected such that the pulse angle θ is equal to 90°/n. At the end, a 90° pulse is achieved. Typical value for Tr is 2 μs. An example is shown in Fig. 10.30 for the following alkenyl ester:

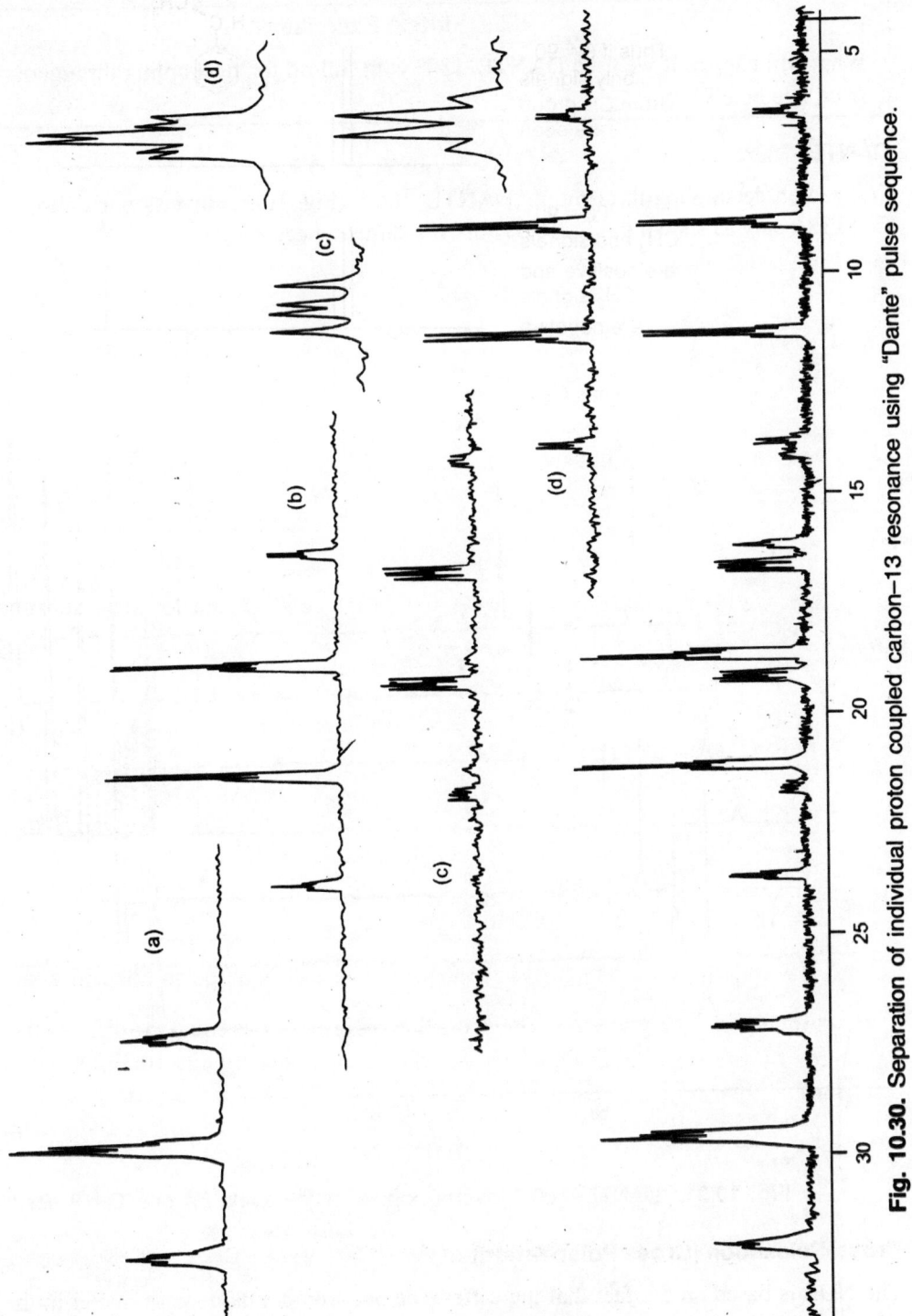

Fig. 10.30. Separation of individual proton coupled carbon–13 resonance using "Dante" pulse sequence.

Intext Exercise

What will happen if we used DANTE–180° with full proton decoupling throughout?
Hint: See below.

DANTE–180°

Full proton decoupling throughout "DANTE–180°" (Fig. 10.31) inverts population of levels for one C–13 site only as shown in Fig. 10.31 for N,N-dimethyl acetamide.

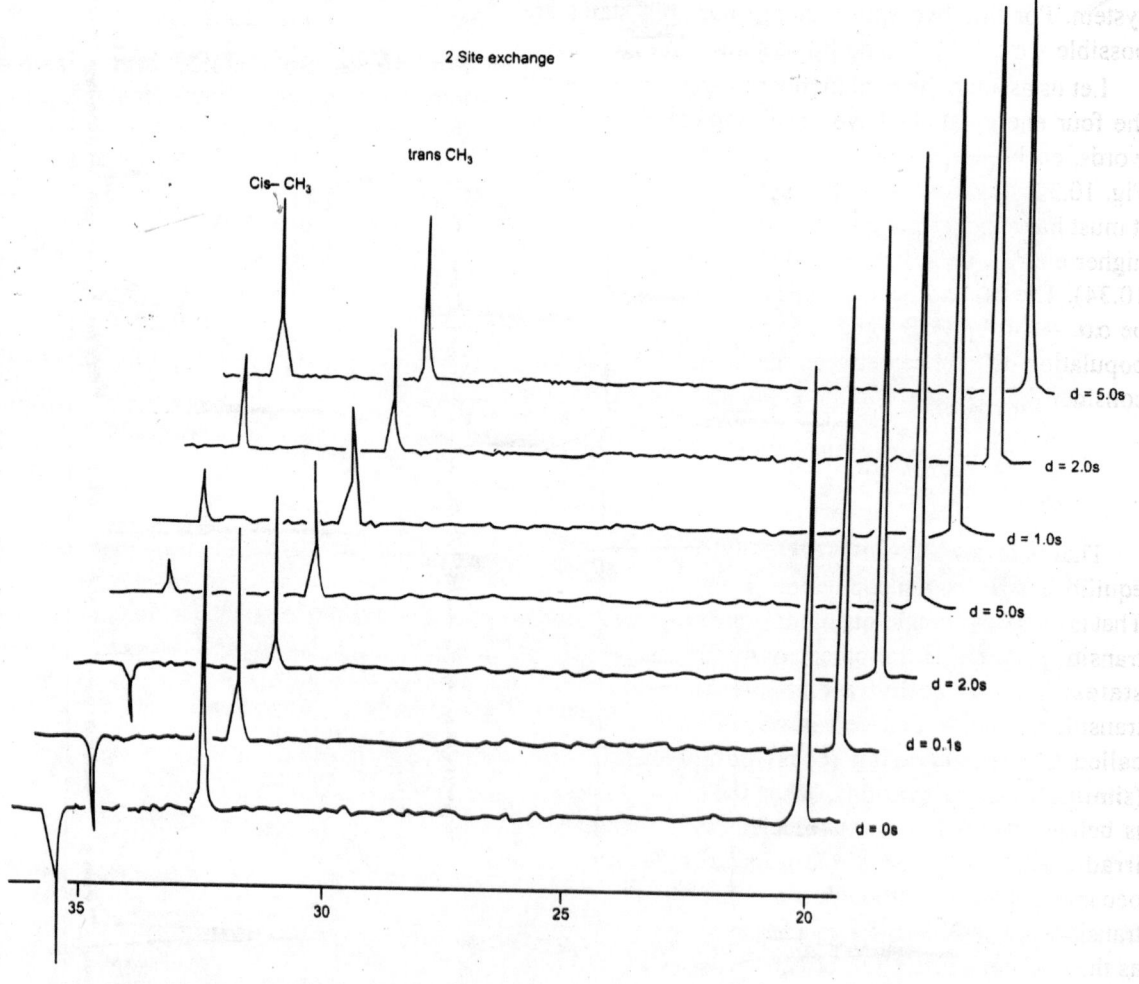

Fig. 10.31. "DANTE–180°" inverts population of levels for one C–13 site only.

Cross-Relaxation (Cross Polarization)

The NOE is based on the fact that the difference between populations of nuclei in the higher-energy state and the lower-energy state is affected by the difference between the populations of (these two) energy states of the nuclei that are situated nearby in space within 5Å. Irradiation and saturation of one nucleus leads to equalization of its two spin states. That causes an enhancement in the population difference between the different energy states of the other interacting nuclei. This enhancement, therefore, leads to an enhancement in the peak intensity of this second nucleus. How does this enhancement occur, can be demonstrated as follows. Let us consider the A–B system. For this two spin system, four spin states are possible – $\alpha\alpha$, $\alpha\beta$, $\beta\alpha$ and $\beta\beta$ as shown in Fig. 10.32.

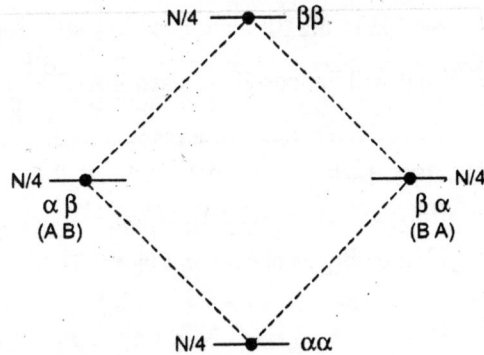

Fig. 10.32. Spin states and possible transitions and their populations. If N is the number of total spins, then each energy state should have N/4 population.

Let us assume the total number of spins as N that all the four energy states have equal population. In other words, each energy state will have N/4 spin-pairs (see Fig. 10.33). As $\alpha\alpha$ energy has lower energy, obviously it must have higher population of spins, say N/4 + δ. On the other hand, the $\beta\beta$ energy state which has higher energy, must have slightly lower population say N/4–δ at Boltzman thermal equilibrium (Fig. 10.34). The $\alpha\beta$ and $\beta\alpha$ energy states have equal energy i.e. N/4 each. The two allowed transitions will be $\alpha\alpha \rightarrow \beta\alpha$ and $\alpha\beta$ to $\alpha\beta$ and the intensity of these allowed transitions will be proportional to the population difference between the involved spin states, $(P_{\alpha\alpha}-P_{\beta\alpha})$ and $(P_{\alpha\beta}-P_{\beta\beta})$ respec-tively. Let us consider the difference in the population of these two states at this point:

$$P_{\alpha\alpha}-P_{\beta\alpha} = N/4 + \delta - N/4 = \delta$$

$$P_{\alpha\beta}-P_{\beta\beta} = N/4 - \delta - N/4 = \delta$$

That is to say DP = d in each tran-sition. After the spin states are perturbed, they try to restore the equilibrium Boltzman population. They can relax by following the reverse path of the transitions shown. That is to say by "single-quantum" transitions in which one nucleus remains the same, the other undergoes transition. There is the other possibility, in which both the $\beta\beta$ spins relax directly back to $\alpha\alpha$ spin states. This is called a "double-quantum" transition, a non-radiative pathway. This is also called **Cross-relaxation (cross-polarization) (simultaneous relaxation)**. When the nucleus A is being observed while the nucleus B is being irradiated, the "double-quantum" relaxation occurs efficiently. Although the single-quantum transitions also occur, we can forget about them as they do not cause NOE effect.

At thermal equilibrium, there will be a slight Boltzman excess of nuclei in the lower energy state, $\alpha\alpha$. That is to say some of $\beta\beta$ spin states have dropped down to the middle equal energy states ($\alpha\beta$ and $\beta\alpha$) such that eventually the

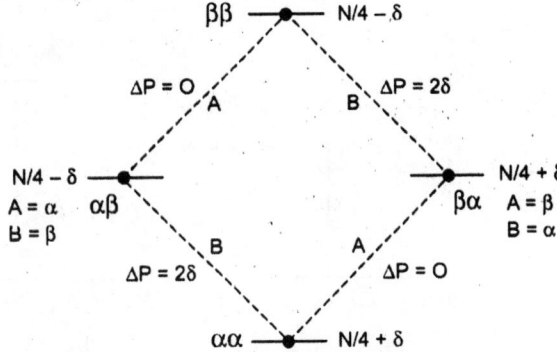

Fig. 10.33. Spin states and possible transitions for a two-spin system and population at Boltzman equilibrium.

population of the ββ state becomes N/2–2δ. The lower spin state will become N/4 + 2δ because the middle energy level spin states which initially become N/4 + δ each, lose δ spins to become N/34 each again. Let us now look at the energy difference between the two spin states:

$$P_{\alpha\alpha} - P_{\beta\alpha} = N/4 + 2\delta - N/4 = 2\delta$$

and

$$P_{\alpha\beta} - P_{\beta\beta} = N/4 - (N/4 - 2\delta)$$
$$= N/4 - N/4 + 2\delta = 2\delta$$

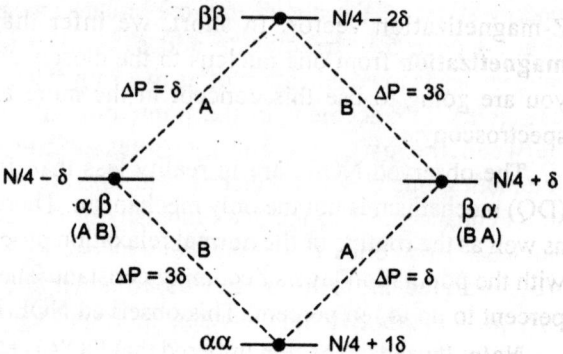

Fig. 10.34. Spin states and possible transitions for a two-spin system and populations after "double quantum" transitions.

Obviously, the population difference ΔP between the two transition states has doubled from δ to 2δ in each transition. So, an enhancement by two fold is expected to occur. This process of pumping up the population of nucleus A by irradiating nucleus B is called **"spin pumping"**. The net change in the NMR spectrum starting from Fig. 10.34 is shown in Fig. 10.35.

As the peak intensity is proportional to the net Mz magnetization vector for each nuclear spin, it is clear from the Fig. 10.35 that in terms of net magnetization, the $M_Z^B = 3/2\, Mo\ (150\%)$ while $M_Z^A = 1/2\, Mo$, it is also clear that M_Z^A is reduced to 1/2 (50%) of M_Z^o (100%). So, while M_Z^B is increased by 50% of its equilibrium value (100%). This means the increase (50%) in M_Z^B is exactly equal to the decrease (50%) in M_Z^A. That also means that the Z-magnetization (Mz) lost by the proton A has actually been transferred on to proton B. Therefore, what does NOE mean in terms of magnetization vector, Mz point of view? This simply means that in NOE experiments, when two nuclei are close enough in space at a distance of < 5°A, irradiation and saturation of one nucleus leads to a transfer of a part of magnetization vector Mz of one nucleus to the other nucleus, thereby increasing the value of its Mz, the

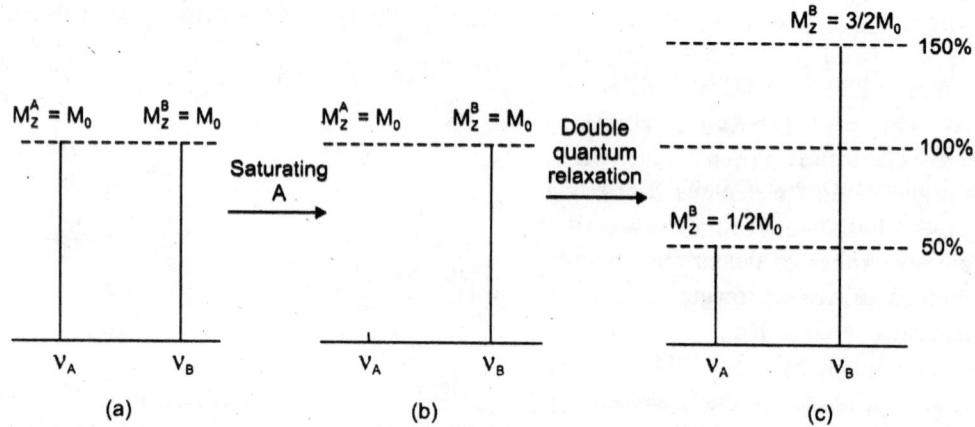

Fig. 10.35. Change in appearance of NMR spectrum of nuclei A and B (say proton), (a) at equilibrium, (b) after saturation of A by continuous irradiation, (c) after double quantum relaxation (DQR) in which the intensity of proton B has enhanced by two times.

Z-magnetization vector. In short, we infer that an NOE experiment leads to a **transfer of Z-magnetization** from one nucleus to the closely situated nucleus. Please remember this conclusion as you are going to use this concept in the more advanced part of the spectroscopy called 2D NMR spectroscopy.

The observed NOEs are in reality less than fifty percent. The reason is that the double-quantum (DQ) mechanism is not the only mechanism. There are other mechanisms in operation as well. The DQ as well as the routine or the normal relaxation processes go on together. In fact, a steady state is reached with the population levels becoming constant. The observable NOE is anything between a fraction of a percent to up to ten percent. This observed NOE is, therefore, also known as steady state NOE.

Note: It needs to be remembered that DQR is effected by magnetic fields that oscillate at a frequency two times that of Larmor frequency of the nucleus. Further, it needed to be noted that DQ relaxation is very significant in case of molecules having low molecular mass, say less than one thousand. The reason for this is that being small, these molecules have very rapid rate of tumbling and they have sufficient populations that tumble at Larmor as well as twice the Larmor frequency. Molecules with MW > 1000, it is the zero-quantum (ZQ) rather than the double-quantum (DQ) relaxation mechanism that is significant. A ZQ transition means one spin droping down and the other spin droping up i.e. $\alpha\beta \rightarrow \beta\alpha$. The large molecules have almost insignificant populations that tumble at single-quantum frequency or at the double quantum frequency. This gives rise to positive NOE, i.e. reduction of peak intensity. For small molecules, the NOE is negative, that is to say the peak intensity is decreased. In fact, molecules having MW 2000–4000 Da exhibit either little or no NOE at all, of course that depends upon the shape of the molecule, rigidity as well as viscosity of the solvent in use. Such molecules show what is called Rotating-Frame Overhauser Effect (ROESY).

PROBLEMS

1. Obtaining a ^{13}C NMR spectrum is much more difficult compared to a ^{1}H NMR spectrum. Explain why?

   Hint: See Section 1.

2. If C–12 were a NMR-active nucleus, then what could have been the disadvantages in CMR spectroscopy?

   Hint: See Section 1.

3. If C–13 had 100% natural abundance like ^{1}H, then what could have been its disadvantages.

   Hint: See Section 1.

4. Write the number of peaks that would be obtained in the CMR spectrum of each of these compounds: (1) Cyclopropane, (2) Cyclobutane, (3) Cyclopentane, (4) Cyclohexane, (5) Benzene, (6) Ethene.

   Hint: See Section 2.

5. Predict the number of peaks in the CMR spectrum of each of these: (1) 1–Chloropentane, (2) Hexyne–1, (3) But–1–ene, (4) Propylene, (5) Oct–1–ene.

   Hint: See Section 2.

6a. How many sets of non-equivalent carbons are present in the following molecules.

6b. Write the expected number of peaks in the CMR (proton decoupled) spectrum of following compounds.

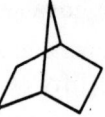

Hind: Three only as explained below.

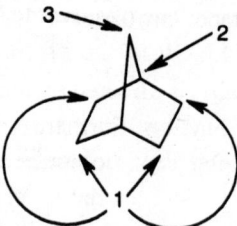

What would be the expected number of peaks in the proton decoupled CMR spectrum of this compound.

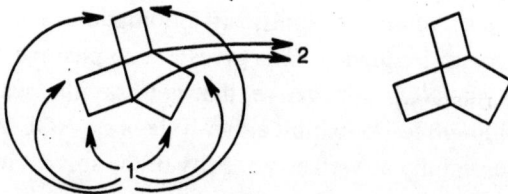

Hint: Two types only as explained above.

6.c How many peaks do you expect in the CMR spectrum of camphor.

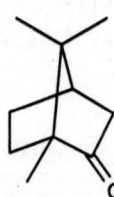

Hint: Ten as the carbons are different in this compound

CMR spectrum of camphor

6d. How will you distinguish between o, m and p-dihydroxy benzenes on the basis of C–13 NMR?
   Hint: See the section "Disubstituted Benzenes" (Aromatic Carbons).

1. Mesitylene, 2. Propane, 3. 2–Chlorobutane, 4. 2–Chloro–2–methyl butane, 5. 2–Methyl pentane, 6. But–3–ene, 7. cis–2–butene.

   Hint: See Section 2.

7. Can we distinguish between 2–bromopropane and 1–bromopropane on the basis of their CMR spectra?

   Hint: See Intext Exercise 1.

8. What is meant by Broad-band or Proton-decoupled spectra? How many signals will be obtained in the Proton-coupled CMR spectra of propanol–1 if only the terminal (C–3) carbon of this molecule were C–13?

   Hint: See Section 4.

9. Explain as to why the routine C–13 NMR spectra are not integrated unlike ^{1}H NMR spectra? Is the principle of CMR spectroscopy different from that of PMR spectroscopy.

   Hint: See Section 6.

10. Why does a quaternary carbon in CMR spectroscopy give a very weak signal?

    Hint: See Section 6.

11. While spin-lattice relaxation times, T_1 are of lattice importance in ^{1}H NMR spectroscopy, they are of great importance in C–13 NMR spectroscopy. Explain.

    Hint: See Section 6.

12. What is the general range of chemical shift in C–13 NMR spectroscopy? Why is it large compared to that in proton NMR spectroscopy? Write approximate shifts for the commonly encountered functional groups carbons.

    Hint: See Section 7.

13. Write the chemical shift (approximate) range for the following selected functional groups: alkanes, acetylenes, olefins, aromatics, carboxyl (acids, esters, amides, aldehydes and ketones).

    Hint: See Table 2.

14. Compare the chemical shifts of protons and C–13 showing the similarities as well as the divergences.

    Hint: See Section 9.

15. Which is a better technique between PMR spectroscopy and CMR spectroscopy for making distinction between alkene and aromatic bonds?

    Hint: See Section 9(b) divergences and Intext question 2.

16. What are the effects or factors in chemical shifts of C–13 nuclei? Enlist these.

    Hint: See Section 10.

17. Enlist the factors that affect chemical shift in CMR spectroscopy. Discuss the following in details: 1. Hyperconjugative effect, 2. Resonance effect, 3. Steric effect, 4. Anisotropy effect.

    Hint: See Section 12, 13, 17 and 18.

18. Explain the hybridisation effects, isotope effects and substituent effects in chemical shifts of C–13.

    Hint: See Section 13–15.

19. Illustrate the γ-effect in cyclohexanes.

    Hint: See Section 16.

20. Explain whereas the CH_2 carbon in ketene, $CH_2=C=O$, absorbs at δ 2.5, the carbonyl carbon resonates at δ 194.0 ppm. Why?

    Hint: See Section 12: Resonance effect.

21. Write a note on substituent effects in ^{13}C chemical shifts: α, β and γ effects.

    Hint: See Section 16.

22. Write a note on γ-effect in CMR spectra of cyclohexanes.

    Hint: See Section 16.

23. Write a note on γ-effect in CMR spectra of alkenes.

    Hint: See Section 16.

24. How will you distinguish between propane and propene on the basis of proton-decoupled CMR spectrum?

    Hint: See Section 19.1 under alkanes.

25. How will you distinguish between the side chains of the rings in the styrene and ethyl benzene on the basis of proton-decoupled CMR spectra.

    Hint: See Section 19.1 under alkanes.

26. Can we distinguish between cis and trans but–2–enes on the basis of their proton-decoupled CMR spectra?

    Hint: Yes, on the basis of γ-effect, see Section 16.

27. Can you distinguish between ethane, ethene and ethyne on the basis of their proton-decoupled CMR spectra?

    Hint: Yes, we can. On the basis of their chemical shifts. See Section 16.3 under alkynes.

28. Where do benzene carbons absorbs in its CMR spectrum?

    Hint: See Section 16.4, aromatic carbons.

29. The central carbon in tert-butyl carbocation absorbs at 328 ppm, that in phenyl dimethyl methane carbocation resonates at 254 ppm. Why?

    Hint: See Section 12 (resonance effects).

30. The central carbon in diphenyl methyl methane carbocation absorbs at 254 ppm while that in phenyl dimethyl methane carbocation resonates at 198 ppm. Why?

$$\overset{\oplus}{Ph\ C(CH_3)_2} \qquad \overset{\oplus}{Ph_2\ C\ CH_3}$$

    Hint: See section 12 (resonance effects).

31. While the central carbon in triphenyl methane carbocation absorbs at 211 ppm, that in diphenyl methyl methane carbocation absorbs at 254 ppm. Why?

$$\overset{\oplus}{Ph\ C} \qquad \overset{\oplus}{Ph_2\ C\ CH_3}$$

    Hint: See section 12 (resonance effect).

32. In cyclopropyl dimethyl methane carbocation, the central carbon absorbs at 280 ppm, while that in trimethyl methane, carbocation resonates at 328 ppm. Why?

    Hint: See Section 12 (resonance effects).

33. Write the general range in which carbonyl carbon of the following compounds absorb in CMR spectra.

    Acid, halides, Acid amides, Esters and Carboxylic acids.

    Hint: See Section 7 and Table 8.1.

34. Write the decreasing order of chemical shift of the carbonyl carbon of the following:

    CH_3COI, CH_3COCl, CH_3COBr

    Hint: See Section 12.

35. Why are the carbonyl carbons of the carbonyl group containing compounds very much deshielded? Explain.

    Hint: See Section 9 and 12.

36. In 2–butanone, the carbonyl carbon absorbs at 207 ppm, whereas in but–1–ene–3 one, the carbonyl carbon resonates at 194 ppm. Why?

    Hint: See Section 12. The positive charge on carbonyl carbon gets reduced due to resonance, in the unsaturated ketone.

37. Can we classify C–13 shifts of hydrocarbons on the basis of their hybridisation? Give the approximate range of the three categories.

    Hint: See Section 15.

38. How many peaks does a monosubstituted benzene ring show in its (proton decoupled) CMR spectrum? Explain. What will be the intensity of the ipso C signal compared to others?

    Hint: See Section 4, monosubstituted benzene.

39. How many peaks do we see in the proton-decoupled CMR spectrum of ethyl benzene? What will be the intensity of the ipso C signal compared to others?

    Hint: See Section 4, ethyl benzene (Fig.).

40. How many signals do we see in the proton-decoupled CMR spectrum of acetophenone? What is the intensity of ipso C signal compared to others?

    Hint: See section 4, acetophenone (Fig.).

41. Can we distinguish three isomeric symmetrically disubstituted benzenes on the basis of their proton-decoupled CMR spectra?

    Hint: Yes, we can. See Section 4.

42. How will you distinguish the three disubstituted dibromobenzenes on the basis of their proton-decoupled CMR spectra.

    Hint: See Intext Exercise 4.

43. Whereas benzene shows only one signal in its proton-decoupled CMR spectrum, replacement of a carbon in benzene by nitrogen produces three signals in its CMR spectrum. Why?

    Hint: Compare Benzene with Pyridine. See Section 5, heteroaromatics.

44. How many signals are expected in the CMR spectrum of indole?

    Hint: Eight. Because all the carbons are non-equivalent. See Section 5.

45. How many signals are expected in the CMR spectrum of iso-quinoline?

    Hint: All 9 carbons are different in this molecule. So, they give rise to their own signals. See Section 6.

46. While the carbon in methanol absorbs at 49 ppm, that in methanamine resonates at 26.9 ppm. Why?

    Hint: The electronegativity of oxygen is more than that of nitrogen. See Intext Exercise and Section 6 and 7.

47. How will you distinguish between the following on the basis of their proton-decoupled CMR spectra?

    Carboxylic acids, esters, amides, anhydrides.

    Hint: See Section 8.

48. What is meant by the Off-Resonance decoupled spectrum in CMR spectroscopy? Explain with the example of 2–Butanone and tert-butyl alcohol. How is the residual splitting J_R related to original $^1J_{CH}$ coupling, J_0 the irradiating power of the decoupler and its separation in Hz, from the proton being decoupled? What is the latest technique which has replaced off resonance?

    Hint: See Section 20.

49. How many groups of spin-spin interactions are observed in CMR spectroscopy?

    Hint: See Section 10.21.

50. Write a note on $^1J_{CH}$ ($^{13}C-^1H$) coupling constants.

    Hint: See Section 10.21.

51. What is meant by $^1J_{CH}$? What is size? What are the factors upon which $^1J_{CH}$ depends?

    Hint: See Section 10.21. Describe and explain hybridisation and electronegativity effects.

52. What is meant by J_{CC} coupling constants? Are they smaller than $^1J_{CH}$ coupling constants? Explain the dependence of $^3J_{CC}$ for $\phi = 0°$ and $180°$, vary from $^3J_{HH}$?

    Hint: see Karplus curve in Section 10.21.

53. What is Gated decoupling? Explain.

    Hint: See Section 10.22.

54. What is Inverse Gated decoupling? When is it used? Illustrate.

    Hint: See Section 10.23.

55. What is DEPT? Is this superior or inferior to INEPT, off-resonance? What are their types? Explain utility of DEPT experiments to explain structure of ethyl benzene, 4–hydroxy–3–methyl–2–butanone or trans–2–methylcyclopentanol.

    Hint: See Section 10.25.

56. Give theory of DEPT in brief.

    Hint: See Section 10.25.

57. Explain the Attached Proton Test (APT) in details.

    Hint: See Section 10.24.

C–13 NMR Relaxation: Factors and Mechanism

11.1 RELAXATION TIMES OF C–13

As we saw in Chapter 1, relaxation is a very important phenomenon in NMR, without which it would have been impossible to get an NMR spectrum. Excitation of spin states from the ground (α in case of ^{13}C, ^1H, ^{19}F, ^{31}P) to the excited state (β in case of ^{13}C, ^1H, ^{19}F, ^{31}P) is important but equally important is the relaxation that restores and maintains the Boltzman population excess. The relaxation times for protons are very small of the order of 1s and the appearance of spectra is in general, unaffected by the differences in the relaxation times of protons. On the other hand, the C–13 nuclei have very long relaxation times having a vast range from a few milliseconds in molecules having higher molecular weight upto several hundred seconds for carbons having no attached protons in small symmetrical molecules. An example is shown in Fig. 11.1.

Carbon No.	T_1	δ_C (CDCl$_3$)
11	1.53	42.9
3	1.82	127.0
14	5.2	141.0
13	8.9	146.6
12	5.1	130.9

Fig. 11.1. Relaxation times of various carbons in the data for Codeine obtained at 25.2 MHz at 1.6 molar concentration at 30° in CDCl$_3$.

11.2 PHYSICAL SIGNIFICANCE OF T_1

Relaxation phenomenon determines as to how long you would have to wait in order to repeat the data acquisition. This phenomenon also governs the decay time of FIDs and as well as the appearance of spectrum i.e. how narrow the lines would be in the NMR spectrum.

Furthermore, relaxation is the basis of NOE effect that is used to determine stereochemistry, the distance between the nuclei.

We require a knowledge of the relaxation time. T_1 values in order to carry out any special repetitive scanning NMR experiments. This is very important indeed.

The relaxation times T_1 in general, do not carry much significance for protons as they do for ^{13}C nuclei. This is because the protons have very small relaxation times usually of the order of 1s. That is to say the excited (β-spin) protons relax to the ground (α-spin) state within a second to restore the "steady-state" Boltzman excess that is needed for the next scan. In other words, the protons relax completely before the next FID is scanned. As the relaxation is complete, the FIDs are complete so that the peak intensities in proton NMR spectra are reliable for quantitative analysis (Fig. 10.4, page 242). In fact, as majority of hydrogens (protons) are bonded to C–12 (99.9%) rather than C–13 (1.1%), therefore, they do not sense any intense oscillating magnetic fields from the C–12 atoms to which they are directly bonded as these C–12 atoms (I = O) are NMR inactive. They, of course, only experience weak oscillating magnetic fields from the nearby vast number of protons present within the molecule.

However, it needs to be noted that as the field strength B_0 increases, the relaxation times T_1 increase as well such that at 600–900 MHz, the protons take 2 to 3 seconds to relax instead of 1s at lower field strengths. Nevertheless, T_1 of ^1H are very small (1–3 s). In the biomedical world, water has different T_1 values in different tissues because of different degree of association with the large biological molecules as well as membranes. So, this phenomenon provides contrast in medical NMR imaging. The contrast agents that are injected in Magnetic Resonance Imaging (MRI) contain paramagnetic ligands – complexed ions having particular affinities for particular tissues like tumors that increase the T_1.

On the other hand, a knowledge of relaxation times for C–13 nuclei has great significance. Why?

We want to ensure that the Boltzman distribution condition has been re-established before the next scan. Such an experiment is a must if we want to carry out quantitative analysis in ^{13}C NMR spectroscopy where the routine CMR spectra are insufficient for knowing the reliable relative ratios of the peak intensities. The major reason there is that the different carbons experience different amounts of peak enhancements due to differential NOE effects. Thus, for quantitative analysis, we require relaxation (pulse) delay of $5 \times T_1$. When we insert such a relaxation delay in ^{13}C along with of course, simultaneous elimination of the NOE, we can get CMR spectra worth quantitative analysis. Complete FIDs give complete relaxation and thus stronger peaks. Incomplete FIDs give incomplete or partial relaxation and thus unreliable peak heights. For routine CMR spectra, we do not spend $5 \times T_1$ times for the relaxation of most slowly relaxing carbon nuclei. That is to say we do not wait in reality for the steady-state Boltzman excess to be re-established before the next scan. In fact, we set up the scanning experiment such that the Boltzman excess is only partially re-established. That is to say for the most slowly relaxing C–13 nuclei the FID is already ceased before they relax to Boltzman excess. That is their FIDs are incomplete. The next scan starts even before the FID is complete! Therefore, the incomplete FID yields partial peak heights in routine CMR spectra. Although those C–13 nuclei in the molecule relax quickly i.e. completely, give reliable peak heights, the ones whose rates of relaxation are very low, they end up giving weak signals.

11.3 STRUCTURAL (CHEMICAL) SIGNIFICANCE OF RELAXATION TIMES

We have become familiar with the physical significance of relaxation times of C–13 nuclei. We also need to know is there any chemical significance of these relaxation times? Are these connected with the chemical structure of the molecule? Can we be in a position to correlate relaxation of a C–13 nucleus with its structural nature i.e. whether it is 1°, 2°, 3° or 4° in nature? Is there any difference in T_1 for protonated and non-protonated carbons? Is there a relation between relaxation times and molecular weight? Is there a relation between relaxation times and molecular symmetry? Similarly, is there any effect of hindered rotation on relaxation times? Is there a relation between T_1 and axes of rotation? What is the effect of rigid position of carbons on their relaxation times? Does association i.e. hydrogen bonding have any effect on T_1? Similarly, we also need to know the relationship between complexation and T_1. Thus, while chemical shifts (as well as coupling constants) give the static picture of a molecule, relaxation times reveal or symbolize molecular dynamics.

11.4 FACTORS AFFECTING C–13 RELAXATION TIMES

11.5 RELATION BETWEEN T_1 AND MOLECULAR WEIGHT

Yes, there is some relationship between the C–13 relaxation times and molecular weights. Thus, bio-polymers and other molecules having high molecular weights have very short T_1, 10^{-3} – 1 second. Molecules which have molecular weight lesser than 1000, have relatively higher T_1 – 0.1 to 300 s. Further among such category of molecules, protonated carbons relax quickly i.e. have T_1 0.1 to 10 s, while non-protonated carbons relax slowly i.e. have T_1 10 to 300 s :

Molecular weight	Relaxation times
Very high	10^3 — 1 s
< 1000	0.1—300 s
Protonated C	0.1 — 10 s
Non-protonated C	10 — 300 s

Molecules that are small, tumble very quickly in solvent. Tumbling leads to higher relaxation times. Thus cyclohexane carbons have a relaxation time of 20 s, benzene carbons have T_1 of 28 s. Other examples include CH_3OH, CH_3I, etc. In sluggish cyclodecane carbons have lower T_1 of 4–5 s.

The local motions of flexible groups in molecule lead to a decrease in correlation time τ_C so that the T_1 values rise. This does not happen in rigid parts of the molecules so that T_1 are small.

Ethyl benzene beautifully demonstrates the different relaxation times for the non-equivalent CH_3, CH_2, quaternary and other carbons.

Thus, while the methyl carbon has a relaxation time T_1 of 9 s, CH_2 13 s, the quaternary (ipso) carbon has 36 s. Similarly, in toluene while CH_3 carbon as T_1 of 16 s, the quaternary (ipso) carbon has T_1 of 38 s.

Carbonyl carbons that are non-protonated have long relaxation times :

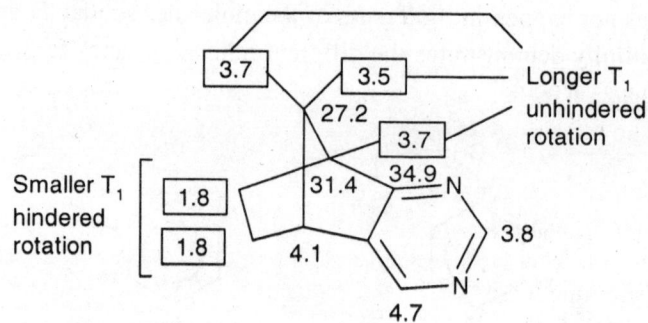

The reason for lower relaxation times of protonated carbons versus non-protonated carbons is that NOE effect helps them in relaxing rapidly.

The effect of protons directly attached to C–13 nuclei dominates over the effect of the distant nuclei. This means that the number of protons attached to C–13 nuclei very much govern their rates of relaxation. Thus, by this argument the relaxation times for CH_3, CH_2 and CH should follow the order:

$$CH_3 < CH_2 < CH$$
Increasing relaxation times $T_1 \longrightarrow$

The carbons which have no attached protons, that is which are quaternary should have even higher T_1 than CH carbons. These carbons experience only very weak oscillating magnetic fields and hence have very high T_1. In fact, that is the reason as to why the CMR experiment requires longer pulse (relaxation) delay for relaxation of quaternary carbons. So we can write :

$$CH_3 < CH_2 < CH < Cq$$
Increasing relaxation times $\longrightarrow$

11.6 RELAXATION TIMES VERSUS RIGID SKELETON (HINDERED ROTATION)

Relaxation times for carbons whose rotation is hindered in a rigid skeleton are smaller than those carbons whose rotation is unhindered.

Examples

1. In quinazoline system shown below, the T_1 values for unhindered methyl groups have longer T_1 versus the T_1 of the methylene carbons:

Thus, the three methyl carbons have $T_1 \sim 3.7$, 3.7 and 3.5. The two CH_2 carbons have T_1 equal to 1.8 s.

2. The T_1 of 9–methyl carbon in 9–methylanthracene is longer (14.8 s) compared to T_1 (5.8 s) of 1–methyl carbon in 1–methylnaphthalene. This is because the methyl carbon in latter molecule is coaxed into a staggered conformation by the peri-proton. Whereas, the methyl of 9–methylanthracene does not have any preferred conformation due to pressure of two peri-hydrogens. That means the 9–methyl carbon has unhindered rotation that enhances its T_1.

3. In N, N–dimethyl formamide, T_1 for the cisoid CH_3 carbon is 28.6 s while that for transoid CH_3 carbon is 13.1 s. This is because the cisoid CH_3 carbon that eclipses the carbonyl oxygen spins more rapidly compared to the transoid methyl carbon. This is because the opposing interaction of the cisoid methyl with the carbonyl oxygen as well as the second methyl group is unfavourable so that there are no favoured rotomeric conformations. However, the transoid methyl faces minimum unfavourable interactions with the other methyl group and the formyl hydrogen :

Intext Exercise

How can we distinguish between the cisoid and transoid methyl carbons in N,N–dimethylformamide by CMR?

Solution : We can imagine a relation between these methyl carbons and their T_1s. CH_3 that is ciscoid eclipses the carbonyl oxygen and the transoid does not. Consequently, the ciscoid methyl should have longer T_1 in N,N–dimethylformamide.

---

4. A structure-spin lattice relaxation time relation has been discovered in a number of variously substituted steroidal molecules. The C–19 methyl group have longer T_1 compared to C–18 in androstane derivatives. This is because the C–19 methyl group spins rapidly owing to larger number of 1,3–steric interaction with axial hydrogens, with the result that this methyl group is not able to assume a preferred conformation.

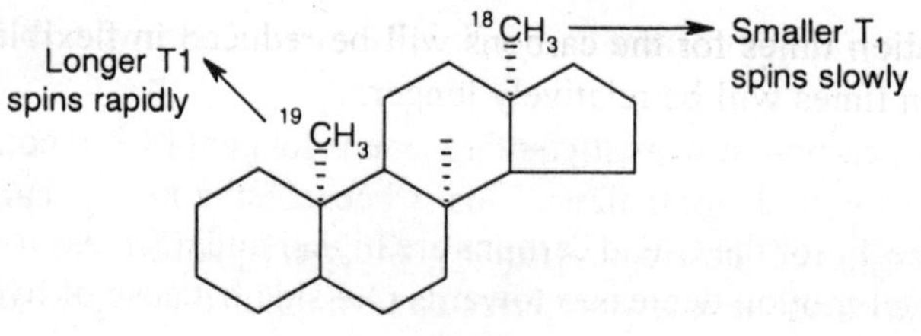

Androstane

Intext Exercise

Should the axial methyl carbons have same T_1 s as equatorial methyls in diterpenoids?

---

5. Similarly, the axial methyl carbons have shorter T_1 compared to equatorial methyl carbons in some diterpenes. This is because of steric crowding of axial methyl carbons.

11.7 RELAXATION TIMES AND PREFERRED AXES OF ROTATION

Unsymmetric molecules have preferred axes of rotation so that the carbons lying along these axes will have short T_1 values. This is because rotation around these axes does not contribute to the correlation times of such carbons.

Examples

1. In nitrobenzene, the carbons C_1 and the para ones lie along the preferred axis of rotation and therefore for the reasons mentioned earlier have shorter relaxation times of 5.6 s and 4.9 s respectively compared to ortho and meta carbons which have longer relaxation times of 6.9 second. The ring rotates relatively easily through this axis.

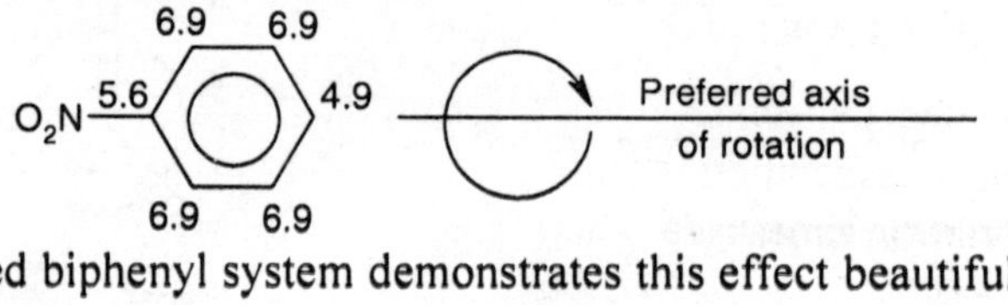

2. The tetramethylated biphenyl system demonstrates this effect beautifully.

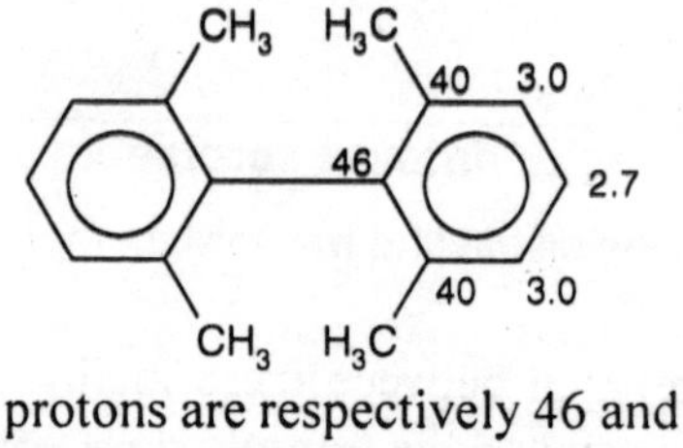

The T_1 for the ortho and meta protons are respectively 46 and 40 s compared to 61 s and 5.9 s for the biphenyl itself. The reason is that while biphenyl has a preferred axis of rotation along the bond that links both the rings, the tetramethyl deriative does not have a preferred axis of rotation due to steric crowding.

11.8 RELAXATION TIMES AND SEGMENTAL MOTION

Some molecules contain flexible as well as non-flexible or rigid systems. Obviously, the local motion or degree of motion in flexible parts will be much more compared to that in the non-flexible parts.

Therefore, the correlation times for the carbons will be reduced in flexible rather than in rigid parts. Hence, their relaxation times will be relatively longer.

Examples

1. In 1–decanol, the T_1 for the C-end carbons are higher and decrease towards OH side. This means that the segmental motion decreases towards OH side because of hydrogen bonding.

$$\underset{3.1}{CH_3} - \underset{2.2}{CH_2} - \underset{1.6}{CH_2} - \underset{1.1}{CH_2} - \underset{0.8}{(CH_2)_5} - \underset{0.7}{CH_2OH}$$

2. In decane, the T_1 of carbons are higher at the end portion and decrease as we move towards the middle.

$$C_5H_{11} - CH_2 - \overset{5.0}{\underset{4.4}{CH_2}} - CH_2 - \overset{6.6}{\underset{8.7}{CH_2}} - CH_3$$

3. T_1 values are of considerable importance in phospholipids and lipid membranes. The differences noted in the T_1 of flexible parts and rigid parts on the basis of segmental motion, provide us with a tool to investigate molecular transport and membrane permeability in these systems of biological importance. An example is dioctanoyl :

$$\underset{3.9}{CH_3} - \underset{1.3}{CH_2} - \underset{0.9}{CH_2} - \underset{0.6}{(CH_2)_4} - \underset{0.5}{CH_2} - \underset{0.3}{CH_2} - \overset{O}{\underset{}{C}} - O - \underset{0.2}{CH} - \underset{0.1}{CH_2} - O - \overset{O}{\underset{O^-}{P}} - \underset{0.6}{CH_2} - \underset{1.0}{CH_2} - \underset{1.2}{N(Me)_3^+}$$

$$CH_3 - CH_2 - CH_2 - (CH_2)_2 - CH_2 - CH_2 - \overset{O}{\underset{}{C}} - O - CH_2$$

11.9 RELAXATION TIMES AND ASSOCIATION

We have already indicated that there exists a relationship between molecular weight and T_1. Some organic compounds show association when dissolved in some solvents. Consequently, their molecular weight as well as correlation times rise. Therefore, their T_1 are lowered.

Example

Carboxylic acids exists as dimers in solution. The T_1 for acetic acid are CH_3 10s, CO 29 s which are lower than those of methyl acetate that does not exist as dimer as shown.

$$\underset{\substack{10}}{CH_3} \overset{29}{-}C \overset{O \cdots H - O}{\underset{O - H \cdots O}{\diagup \diagdown}} \overset{29}{C} - \underset{10}{CH_3}$$

Acetic acid

$$\underset{16}{CH_3} - \overset{O}{\underset{}{C}} - O - \underset{35}{\overset{17}{CH_3}}$$

Methyl acetate

11.10 RELAXATION TIMES AND COMPLEXATION

Relaxation times are also related to complexation of ions. This is because when an organic molecule undergoes complexation, then its effective molecular mass increases. Obviously, the correlation times are lowered. However, depending upon the mechanism of relaxation, the T_1 will either be lowered (paramagnetic relaxation) or increased (diamagnetic relaxation).

Further, the T_1 are also dependent upon the concentration of the metallic ion with which the ion complexes.

11.11 C–13 RELAXATION MECHANISM

Many pathways have been observed to be responsible for relaxation of C–13 nuclei, the main being as follows :

1. Dipole-dipole
2. Spin-rotation
3. Quadrupolar
4. Chemical shift anisotropy
5. Scalar
6. Electron-nuclear

The overall spin-lattice relaxation, characterised by time T_1 is given by :

$$\frac{1}{T_1} = \frac{1}{T_1^{DD}} + \frac{1}{T_1^{Q}} + \frac{1}{T_1^{SR}} + \frac{1}{T_1^{CSA}} + \frac{1}{T_1^{e}}$$

11.12 DIPOLE-DIPOLE RELAXATION

This term is used when relaxation of a nuclear dipole is caused due to magnetic field of nearby nuclear dipoles. This is denoted as $T_1 DD$.

The relaxation of ^{13}C nuclei occurs due to the presence of nearby nuclear dipoles which means the protons.

As majority of carbons in molecules are attached directly to protons, therefore, this mechanism of relaxation is of great importance. In fact, this then constitutes the **single significant mechanism** in such cases.

When the molecule tumbles, the proton attached to the ^{13}C nucleus (let us way in a –CH– group) retains its rigid orientation with respect to the applied field B_0 and this helps in the relaxation of the ^{13}C nucleus.

The ^{13}C nucleus will experience a magnetic field B^{DD} that will depend on magnitudes of μC and μH as well as their orientation θ along ^{13}C–H with respect to the applied field B_0 as shown in Fig. 11.2.

$$B^{DD} = \frac{\gamma_H \, h}{4\pi r^3} (3 \cos^2 \theta - 1)$$

Because of tumbling, the angle θ causes fluctuation in B^{DD}. The effective magnetic field (B_{eff}) sensed by the ^{13}C nucleus is thus modulated by a sinusoidal variation (see Fig. 11.2 having frequency

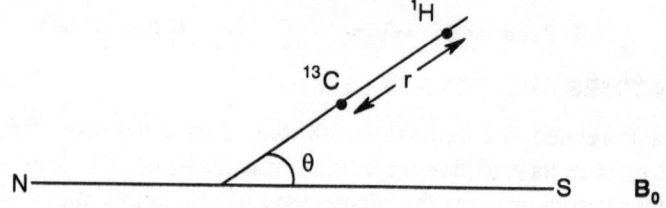

Fig. 11.2. Representation of orientation of nuclear dipoles ^{13}C and ^1H w.r. to B_0.

equal to the rate of tumbling of the molecule. And its amplitude is proportional to magnet strength i.e. r_H and to r^{-3}, the distance between ^{13}C and ^1H, γ_{CH} being 1.1 Å. Only if the frequency exactly matches the larmor frequency for the ^{13}C nucleus that is equal to Y_C. $B_0/2\pi$, then this would stimulate the ^{13}C nuclei to relax from the β-spin state to the α-spin state. The energy involved is coupled to rotational motion of the sample molecule and is therefore released as thermal energy. The rate of these stimulated transitions is proportional to r^{-6}, the distance between ^{13}C and ^1H in C—H bond. In fact, the dipole-dipole interaction is responsible for NOE that is also proportional to r^{-6}.

The rate of dipolar relaxation R_1^{DD} $(1/T_1)^{DD}$ after theoretical consideration has been shown to be dependent upon correlation time τ_C as well :

$$R_1^{DD} = y_H^2 y_C^2 h^2 r^{-6} \tau_C \qquad \qquad ....(A)$$

where h is the Planck's constant, τ_C is the time that characterizes reorientation of a molecule in liquid. This is essentially the average tumbling time of a molecule required to change its orientation relative to the direction of B_0. Molecules that are small have small τ_C as they tumble rapidly. On the other hand, larger molecules tumble slowly and consequently have a long τ_C.

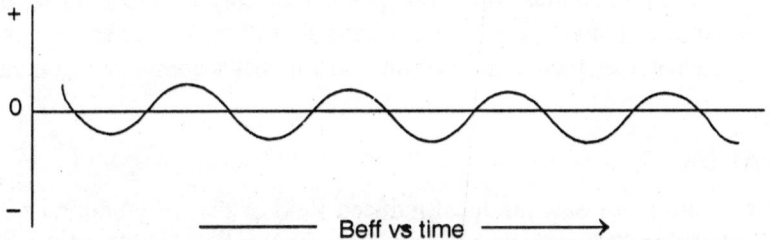

Fig. 11.3. The sinusoidal B_{eff} versus time in dipolar-dipolar relaxation.

Evidently, it is clear from equation, the dipolar-dipolar interaction rate is dependent to r^{-6}, and should therefore, drop off rapidly with distance. That is why, this is the major mechanism for relaxation for ^{13}C nuclei attached to protons (CH_3, CH_2, CH). If the ^{13}C nuclei are not attached to protons directly, this mechanism would not be efficient for relaxation of such nuclei and therefore such carbons are expected to have longer relaxation times. This also means that such carbons will also contribute weaker signals in routine CMR spectra wherein we do not use relaxation delays of the orders of $5XT_1$, a time consuming process as explained earlier.

The equation has got a great significance as it can give us information regarding the internuclear distances, r as well as molecular dynamics in the liquid state.

The fractional dipolar relaxation rate is related to NOE as follows :

$$\text{Dipolar relaxation} = \frac{ni}{Y_H / 2Y_C} \times 100$$

$$= \frac{n_i}{1.988} \times 100 \text{ as } \frac{Y_H}{2Y_C} = 1.988$$

n_i is the NOE factor for a specific ^{13}C nucleus $Y_H/2 \, Y_C$ = max value of NOE = 1.988

The quaternary carbons can be characterized by the fact that they have about 10X to 20X longer T_1s compared to protonated carbons. This can be understood in terms of the inverse sixth power relation of the internuclear C, H distance, r_{CH}^6. Therefore, it is easy to distinguish the quaternary carbons (Cq) as a whole from a non-quantitative relaxation time measurement experiment.

Carbon	T_1s
C_9	66
C_{11}	112
C_{12}	72

Acenaphthene

C-11 has longer T_1 of 112 s compared to C_{12} (72 s) and C_9, C_{10} (66 s). This is because C-11 is separated from the nearest protons by three bonds. C-12 and C-9, 10 are aided in relaxation by geminal protons.

Further, it needs to be noted that the dipole-dipole mechanism is of significance not only for C-13 but for nuclei that are close to hydrogen or fluorine and particularly so for the directly bonded ones. It is therefore, expected as already stated that nuclei away from hydrogen should relatively have higher T_1 compared to protonated compounds. However, this is true only for those nuclei that have I = 1/2. The relaxation times for nuclei having I > 1/2 are always shorter by factors as high as 10^8 on the basis of T_1^{DD}. Obviously in such nuclei, there is another mechanism that is dominant that is called quadrupolar relaxation.

11.13 SPIN ROTATION

In dipolar-dipolar relaxation, we saw the local induced field of the neighbouring nuclei having non-zero spin aiding in relaxation. But sometimes, the sample molecule is itself associated with a magnetic moment. Such a magnetic moment occurs as a consequence of the modulation of the magnitude as well as the direction of the angular momentum vector with the rotation of the sample molecule. The result is the generation of molecular magnetism that does not depend upon the electronic charge distribution when the molecular motion increases, so does the induced magnetic moment. Therefore, small, rapidly tumbling molecules will also relax via this mechanism. Relaxation via this mechanism is likely to increase with increase in temperature as well as in the vapour phase.

The rate of dipolar-dipolar relaxation is equal to :

$$R_1^{DD} = 1/T_1^{DD} = h^2 Y_H^2 Y_C^2 \sum_i Y_{CH}^{-6} \times \tau_C$$

where X is equal to :

$$\chi = \frac{1}{4}(3\cos^2 \theta - 1) + 18(5 + P)^{-1} \sin^2 \theta \cos^2 \theta + \frac{9}{4}(1 + 2p)^{-1} \sin^4 \theta$$

where

θ represents the angle between the axis for internal rotation and the C—H bond vector
$P = D_{11}/D_1$ $D_{11} = (6\tau_C)^{-1} + (5\tau_G)^{-1}$
$D_\perp = (\tau_C)^{-1}$

$D_\perp$ is the diffusion constant for rotational diffusion parallel to the axis for internal motion. D_{11} being the diffusion constant for the rotational diffusion that is anti-parallel to the axis for internal motion. τ_C the correlation time for overall reorientation. τ_G is correlation time for group rotation.

When the rotation is much faster (limiting case) which means $\tau_G \ll \tau_C$, the equation becomes simplified :

$$X = \left(\frac{3}{2}\cos^2\theta - \frac{1}{2}\right)^2$$

For a methyl group, CH_3 (with $\theta = 109°$) present in the molecule that rotates very rapidly, the carbon will relax about nine times more slowly compared to when such as internal motion is non-existent. From the above equation, it is also evident that when segmental motion is possible about several axes, the carbon nuclei will relax even more slowly.

T_1^{SR} or T_1^{DD} is dominantly causing relaxation. Spin rotation relaxation mechanism is responsible for causing broad resonances in gaseous samples. It should be noted that the spin-rotation relaxation has been found not to lead to NOE effect in peaks in CMR spectra. This means that the C–13 nuclei that relax dominantly by spin-rotation mechanism contribute weak signals, that serves as an aid for us in their assignment. Thus, the methyl carbon signal in CMR spectrum of toluene shows a very weak signal as shown in Fig. 11.4.

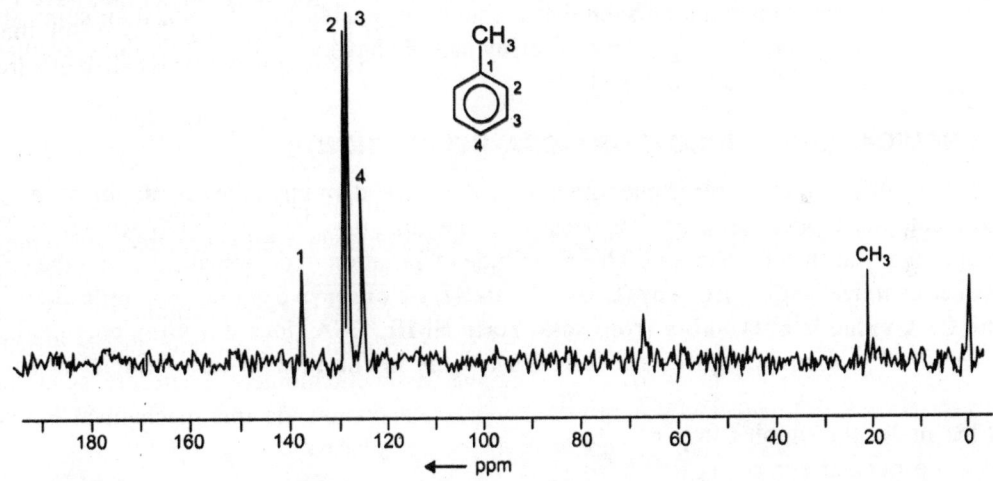

Fig. 11.4. Spin-rotation relaxation stands responsible for low-intensity of the C-13 of CH_3 group in toluene.

11.14 QUADRUPOLAR RELAXATION

This is a mechanism that for many nuclei is the sole mode of relaxation. Nuclei that have I > 1/2 possess a quadrupole moment Q. Examples include N–14, H–2, B–11. The quadrupole moment in such a nuclei arises due to unequal distribution of charge as the nucleus is ellipsoidal rather than spherical as shown in Fig. 11.5.

There occurs disposition of the electric quadrupole. Electric field gradients are generated at the nuclei

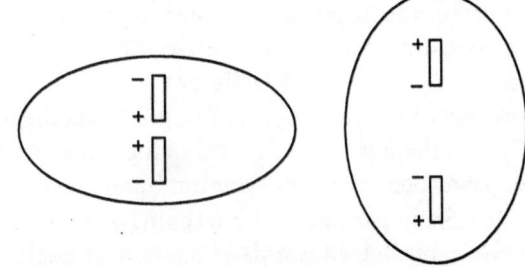

Fig. 11.5. Uneven charge distribution in nuclei having I > 1.2

because of asymmetries in the spatial arrangement of the bounding electrons. When the molecule tumbles, the direction of the resulting electric quadrupole torque changes in random manner about the nucleus. This can be thought to occur in a manner similar to that in which the torque due to magnetic relaxation field occurs around the nucleus. Thus, rotating electric torque components exist which have frequency equal to the nuclear larmor frequency that allow transfer of energy between nucleus and the lattice, causing spin-lattice relaxation.

The value of relaxation time for a particular nuclear species is governed by the electric field gradient. The latter primarily depends on the electronic symmetry about the nucleus, it does wholly upon the symmetry of the molecule.

The quadrupole mechanism is very effective relaxation both for the nucleus with a quadrupole moment as well as the neighbouring ^{13}C nuclei. Thus, the T_1 of C in $C \overset{\ominus}{N}^{14}$ ion is 8.3 which is much smaller than the T_1 of C in $C \overset{\ominus}{N}^{15}$ ion. N–15 nucleus does not have a quadrupole moment unlike N–14. Further, this mechanism is so efficient that no ^1H or ^{13}C coupling to Br or Cl is observed even though both these halogens have nuclear spin. Br, Cl have large values of quadrupole moment. These nuclei undergo rapid nuclear transitions on such that the adjacent nuclei do not sense their spins and hence donot show any spin-spin splittings. That is to say as they have very short T_1 values, so they do not show any coupling with the adjacent nuclei.

11.15 CHEMICAL SHIFT ANISOTROPY (CSA) RELAXATION

The chemical shift is an anisotropic phenomenon as it is dependent upon the orientation of the molecule with respect to the applied field, B_0. It is because of the rapid tumbling of the molecule in solution that an average chemical shift is observed. The magnitude of variation in chemical shift with the orientation is known as chemical shift anisotropy (CSA). **Actually, we observe δ iso i.e. isotropic chemical shift and the CSA value is obtainable from solid state NMR. CSA does not alter chemical shifts of nuclei in solution form. Despite this fact, CSA helps in the relaxation of nuclei in solution in NMR.**

As the molecule tumbles in solution, the nuclear screening gets changed. Due to this, a small fluctuation in magnetic field at the nucleus exists which contributes towards nuclear relaxation. As the molecule tumbles and samples different

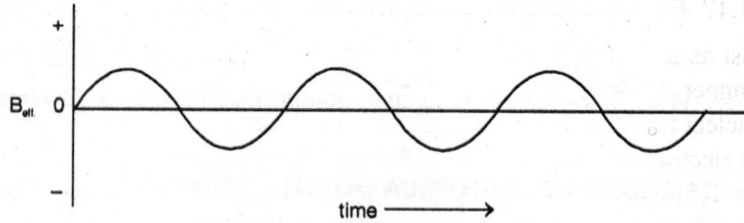

Fig. 11.6. B_{eff} versus time in CSA.

orientations with respect to Bo, the B_{eff} at the nucleus is modulated in a sinusoidal form (see Fig. 11.6). The oscillating magnetic field induces nuclear transitions and thus causes nuclear relaxation. The CSA depends upon the molecular tumbling rate as well as molecular size as happens in dipole-dipole effect. The CSA in parts per million (ppm) is independent of Bo, but is proportional to Bo^2 in hertz. Therefore, CSA contributes towards relaxation in nuclei in a rather highly anisotropic environment and which have large chemical shift ranges. CSA is used to sharpen peaks of large protein types molecules in solution, although it does not affect chemical shift.

10.16 THE SCALAR RELAXATION, $T_1{}^S$

This relaxation mode is a result of scalar coupling of a carbon to a rapidly relaxing nucleus. The $T_1{}^3$ is only significant in case the resonance frequencies of the two interacting nuclei are similar as per example in ^{13}C–Br^{79}. When the life time of the coupled nucleus is sufficiently short because of quadrupolar relaxation, rapid chemical exchange etc., fluctuating magnetic fields are induced that cause relaxation. It should be noted that spin-spin relaxation (T_2) of carbons banded to a quadrupolar nucleus predominantly relaxes by scalar relaxation mechanism.

R_1^S is given by :

$$R_1^S \; (1/T_1^S) \propto J^2 S(S+1) \, f(\omega \tau)^*$$

* assuming a cylindrical symmetry
S = spin number of nucleus to which ^{13}C is coupled
ω = Larmor frequency
τ = correlation time

In p-bromobenzonitrile, the quaternary carbon Cp has T_1 of 47 s, while the carbon–4 adjacent to bromine has a considerably shorter T_1 of just 8 s that is close to 6 s T_1 of the protonated carbons in the molecule. Scalar relaxation mechanism is the major contributor here as Br–^{13}C dipolar is ruled out to be a major mechanism.

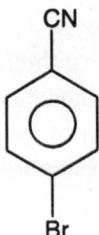

11.17 ELECTRON-NUCLEAR RELAXATION, $T_1{}^e$

Just as a neighbouring proton's magnetic dipole induces relaxation (dipolar relaxation), in a similar manner, an electron's magnetic dipole also causes relaxation of the C–13 nucleus. This is called electron-nuclear relaxation characterised by relaxation time $T_1{}^e$. It should be noted that the magnetic moment of an electron is larger than that of a proton by about three orders of magnitude (Ye/YH = 65.7). Obviously, for $T_1{}^e$ to occur, the presence of a spec is having non-zero spin such as free radicals is essential, even though in low amounts. The rate of this electron-nuclear dipole-dipole relaxation is given by :

$$R^e = \frac{1}{T_1^e} = 16M^2 /15 \; Nsh^2 S(S+1) Y_S^2 Y_C^2 X / kT$$

where X. is solution viscosity, S stands for total electron spin quantum number. k is the Boltzman constant. Ns means the concentration of the present paramagnetic species per cubic cm. Ys is the gyromagneto ratio of the electron. It is clear from the equation that the $T_1{}^e$ depends upon concentration (Ns), solution viscosity X and absolute temperature T for a paramagnetic relaxation species present in the sample solution. Obviously, the paramagnetic species must be chemically inert.

11.18 SEPARATION OF RELAXATION MODES FROM OVERALL RELAXATION TIME

Dipole-Dipole mechanism is the predominant relaxation mechanism for the protonated carbons. Other mechanisms, in particular, the spin-rotation becomes significantly competitive in smaller molecules. The scalar coupling and the chemical shift anisotropy contribute significantly to the overall T_1, only in a few cases. The T_1^{CSA} can be readily separated by observing its dependance on the field strength B_0 (CSA $\propto B_0^2$). In fact, the CSA becomes significantly competitive either at high magnetic field strengths or at low temperatures. It should be noted that the T_1 originating from other mechanisms except dipolar-dipolar is irrelevant in assignments, only the T_1^{DP} serves an aid in this taste.

11.19 DEUTERIUM ISOTOPE EFFECTS ON RELAXATION TIMES

This is used for assignment of relaxation time :

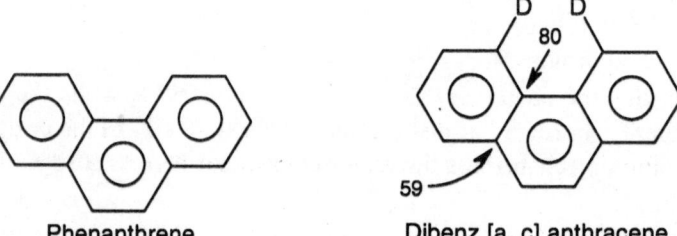

Phenanthrene   Dibenz [a, c] anthracene

While one type of quaternary carbon in phenanthrene which have two geminal protons each, have T_1 of 51s, the other set of quaternary carbons which have only one geminal proton each have T_1 of 59 s. If in the later set, of the α protons are replaced by deuterium, then the T_1 of those carbons increases from 59 to 80s, which proves the existence of a substantial dipolar relaxation for carbons that are attached to protons.

11.20 ASSIGNMENT OF C–13 RESONANCE WITH RELAXATION TIMES, T_1s

Let us consider codeine. The T_1 and chemical shifts for the various carbons are as follows at 30°C, 1.6 molar in $CDCl_3$ and at 25.2 MHz (see Fig. 11.7).

	$T_1 s$	$\delta\ ppm$	Geminal protons
C–11	1.53	42.9	4
C–3	1.82	127.04	3
C–14	5.2	141.73	1
C–13	8.9	146.6	0
C–12	5.1	130.9	0

As per the equation :

$$\frac{1}{T_1^{DD}} = h^2\ Y_C^2\ Y_H^2\ Nr_{CH}^-\ \tau_C$$

it is evident that the T_1 would be proportional to the sum of r_{CH}^{-6} internuclear distances.

Therefore, of the four aromatic carbons that appear at 127, 141.7, 146.6 and 130.9, we can easily assign signal at 127.04 ppm to C–3 as it has three α-CHs. The signal at 146.6 ppm that has T_1 of 8.9 s can be assigned to C–13 as it has no α CH protons. As C–14 has one α-proton, therefore, it should relax faster than C–13. Hence, the carbon with T_1 of 5.2 s is assigned the signal at 141.7.

As C–13 is assigned at 146.6 ppm, the C–12 is, therefore, assigned at 130.9 ppm. That is to say that although C–12 and C–13 have zero α-protons, the C–12 relaxes faster (T_1 5.1) compared to C–13 (T_1 8.9 s). This is because the C–15 methylene protons being in closer proximity did in its faster relaxation.

The C–11 has the shortest T_1 of all 1.53 s and is therefore, assigned the peak at 42.9. It is expected to show small T_1 because it has no directly attached protons, it is sp^3 hybridized.

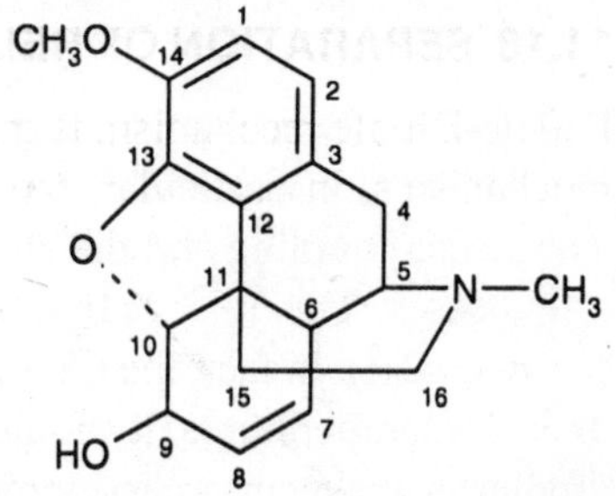

Carbon No.	T_1	δ_C (CDCl$_3$)
11	1.53	42.9
3	1.82	127.0
14	5.2	141.0
13	8.9	146.6
12	5.1	130.9

Fig. 11.7. Relaxation times of various carbons in the data for Codeine obtained at 25.2 MHz at 1.6 molar concentration at 30° in CDCl$_3$.

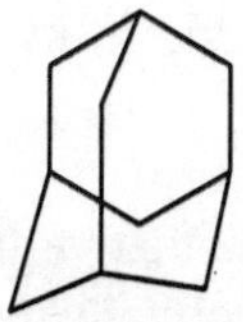

$T_1CH_2 = 11.4$ s
$T_1CH = 20.5$ s

The requirement of a single correlation time τ_c for all carbons in a molecule applies only when the molecule rotates isotropically. That means when there are no preferred axes for reorientation as in adamantane. This molecule has a tetrahedral symmetry and tumbles isotropically with the consequence that τ_C is identical for each C—H of the two non-equivalent carbon nuclei.

As per the equation :

$$\frac{1}{T_1^{DD}} = h^2 Y_C^2 Y_H^2 N r_{CH}^{-6} \tau_C$$

the $T_1CH : T_1CH_2$ ratio should be 2:1. But taking into account the next nearest protons, the expected ratio would be 1.82:1. The experimental ratio is 20.5:11.4 or 1.80:1. Thus, the two values are close enough to prove the validity of the equation.

Brucine

The T_1s and peak positions of various carbons are as follows (at 25.2 MHz, in 1.2 M in CDCl$_3$ at 30°C.

C	T_1	δ_C	Geminal protons
C–8	2.6	51.83	4
C–20	2.92	140.29	4
C–15	4.30	168.64	2
C–2 or C–3	9.35	149.13	1
C–2 or C–3	10.70	146.14	1
C–5	7.25	136.00	1
C–6	11.75	123.45	1

Brucine

The aromatic carbons, C–2/3, C–5, C–6 show T_1s, nearly of 10s average value. All of them have one geminal proton each for relaxation. The olefinic carbon C–20 having four geminal protons has T_1 of 2.92 s and contributes a signal at 140.29 pm. C–8, that is a quaternary sp^3 carbon and has four α-protons to aid in its relaxation has T_1 of 2.6s and contributes a signal at S 51.83. The C–15 carbonyl carbon as T_1 of 4.30s and appear at 168.64 ppm. It has two α-protons to assist in its relaxation.

11.21 RELAXATION REAGENTS

As we have already learnt that in order to have CMR spectra worth quantitative interpretation, we require inverse-gated-CMR spectra in which a relaxation delay of $5 \times T_1$ is normally required. However, price paid in terms of time is too much. For instance, it requires about 18 h to have a quantitative CMR analysis for acenapthene in which relaxation times for C–9, C–11 and C–12 are 66s, 112s and 72s respectively, while the normal CMR of this molecule just requires just min.

Therefore, it became essential to find out alternatives to save time. Fortunately, it was discovered that there are certain reagents which when added into the solution in the nmr tube could lower down the relaxation times drastically so that these could be used both for qualitative as well as quantitative CMR analysis. An example is the complex Cr(acac)$_3$. The T_1 for protonated carbons and quaternary carbons are generally 1s and 10s respectively. When a paramagnetic relaxation reagent such as Cr (acac)$_3$ is added at concentration of ca 5×10^{-2} molar metal concentration, the relaxation times of protonated carbons are reduced to a mere 0.09 s and 0.18 for the protonated and quaternary (non-protonated) carbons respectively:

Type of carbons	Relaxation times (T_1)	
	No Cr(acac)$_3$	Cr(acac)$_3$
Protonated	1s	0.09s
Non-protonated quaternary	10s	0.1s

11.22 APPLICATIONS OF C–13 NMR SPECTROSCOPY

11.22.1 Stereochemistry

1. Syn-anti isomerism

Ketoximes could be easily differentiated on the basis of their CMR spectra. Thus, steric compression shifts are observed for the syn-isomer.

Examples

1. Oxime of ethyl methyl ketone

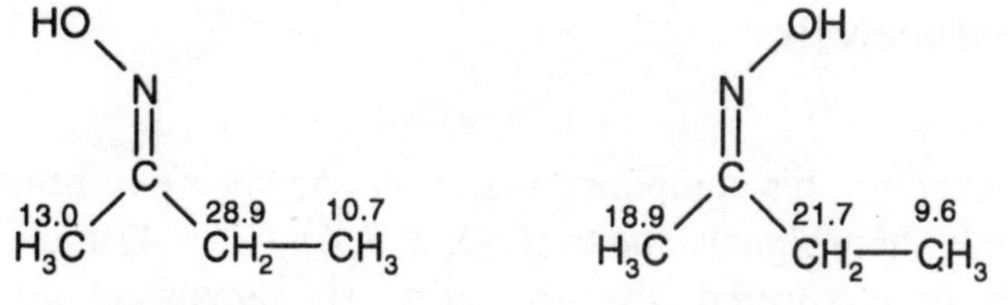

anti

syn

2. Oxime of [2, 2, 1] bicyclohexanone: steric compression is quite evident here as well.

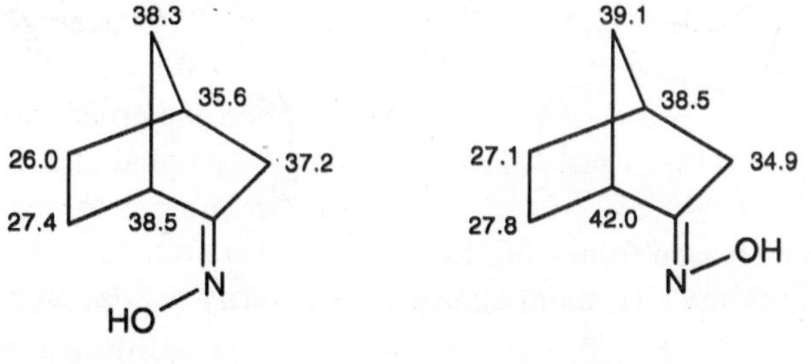

3. Diastereoconversion: Diastereomeric DL-N-formyl–4–carboxythiazolidines: The following two diastereomer thiazolidines could be easily distinguished on the basis of the CMR spectra.

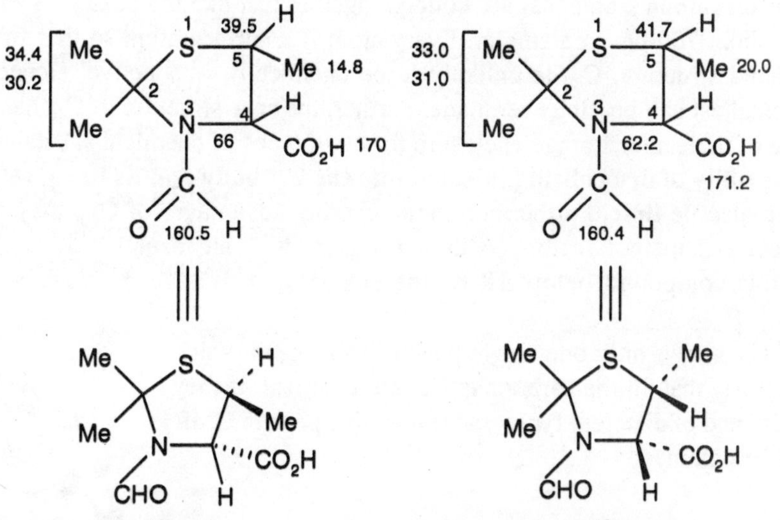

threo

erythro

It is clear that in the erythro form, the CO group is cis to C–4 that faces steric compression and resonates at 62.2. In the threo form, the C–4 resonates downfield at 66.0 which indicates that the CO group is trans w.r. to C–4.

The C–5 methyl absorbs at 20 ppm in erythro while in threo it absorbs at 14.8 ppm. The C_5–Me and the CO_2H are trans in threo while they are cis in erythro. Hence, the threo and erythro diastereomeric isomers are easily distinguished.

11.22.2 Conformational analysis

Example

Cis–1,4–dimethylcyclohexanol: This compound occurs in two chair conformations which interconvert rapidly at r.t. so that at only three signals due to (C–2, 3, 5, 6), (C–1, 4) and CH_3 carbons are obtained. However, as the temperature is lowered down to – 60°C, six signals are seen, the two at 23 ppm and 17.5 ppm being due to the equatorial and axial methyls respectively.

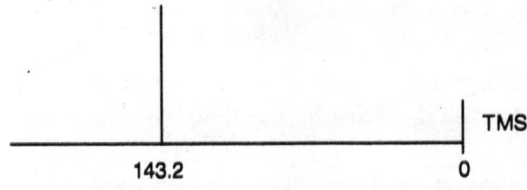

As the temperature is increased from – 60° to – 15°, the peaks due to C–2 and C–3 carbons coalesce, although the CH_3 equatorial and CH_3 axial appear as two partly overlapping broad resonances.

11.22.3 Nanotechnology application

CMR Spectrum of C_{60} Fullerene

C_{60} Fullerene has 60 carbon atoms that are bonded together just like the hexagons and pentagous on a soccer ball. It is about 700 pm in diameter. Every atom is a surface atom so that fullerene is hollow. Because of its bond structure, C_{60} is unlikely to be chemically very active. Hence, it is a possible lubricant or the smallest ball bearing ever made. Further, the cage structure of C_{60} has great potential to be used as a type of molecular storage enclosure for other types of chemical substances such as drugs. **There is the possibility of drugs being injected into the C_{60} body and its being released later on at a specific site at specific time.** Furthermore, among other advantages of C_{60}, they can in chemically modified form act as superconductors. Although C_{60} is itself an insulator, K_3C_{60}, its derivative is conductive. In this compound below 18 K, the electrical resistance becomes zero! Thus, it is a superconductor.

^{13}C NMR of C_{60} shows only one single peak at 143.2 ppm which indicates quite clearly that all the carbons in C_{60} are identical. If they were non-identical and of different types, more than one peak in CMR spectrum would be obtained:

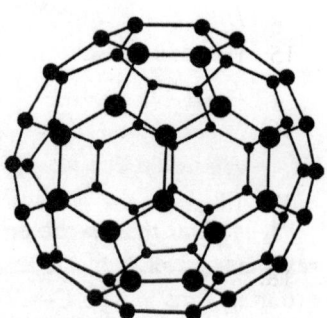

Fig. 11.8. C_{60} fullerene.

TMS

143.2   0

^{1}H-decoupled CMR spectrum of C_{60} fullerene

PROBLEMS

1. What are the factors that affect C–13 Relaxation Times? Discuss in details.
   Hint: See Section 11.1.

2. Enlist the C–13 relaxation mechanisms. Which is the single significant mechanism in C–13 relaxation?
   Hint: See Section 11.4.

3. Explain dipole-dipole relaxation in details. On what factors, the rate of dipolar relaxation depend?
   Hint: See Section 11.12.

4. What is spin-rotation C–13 relaxation mechanism?
   Hint: See Section 11.13.

5. Illustrate the quadrupole relaxation mechanism for C–13 nuclei.
   Hint: See Section 11.14.

6. Write a note on relaxation by chemical shift anisotropy.
   Hint: See Section 11.15 and Section 2.5.2.4, subpoint 15.

7. What is Scalar relaxation?
   Hint: See Section 11.16.

8. What is electron-nuclear relaxation?
   Hint: See Section 11.17.

9. How can you separate relaxation modes from overall relaxation time?
   Hint: See Section 11.18.

10. Illustrate isotope effects on relaxation times.
    Hint: See Section 11.19.

11. Give some applications of CMR spectroscopy with respect to stereochemistry, syn-anti isomerism, conformational analysis and nanotechnology.
    Hint: See Section 11.22.

12. What is the physical significance of T_1?
    Hint: See Section 11.2.

13. What is the structural significance of relaxation times?
    Hint: See Section 11.3.

14. What is the relation between T_1 and molecular weight.
    Hint: See Section 11.5.

15. How do relaxation times correlate with rigid skeleton (hindered rotation)? Give examples.
    Hint: See Section 11.6.

16. What is the relation between relaxation times and preferred axes of rotation?
    Hint: See Section 11.7.

17. Illustrate the relation between relaxation times and segmental motion with few examples.
    Hint: See Section 11.8.

18. What is the relation between relaxation times and association?
    Hint: See Section 11.9.

12

Coherence Transfer and INEPT

Before we learn about 2D NMR spectroscopy, it will be better if we first learn about coherence transfer, the transfer of magnetization from one spin to another and INEPT which are used in 2D NMR experiments. We will study **transfer of magnetiztion from ^{1}H(I) to ^{13}C(S)**.

12.1 INEPT AND SPIN OPERATORS

Magnetization transfer occurs not only through NOE, but can also occur through J coupling i.e. via bonds. Let us consider a $^1J_{CH}$ coupling i.e. one proton attached to a $C-13$ nucleus. For simplicity, we will assume that the ^1H as well as the ^{13}C frequencies are precisely on-resonance. The **'spin operator''** **notation is just a shorthand notation that allows us to succinctly define or specify the net** **magnetization state.** We usually use I for ^1H and S for ^{13}C or ^{15}N i.e. the second nucleus. Thus when ^1H and ^{13}C or ^{15}N spins tend to align with the z-direction, using spin operator notation, we will specify the states of ^1H and ^{13}C (or ^{15}N) nuclei as $+I_z$ (or $+$ Hz) and $+S_z$ ($+$ $^{13}C_z$ or $^{15}N_z$) respectively.

When we apply a 90° pulse, we will now specify the state of ^1H as $-H_y$ ($-Iy$). There are two spin states of ^1H - the α and β attached to ^{13}C (or ^{15}N) in the x-y plane. It is these two spin states that split the $C-13$ signal into a doublet with J coupling. The α state giving the downfield (left hand) peak and the β state the upfield (right hand) peak of the doublet.

Let us now allow the α and β spin population to process for $1/(2J)$ i.e. one fourth of a period. The result will be the α and β states rotate around Z axis by 90° in opposite directions. That is to say the downfield peak component of ^{13}C arising due to ^1H nuclei in the α spin state rotates counterclockwise in the $x'-y'$ plane towards the $-x'$ axis with an angular frequency of $J^-/2$ Hz. Obviously, the upfield peak component of C arising due to ^1H nuclei in β spin-state will rotate in the clockwise direction towards $+x'$ axis with an angular frequency of $-J/2$ Hz. When the two vectors are oriented 180° apart, there will be no net magnetization vector as the α and β populations of ^1H cancel out each other like the two populations α and β of ^{13}C. We call the state as antiphase magnetization represented as $-2H_xC_z$ ($-2I_xS_z$).

Intext Exercise

1. What does the product operator notation $-2I_x S_z$ specify?

   Hint : This means I spin magnetization vector is along the $-x'$ axis while that of the spin S is along the $+x$ axis that is to say, the I spin state is antiphase with respect to the Z-orientation of the individual S spins. And both the receivers are equal in magnitude.

In other words, because the two spin states of ^1H nuclei are out of phase with respect to each other, being at 180° apart, the $-2H_x C_z$ term means anti-phase or more explicitly, 'H anti-phase and w.r. to C' (I anti-phase w.r. to spin S). The negative sign means both these types of magnetization vectors are equal in magnitude. If we were to record the spectrum now taking $+x$-axis saw the reference axis, we will get a doublet with downfield peak being negative absorptive, while the upfield peak will be positive absorptive as shown in Fig. 12.1.

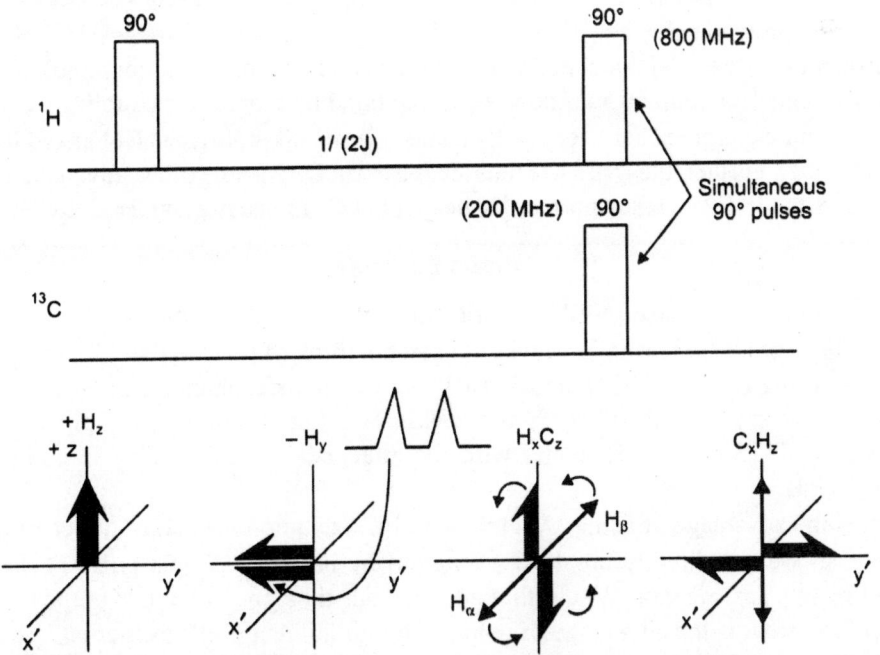

Fig. 12.1. Simultaneous ^1H and ^{13}C 90° pulses. ^1H magnetization has been converted to transverse ^{13}C magnetization.

If we simultaneously apply, a 90° pulse at the ^1H-frequency and another 90° pulse at the ^{13}C frequency, something not less than a magic occurs! That is to say, the ^1H magnetization that was antiphase to the C–13 nucleus, has been converted into ^{13}C magnetization that is antiphase to the attached ^1H. In other words, the x-y plane detectable magnetization has jumped onto the ^{13}C nucleus from the ^1H because of this special pulse sequence! **Or we can say the C–13 magnetization has magically been created from ^1H magnetization (Fig. 12.1)!**

In conclusion, we have created coherence on ^1H with a 90° pulse and then waited for a period of time, $-1/(2J)$ till the two components of the doublet become opposite in phase i.e. "antiphase". The antiphase has a characteristic property in the sense that when subjected to 90° pulses simultaneously affecting ^1H as well as ^{13}C involved in J-coupling, the coherence "jumps" from ^1H to ^{13}C. That is to say there is no antiphase coherence on the starting ^1H nucleus, rather it is now present on the ^{13}C nucleus, J-coupled to ^1H. In fact, this principle of INEPT transfer can be operated upon any J-coupled nuclei such as ^1H and ^{15}N etc. Further, this principle can be

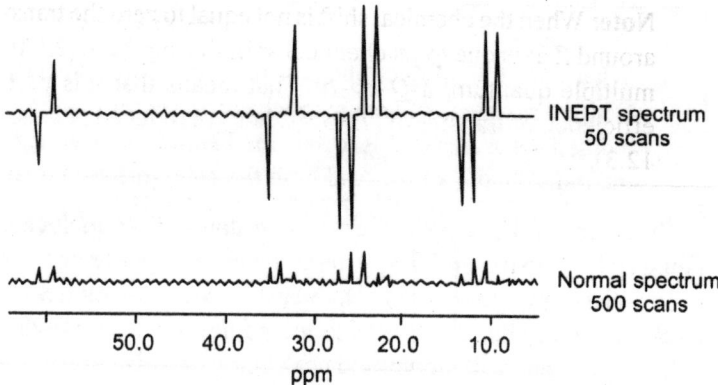

Fig. 12.2. The INEPT and normal ^1H-decoupled C–13 spectra of $CH_3CH_2CHClCH_3$.

applied not only to those nuclei that are ^1J-coupled (one bond heteronuclear coupling), but to ^2J-coupled (two bond heteronuclear coupling), ^3J-coupled (three bond heteronuclear coupling) and so on.

That is why, the experiment has been rightly named - **Insensitive Nucleus Enhanced by Polarization Transfer (INEPT)**. Further, the INEPT technique is used in DEPT, one of the advanced 1D experiment. Fig. 12.2 shows the INEPT versus normal ^1H-decoupled C–13 spectra of $CH_3CH_2CHClCH_3$.

Intext Exercises

2. Can we think of a reverse INEPT experiment? What use can we put it to?

   Ans. Yes, there is no reason as to why we can not think of reverse INEPT. It is possible to do that. By using reverse INEPT and INEPT, we can transfer magnetization back-and-forth at will between say ^1H and ^{13}C or ^1H and ^{15}N. In fact, this technique can help us in correlating individual C–13 (or N–15) nuclei with the attached ^1H nuclei. This is done through 2D experiments.

3. What is the advantage of using $^1J_{CH}$ to create ^{13}C excitation instead of direct ^{13}C excitation?

   Ans. Can we not directly create C excitation by using a ^{13}C 90° pulse at the start of an experiment? Yes, we can. Would that not save our time and serve our purpose? Yes, it can. Therefore, what is the advantage of going in for an indirect C–13 excitation? This is because the magnitude of the C–13 magnetization generated in an indirect manner is four times more compared to that generated directly. The reason for this is the C–13 is four times less than that of γ-H. This γ precession frequencies but also a difference in population. Thus, while the excess of protons from the upper cone at equilibrium is 1/1 million, the excess of C–13 from the upper cone is just (1/4) million.. This causes four times more C–13 nuclei to get excited due to transfer of 1/1 million excess of protons to C–13. Similarly, the magnitude of N–15 magnetization generated via INEPT experiment is about 10 times more than that generated directly as γ_N is 1/1 million of γ_H. Further, while the excess of protons from the upper cone is 1/1 million at equilibrium, the excess of N–15 from the upper cone is 1/10 million. This is how 10 times more N–15 nuclei are excited as a result of transference of 1/1 million excess of protons to N–15.

Note: When the chemical shift is not equal to zero the transverse ^1H magnetization also precesses around Z axis due to its chemical shift during the $1/(2J)$ time period. ^1H chemical shift leads to multiple quantum, *MQ–cy–ty*. That means that this part of magnetization is lost and so the efficiency of transfer of ^1H to ^{13}C has got reduced because of ^1H chemical shift evolution (Fig. 12.3).

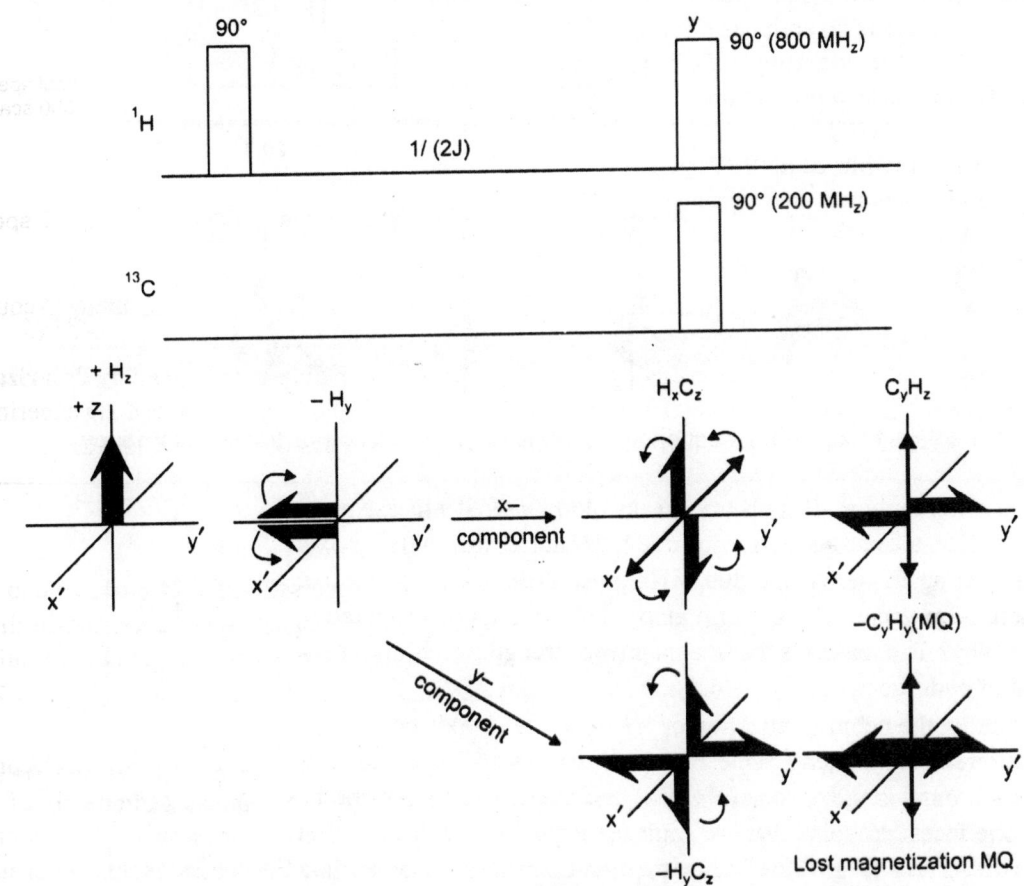

Fig. 12.3. When chemical shift is not zero, some magnetization (MQ) is lost.

The above reduction in transfer efficiency can be eliminated by simultaneous 180° pulses at the centre of the $1/(2J)$ period i.e. after $1/(4J)$ as shown in Fig. 12.4.

12.2 $^1J_{CH}$ COUPLING: THE CAUSE AND UTILITY IN MAGNETIZATION TRANSFER

Let us consider a methine carbon.

At the Boltzman equilibrium excess, the ^1H as well as ^{13}C nuclear spins start precessing around the Bo field along the z-axis (Fig. 12.5). The α state of both these nuclei is more populated compared to the β-spin state. This leads to a net magnetization vector in the z direction for both ^1H as well as ^{13}C nucleus.

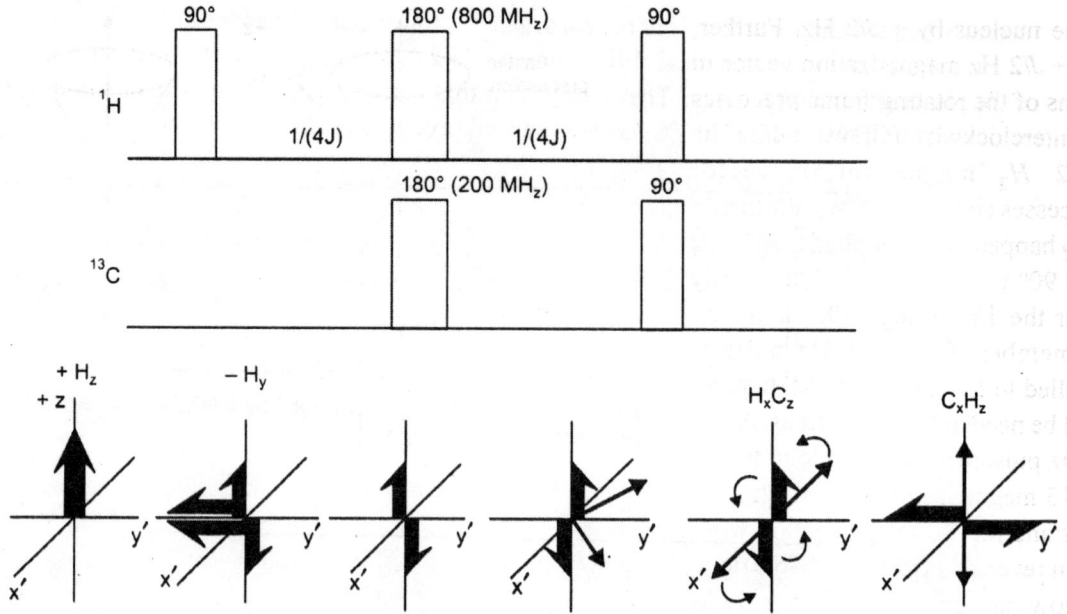

Fig. 12.4. INEPT sequence : elimination of reduction in transfer efficiency.

When we apply a 90° pulse (x means along x-axis) precessing at say 800 MHz, the net magnetization due to ^1H nuclei tips to the $-y$ axis of the rotating frame. At the 800 MHz pulse does not cause the net magnetization vector of ^{13}C to tip along the $-y'$ axis of the rotating frame. Why? The reason is that the magnetic strength, Y_C is about 1/4 of that of hydrogen, Y_H ($Y_C = 1/4Y_H$).

Actually, the net magnetization of ^1H along the $-y$ axis consists of two different components. One component faces ^{13}C spin that are spinning around in the α-cone (+ z axis), and the other component the other one faces ^{13}C spins that are spinning around in the β-cone that

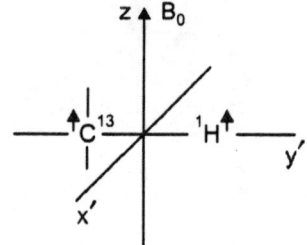

Fig. 12.5. Net magnetization along Z-direction.

lies in the $-z$ axis (Fig. 12.6). While the first component is downfield the second is upfield. That is to say that the first component magnetization vector precesses at a slightly higher speed compared to second one and the ^1H spectrum shows a doublet. As the population of ^1H nuclei in α state is slightly larger by one part in ten million, so the downfield peak is more intense then the upfield peak by almost 1/10 million part. Of course, that difference is too tiny to be measured. Anyway, the doublet obtained is actually centered about δ, the chemical shift of the proton. We say the separation or the coupling constant between the two component peaks is around 150 Hz that is $^1J_{CH}$ is 150 Hz. What does this coupling or separation indicate? It has no meaning in itself. But when we consider the chemical shift, it has got great meaning. Then it tells us that while the α-population of ^1H nuclei precesses 75 Hz more rapidly around the +Z axis compared to the β-population of ^1H nuclei that precesses 75 Hz more slowly around the $-Z$ axis. So, instead of writing $J = 150$ Hz, we need to write that coupling is ± 75 Hz ($J \pm 75$ Hz). So, the effect of coupling J is to alter the rate of precession of the two involved populations of the same nucleus by $\pm J/2$ Hz. Further, the $+ J/2$ Hz magnetization vector in terms of the rotating frame precesses counterclockwise (CCW), while the $-J/2$ H_2 magnetization vector precesses clockwise (CW). Further, it also happens if we applied a $90°\, y\, {}^1H$ and $90°\, x\, {}^{13}C$ pulses simultaneously after the $1/(2J)$ delay ($90°$ about z). Remember if a 800 MHz pulse is applied to ${}^1H$, then a 200 MHz pulse will be needed for ${}^{13}C$ nucleus. A 800 MHz pulse will not be able to tip the

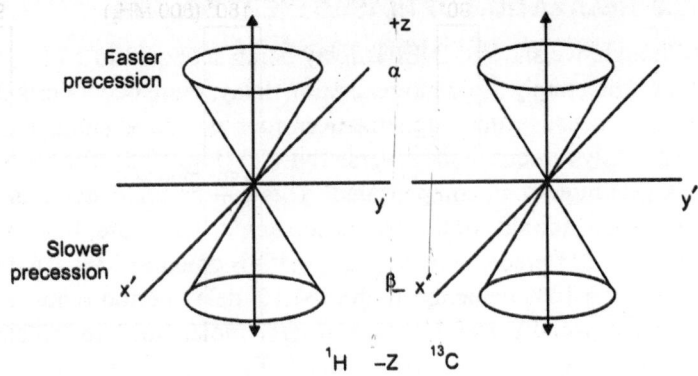

Fig. 12.6. Faster precession (α-spin state) and slower precession (β-spin state).

C–13 magnetization vector. Thus, as a result of $90°\, y$ pulse, the ${}^1H$ magnetization rotates in to the $\pm Z$ axis and the ${}^{13}C$ magnetization will rotate to the $\pm y$ axis. That means the roles of the ${}^1H$ and ${}^{13}C$ have been reversed effectively! How do we now describe the state of the system? We will say that the system is now 'anti-phase' C–13 (Fig. 12.7).

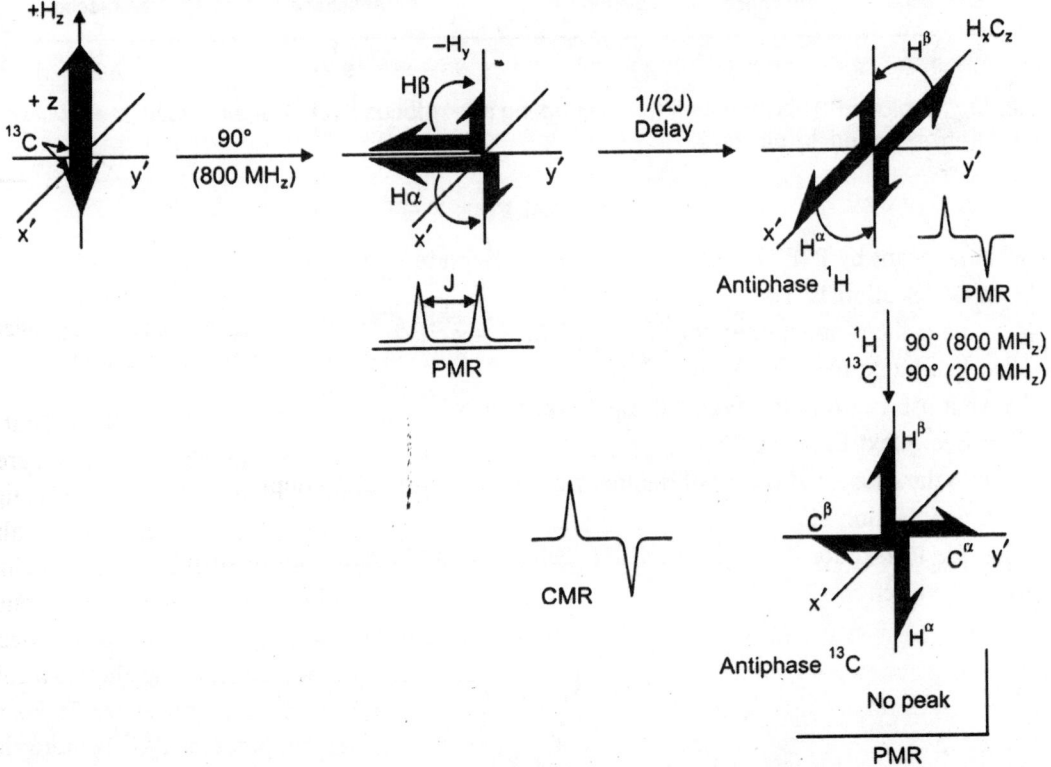

Fig. 12.7. Conversion of all the available ${}^1H$ magnetization into transverse ${}^{13}C$ magnetization (C_y Hz).

12.3 RELAXATION-OPTIMISED INEPT DELAYS

Although, we showed INEPT delay being set equal to $1/(4J)$, it is in reality somewhat shorter. This is done deliberately as due to relaxation delay, there occurs less than one hundred per cent magnetization transfer because the magnetization does not have enough time to be completely anti-phase (or to completely refocus in the reverse INEPT) (Fig. 12.8). But by bringing in reduction in relaxation losses, this gets more than compensated! This can be understood as follows : The anti-phase magnetization develops as the sine of the precession angle. Therefore, if we reduce the delays by ten per cent, then we will have 81° precession. Nine sin (81°) is equal to 0.99. That means a loss of just 1%. Thus, we have seen that a 10% reduction in the INEPT delay period reduces the relaxation losses by more than 1%. This is especially useful in case of large molecules like proteins.

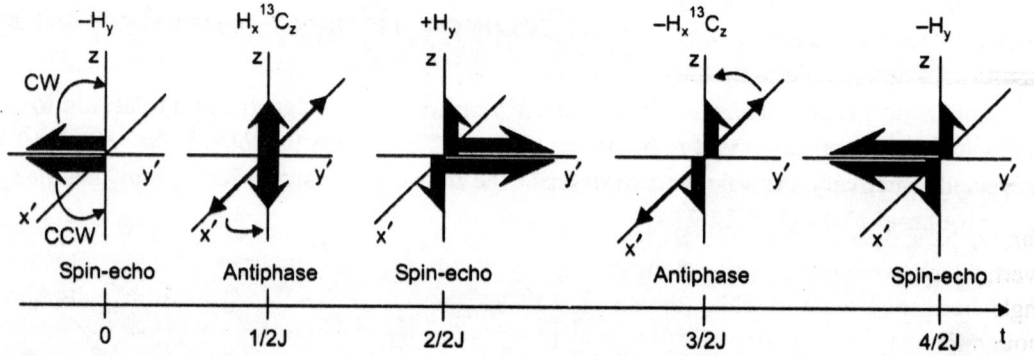

Fig. 12.8. $^1J_{CH}$ evolution. This indicates that J coupling can refocus itself. For simplicity, the ^1H chemical shift has been assumed to be zero.

PROBLEMS

1. What is meant by INEPT and Spin Operators? Explain in details.
   Hint: See Section 12.1.

2. What does the product operator notation $-2I_xS_z$ specify?
   Hint: See Intext Exercise 1.

3. To what use can we put reverse INEPT experiment?
   Hint: See Intext Exercise 2.

4. Explain the cause and utility of magnetization transfer in $^1J_{CH}$ coupling.
   Hint: See Section 12.2.

5. What are Relaxation-Optimized INEPT Delays? What is their significance?
   Hint: See Section 12.3.

13

Two- and Three-Dimensional NMR Correlation Spectroscopy

13.1 TWO-DIMENSIONAL NMR SPECTROSCOPY

So far, we have discussed 1–D NMR spectroscopy. A 1–D NMR spectrum is a graph of intensity along the vertical axis versus frequency along the horizontal chemical shift scale (Fig. 13.1a). This we call as a single-frequency scale in which the signal is a function of one parameter called the chemical shift. Although the single frequency NMR spectrum gives us sufficient information regarding the structure elucidation of simple molecules, we are unable to obtain that in case of molecules having complex spectra wherein we are not able to resolve many peaks. If you look at the 1D spectra of proteins, you find that they are too complex as most of the peaks overlap heavily. Those problems can be overcome if we get 2–D NMR spectra in such cases.

What is done in a 2–D NMR spectrum is that the spectrum is recorded as a graph of two coordinate

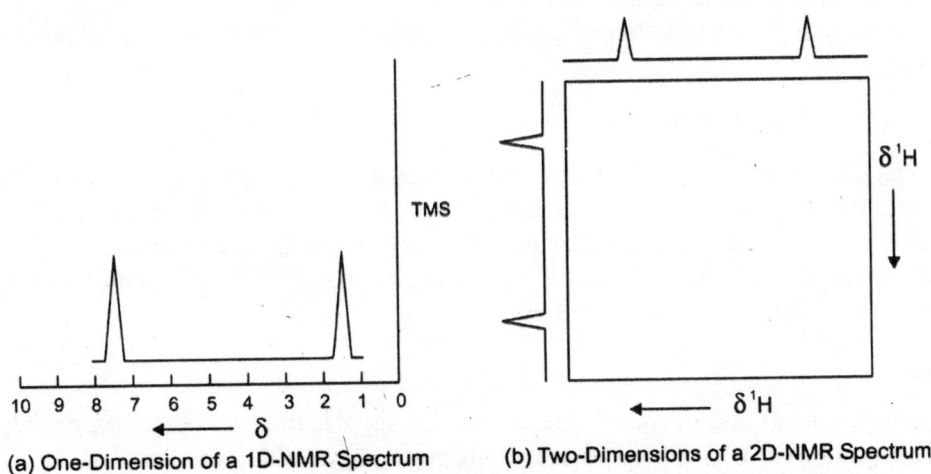

(a) One-Dimension of a 1D-NMR Spectrum   (b) Two-Dimensions of a 2D-NMR Spectrum

Fig. 13.1. (a) One dimensional and (b) two-dimensional spectra.

axes, two frequency scales – one along the vertical scale and another on the horizontal scale (Fig. 13.1b). The result is that the signal is now a function of two chemical shift ranges. A 2D NMR spectrum is actually a three-dimensional spectrum. The third axis is intensity or the magnitude of the signal that comes out of the paper either as a **contour** or **tomographic map** or as **colour coding** also called intensity plot.

13.2 THE ANATOMY OF A 2D EXPERIMENT

The prototype of a 2D experiment always involves four steps as shown in Fig. 13.2(a) and (b).

Preparation	Evolution	Mixing	Detection	2D spectrum

(a)

Exciting spin A shift of spin A	Measuring chemical shift of spin A	Transferring M_Z^A to spin B	Measure chemical shift of of spin B	2D spectrum

(b)

Fig. 13.2. Schematic prototype of a 2D–NMR spectrum, (a) terminology, (b) functions of different terms used in (a).

1. Preparation

It means doing something on a spin (nucleus). Usually a 90° ($\pi/2$) pulse is used to excite all the desired nuclei i.e. ^1H or ^{13}C, simultaneously.

2. Evolution

This step involves measurement of chemical shift of spin A indirectly before this spin A transfers its magnetization, M_Z^A on to spin B. The spins A and B are allowed to precess freely for a time t_1, the magnetization is labelled with the chemical shift of spin A. The coherence of spin A rotates in the x–y plane. This is done for say about 512 times. The FID is recorded each time with t_1 delay being incremented each time by a fixed amount. A second Fourier transform reveals the time course of motion of magnetization of spin A as a function of delay t_1. Usually t_1 is of the order of microseconds (μs) or milliseconds (ms).

3. Mixing

During mixing the magnetization of nucleus of A is allowed to jump on to spin B by application of a combination of RF pulses and/or delay periods (t_2). While t_1 is of the order of microseconds, t_2 is of the order of seconds. The transfer of magnetization either occurs via dipolar mechanism (NOE) or scalar coupling (J coupling). The different 2D NMR experiments such as COSY, HETCOR, NOESY, ROESY, TOCSY etc. have different mixing sequences.

4. Detection

In this step, the chemical shift of spin B is measured. During this time period i.e. the chemical shift of the nucleus B is labelled. We can now represent the prototype of a 2D experiment as Fig. 13.2b.

In a 2–D NMR spectrum, a diagonal of signals A and B partitions the spectrum in two equal halves. There are more signals, called cross signals (X) symmetrical to this diagonal. It is these cross signals that contain the really important information of 2D spectra. These arises from spins that exchanged magnetization during the mixing step (Fig. 13.3a).

If the interacting nuclei are the same, the 2D–spectrum is called homonuclear. If, they are of different types, the spectrum is called heteronuclear. The heteronuclear 2D spectra do not have a diagonal and diagonal symmetry.

13.3A 2D–HETCOR SPECTRUM (^{1}H–^{13}C COSY)

A 2D–HETCOR spectrum is a spectrum of two-frequencies, one a ^{1}H vertical or F_1 dimension and the other, the horizontal or F_2 dimension of C–13. In other words, this spectrum allows us to correlate C–13 nuclei that are directly coupled or bonded to protons. This spectrum allows us to pair up each proton seen in proton nmr spectrum with a carbon to which it is attached in the CMR spectrum.

A schematic HETCOR 2D is shown in Fig. 13.3b.

In order to correlate a peak in the ^{1}H spectrum, with a peak in the CMR spectrum, a horizontal line is followed till it meets a spot. Then from the spot we follow a vertical line that joins it with a peak in the CMR spectrum. Thus, it becomes possible to have complete assignment of both the ^{1}H as well as ^{13}C spectra, without an iota of doubt.

Example

2D HETCOR of Ethylacetate.

Ethylacetate is

$$\overset{1}{C}H_3-\overset{2}{\underset{\underset{O}{\|}}{C}}-O-\overset{3}{C}H_2-\overset{4}{C}H_3$$

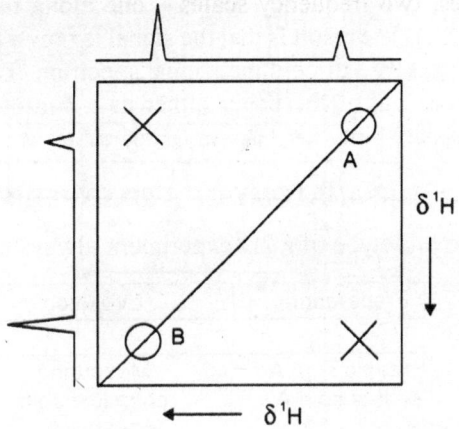

Fig. 13.3a. A schematic 2D NMR spectrum.

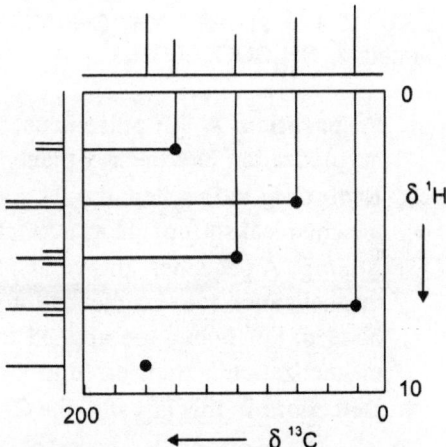

Fig. 13.3b. A schematic 2D HETCOR spectrum.

Its 2D HETCOR spectrum is shown in Fig. 13.4. It contains four carbons marked 1, 2, 3 and 4, all appearing as singlets in the horizontal CMR spectrum as shown. The ^{1}H spectrum is drawn along the vertical axes. The triplet at δ1.3 gets paired up with carbon C_4. The CH_3 singlet at 2.1 pairs up with carbon C_1. Similarly the quartet at 4.1 ppm pairs up with the signal due to C–3. Obviously, the C_2 carbon which is not attached to a hydrogen does not get paired up with a peak in NMR spectrum.

2D COSY of proteins is very important. Crosspeaks between NH and H^α have great significance attached to them. This is because the ^3J value between these nuclei can lead to the derivation of the Phi torsion angle of protein backbone. Fig. 13.5 shows the 2D ($H_\alpha N_H$) COSY of a protein.

13.3B ANATOMY OF A HETCOR EXPERIMENT (CREATION OF A 2D FROM A 1D EXPERIMENT)

As already discussed any 2D NMR experiment consists of four steps:

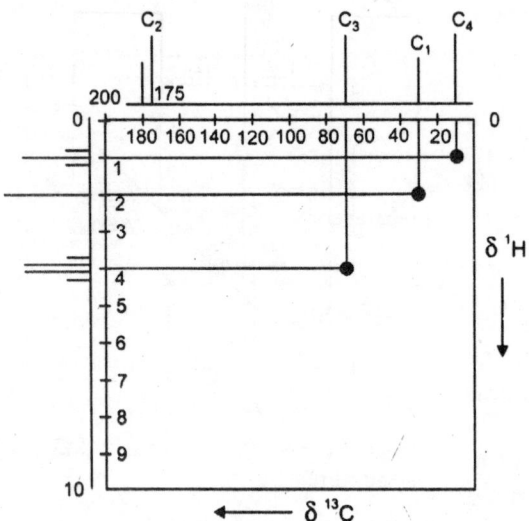

Fig. 13.4. A 2D HETCOR CH COSY of ethyl acetate, $CH_3COOCH_2CH_3$.

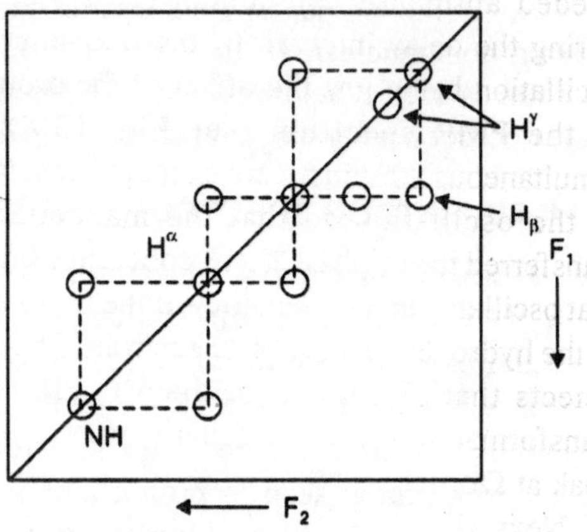

Fig. 13.5. 2D COSY of a protein.

1. **Preparation:** A 90° pulse is used to excite all the desired nuclei – ^1H and this rotates the M_z magnetization into the x–y plane.

2. **Evolution:** In this step, the ^1H magnetization precesses in the x–y plane for time t_1 and encodes the chemical shift of ^1H as a function of time t_1.

3. **Mixing:** A sequence known as **INEPT** (see preceeding Chapter) is used that converts the ^1H magnetization into magnetization that is antiphase with respect to the C–13 to which the ^1H is bonded. 90° pulses are applied to ^1H as well as ^{13}C channels as a consequence of which ^1H magnetization is transferred to ^{13}C magnetization as shown in Fig. 13.6–13.9.

4. **Detection:** In this last step the C–13 FID is detected during time t_2.

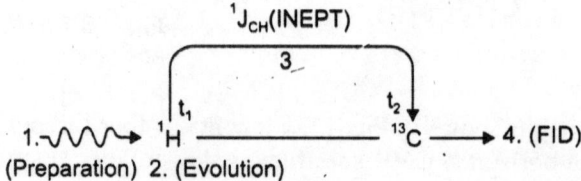

Fig. 13.6. Flow of magnetization from ^1H to ^{13}C in a HETCOR experiment.

The simplest **pulse sequence** in HETCOR experiment is as follows (Fig. 13.6–13.9):

That consists of a 90° pulse, a delay of time t_1 (evolution), an INEPT sequence (mixing) followed by detection. The most simple INEPT sequence is 90° (^1H)–τ–90° (^1H)/90° (^{13}C). τ is the delay period for J-coupling evolution of the ^1H doublet into antiphase. The simultaneous 90° pulses transfer coherence to ^{13}C from ^1H. Often, t is put equal to $1/(2J)$ for complete conversion of coherence from in-phase to antiphase (i.e. $I_x \rightarrow 2I_yS_z$). Simultaneous 180° pulses are applied on ^1H and ^{13}C in the centre of the delay to refocus the proton chemical shift evolution. As we require ^1H chemical shift evolution for a 2D

NMR experiment, hence the delay t is made into the simple evolution delay t_1. As a result of the evolution of the chemical shift of the I_y part, the needed antiphase component $(2I_yS_z)$ oscillates during the delay interval, t_1, the frequency of this oscillation being just the offset of the proton (Ωa) in the PMR spectrum (see Fig. 13.8). Next, simultaneous 90° pulses are executed at some point in the oscillation so that the magnetization is transferred to antiphase C–13 coherence (i.e. $2S_yI_z$) that oscillated at the frequency of the C–13 attached to the hydrogen in the CMR spectrum. The detector detects that oscillation in the ^{13}C FID. Fourier transformation yields a frequency spectrum with a peak at Ωb frequency.

Next, the above experiment is repeated, value of t_1 being slightly longer say 5 ms instead of 4 ms such that only when the ^1H coherence transfer is nil, the coherence transfer occurs. As C–13 coherence is zero, the detected FID is merely noise in nature so that no peak is observed in CMR spectrum. Next the experiment is repeated with the t_1 interval delay being, slightly longer (say 6 ms) such that the H coherence has a negative maximum value and the fourier transformation of the detected FID gives an inverted C–13 peak in the CMR spectrum (Fig. 13.9).

From the above, it is clear that the peak intensity in the CMR spectrum oscillates such that it exactly follows the oscillation of proton coherence during the t_1 delay period. Thus, the intensity of the C–13 peak can be plotted as a ^1H FID with the timescale called the 'indirect time domain' as t_1. **This idea is very important in 2D NMR as it helps us in creating a "fake" time domain with a delay period, that is to say it enables us to generate a second "indirect" frequency scale.** It is the fourier transformation of these collected ^1H FIDs that yields a ^1H NMR spectrum with a peak at the frequency of the original ^1H, Ωa as shown in Fig. 13.8. The second fourier transform actually traces backward from the variation in the C–13 peak to the history of the ^1H during t_1 delay while it is undergoing chemical shift evolution. That is why, it is

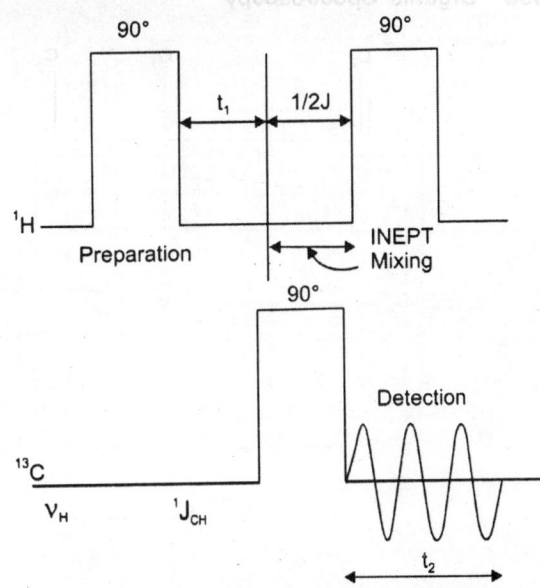

Fig. 13.7. Pulse sequence in HETCOR.

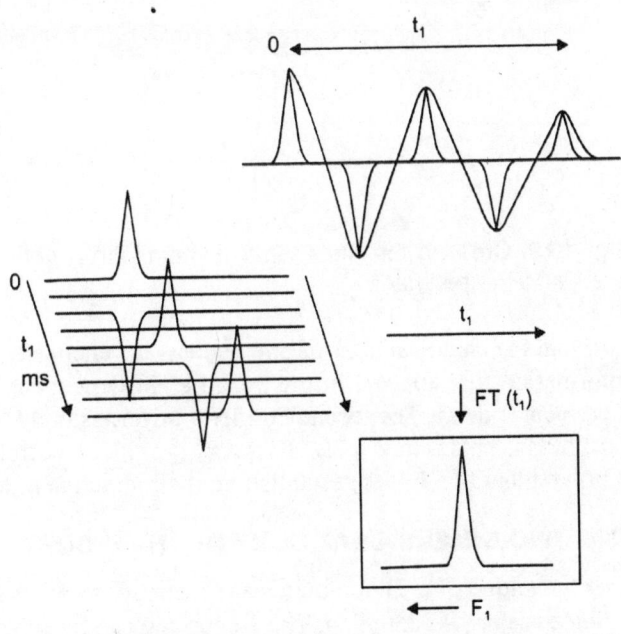

Fig. 13.8. Oscillation of ^{13}C coherence with that of ^1H.

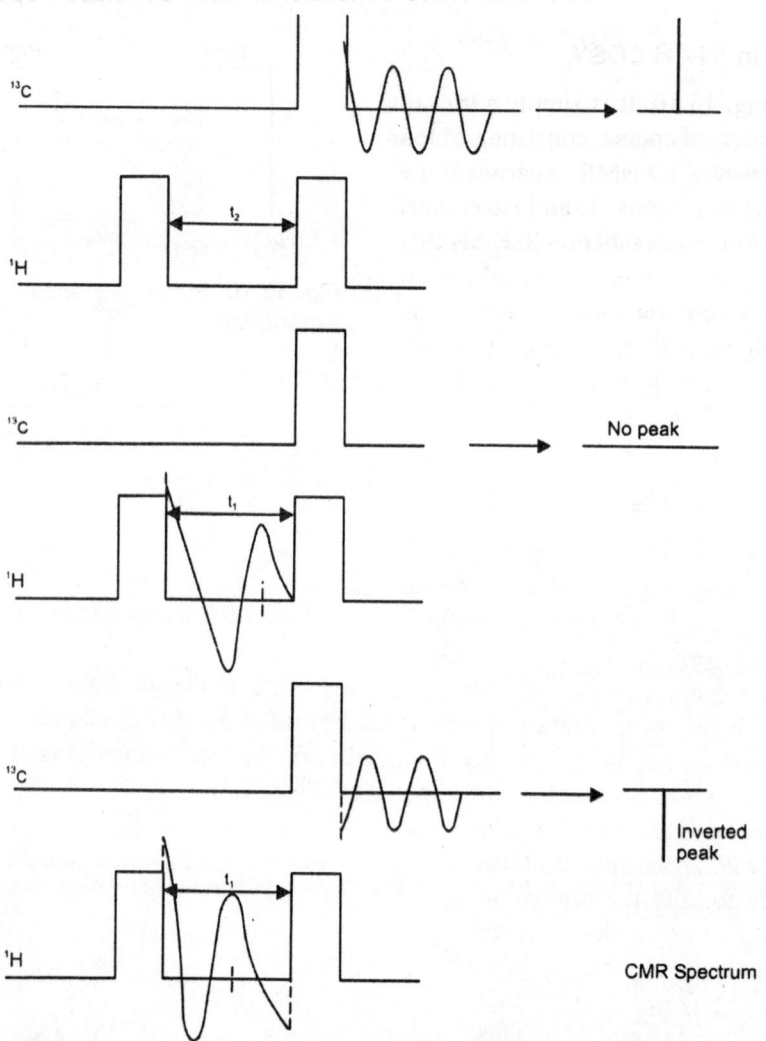

Fig. 13.9. Creating the "fake" time domain with a delay to generate a second "indirect" frequency in a 2D NMR experiment.

said that the chemical shift of one nucleus is "encoded" (labelled) during t_1 and that it is this encoded information that appears in the peak height dependence of the Cb peak on t_1, the magnitude of the incremented delay. The second Fourier transform simply "decodes" this information to yield the chemical shift of Ha. This is how a 2D HETCOR provides a correlation between the chemical shift of proton Ha (Ωa) and that of Cb (Ωb) establishing their attachment to each other.

13.4 TWO-DIMENSIONAL COSY OR ^{1}H–^{1}H COSY

This technique of 2–D homonuclear spectroscopy allows us to correlate one proton to another through a single scalar (J–) coupling. The J-coupling can be either two-bond or three-bond or four or five-bond long range coupling rarely.

Pulse-sequence in ¹H–¹H COSY

This is shown in Fig. 13.10. It is simply a $90°$–t_1–$90°$–t_2 (FID) sequence, of course, consisting of four usual steps just as in any 2D NMR experiment. Let us consider two vicinal protons Ha and Hb coupled to each other. The four steps function like this (Fig. 13.10).

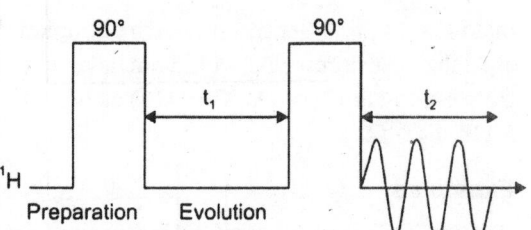

Fig. 13.10. Pulse sequence in a ¹H–¹H COSY experiment.

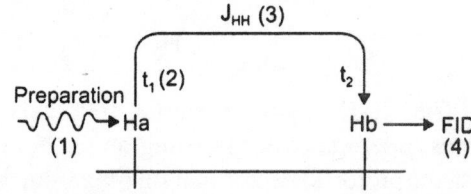

Fig. 13.11. Flow of magnetization in the ¹H–¹H COSY experiment.

1. Preparation

A $90°$ pulse is applied that rotates the magnetization vector M_z of Ha into the x–y plane i.e. by $90°$.

2. Evolution

Magnetization of Ha precesses in the rotating time-frame, the rate of the precession being dependent upon its chemical-shift offset (Ωa). Simultaneously, the evolution of J-coupling also takes place to generate magnetization Ha such that it is anti-phase with regards to its J-coupling with the second proton, Hb.

3. Mixing

Now a second non-selective $90°$ ¹H pulse is applied. This has the effect of transferring antiphase Ha magnetization to anti-phase magnetization of Hb.

The flow of magnetization from Ha to Hb in this COSY experiment can be represented by the Fig. 13.11.

4. Detection

In this final step, the magnetization of Hb precesses at its characteristic rate (Ωb) in the rotating frame. This induces a voltage that is detected by the probe coil as the FID. Fourier transformation in F_2 followed by fourier transformation in F_1 gives the 2D NMR spectrum with a crosspeak at $F_1 = \Omega a$, and $F_2 = \Omega b$ as shown in Fig. 13.12.

The cross-signals or peaks arise from nuclei Ha and Hb that exchanged magnetization during the mixing sequence. These indicate that an interaction has taken place between Ha and Hb

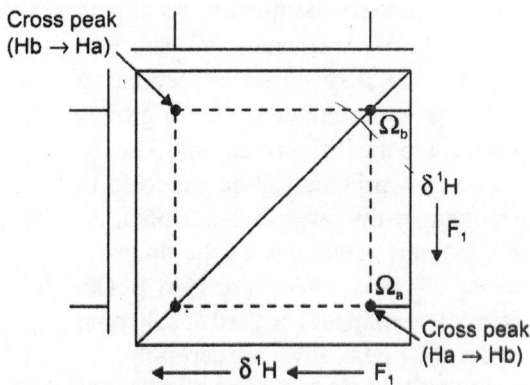

Fig. 13.12. A COSY ¹H–¹H 2D spectrum. A diagonal of signals divides the spectrum into two equal halves. Symmetrical to the diagonal are more signals called cross-signals or peaks. The diagonal arises due to contributions of the magnetization that was not affected by the mixing sequence. In other words, it arises from contributions that remained on the same nucleus during both the evolution times t_1 and t_2. This occurs because coherence transfer is never 100% complete at the end of the mixing sequence.

that is to say, that the two nuclei are coupled. If there were no J-coupling between these two nuclei, Ha and Hb, these crosspeaks would not have been obtained. The crosspeaks indicate the transfer of coherence from Ha to Hb ($F_1 = \Omega a$, $F_2 = \Omega b$) as well as the opposite i.e. transfer of coherence from Hb to Ha ($F_1 = \Omega b$, $F_2 = \Omega a$).

Examples

^{1}H–^{1}H-COSY spectrum of 3-Heptanone.

3–Heptanone is:

$$\overset{1}{C}H_3—\overset{2}{C}H_2—\overset{3}{\underset{\displaystyle \quad}{C}}\overset{\displaystyle O}{\overset{\|}{}}—\overset{4}{C}H_2—\overset{5}{C}H_2—\overset{6}{C}H_2—\overset{7}{C}H_3$$

The ^{1}H–^{1}H COSY spectrum (600 MHz) of this molecule is shown in Fig. 13.13. This has the typical presentation of F_2 being on the bottom with the proton scale. F_1 axis is displayed on the right with the proton scale as usual running from top to bottom. Note that the proton spectrum is not displayed either along the F–1 or the F–2 axis. These 1D spectra are displayed merely for the sake of convenience and are not a part of the usual ^{1}H–^{1}H COSY spectrum. Do not worry. You have the diagonal as your ID spectrum. You can trace along the diagonal line from the lower left to the upper right and you will trace out the 1D ^{1}H spectrum.

In order to interpret the 2D COSY spectrum successfully, a point of distinctive absorption is required as an entry point. That is you require a proton peak that is resolved and that can be unambiguously assigned to its chemical shift based upon its coupling pattern.

In case of 3–heptanone, we can enter its 2D COSY spectrum by beginning with the two methylene (CH_2) groups adjacent to the carbonyl carbon. The H–2 and H–4 protons can be expected to resonate in the range δ 2–2.5 ppm. At the extreme lower end of the diagonal along F_2 axis, there are two peaks (almost overlapped) centred at 2.30 ppm and at 2.27 ppm. If we see carefully, the peak at 2.30 ppm lines up with the crosspeak at 0.90 ppm along the F_1 axis, which means that the peak at 0.90 ppm is due to CH_3 (1) protons, thus indicating that the two peaks at 2.30 ppm and 0.90 ppm are due to $\underset{1}{C}H_3—\underset{2}{C}H_2—CO$ spin system.

Obviously, other peak at the diagonal at 2.27 ppm must be due to the other CH_2 (4) group protons. This peak meets the

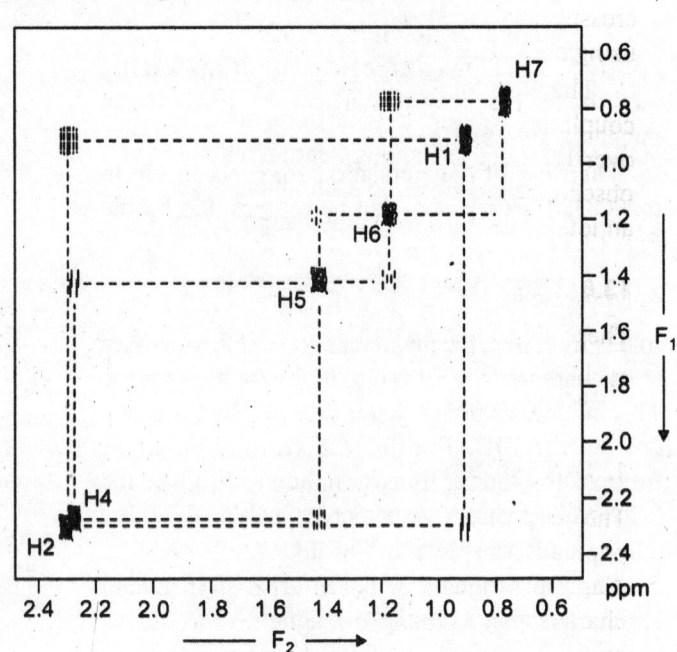

Fig. 13.13. ^{1}H–^{1}H COSY of 3–Heptanone.

crosspeak due to CH_2 (5) at δ 1.42 ppm, which in turn meets the crosspeak at 1.2 ppm due to H–6 and if we move H–6 up, we get a crosspeak at δ 0.77 ppm which must be due to H–7. **See more solved examples in Problems 13.13–13.14.**

13.5 CROSS PEAKS: THE FINE STRUCTURE AND J VALUE

Cross peaks can be anticipated to have fine structure. Why? Our previous discussion, gives the impression that the crosspeaks are simply "blobs" of intensity that correlate Ha, a proton in F_1 axis with Hb, another proton in F_2 axis, of course, at the intersection of their chemical shift positions i.e. $F_1 = \Omega a$ and $F_2 = \Omega b$). This impression can not reflect the true picture as we know the protons may be coupled, not only to one

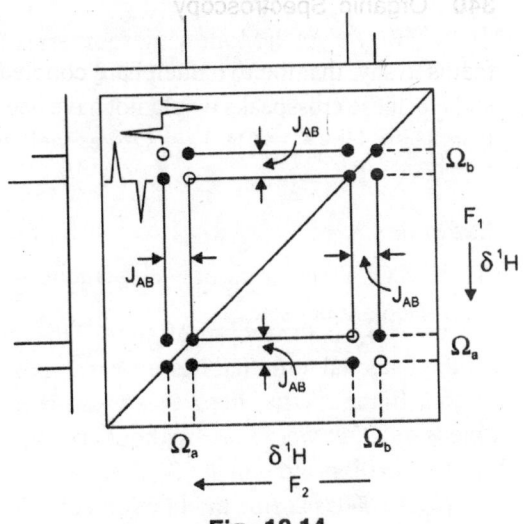

Fig. 13.14.

another but also to other protons. This means at least, we can expect to get a doublet for each if they are not coupled to other protons. So, instead of two single lines, for the two protons Ha and Hb, we should expect two doublets, for each of these protons. If that is so, the cross peaks must have fine structure. Indeed, that is so as shown in Fig. 13.14. We get four peaks in each cross peak as well as in each diagonal peak i.e. there are four circles in each of the two crosspeaks as well four circles in each of the two diagonal peaks. The closed circles represent the positive intensities while the unfilled open circles represent the negative intensities. The intensities are antiphase (+/–) in each dimensions because the crosspeaks originate due to transfer of antiphase coherence to antiphase coherence by the mixing sequence using a 90° pulse.

The value of J_{ab} can be measured by making a slice through the crosspeak. The J_{ab} corresponds to coupling between Ha with frequency Ωa and Hb having frequency Ωb. The advantage of 2D spectra over 1D spectrum is thus clear. When it becomes difficult to assign which of the peaks in the multiplets observed are coupled to each other, in the 1D spectrum, the 2D spectra can sort this out clearly, without an iota of doubt. That is the beauty of the crosspeaks obtained in the 2D spectra.

13.6 TYPES OF COSY EXPERIMENTS: DQF-COSY AND COSY–35

These are of two types
1. DQF–COSY
2. COSY–35

1. DQF–COSY

The basic COSY sequence we learnt earlier is no longer in use. Instead it has been replaced by the very popular DQF–COSY. This means Double Quantum Filtered COSY. This variant of COSY gives reduced diagonal intensity but improved phase properties. COSY sequence has some associated phase characteristics problems. The COSY pulse sequence involves two 90° pulses separated by the required evolution period t_1 and the acquisition time t_2 i.e. 90°–t_1–90°. When we consider two vicinal protons

Ha and Hb, we get the following four terms for the detected magnetization of this vicinal system of Ha and Hb.

$$
\begin{array}{cc}
\text{Ha} & \text{Hb} \\
| & | \\
-\text{C} & -\text{C} \\
| & |
\end{array}
$$

$$-I_z^a cc', - 2I_x^a I_y^b cs', + I_x^a sc', - 2I_y^b I_z^a ss'$$

where $-2I_y^b I_z^a$ is the crosspeak term. This term in the COSY sequence lies on the y' axis compared to I_x^a, the diagonal term that lies on the x' axis (remember x', y', z' terms represent the coordinates in the rotating frame). What does that mean regarding phasing of the crosspeaks to absorption in the F_2 dimension? Can we do that without having the diagonal peaks in the dispersion mode? Obviously not. Similar situation exists in the F_1 dimension as well wherein while the diagonal peak has sine modulation, the crosspeak has cosine modulation in t_1. So, in order to get a phase correct 2D COSY spectrum, either we have to have absorptive crosspeaks or the dispersive diagonal peaks, the opposite being true as well. Unlike, the absorptive crosspeaks, the dispersive signals do not become zero quickly as you move away from the centre of the resonance. The result is that you have long streaks extending above and below as well as to the left and right of the diagonal peaks. That is to say you see long streaks stretching out in F_1 as well as F_2 that interfere with the observation of crosspeaks. So, how to simplify the fine structure of crosspeaks?

This phase problem is avoided by the DQF–COSY experiment as the phase of the diagonal is the same as that of the crosspeaks. What is done in this experiment is that we simply add a 90° pulse immediately following the second 90° pulse used in simple COSY experiment sequence.

The introduction of the third 90° pulse achieves the phase correction as follows (Fig. 13.15). The antiphase Ha magnetization is not transferred into antiphase Hb magnetization directly with the second 90° pulse. Rather, it converts the Ha magnetization into DQC i.e. H_a^α, $H_b^\alpha \leftrightarrow H_a^\beta H_b^\beta$, the intermediate state in coherence transfer first of all. This is then filtered by removing all other coherences such as single transition coherence (SQC), zero quantum transition coherence (ZQC) and I_z with a single phase. The third 90° pulse then immediately converts the "filtered" DQC into antiphase Hb magnetization and is then detected as FID. This filtering technique ensures that only the magnetization passing briefly

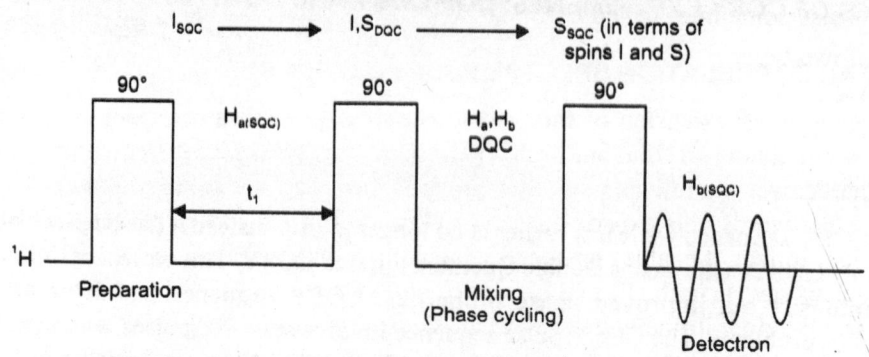

Fig. 13.15. The pulse sequence in DFQ–COSY experiment.

through the double-quantum state (DQS) between the 2nd and the 3rd pulse is observed in the FID.

The filtration is achieved as follows: The phase of the 3rd pulse is varied by 90° on each successive transient for example x′, y′, –x⁻, –y′, etc. and by varying the receiver phase or the reference axis such that it selects only magnetization that is converted from DQC to SQC on application of the 3rd 90° pulse. This is shown in Fig. 13.16.

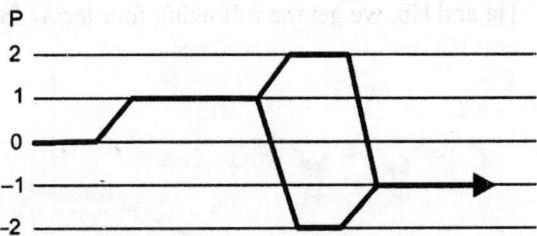

Fig. 13.16. Conversion of DQC to SQC by the 3rd 90° pulse in DQF–COSY experiment.

This spectrum leads to a very simple 2D spectrum reducing the number of peaks within a crosspeak to about half. Consequently, it becomes much easy to correlate the coupling patterns in the F_1 and F_2 dimensions.

The DFQ–COSY sequence is depicted in the Fig. 13.17.

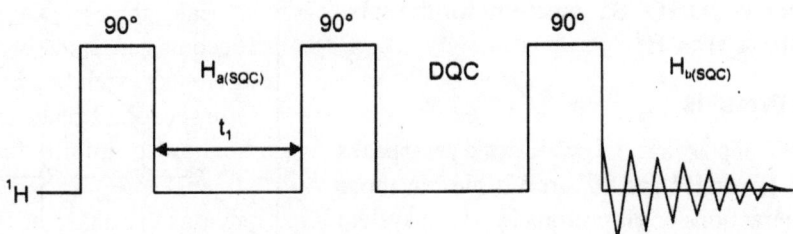

Fig. 13.17. The pulse-sequence in DFQ–COSY experiment.

Example of DFQ–COSY experiment

The 2D–COSY spectrum shown in Fig. 13.13 is actually a DFQ–COSY 2D spectrum! COSY is no longer in use!

2. COSY–35

The COSY–35 sequence is shown in Fig. 13.18. The COSY–35 is also sometimes called COSY–45.

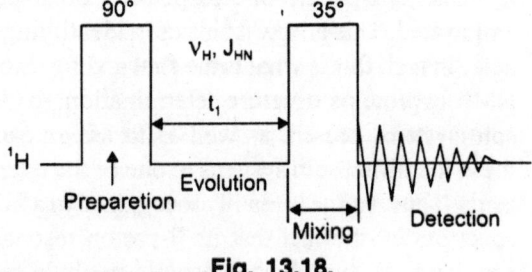

Fig. 13.18.

13.6B TOTAL CORRELATION SPECTROSCOPY (2D TOCSY)

This experiment is an extension of the COSY experiment which arose from the need to allow the transfer of coupling not just from one proton to another through scalar or J-coupling but to all over the molecule, that is over the full spin-system that would cover all the group of protons coupled through bonds J. In other words, this experiment is based upon **multiple jumps rather than single jump of magnetization.** In fact, it enables us to allow jumping of magnetization, of course through J-coupling from one nucleus say Ha in the F_1 axis to intermediate nucleus (say C or D) or other undetected nuclei say C or D and E before it finally transfers it to another nucleus in the F_2 axis, thus covering the entire spin system (Fig. 13.19). That is why, it is called total correlation spectroscopy experiment. The TOCSY sequence is shown in Fig. 13.20.

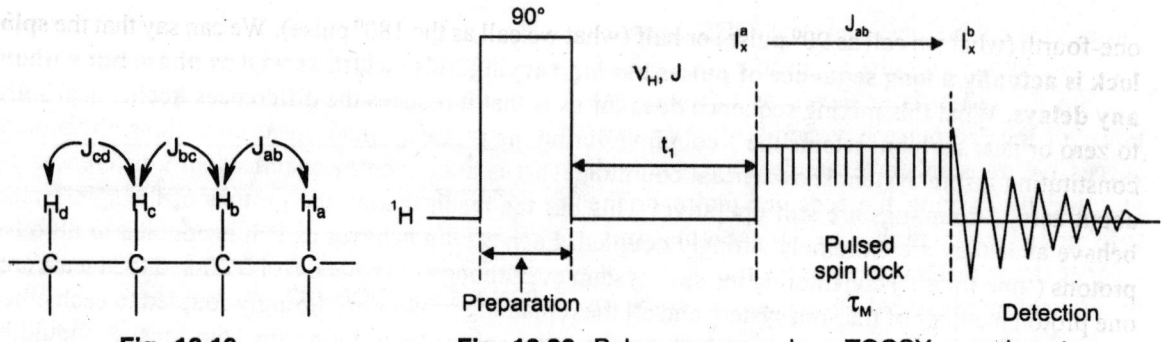

Fig. 13.19.

Fig. 13.20. Pulse sequence in a TOCSY experiments.

Thus, the 2D TOCSY spectrum obtained for 3–hepta-none spin system clearly shows that it contains more cross peaks compared to COSY spectrum (Fig. 13.13).

Fig. 13.21 shows 2D TOCSY spectrum for the spin-system $CH^a–CH^b–CH^c–CH^d$.

2D TOCSY of Proteins

In the 2D TOCSY of proteins, not only are the crosspeaks due to NH and H^α or H^α and H^β are visible but those arising from interactions of all protons in a spin system that are not directly connected through three-chemical bonds are also seen (Fig. 13.22). In other words, a characteristic pattern of crosspeaks is obtained from an amino acid. This is how it aids us in identifying an amino acid. In fact, this is what is the first and foremost, aim of NMR in proteins structure determination: to identify the spin systems present as well as to assign each one of these identified spin systems to one of the twenty amino acids. Thus, valine is readily recognized in a 2D TOCSY spectrum by the fact that its β-proton resonates at 2.1 ppm and the two diastereotropic methyls resonate at about 0.8 ppm.

Anatomy of a 2D TOCSY Experiment

The TOCSY like any 2D NMR spectrum consists of four steps – preparation (90° pulse), evolution over period t_1, mixing followed by detection of FID.

The mixing sequence is actually a **spin-lock** i.e. a long RF pulse that gives a very large number of rotations of M_Z, the net magnetization vector of a nucleus. The number may run into hundreds or thousands instead of

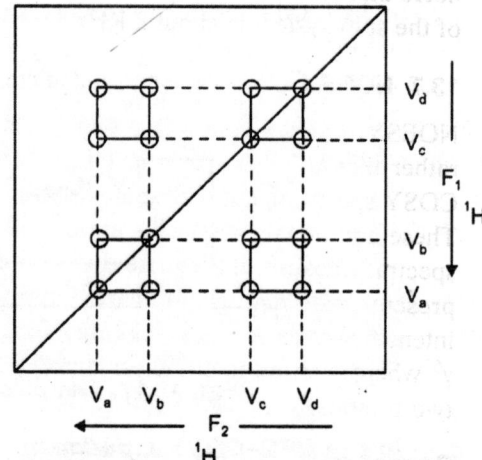

Fig. 13.21. TOCSY spectrum for spin system $CH^a–CH^b–CH^c–CH^d$.

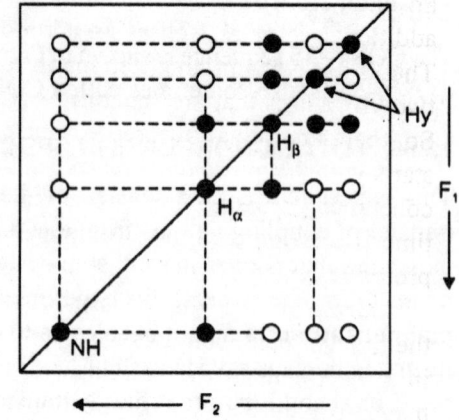

Fig. 13.22. 2D TOCSY spectrum of proteins.

one-fourth (what we call as 90° pulse) or half (what we call as the 180° pulse). We can say that the **spin-lock is actually a long sequence of pulses having varying pulse width as well as phase but without any delays.** What this mixing sequence does for us is that it reduces the differences in chemical shifts to zero or near zero but retains the J-coupling during the process. Under these conditions, the protons constituting a spin system show virtual coupling. That is although, the chemical shift differences are about zero, J-couplings are still operative! This has the result that all the protons of the spin system behave as if they are extremely strongly coupled. Each proton behaves as if it is coupled to all other protons ('one for all') constituting the spin system even though or rather as it is coupled to at least only one proton member of the spin system and all the remaining protons are strongly coupled to each other. In other words, the coherence spreads throughout the spin system during the spin lock. It should be noted that the duration of the spin lock is a very important factor equal to about 70 ms and the amplitude of the spin-system is about 8 KHz.

13.7 NOESY

NOESY means Nuclear Overhauser and Exchange Spectroscopy. This is a Z-magnetization transfer rather than a coherence transfer experiment. In appearance, 2D NOESY spectrum resembles a 2D COSY spectrum, but with some differences in that it contains some additional peaks rather crosspeaks. These additional crosspeaks are the ones which are not seen in the COSY spectra or even TOCSY spectra. Because, these arise due to those pairs of protons that are not directly bonded but they are present close enough in space within 0.5 Å. The intensities of these crosspeaks are a function of the $1/\gamma^6$ where γ is the internuclear distance between the two protons (Figs. 13.23 and 13.24).

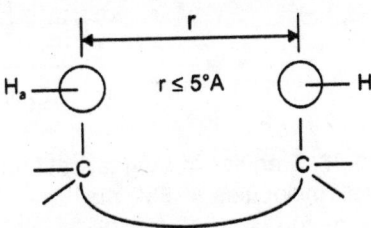

Fig. 13.23. NOE between Ha and Hb situated at a distance $\gamma \leq 5\text{Å}$.

Sequence

Just like any 2D NMR sequence, it consists of four steps – the preparation (a 90° pulse), evolution t_1, mixing followed by detection. Basically, NOESY is an extension of COSY pulse sequence plus one additional delay as well as an additional 90° pulse. That is to say the mixing step involves application of two 90° pulses that are separated by a delay period. So, there are a total of three 90° pulses. Preparation starts with 90° pulse that creates Ha coherence. This coherence precesses during the evolution step over time t_1 and indirectly records the chemical shift of proton Ha.

During mixing (that consists of two 90° pulses), the first 90° pulse converts the magnetization rotating in x'–y' plane in the rotating frame back into z-magnetization. The z-magnetization can lie anywhere between +Mo to –Mo that, of course, depends upon the precession in evolution step. This z-magnetization

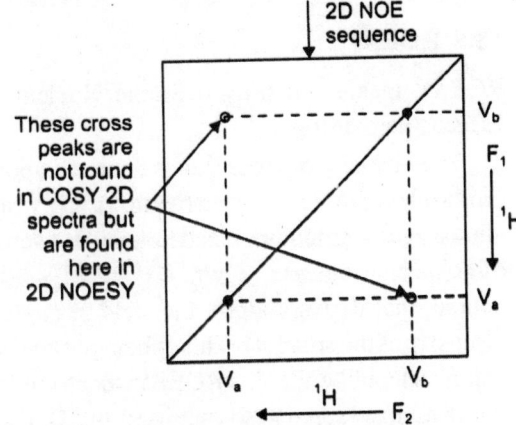

Fig. 13.24. A 2D NOESY spectrum.

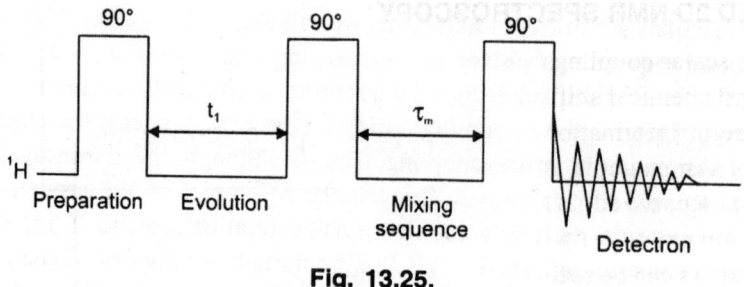

Fig. 13.25.

during the mixing delay τm, alters the population difference of the nearby proton Hb due to cross-relaxation with the result that Z-magnetization of Hb is enhanced. Now this has to be recorded. Obviously, this is done by applying the additional 90° pulse that transfers the Hb-z-magnetization into x'–y' plane that precesses during t_2 and is detected as shown in Fig. 13.25 and Fig. 13.26.

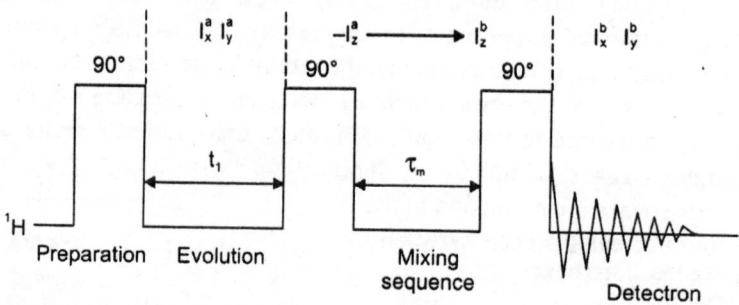

Fig. 13.26. Transfer of magnetization in NOESY. It should be noted that a typical optimal mixing time for small molecules is 350 ms.

The intensity of crosspeaks depends upon the rate of cross-relaxation ("cross-polarization") for the NOE paired protons.

13.8 ROESY

ROESY means Rotating – Frame Nuclear Overhauser Effect Spectroscopy.

The intensity of cross-peaks depends upon the rate of cross-relaxation (cross polarization). This rate becomes almost zero for medium-sized molecules such as peptides, oligosaccharides etc. ($(w\tau_c \cong 1)$ MW ~ 2000 Da), of course, that depends upon the field strength as well as

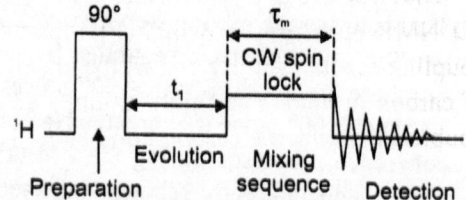

Fig. 13.27. The pulse sequence in ROESY experiment.

viscosity of the solvent). This is because the NOE changes from negative to positive. It is for such cases that instead of NOESY, a ROESY spectrum is the solution. The ROESY differs from NOESY sequence but is almost identical to that used in 2D TOCSY as shown in Fig. 13.27. A typical τm is 200 ms for small organic molecules.

13.9 J. RESOLVED 2D NMR SPECTROSCOPY

In such spectra, the scalar couplings (J) are plotted against chemical shift. This yields very useful information regarding couplings. An example is provided by the J. Resolved 2D spectrum of ethyl ethanoate (ethyl acetate) (Fig. 13.28a). As can be seen the mid points of the multiplets are present in the middle row of the stack and J can be measured around the zero datum. This representation leads to a decoupled ^1H NMR spectrum as a bonus.

It should be noted that this type of spectroscopy can be homonuclear ($^1H-^1H$) and heteronuclear ($^{13}C-^1H$ or $^{15}N-^1H$).

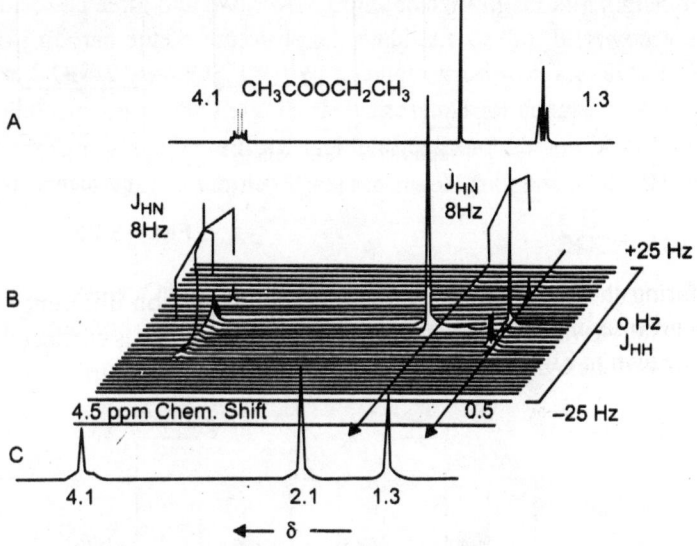

Fig. 13.28a. A J. Resolved 2D spectrum of ethyl acetate.

Example: 2D J resolved NMR of C_{70} fullerene

C_{70} is rugby ball shaped and contains 12 pentagons (2 regular) and 25 hexagons. This has five different types of carbons as it shows five lines in its CMR spectrum as shown in Fig. 13.28b. These are indicated as b, b, c, d and e. Their integral ratios are 10:10:20:20:10 which makes the total number of carbons as seventy. That is why it is called C_{70}.

The structure of C_{70} is further confirmed via its 2D NMR spectrum in which F_1 represents the coupling constants in Hz and F_2 the chemical shift of carbon in ppm. The figure exhibits clearly the doublets that link the carbon bond pairs.

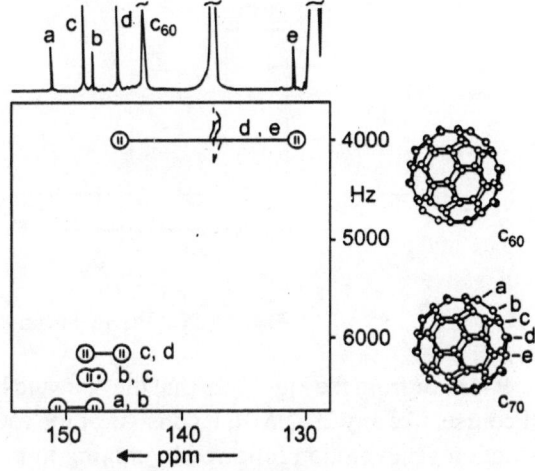

Fig. 13.28b. A J. Resolved 2D spectrum of C_{70}.

13.10 INVERSE HETERONUCLEAR 2D SPECTROSCOPY HSQC, HMQC AND HMBC

Unlike the Heteronuclear COSY (HETCOR) spectra these three 2D experiments also correlate ^{13}C with ^1H nuclei but they differ from HETCOR in that they are "Inverse" in nature. They differ from HETCOR in the sense that while in HETCOR we have ^1H in F_1 dimension and ^{13}C in F_2 dimension, in these experiments, we have ^{13}C in F_1 and ^1H in F_2 dimension. In fact, an HSQC spectrum looks as though it is a HETCOR 2D spectrum turned on its side by 90°.

These three experiments also have better sensitivity compared to HETCOR. Further, they give us an insight into long-range couplings over two and three bonds. In fact, HSQC and HMBC together give us a powerful tool to elucidate the structure of the carbon skeleton of an organic molecule. In fact, HETCOR has now been replaced by the HSQC and HMQC experiments because of these reasons.

HSQC stands for Heteronuclear Single Quantum Correlation.

HMQC stands for Heteronuclear Multiple Quantum Correlation.

HMBC stands for Heteronuclear Multiple Bond Correlation.

13.11 HSQC

The basis of correlation in Heteronuclear Single Quantum Correlation, HSQC, is the $^1J_{CH}$ i.e. the one-bond coupling between ^{13}C and ^1H that are directly bonded. The pulse sequence for HSQC experiment is shown in Fig. 13.29.

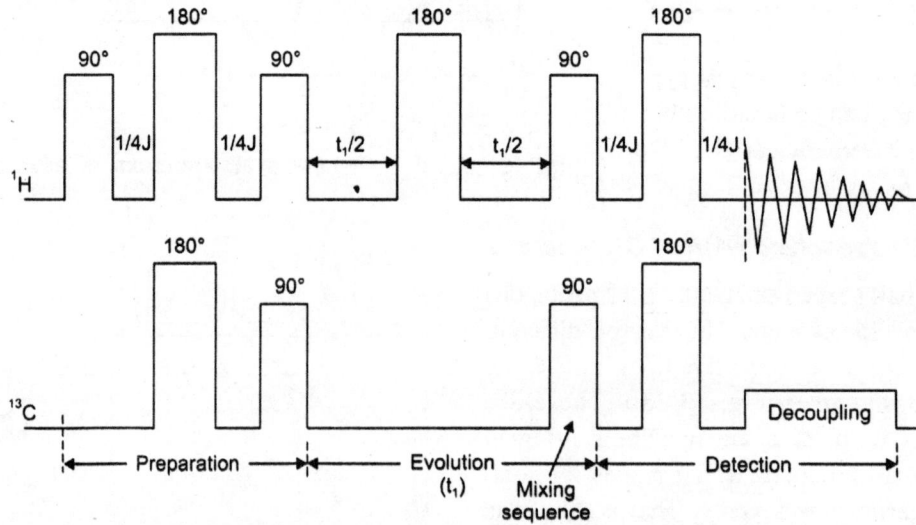

Fig. 13.29. Pulse sequence in an HSQC experiment.

It is clear from the Fig. 13.29 that the "out and back" coherence transfer is employed in this technique. Of course, like any 2D NMR, it consists of the four usual steps beginning with preparation, ending with detection via evolution followed by mixing in between.

The single quantum coherence SQC for ^1H that is created evolves into antiphase w.r. to the ^{13}C (1/ 2J for about 3.3 ms) to which it is directly bonded. Simultaneously ^1H and ^{13}C 90° pulses are used to transfer coherence from ^1H and ^{13}C. During evolution (t_1) the ^{13}C SQC that is antiphase w.r. to ^1H that is directly attached to it undergoes precession at the frequency of the ^{13}C chemical shift. A ^1H 180° pulse in the middle is used to reform any J-coupling evolution. Simultaneously application of ^1H and ^{13}C 90° pulses after t_1 transfers the coherence back to ^1H SQC, of course, antiphase with regards to ^{13}C. A refocussing period 1/(2J) is inserted to permit J-coupling evolution back to in-phase ^1H SQC from antiphase. ^{13}C decoupling is done during recording of FID that collapses the very wide ^1H doublets into normal proton peaks. You might wonder to what is the use of simultaneous 180° pulses on ^1H and

^{13}C in the middle of 1/(2J) delay periods? This sequence prevents any ^{1}H chemical-shift evolution so that only J-coupling evolution occurs during dephasing and refocussing periods. $^1J_{CH}$ value is the important parameter to be adjusted as it depends upon the state of hybridisation of the involved carbon.

The HSQC is so called as it involves ^{13}C SQC during evolution (t_1). As mentioned earlier, a 2D HSQC spectrum of a molecule looks like the HETCOR spectrum that has been turned on its side by 90° as shown in Fig. 13.30 and Fig. 13.31.

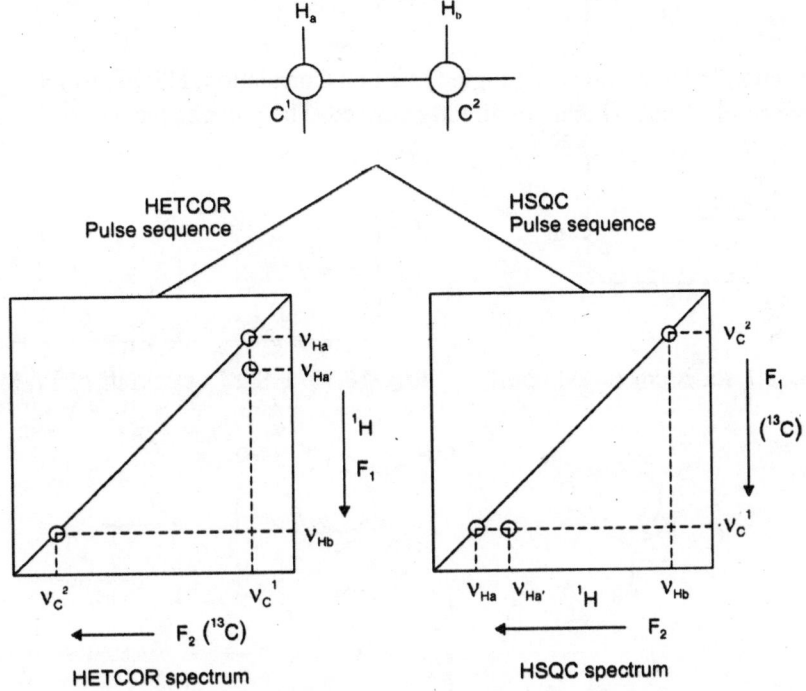

Figs. 13.30 and 13.31. HSQC versus HETCOR for the same molecule bond.

Examples

1. HSQC of 3–heptanone: 2D HSQC of 3–heptanone is shown in Fig. 13.32. There are a total of six crosspeaks. The 7th crosspeak due to carboxyl carbon is not expected anyway as it is not attached to a proton. The six peaks along the F_2 axis line up with the corresponding ^{1}H peaks in the F_1 axis, very clearly. The crosspeaks have been numbered as per the numbering of the proton they correspond to. The two peaks at the lower left numbered 2 and 4 respectively, which could be assigned to CH_2^2 and CH_2^4 respectively as carbon in CH_2^4 is expected to be more deshielded than carbon in CH_2^2. The crosspeak –1 is assigned to CH_3^1 rather than CH_3^7 as the carbon in CH_3^1 is expected to be shielded relative to the carbon in CH_3^7. As CH_2^5 is expected to be deshielded due to its close proximity to CO than CH_2^6, so that makes the assignment unambiguous.

2. HSQC spectrum of Wheland-Meisenheimer (W–M) complex in CD_2Cl_2 obtained by reaction between 1,3,5–tris (N-dipiperidinylamino)benz–4,6–dinitrotetrazolopyridine is shown in Fig. 13.33.

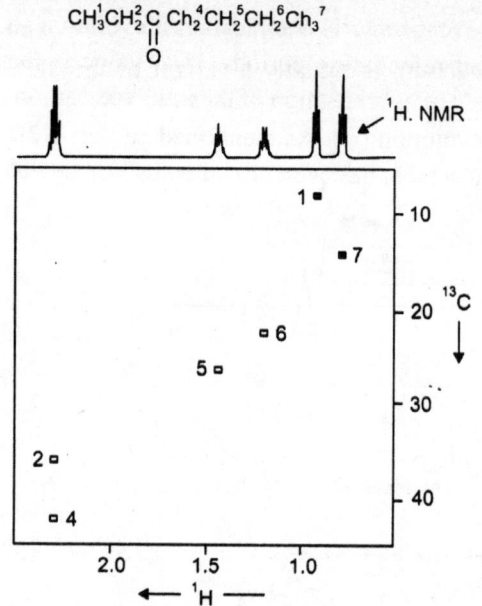

$CH_3^1CH_2^2\overset{\|}{\underset{O}{C}}\,Ch_2^4CH_2^5CH_2^6Ch_3^7$

¹H. NMR

10
20 ¹³C
30
40

2.0   1.5   1.0

← ¹H —

Fig. 13.32. HSQC 2D spectrum of 3–hepta-none.

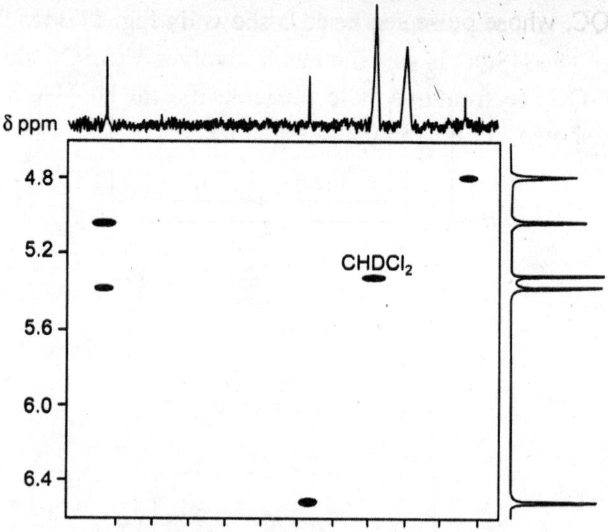

δ ppm

4.8
5.2   CHDCl₂
5.6
6.0
6.4

Fig. 13.33. HSQC spectrum of W–M complex A.

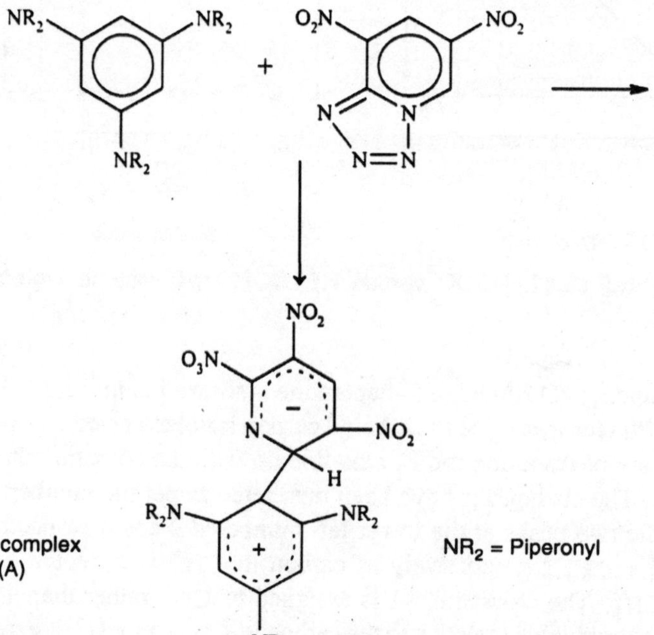

NR₂ = Piperonyl

W.M. complex
(A)

Thus, it is clear that the ¹H signals at 5.01 and 5.35 ppm show connectivity with C–12 and C–14 that resonate at 91.5 ppm. The proton signals that appear at 6.47 and 4.76 ppm are connected to the carbon at 63.38 ppm and 41.63 ppm respectively.

13.12 HMQC

The heteronuclear multiple quantum correlation (HMQC) spectrum is actually a variant of the 2D HSQC, whose pulse sequence is shown in Fig. 13.34a.

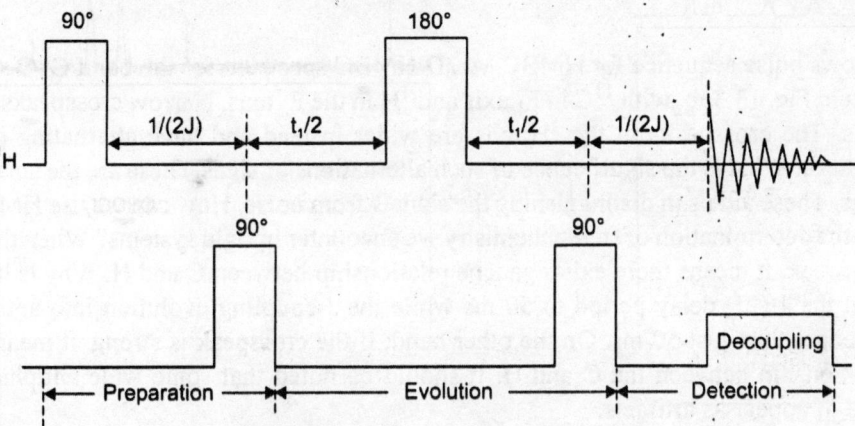

Fig. 13.34a. Pulse-sequence in HMQC.

Example: HMQC spectrum of 3–heptanone

The HMQC spectrum of 3–heptanone is shown in Fig. 13.34b.

The most intense ^{1}H peaks appear at 0.78 ppm (H–7), 0.93 ppm (H–1) and 2.30 ppm (H–2 and H–4). The contour-threshold in this experiment was set high in order to minimize the ^{12}C–^{1}H artifacts so that only the most intense peaks are seen. These are the triplets due to H–1, H–7 and H–4, only the

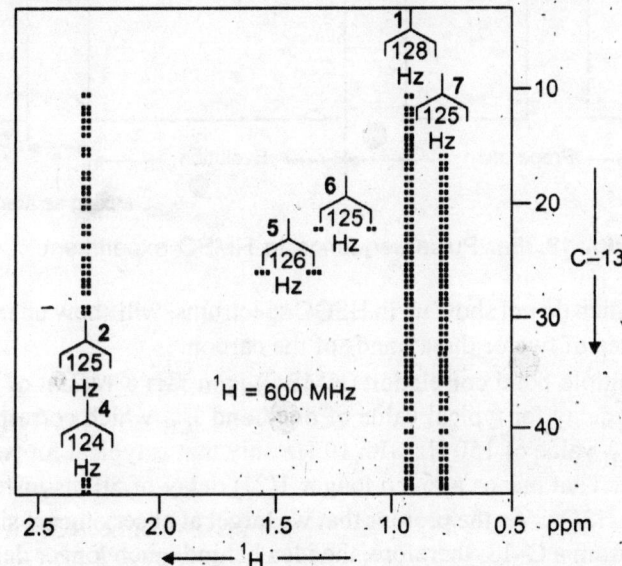

Fig. 13.34b. HMQC for 3–Heptanone.

central doublets of the H–6 sextet and the H–2 quartet as well as the central triplet of the H–5 quintet. The $^1J_{CH}$ can be readily measured from the crosspeak separations as shown. These lie in the typical range 125–128 Hz as expected for the sp^3–hybridised carbons.

13.13 HMBC

Fig. 13.35a shows pulse sequence for HMBC. A 2D HMBC spectrum for the bond C–C–C–H system looks as shown in Fig. 13.35b, with ^{13}C in F_1 axis and ^1H in the F_2 axis. Narrow crosspeaks can be seen in the ^{13}C axis. The crosspeaks in the ^1H axis are wider instead and have alternating positive and negative intensities. What is the significance of such alternations of sign? These are the small antiphase $^{23}J_{CH}$ couplings. These aid us in distinguishing the signals from noise. How can we use HMBC spectral data regarding the determination of stereochemistry we encounter in rigid systems? When the crosspeak is missing or a weak, it means there exists gauche relationship between C and H. Why is it so? This is because we set the 1/(2J) delay period to 50 ms while the J-coupling evolution into antiphase takes considerably longer than just 50 ms. On the other hand, if the crosspeak is strong, it means that there exists anti-relationship between the C and H. It should be noted that some wide antiphase doublets separated by $^1J_{CH}$ appear as artifacts.

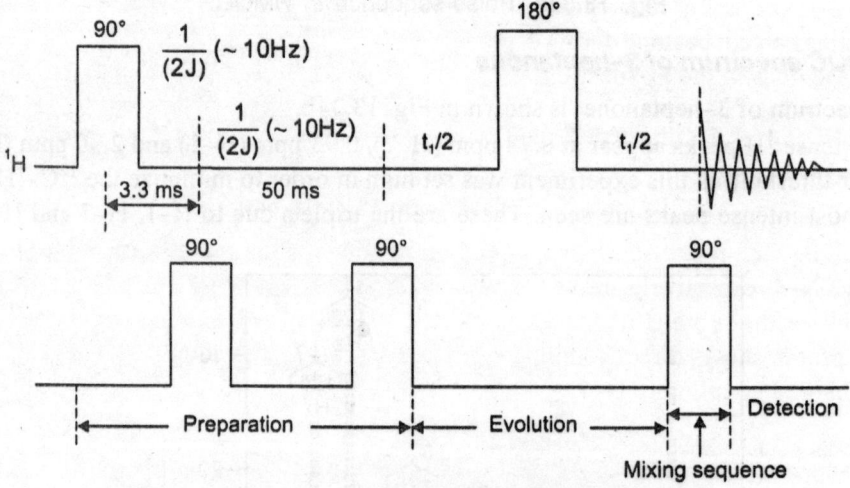

Fig. 13.35a. Pulse sequence in HMBC experiment.

Quaternary carbons which do not show up in HSQC spectrums, will show up in the HMBC spectrum if they are within a distance of two or three bonds of the carbon.

The heteronuclear multiple bond correlation (HMBC) is in fact a variant of the HMQC. While in HMBC, we set the 1/(2J) delay for typical value of one-bond J_{CH} which corresponds to ~ 150 Hz, in HMBC, we replace the J_{CH} value of 150 Hz with 10 Hz only that is typical for two and three bond J_{CH} (the long-range coupling). That means a much longer 1(2J) delay of 50 ms instead of 3.33 ms that is done in HMQC as well as HSQC. As the protons that we target at observing are situated at a distance of two or three bonds away from a C–13, therefore, the idea behind much longer delay is to maximize the coherence transfer from ^1H to the C–13 located at a distance of two or three bonds. At the same time,

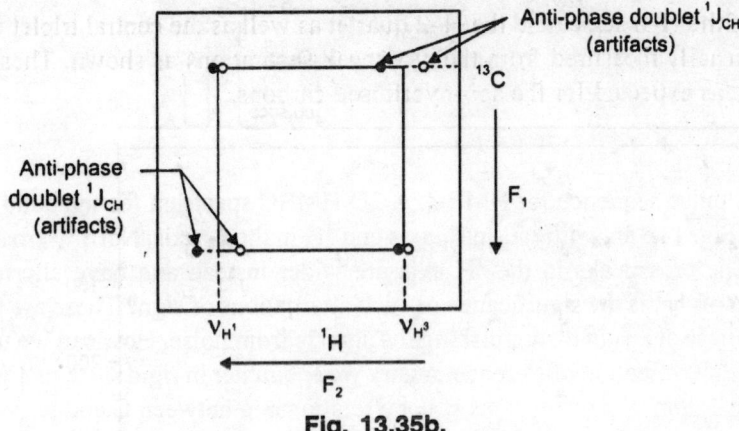

Fig. 13.35b.

we are interested in doing away with any coherence transfer from ^1H to the carbon–13 that is one-bond away. As the $1/(2J)$ defocussing delay is long, so signal loss due to T_2 relaxation is the likely result. However, in order to minimize such losses, the $1/(2J)$ refocussing delay is emitted and the antiphase ^1H coherence (SQC) is directly recorded in FID (remember this is done in DFQ–COSY). As a result, the C–13 decoupling can not be done during acquisition, otherwise the signal would be lost due to cancelling of the antiphase lines in the F_2 spectrum.

Example: HMBC of 4,5–Dihydro–2H–1,2,4–triazine–3–thione

(^1H, ^{15}N) HMBC of this compound (along with ^1H NMR) is shown in Fig. 13.37. In fact, this served as an important tool for its structure determination. Crosspeaks of all expected ^nJ (^1H, ^{15}N) couplings for n = 1, 2, 3 can be seen in the spectrum. Direct, geminal, and vicinal couplings can be seen for 2–H to N–2, N–1, and N–4 respectively. As can be seen both the diastereotopic methylene protons of the ethyl groups as well as the protons of the CH_3 group attached to C–5 exhibit vicinal couplings to N–4. Further N–4 proton shows direct coupling (^1J) to N–4 and a vicinal coupling (^2J) to N–2. The 6–CH_3 protons exhibit a ^3J coupling to N–1:

(121) 8.60 HN_4 3 2 NH 10.75 (162)

(24.9) 1.23 H_3C 5 6 1 N 301

(31.2) 1.43/1.60 CH_2 CH_3 1.83 (17.3)

(8.61) 0.77 CH_3

13.14 THREE-DIMENSIONAL AND FOUR-DIMENSIONAL NMR (BIOLOGICAL NMR) SPECTROSCOPY

With 1D and 2D NMR we could determine the covalent structure of molecules from the point of view of bonding network within small molecules. These techniques can be utilized to reveal as to what

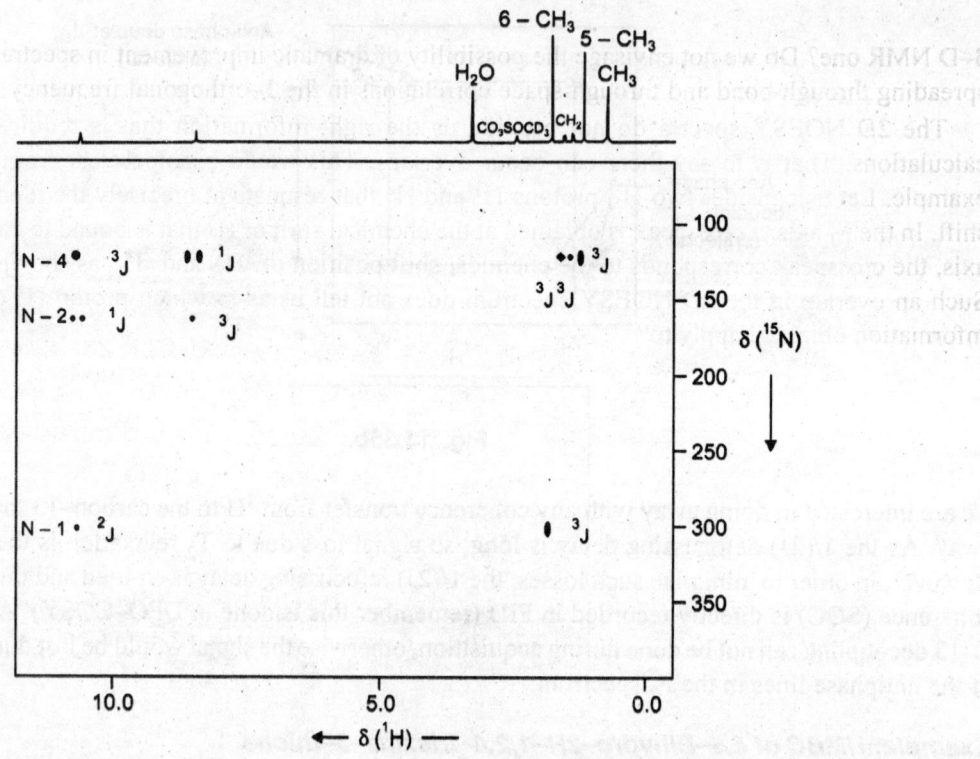

Fig. 13.37. (^{1}H, ^{15}N) HMBC spectrum of 4,5–Dihydro–2H–1,2,4–triazine–3–thione.

nuclei within a molecule are joined to each other, and what is their stereochemical disposition. In other words, we could discover whether they are axial or equatorial, α or β or E or Z.

However, the above techniques suffer from serious limitations – first these apply efficiently only to small-size molecules. These do not do well in case of large molecules like proteins, DNAs, RNAs etc. Further, these fail to address the three-dimensional structure or fold of the large molecules – the biopolymers.

We have already become familiar with 2D–NMR spectroscopy in the preceeding chapter. Increased resolution could be achieved by extending one dimensional NMR experiments into a second dimension. Consequently, we were able to detect as well as interpret the effects which we could not do in one-dimensional NMR spectra as they were highly crowded and provided much reduced information. Following that technique, we were able to elucidate the structure of smaller proteins.

When we consider the 2D spectra of relatively higher proteins (in the 150–300 residue range), for example interleutin–1–beta, we find that these are difficult to interpret due to large overlap of cross-peaks. In fact, this overlapping of cross-peaks in the 2D spectra of large proteins present before us a major barrier to their unambiguous identification. Therefore, a question arises as to how to achieve still higher resolution. A little think and we have the solution to this problem. Recall that this problem is analogous to that we encountered while dealing with 1D–NMR spectra. The problem was eliminated by devising 2D–NMR technique. Therefore, why not extend the 2D–NMR spectral technique into a

3–D NMR one? Do we not envisage the possibility of dramatic improvement in spectral resolution by spreading through-bond and through-space correlations in the 3–orthogonal frequency axis?

The 2D NOESY spectra do not provide us the right information that is required in structure calculations. That is to say there can occur overlaps. This would become clear from the following example. Let us consider two H_N protons H^1 and H^2 that resonate at precisely the identical chemical shift. In the F_1 axis, a crosspeak is obtained at the chemical shift of H^3 that is bound to carbon. In the F_2 axis, the crosspeak corresponds to the chemical shift position of ^1H_N and ^2H_N as shown in Fig. 13.38. Such an overlap in the 2D NOESY spectrum does not tell us as to which proton H^1 or H^2 does the information obtained apply to?

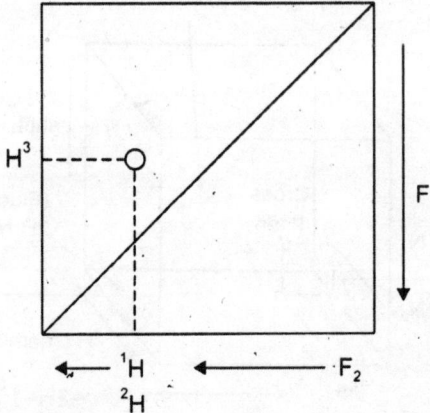

Fig. 13.38. A 2D NOESY spectrum that shows overlap with regards to H_N^1 and H_N^2.

This resonance overlap, however, can be done away with the isotopic labelling – that is to say if the protein sample in question is ^{15}N-labelled. The result will be that $^1H–^{15}N$ and $^2H–^{15}N$ will now be distinguishable, they will now have different chemical shifts as ^{15}N will have different chemical shifts for N_1 and N_2 as shown:

$$
\begin{array}{ccc}
\text{N—H}^1 & & \text{N—H}^1 \\
?\uparrow & & \uparrow \text{NOE} \\
\text{NOE}\quad \text{H}^3\text{—C} \longrightarrow & \text{NOE}\quad & \text{H}^3\text{—C} \\
?\downarrow & & \downarrow \text{No NOE} \\
\text{N—H}^2 & ^{15}\text{N—H}^2 &
\end{array}
$$

Therefore, we can imagine using the spin of naturally occurring ^{14}N isotopes for our 3rd dimensional i.e. 3rd Orthogonal frequency axis, as it has a spin number, l equal to 1 and hence it should be NMR-active. However, there is a problem as we recall from our studies of NQR that ^{14}N, is associated with a nuclear quadrupole moment that leads to peak broadening and hence is likely not to serve the desired purpose of achieving the increased resolution through this experiment. Fortunately, however, the hope is not lost as we know that ^{15}N isotope is NMR-active. Therefore, we can visualize labelling the protein in question with ^{15}N isotope and then devising a 3D experiment.

In a 3D–NMR spectrum, ^{15}N or ^{13}C are distributed in a cube rather than in a plane.

The 2D–NOESY spectrum can be made the floor of the cube. The ^{15}N–chemical shift can be made the third dimension as shown in Fig. 13.39. Consequently, all the 2D crosspeaks are lifted above the floor, of course, by a distance that will correspond to the N–15 chemical shift of the NH group nitrogen. So, you can see that the crosspeak is now vertically positioned at the $^{15}N–H^2$. What does that tell us? It is giving us the message that it is the $^{15}NH^2$. That is involved in NOE relation w.r. to C–H^3. As the J coupling between ^1H and ^1N is a one-bond correlation, so it represents a 2D HSQC spectrum from the front. So, the 3–D spectra can be regarded as combination of the 2–D methods.

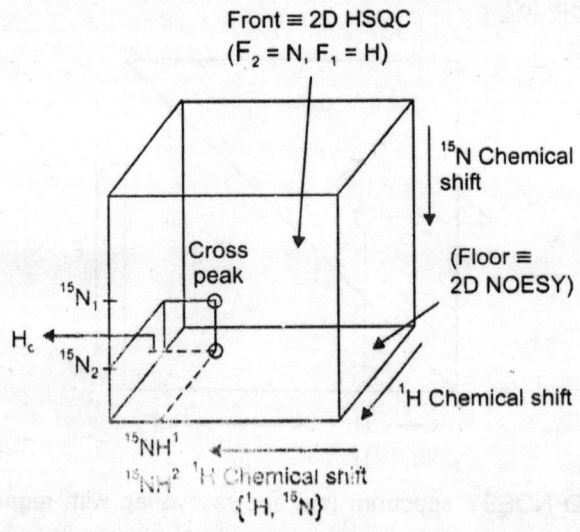

Fig. 13.39. A 3D chemical shift {^1H, ^{15}N} NOESY HMQC spectrum.

It should be noted that the protein sample is labelled with N–15 by what is called expression. The bacterial growth medium contains $^{15}NH_4Cl$ as the only source of nitrogen. So, the protein sample is then we can say is produced as its ^{15}N-enriched analogue (Fig. 13.40):

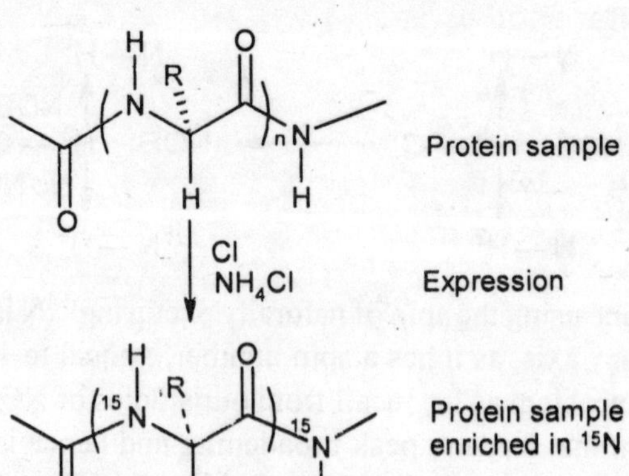

Fig. 13.40.

13.15 CONSTRUCTING A 3D–NMR EXPERIMENT FROM A 2-DIMENSIONAL ONE

Based upon the knowledge we acquired by constructing a 2D–NMR experiment from a 1D–NMR experiment, we can readily extend a 2D–experiment into a 3D–experiment as shown in Fig. 13.41. Instead of one evolution time, we require two evolution times (t_1 and t_2) i.e. one evolution time (t_1) followed by a second evolution time (t_2) after the mixing period (call it first mixing period). The second evolution time (t_2), of course, has to be followed by a second mixing period before the direct data acquisition of the obtained FID (detection phase) is done. Each of the indirect line.

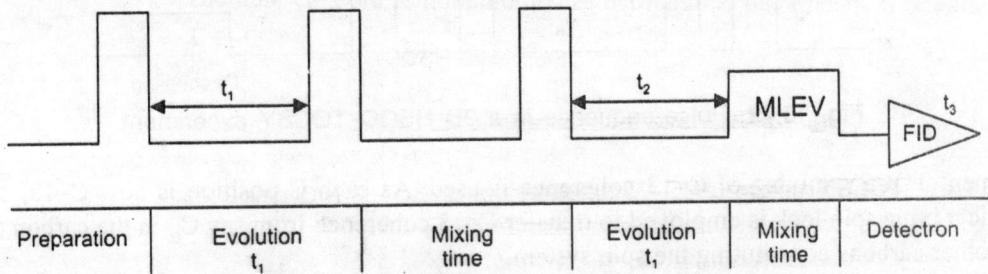

Fig. 13.41. Pulse sequence in a 3D NMR experiment.

13.16 TYPES OF 3D EXPERIMENTS

Broadly these are categorized into two types:
1. 'Two–2D experiments after another'. These are further classified as:
   (a) NOESY–HSQC
   (b) TOCSY–HSQC
   (c) HCCH–TOCSY
2. The Tripple Resonance Experiments for which proteins have to be doubly labelled with ^{13}C and ^{15}N. These experiments are so called as they correlate three different nuclei (^1H, ^{13}C, ^{15}N) instead of two (^1H and ^{13}C).

1. Two 2D Experiments after another 3D Experiment

(a) NOESY–HSQC

In 3D NOESY–HSQC experiments the NOESY experiment is extended by an HSQC step and the acquisition begins after HSQC step rather than at the end of the NOESY mixing time.

(b) TOCSY–HSQC

This is done by combining a TOCSY and the HSQC experiment in a way similar to that for NOESY–HSQC experiment. The pulse sequence for this experiment is shown in Fig. 13.42.

(c) HCCH–TOCSY

This 3D experiment is done when the carbon in protein is no longer dilute – that is to say when the protein has been enriched with ^{13}C in U–^{13}C glucose (or U–^{13}C acetate) medium only. In this 3D

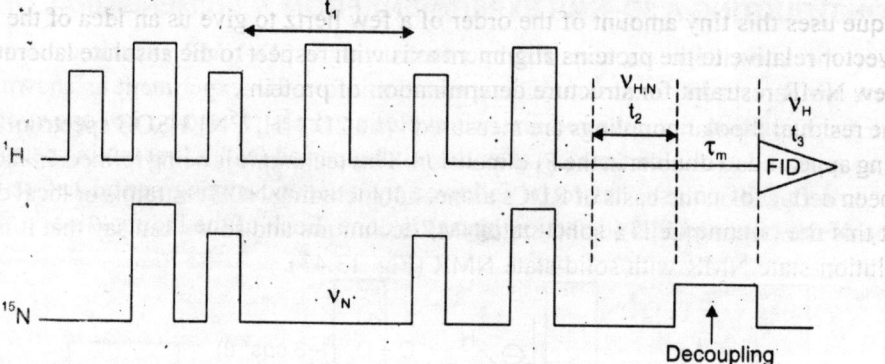

Fig. 13.42. Pulse sequence in a 3D HSQC–TOCSY experiment.

experiment TOCSY mixing of C–13 coherence is used. As each C position is now C–13, so C–13 isotropic mixing spin lock is employed to transfer C–13 coherence from say C_α in the carbon chain to all the other carbons constituting the spin system.

$$\begin{array}{cccc} \text{H} & \text{H} & \text{H} & \text{H} \\ |\alpha & |\beta & |\gamma & |\delta \\ -\text{C}- & \text{C}- & \text{C}- & \text{C}- \\ | & | & | & | \end{array}$$

So beginning with H_α, after preparation, the evolution period records its chemical shift. Now INEPT is used to transfer coherence to the C–13 to which it is attached. This is followed by C–13 evolution time which measures the C–13 chemical shift of the carbon to which it is directly attached. The mixing period (TOCSY) spreads the C–13 coherence on to another carbon–13. The final INEPT transfer transfers the coherence to the last H i.e. the H that is present on this last carbon. That is why, it is called H→C→C→H or HCCH. The ^{1}H FID gives the ^{1}H chemical shift of this last proton. It needs to be noted that the coherence transfer via $^1J_{CC}$ that is equal to about 33 Hz is much more efficient compared to that via H–H TOCSY transfer as $^3J_{HH}$ is small, only a mere 7 Hz.

2. Tripple-Resonance 3D Experiments

The tripple resonance experiments (^{15}N, ^{13}C, ^{1}H) are the methods of choice for the sequential assignment of larger proteins having more than 150 AA. These are so named as they correlate three different nuclei ^{1}H, ^{13}C, ^{15}N. That is to say, these experiments employ pulses on three channels – ^{1}H (say 600 MHz), ^{13}C (150 MHz) and ^{15}N (60 MHz) of course, with appropriate delays to allow INEPT transfer along the protein chain. The tripple resonance experiments are carried out on doubly labelled (^{13}C, ^{15}N) proteins. These are of three types: HNCO, HN(CA)CO and HNCA.

13.17 RDC AND TROSY – THE NEW TECHNIQUES FOR PROTEINS

1. RDC

This means Residual Dipolar Coupling. It is indeed dipolar coupling but as the name implies, it is reduced. By reduced, we mean only about small fraction of 1% of the total dipolar coupling. The new technique uses this tiny amount of the order of a few hertz to give us an idea of the orientation of the N–H vector relative to the proteins alignment axis with respect to the absolute laboratory frame, giving us a new NMR restraint for structure determination of protein.

The residual dipolar couplings are measured via a 2D {^{1}H, ^{15}N} HSQC spectrum such that the $^1J_{NH}$ coupling appears as a doublet in the F_1 dimension. This technique is being refined. In fact, some structures have been deduced on the basis of RDCs alone, not including NOE restraints or local dihedral restraints. In fact this new technique is a solid-state NMR technique and so we can say that it is inter-connecting the solution-state NMR with solid-state NMR (Fig. 13.43).

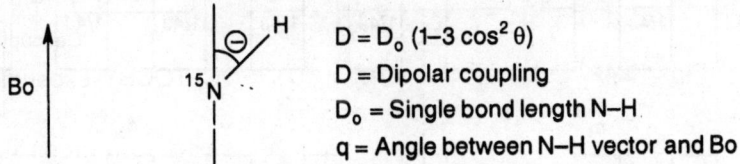

$$D = D_o (1 - 3 \cos^2 \theta)$$

D = Dipolar coupling

D_o = Single bond length N–H

q = Angle between N–H vector and Bo

Fig. 13.43.

2. TROSY

This means Transverse Relaxation Optimized Spectroscopy and is used for improving the resolution and sensitivity of the HSQC spectrum.

Line width is a serious problem in NMR that along with other factors limits the size of the proteins whose structure can be investigated. In this new technique the decoupling is turned off in F_1 and F_2 dimensions of an HSQC experiment such that of the four components of each crosspeak three disappear and only one most narrow peak is selected and converted into a sharp, a very sharp peak (Fig. 13.44).

These peaks were earlier present in coupled HSQC spectrum but are not present in this TROSY spectrum. That is why these have been shown as dotted

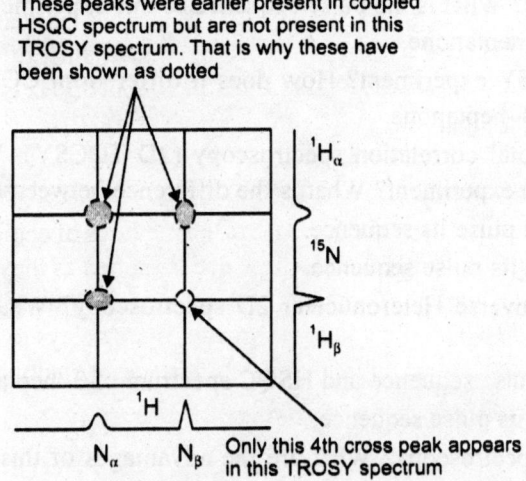

Only this 4th cross peak appears in this TROSY spectrum

Fig. 13.44. The sharp crosspeak in the new TROSY technique.

In other words words, in the ^{1}H, ^{15}N TROSY HSQC spectrum only one crosspeak of a quartet characterizing an amino acid is obtained. Using TROSY, an 800 KD symmetrical complex molecule consisting of 14 identical subunits has been investigated. As all 3D experiments are based on HSQC experiment, so TROSY versions of all these 3D techniques can be tailored which can give much better line width even for the complicated proteins.

What is done in TROSY is that decoupling pulses are removed in each dimension in order to prevent mixing of sharp and broad components. This way the sharp component is selectively detected by phase cycling. This is shown in Fig. 13.45.

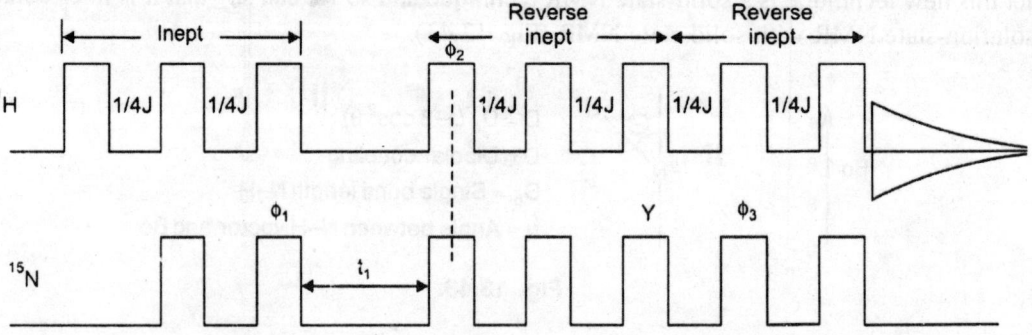

Fig. 13.45. TROSY pulse sequence. Pulses ϕ_1, ϕ_2, ϕ_3 are phase cycled.

PROBLEMS

1. What is two-dimensional NMR spectroscopy? Explain the anatomy of a 2D experiment.
2. Explain 2D-HECTOR spectrum by a schematic spectrum as well as by the spectrum of ethylacetate. What is the anatomy of a 2D-HETCOR experiment i.e. how will you create a 2D from 1D experiment?
3. What is $^1H^1H$ COSY? What is the pulse-sequence of this experiment? Explain the $^1H^1H$ COSY of 2–hexanone or 3–heptanone.
4. What is a DQF-COSY experiment? How does it differ from COSY? Explain the 2-D DQF-COSY spectrum of 3–heptanone.
5. What is meant by total correlation spectroscopy (2D TOCSY). What is the anatomy (pulse sequence) of such an experiment? What is the difference between COSY and TOCSY?
6. Explain NOESY and pulse its sequence.
7. Explain ROESY and its pulse sequence.
8. What is meant by Inverse Heteronuclear 2D spectroscopy? What are their advantages over HETCOR?
9. Explain HSQC, its pulse sequence and HSQC spectrum of 3–heptanone.
10. Explain HMQC and its pulse sequence.
11. What is 3D NMR spectroscopy? What are the advantages of this technique over 1D and 2D NMR experiments? Draw a schematic 3D NMR spectrum. How can you construct a 3D-NMR experiment from a 2D one? What are the two broad 3D experiments?
12. Explain RDC and TROSY, the new techniques for proteins. What is the pulse sequence in TROSY?

13. Explain the $^1H–^1H$ COSY spectrum of 2–hexanone recorded below (Fig. 13.46).

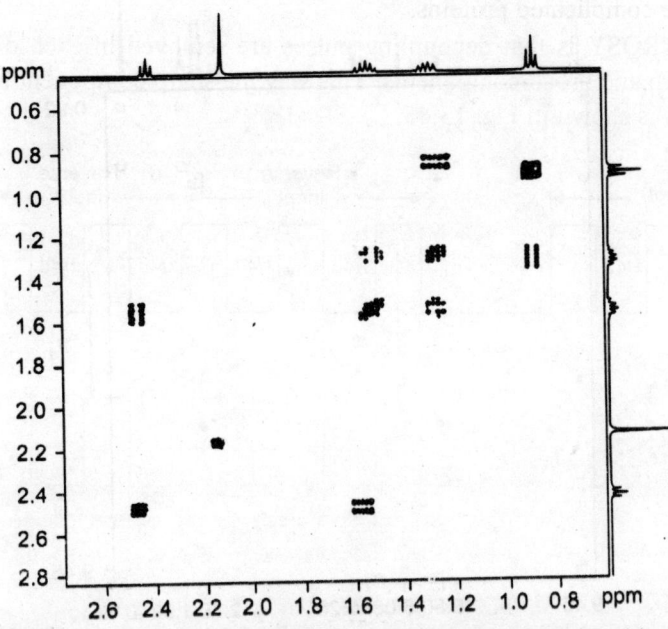

Fig. 13.46. $^1H^1H$ COSY spectrum of 2–hexanone for Problem 13.

Hint: The best entry point in this COSY spectrum can be the CH$_3$ (1) group and the CH$_2$ (3) group around the carbonyl group. The peak at the lower end of the diagonal along the F$_2$ axis does not line up with a cross peak along the F$_1$ axis. This means these are the methyl, CH$_3$ (I) protons. The peak at the extreme lower end of the diagonal along the F$_2$ axis at 2.4 ppm lines up with the cross peak at 1.6 ppm along the F$_1$ axis. So far, we have accounted for the CH$_3$COCH$_2$ spin system. As we move up along the diagonal, we find that the peak at 1.6 ppm also lines up with the cross peak at 1.3 ppm along the F$_1$ axis as well. This means we have accounted for the following unit in the molecule:

CH$_3$ CO   CH$_2$ CH$_2$ CH$_2$—

2.1   2.4   1.6   1.3

As we move up towards right, along the diagonal, we encounter a peak at 1.3 ppm that also lines up with the cross peak at 0.9 ppm. Thus, the total connectivity and assignment of protons chemical shifts is as follows:

2.1   2.4   1.6   1.3   0.9   (chemical shifts)

CH$_3$ CO   CH$_2$ CH$_2$ CH$_2$ CH$_3$

1   2   3   4   5   6   (numbering)

14. Interpret the $^1H^1H$ COSY spectrum of nona–2–trans–6–cis-dienal shown in Fig. 13.47.

Hint: Nona–2–trans–6–cis-dienal is:

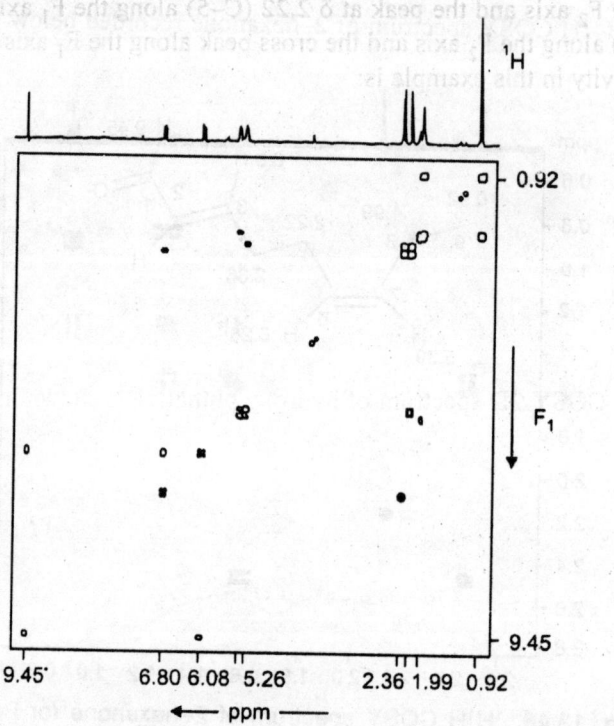

Fig. 13.47. ¹H¹H COSY 2D spectrum of nona–2–trans–6–cis–dienal.

As already discussed in order to interpret a 2D COSY spectrum successfully, a point of distinctive absorption is required as an entry point. That is we require a proton peak that is resolved and that can be unambiguously assigned based upon its coupling pattern and or its chemical shift.

In the present case, we can enter the 2D spectrum by beginning with the aldehydic proton C–1, C–9 and C–2 protons. At the extreme lower end of the diagonal, we find along the F_1 axis a peak at 9.45 ppm (CHO) that lines up with the cross peak at δ 6.8 (H–2). This means that the aldehydic proton is coupled to the olefinic proton C–2 at δ 6.8.

As we move up the diagonal, we find a peak that lines up with the cross peak at 6.80 along the F_2 axis and with the cross peak at 6.08 along the F_1 axis. This means that the C–2 aldehydic proton is coupled to the olefinic proton at C–3. Further up the diagonal, the peak at 5.39 meets the cross peak at 5.39 along the F_2 axis and the cross peak along the F_1 axis at δ 5.26 ppm. C–8 meets the cross peak at δ 1.99 ppm along the 1 axis. The diagonal at δ 5.26 meets the cross peak at 5.26

(C–6) along the F_2 axis and the peak at δ 2.22 (C–5) along the F_1 axis. Further up, the peak at 0.99 ppm (C–8) along the F_2 axis and the cross peak along the F_1 axis at 0.92 ppm (C–9). Thus, the ^{1}H connectivity in this example is:

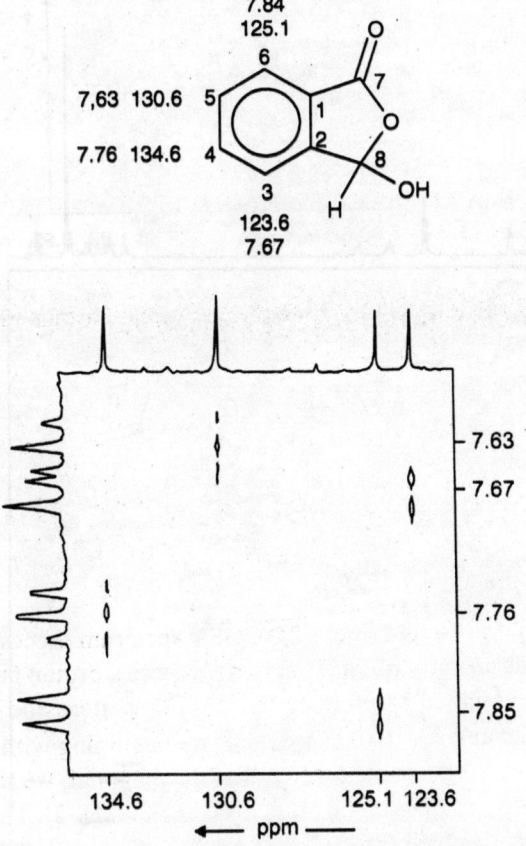

15. Explain the CH COSY 2D spectrum of hydroxy phthalide is shown in Fig. 13.48.

Fig. 13.48. CH COSY 2D spectrum of hydroxy phthalide.

Hint: The C–4 (134.6 ppm) is coupled to proton with δ 7.76 ppm. The C–3 (123.6 ppm) is connected with proton at 7.67 ppm. C–5 (130.6 ppm) is coupled to hydrogen at 7.63 ppm and C–6 (125.1 ppm) is coupled to hydrogen at δ 7.84 ppm.

16. Explain the CH COSY of carveol.

CH COSY of carveol, cis–6–hydroxy–1–methyl–4–isopropylcyclohexene is shown in Fig. 13.49.

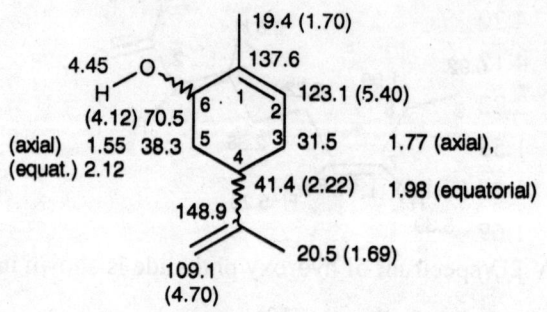

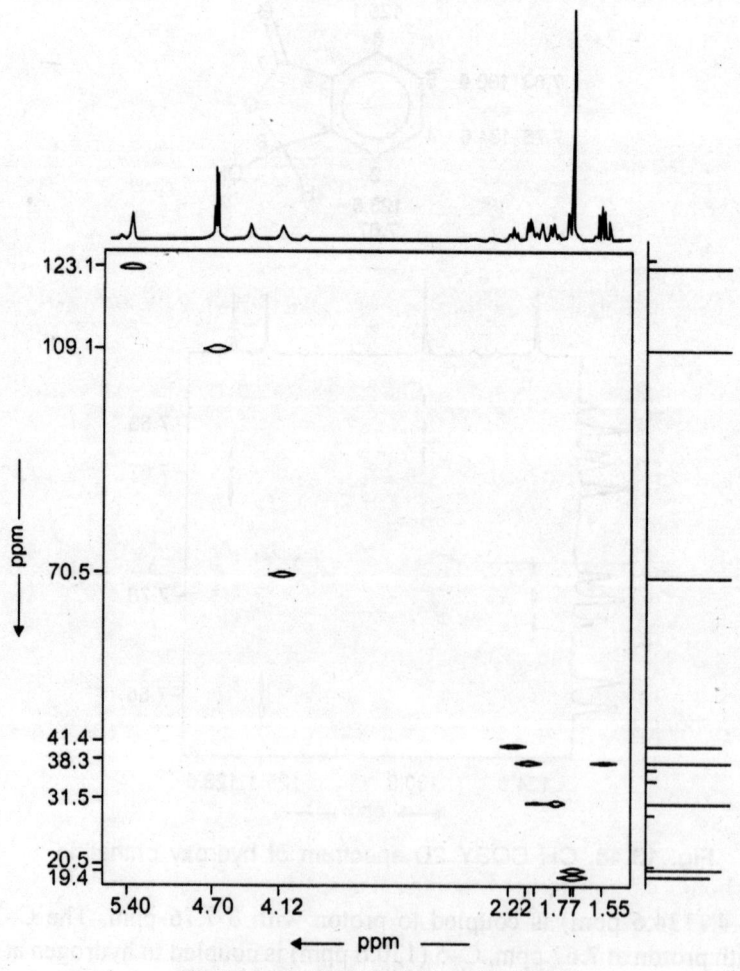

Fig. 13.49. CH COSY spectrum.

From the Figure, the following C–H connectivities are quite clear:

C	—	H
123.1		5.40
109.1		4.70
70.5		4.12
41.4		2.22
38.3		1.55
31.5		1.77 (axial), 1.98 (eq.)
20.5		1.69
19.4		1.70

17. Interpret the CH COSY of 2–hexanone shown below:

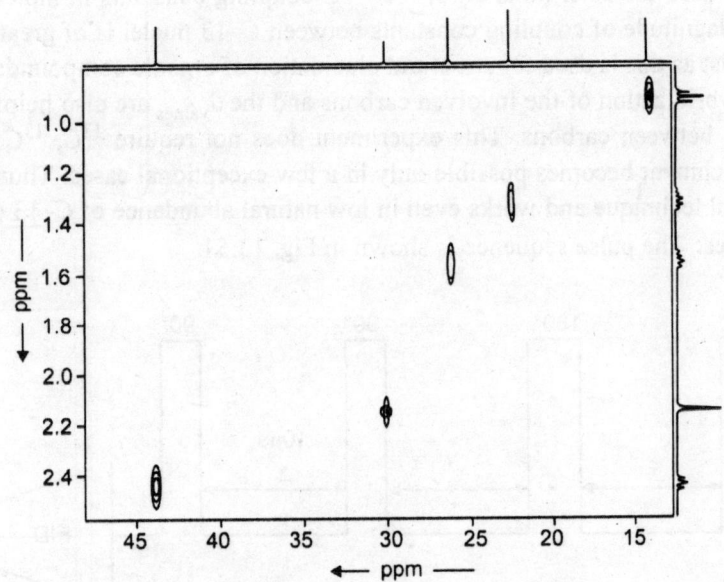

Fig. 13.50. CH COSY of 2–hexanone.

Hint: 2–Hexanone is:

$$CH_3\text{—}\overset{\displaystyle O}{\underset{\displaystyle \|}{C}}\text{—}CH_2\text{—}CH_2\text{—}CH_2\text{—}CH_3$$

As the carbonyl carbon is not attached to a hydrogen, therefore, it does not show up in the spectrum. The crosspeak at 30 ppm is coupled to the proton at 2.1 ppm. As this proton is a singlet, so it must be due to 1–CH_3 protons. The crosspeak at δ 43.7 ppm lines up with the proton (triplet) at 2.4 ppm. Clearly, this must be the deshielded –CH_2– carbon (i.e. C–3). The crosspeak at 26 ppm corresponds to a proton which is present at δ 1.6 ppm. So, this carbon must be C–4. The crosspeak at δ 22 that connects to proton (a multiplet) at δ 1–3 ppm must be the C–5. The crosspeak at δ 14 ppm connects to the proton, a triplet at δ 0.7 ppm. Obviously, this must be the methyl (C–6) at the other end of the molecule. Thus, the connectivities are:

C–No	δ C	δ H
C–3	43	2.4
C–1	30	2.1
C–4	26	1.6
C–5	22	1.3
C–6	14	0.7

18. **What is INADEQUATE?**

This stands for **Incredible Natural Abundance Double Quantum Transfer Experiment.** This experiment is used for determination of ^{13}C–^{13}C coupling constants in molecules with natural abundance. Magnitude of coupling constants between C–13 nuclei is of great importance to an organic chemist as this is used for structural elucidation of organic compounds. $^1J(^{13}C, {}^{13}C)$ is a function of hybridization of the involved carbons and the J_{values} are also helpful in establishing connectivities between carbons. This experiment does not require ^{13}C, ^{13}C double labelling. Synthetic enrichment becomes possible only in a few exceptional cases. Thus, INADEQUATE is a very useful technique and works even in low natural abundance of C–13 (1.10%).

Pulse sequence: The pulse sequence is shown in Fig. 13.51.

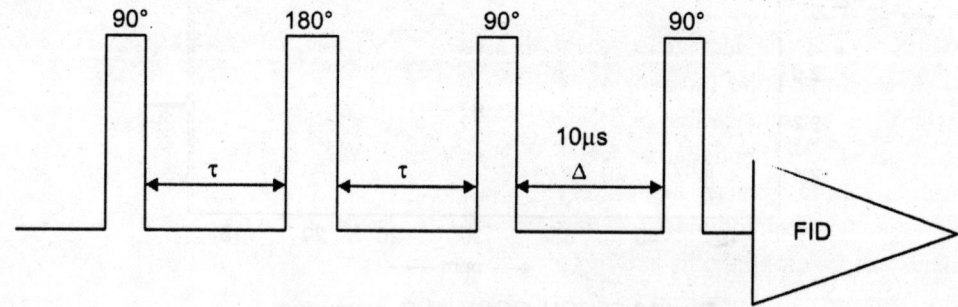

Fig. 13.51. Pulse sequence in 1D INADEQUATE.

The basis of the pulse sequence is that by appropriate treatment of the spin system that consists of the AX system of the coupled C–13 nuclei and the intense signal of the parent organic compound with just one C–13, the principal signal can be suppressed. Obviously, this requires a 90° phase difference between the transverse magnetization of the satellites as well as that of the main signal which allows the selection of the AX magnetization for detection.

Fig. 13.52 shows the result of INADEQUATE for (η^5–cyclopentadienyl)–η^1, η^2–2,2–dimethyl–3–butenylnickel.

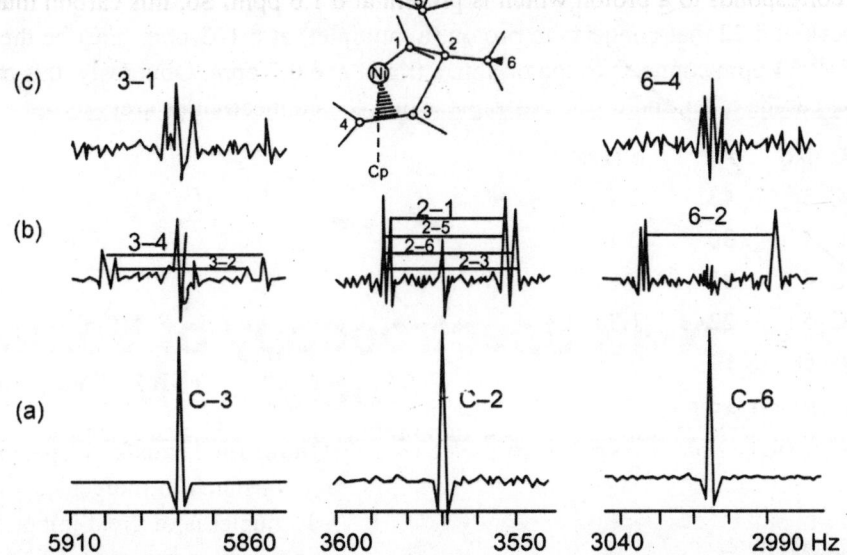

Fig. 13.52. Determination of ^{13}C, ^{13}C coupling constants of (η^3–cyclopentadienyl)–η^1, η^2–2,2–dimethyl– 3–butenylnickel [72] by INADEQUATE (a) signal of C atoms 3, 2 and 6; (b) INADEQUATE spectra with $r \approx 6.2$ ms or $^1J(^{13}C, {}^{13}C) \approx 40$ Hz; (c) as (b) with $t = 0.88$ s for geminal and vicinal $J(^{13}C, {}^{13}C)$ coupling constants; spectral width 5000 Hz, 1600 transients, FID-Gauss multiplication that yielded $^1J(1,2) = 32.1$, $^1J(2,3) = 37.1$, $^1J(2,5) = 34.7$, $^1J(2,6) = 37.1$, $^1J(3,4) = 44.7$, $^2J(1,3) = 8.5$, $^1J(4,6) = 3.2$ Hz.

19. What is 2D-INADEQUATE?

Thus, while the 1–D Inadequate experiments lead to the suppression of the intense ^{13}C–^{12}C main signal with the consequence that both AX and AB systems for all ^{13}C–^{13}C bonds can be seen in a single spectrum, the 2–D version segregates the AB systems based upon their individual double quantum frequencies (DQF) along the F_2 axis.

Example: Inadequate spectrum of n-butanol is shown below. We can clearly see the segregated AB systems for every C–C bond. The arrows enable us to establish the C–C bonds in the molecule from C–1 (62.9 ppm) → C–2 (36.0 ppm) → C–3 (20.3 ppm) → C–4 (15.2 ppm).

$$HOCH_2 - CH_2 - CH_2 - CH_3$$
$$62.9 \quad\quad 36.0 \quad\quad 20.3 \quad\quad 15.2$$

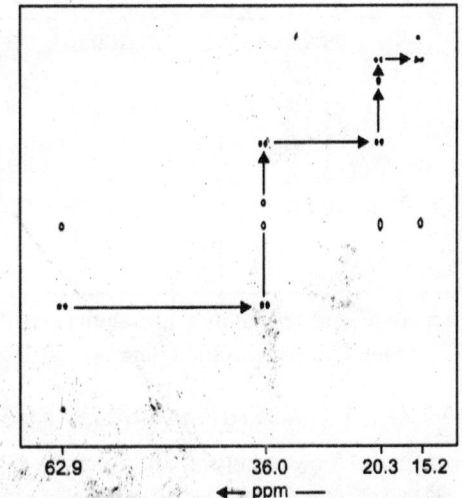

Fig. 13.53. 2D INADEQUATE of n-butanol.

NMR Spectroscopy of Some Other Nuclei – ^{15}N, ^{19}F, ^{31}P, ^{11}B

14.1 INTRODUCTION

In this chapter, we will learn NMR phenomenon with respect to nuclei other than ^1H and ^{13}C. Table 14.1 lists chemical shift range range, coupling constant and T_1 values of these nuclei.

Table 14.1. Magnetic properties of some nuclei

Isotope	Natural abundance (%)	Spin	Res. freq. at 2.35 T (MHz)	Receptivity cf. Carbon–13	Chem. shift range (ppm)	Reference	$^4J_{X-H}$ (Hz)	T_1*
^{1}H	99.98	1/2	100.0	5677	15	TMS	–	m
^{2}D	0.02	1	15.4	8×10^{-3}	15	d-TMS	–	m–s
^{11}B	81.17	3/2	31.2	754	220	BF$_3$Et$_2$O	30–180	s
^{13}C	1.11	1/2	25.2	1	250	TMS	125–250	1
^{15}N	0.37	1/2	10.1	2×10^{-2}	700	Liquid NH$_3$	60–140	vl
^{17}O	0.04	5/2	13.6	6×10^{-2}	900	H$_2$O	80 ± 5	vs
^{19}F	100	1/2	94.1	4728	500	CFCL$_3$	–	m
^{31}P	100	1/2	40.5	377	800	85% H$_3$PO$_4$	30–1100	m–l

Receptivity and sensitivity × nat. abundance (sensitivity to detection of a nucleus, a $Y^3I(I+1)$

* T_1 – longitudinal relaxation times : m (0.1–5); s (0.01–1); 1 (1–100) in seconds

14.2 N–15 NUCLEAR MAGNETIC RESONANCE

Nitrogen–15 has a natural abundance of 0.37% and spin = 1/2. Its relative sensitivity w.r. to proton is 1.04×10^{-3} i.e. its about an order of magnitude less sensitive than carbon–13 (1.59×10^{-2}). The γ for nitrogen is small and negative, –2712. So, γ for nitrogen is 1/10th of that of γ_H.

The chemical shift of common N-containing organic compound is about 600 ppm (Fig. 14.1) and this is 3 times that of C–13 (which is about 200 ppm). The standard reference used is liquid ammonia. This is shown in Fig. 14.1.

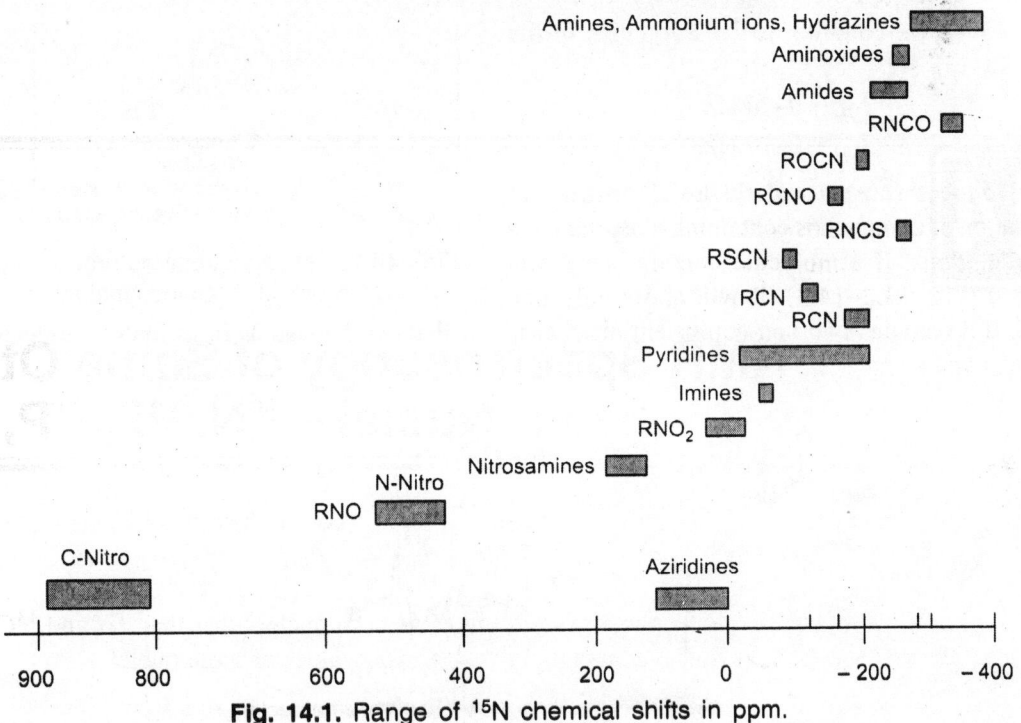

Fig. 14.1. Range of ^{15}N chemical shifts in ppm.

(i) There seem to occur some parallels with the CMR spectroscopy. We have seen that, chemical shift of carbonyl follow the order :

Carbonyl > Carboxy > Alkenyl > Alkyl

CO   COO$^-$ $-\overset{|}{C}=\overset{|}{C}-$ $-\overset{|}{\underset{|}{C}}-$

The same order is observed for the corresponding N-containing compounds – nitroso, nitro, imino and amino compounds :

Nitroso > Nitro > Imino > Alkyl

N–N = O   – NO$_2$ $-C=\overset{|}{N}-$ $-\overset{|}{\underset{|}{N}}-$

590–520   400–320   340–250   100–0

(ii) Another parallel is found among (imines, pyridine), nitriles, amines and aziridines :

Imines, pyridines > Nitriles > Amines > Aziridines

C = NH   ⬡N   –C ≡ N   – NH$_2$ △—NH

which is similar to that observed for the corresponding compounds in CMR

alkenes, aromatics > Alkynes > Alkanes > Cyclopropanes

C = C   ⬡   C ≡ C   –CH$_2$–   △

N–15 shows coupling to ^1H. $^1J_{NH}$ lies in the range 75–135 Hz.

$$^2J_{NH} = 0\text{--}20 \text{ Hz}$$
$$^3J_{NH} = 0\text{--}10 \text{ Hz}$$

N–15 spectra are particularly useful for structure elucidation of compounds containing more than one nitrogen. Thus, if a molecule contains only one nitrogen (Fig. 14.2–14.3), it will show only one

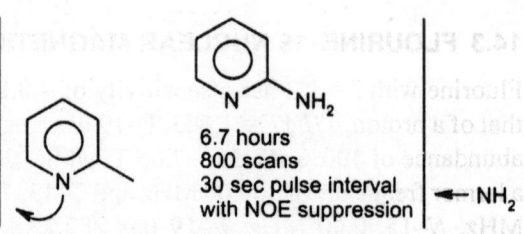

6.7 hours
800 scans
30 sec pulse interval
with NOE suppression

Fig. 14.2. ^{15}N spectrum natural abundance (^1H-decoupled) of 2–aminopyridine.

signal. If it contains two non-equivalent nitrogens, it will show the signals in its hydrogen-decoupled spectrum and so on.

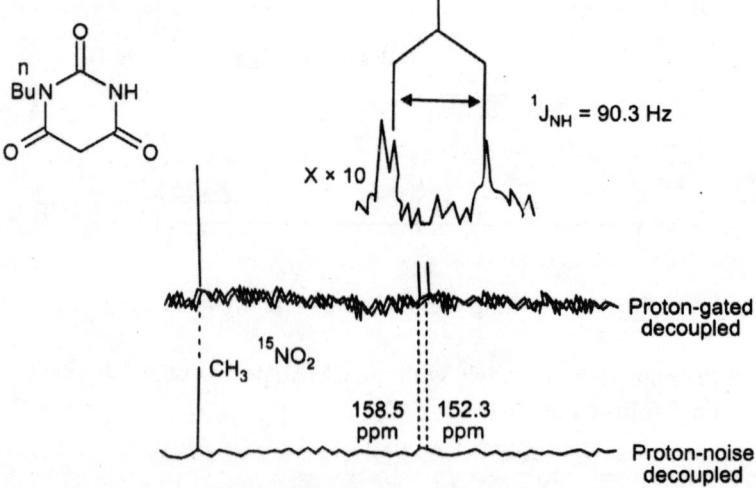

Fig. 14.3. ^{15}N NMR spectrum of 1–n-butylbarbituric acid.

Chemical shifts of some N-containing compounds is as under:

Compound	δ w.r. to liquid NH_3
CH_3NH_2	1.3
$CH_3CH_2CH_2NH_2$	19.8
$CH_3\text{--}CH\text{--}NH_2$ $\quad\;\;|$ $\quad\; CH_3$	43.6
$CH_3\text{--}(CH_2)_3NH_2$	21.0
$CH_3(CH_2)_4\text{--}NH_2$	43.6
(cyclohexyl-NH_2)	42.5
$CH_3\text{--}CH_2\text{--}NH$ $\qquad\qquad\;\;|$ $\qquad\qquad\; CH_3$	27.7

14.3 FLOURINE–19 NUCLEAR MAGNETIC RESONANCE

Fluorine with $I = 1/2$ has a sensitivity of ~ 0.83 of that of a proton. $YH/YF = 1.063$. F–19 has a natural abundance of 100%. At Bo = 7.05 T, while ^1H has a larmor frequency of 300.00 MHz and C–13, 75.43 MHz, N–15, 0.40 MHz, F–19 has 282.23 MHz. $CFCl_3$ is the standard reference used.

Fluorine–19 shows coupling to both H and ^{13}C.

$^2J_{FH}$ for $H-C-F$ unit = 60 Hz

$^3J_{FH}$ for $H-C-C-F$ unit = 20 Hz

The splitting of CH_2 group in 2,2,2– Trifluoroethanol is shown in Fig. 14.4. The CH_2

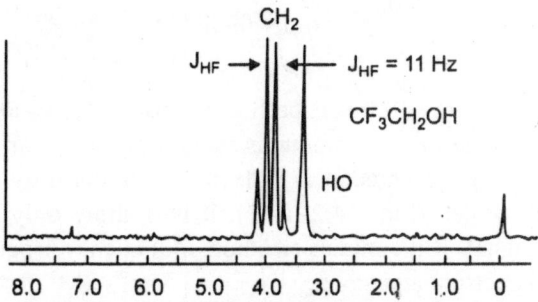

Fig. 14.4. The splitting of CH_2 group in the PMR spectrum of 2,2,2–Trifluoroethanol.

group is split into a quartet by the three neighbouring F–19 nuclei with $^3J_{FH}$ = 11 Hz.

In β-fluoropropionic acid $F-CH_2-CH_2-COOH$ (Fig. 14.5), the $^2J_{FH}$ ($F-CH_2$) is 45 Hz while $^3J_{FH}$ ($F-CH_2-CH_2$) is 24 Hz. As the chain length increases, coupling of fluorine to protons of third methylene group becomes very small, 0–3 Hz. No coupling is observed beyond that.

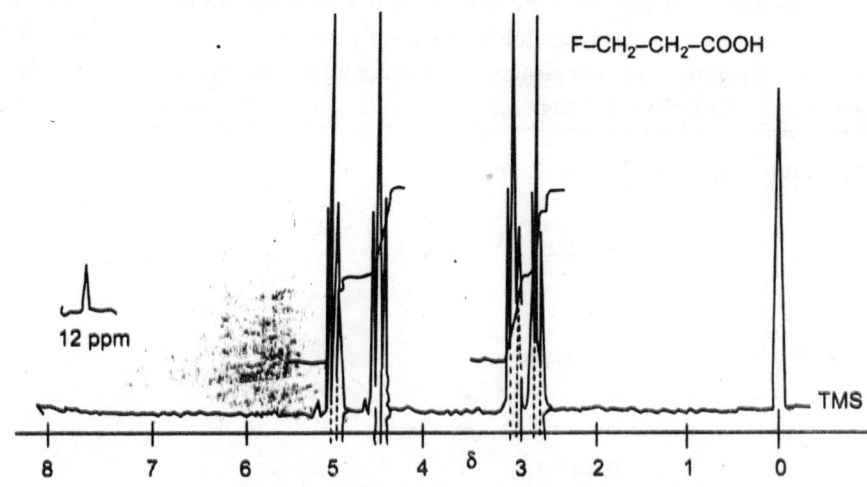

Fig. 14.5. Proton NMR spectrum of 3–fluoropropionic acid.

Intext Exercise

1. Can we distinguish the unsymmetrical "*T*-shaped" structure of ClF_3 from its probable trigonal planar and trigonal-bipyramidal structures on the basis of ^{19}F NMR spectrum?

   Solution : Yes, we can. If ClF_3 were to assume the structures – trigonal planar and trigonal bipyramidal, then all the fluorine atoms would be equivalent and would give us only one peak in the ^{19}F NMR spectrum. The real spectrum has more than one peak (Fig. 14.6). So, these two structures are ruled out. The spectrum actually shows a doublet and a triplet in the integral ratio of 2:1. This tells us the right structure of ClF_3 being two axial flourines and one equatorial around Cl. The singlet due to two equivalent F is split into a doublet by coupling with the equatorial F. The equatorial F is in turn split into a triplet by the two equivalent F as per the N + 1 rule.

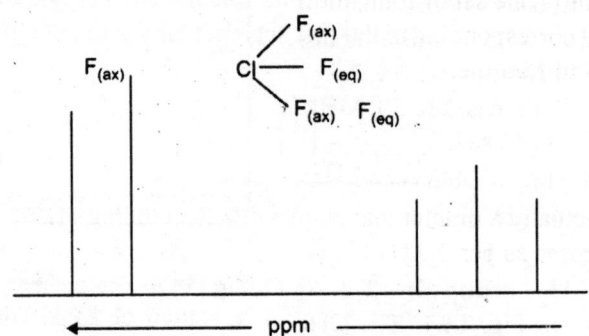

Fig. 14.6. ^{19}F (100% abundance) NMR spectrum of ClF_3.

2. Can you prove with the help of F–19 NMR spectroscopy the trigonal bipyramidal structure of SF_4?

Solution : Yes we can. If the two F atoms occupy the axial positions and the remaining two the equatorial positions, then the lone pair of electrons would occupy an equatorial site. In this geometry, we therefore have two groups of Fluorine atoms and we should, therefore, expect to see two triplets in the ratio 1:2:1 as per the N + 1 rule. This is indeed seen in the F–19 spectrum.

Some more typical J_{HF} values are as follows :

$$H_2C-C-CF$$ 0–4 Hz

$$\underset{H}{\overset{}{}}C=C\underset{F}{\overset{}{}}$$ 1–8 Hz

$$\underset{}{\overset{H}{}}C=C\underset{F}{\overset{}{}}$$ 12–40 Hz

---

Intext Exercise

3. How will you distinguish the following olefinic compounds?

$$\underset{}{\overset{H}{}}C=C\underset{F}{\overset{}{}} \qquad \underset{H}{\overset{}{}}C=C\underset{F}{\overset{}{}}$$

Answer : We can do that on the basis of J_{FH} :

For cis J_{HF} = 1–8 Hz

For trans J_{HF} = 12–40 Hz

Structure determination of BrF₅ using F–19

The F–19 NMR spectrum of BrF_5 shows two signals in the ratio 4:1. This shows that there are two sets of fluorines in the molecule – one set of four fluorines and the another one of the remaining fluorine. Further, the stronger signal corresponding to the first set is actually a doublet, that arises due to coupling with the other set of the fifth fluorine:

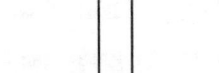

The weaker signal is actually a quintet that results due to coupling of one unique fluorine with the four equivalent fluorine atoms as per the N+1 rule:

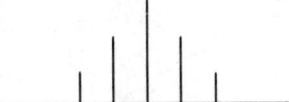

14.4 PHOSPHORUS–31 NMR SPECTROSCOPY

Phosphorus–31 with $I = 1/2$ has a natural abundance of 100% which makes it particularly suitable for analytical and NMR studies, despite its low sensitivity which is just 6.6% of that of hydrogen. If the ^1H resonance frequency is 100 MHz, that of P–31 is 40.48 MHz. $\gamma_P = 10840$.

The chemical shift of phosphorus is over 700 ppm (Fig. 14.7). The standard reference used is 85% H_3PO_4. Generally, the shielding decreases i.e. chemical shift increases with lowering of coordination

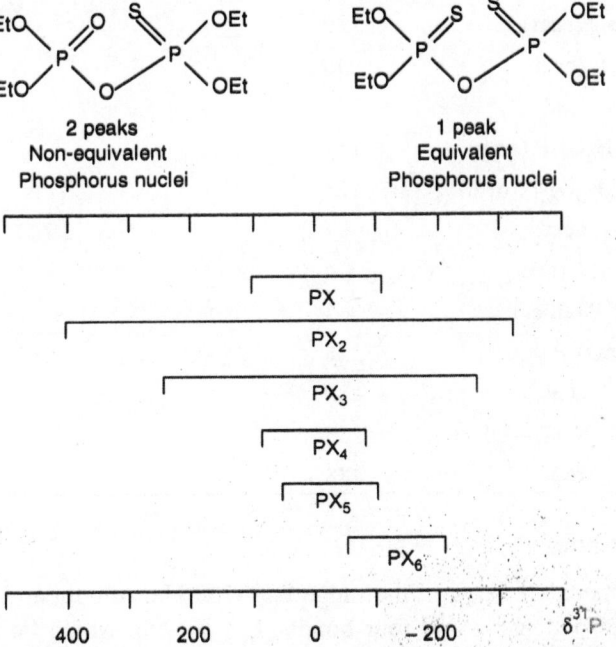

Fig. 14.7. The dependence of $\delta^{31}p$ on the coordination number of phosphorus.

number (some primary and secondary phosphines and two coordinated compounds are exceptional as they have negative chemical shift). The paramagnetic term is dominant in phosphorus compounds. The shielding is mainly caused by the electron localized on the different orbitals of the phosphorus atom. Further, the intermolecular effects like solvent effects are generally small as substituents isolate the phosphorus nucleus effectively from the surrounding molecules (Fig. 14.7).

14.4.1 Equivalent Phosphorous nuclei

The hydrogen-decoupled P–31 spectrum are of great use in compounds containing more than one phosphorus nucleus. If a compound shows only one signal in its proton decoupled spectrum, it contains only one phosphorus e.g.

H_3PO_3,	H_3PO_4,	$(EtO)_2P(O)OH$
1 peak	1 peak	1 peak
$(EtO)_3P$	$(EtO)_2P(S)SH$	$(Ph_3O)_3P$
1 peak	1 peak	1 peak

14.4.2 Non-equivalent P nuclei

If there are two peaks in the ^1H-decoupled P–31 spectrum, there are present two non-equivalent phosphorus nuclei in the molecule.

Table 14.2. δP shifts of some compounds w.r. to 85% H_3PO_4 (δ 0.0 ppm)

Compound	Sp	^{31}P couplings (CPS)
PBr_3 (neat)	− 229	
PCl_3 (neat)	− 220	
PI_3 (neat)	− 178	
$(CH_3O)_3P$ (neat)	+ 141	
$(C_6H_5O)_3P$ (neat)	+ 128	
PF_3 (neat)	− 97	1410
$POCl_3$ (neat)	− 5.4	
Ph_3P (ether)	− 4.5	
$(PhO)_3P$ (ether)	+ 18	
PCl_5 (CS_2)	+ 80	
PH_3 Neat, − 90°	+ 238	179
P_4 (CS_2)	+ 488	

14.4.3 Coupling constants

The J_{H-P} coupling constants are large in the range 200–700 Hz, of course, ^1J-bond (direct) coupling constants are larger than two, three and four bonds (J_{HC-PC}) etc. which lie in the range 0.5–20 Hz, which are similar to ^1H–^1H couplings in magnitude for 2 and 3–bond relationships.

$$\begin{array}{c} >P-H \\ \parallel \\ O \end{array}$$ J = 630–707 Hz

$(CH_3–CH_2)_3P$ $^3J_{HCCP} = 0.5$ Hz
                                         $^2J_{HCP} = 13.7$ Hz

$(CH_3–CH_2)_3PO$ $^3J_{(HCCP)} = 11.9$ Hz
                                         $^2J_{(HCP)} = 16.3$ Hz

$$\begin{array}{c} O \\ \parallel \\ CH_3 — P - (OR)_2 \end{array}$$ $^3J_{HP} = 10–13$ Hz

Examples

1. Dimethylmethylphosphonate:

$$\begin{array}{c} O \\ \parallel \quad /OCH_3 \\ CH_3 — P \\ \qquad \backslash OCH_3 \end{array}$$

The ^{1}H NMR spectrum of this compound shows a doublet (3H) due to CH_3P at δ 1.481 ppm with $^2J_{HP} = 17.4$ Hz and another doublet (6H) centred at d 3.741 ppm due to 2 × CH_3O protons with $^3J_{HP} = 11.0$ Hz.

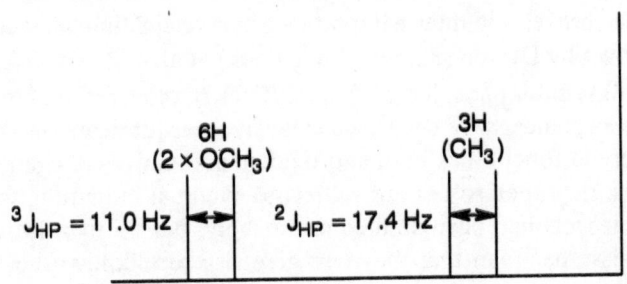

2. NMR spectrum of trimethyl phosphine, $(P(CH_3)_3$. The ^{31}P NMR spectrum of this molecule shows a doublet due to coupling with the methyl protons. The $^2J_{PH}$ is found to be 3.0Hz:

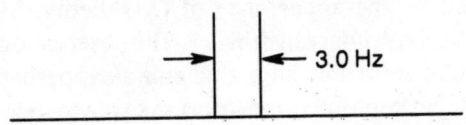

Coupling constants observed in some common compounds are collected in Table 14.3.

Table 14.3. ^{31}P coupling constants (cps) of some common compounds

1. PH_3	179	P-H
2. PF_3	1410	P-F
3. CH_3PH_2	207	P-H
4. $(CH_3)_2PH$	207	P-H
5. $(CH_3O)_2HPO$	690.3	P-H
6. $(CH_3)_3PO$	11.19	$P-H(CH_3)$
7. $(CH_3CH_2O)O$	8.38	$P-H(CH_2)$
8. ATP	480	P-P
	19.3	$P\alpha-P\beta$
	19.3	$P\beta-Py$
	0.0	$P\alpha-Py$

14.4.4 Applications of P–31 NMR Spectroscopy

P–31 NMR has many applications, some of which are as follows:

14.4.5 Elucidation of Mechanism of Reactions

14.4.6 Hydrolysis of Zinc (II) O,O-Dialkyl dithiophosphates (ZDTPs)

P–31 has been used to investigate the mechanism of Zinc (II) O,O–dialkyl dithiophosphates. This is represented by the hydrolysis of the corresponding diethyl derivative. This example shows that how P–31 NMR spectroscopy can prove of immense importance in investigating the mechanism of complicated molecules. This was shown by Dewan (author of this book) et al.

Zinc (II) bis (O,O-dialkyl dithiophosphates), $Zn[S_2P(OR)_2]_2$, often referred to as 'normal' or 'neutral' zinc O,O-dialkyl dithiophosphates, have been used extensively as lubricant oil-additives for many years, owing to their dual ability to function as both anti-oxidant and anti-wear agents. While improving the performance of base oils, they themselves are subject to eventual oxidation, thermal degradation and hydrolysis. The former aspects had been studied extensively, but till then little was known about the nature of their hydrolysis other than that they can give rise to unknown acidic oil-soluble and oil-insoluble products which lead to degradation and loss of performance.

Mechanistically, it can be assumed that attack by water on ZDTP (1) (+ 101 ppm) could occur at one or more sites, including the α-carbon of the ethyl group, the phosphorus atom, and the metal atom. From ^{31}P NMR spectra of the hydrolysis (Fig. 14.8) initial attack of water was found to occur exclusively at the metal atom as evidenced by the appearance of O,O-diethyl S-hydrogen phosphorodithioate, $(EtO)_2P(S)SH$ (3) (+ 84.6 ppm) as the primary hydrolysis. The observation of (3) as the primary hydrolysis product points to the concomitant formation of a zinc complex, perhaps (2), (see Fig. 14.9) although the latter was not detected per se, in solution (vide infra). As shown in Fig. 14.10 subsequent hydrolysis of (3) yielded firstly phosphorothioic O,O,O-acid (6) (+ 58.7 ppm), and then phosphoric acid (7) (0.0 ppm), followed by O-ethyl O,O-dihydrogen phosphorothioate (9) (+ 64.1 ppm) and ethyl dihydrogen phosphate (10) (− 0.3 ppm), in that order.

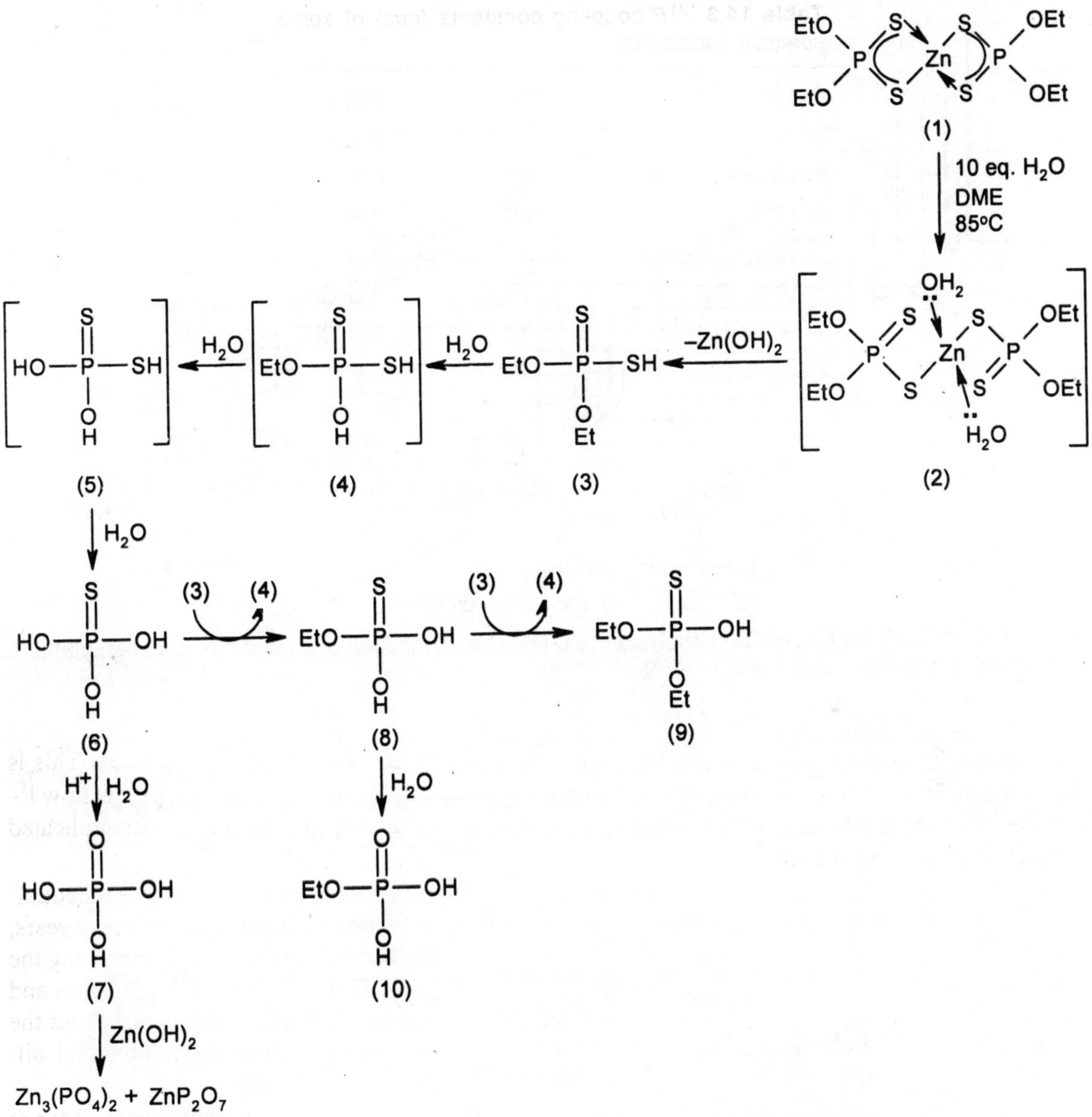

Fig. 14.9. Mechanism for the hydrolysis of zinc(II) O,O-diethyl dithiophosphate (1).

Formation of (3) as the key intermediate in the hydrolysis of (1) was confirmed by the fact that under the same conditions of hydrolysis, an authentic sample of (3) produced the same products in identical proportions. Since the conversion of (3) into (6) involves a radical change of structure, it was reasonable to assume that the stepwise loss of the functional groups occured as shown in Fig. 14.11 whereby O-ethyl O,S-dihydrogen phosphorodithioate (4) and phosphorodithioic O,O,S-acid (5) are formed as intermediates. Under the original conditions of hydrolysis (85°C and 10 equiv. of water) these compounds (4) and (5) were not observed by ^{31}P NMR spectroscopy as intermediates, but

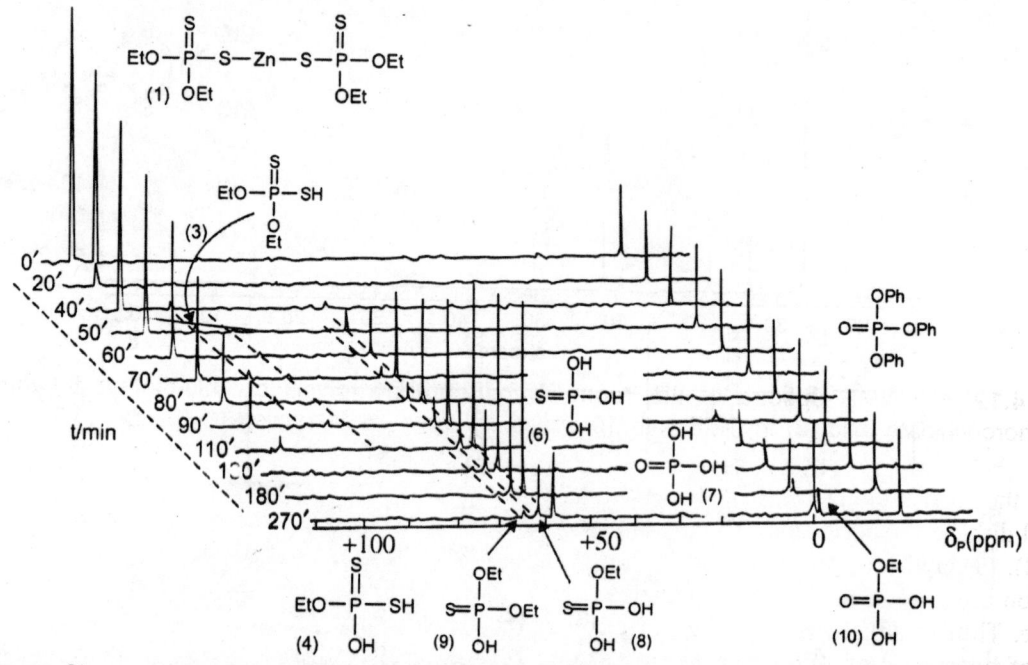

Fig. 14.10. ^{31}P NMR spectra of the hydrolysis of ZDTP (1) as a function of time in 1,2–dimethoxyethane, DME at 85 ± 1°C with equivalent of water.

monitoring of the hydrolysis of (3) to (6) at a lower temperature (25°C) revealed the involvement of two phosphorus-containing species at +78.1 and + 71.3 ppm [Fig. 14.12a]. The identity of these two intermediates as the dithiophosphate (4), and dithiophosphoric acid (5), respectively, was established from the ^1H-coupled spectrum which showed a quintet for (3), triplet for (4) and singlets for (5) and (6) as expected ($^3J_{PH}$ = *ca.* 10 Hz).

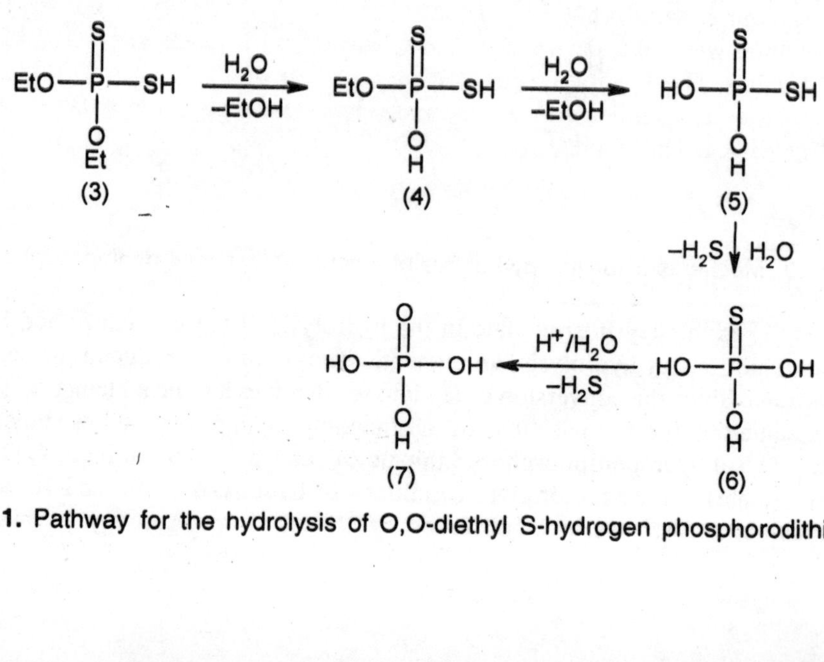

Fig. 14.11. Pathway for the hydrolysis of O,O-diethyl S-hydrogen phosphorodithioate (3).

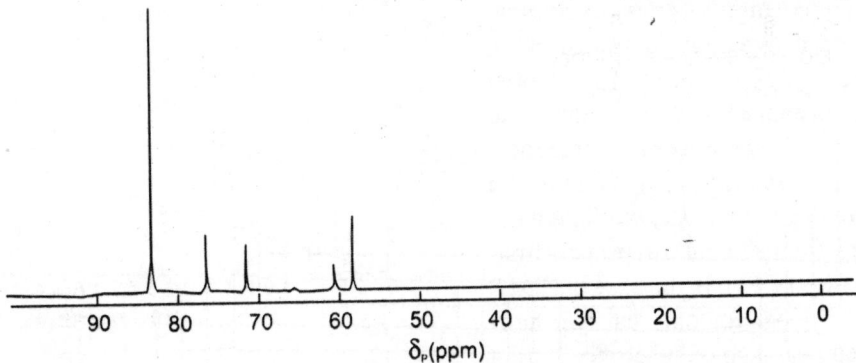

Fig. 14.12. ^{31}P NMR spectra of the room temperature hydrolysis of O,O-diethyl S-hydrogen phosphorodithioate acid (3) in DME with 10 equiv. of water: [1]H-decoupled.

Of the final product (7), (8), (9), and (10) obtained from the hydrolyses of both ZDTP (1) and diethyl dithiophosphoric acid (3), only (7) arises directly by hydrolysis. Reference to Fig. 14.3 shows that (8), (9), and (10) are produced in that order i.e. (8)→(9)→(10) but so far, so good. But now a question arises as to how do intermediates (8), (9) and (10) arise? This is where kinetics comes into picture. Thus the question as to their origin was answered by kinetic investigations into the relative rates of hydrolysis of ZDTP (1), its primary hydrolysis product (3) and the subsequently obtained phosphorothioic acid (6) as explained next.

Kinetic studies: Kinetic analyses for the hydrolyses of ZDTP (1), diethyl phosphorodithioate (3) and phosphorothioic acid (6) were carried out individually under identical conditions, viz. 85°C/DME and 10 equivalent of water, by monitoring their respective rates of disappearance using ^{31}P NMR spectroscopy. It was necessary to use triphenyl phosphate as an inert internal standard control. Experiments showed that triphenyl phosphate is not hydrolysed under the kinetic conditions. The [1]H-decoupled spectra were obtained under conditions in which the T_1 values of the various species were taken into account. [31]P spin-lattice (T_1) relaxation times were determined from proton-decoupled inversion-recovery Fourier transform (IRFT) spectra using a $(-T-180°-\tau-90°-)_n$ pulse sequence. The 90 and 180° pulse times were 20.5 and 41 μs; T was 60s; and typical values of τ were 0.02, 0.08, 0.5, 1, 2, 3, 4, 5, 7, 15, and 20 s. The T_1 values were calculated with the JEOL T_1 program which uses a least-squares fit to equation (1). Duplicate measurements suggest a precision of ± 10%. The results are summarised in Table 14.4. Thus, under these conditions, the:

$$(M_o - M_z)/2M_o = \exp(-t/T_1)$$ (1)

Table 14.4. [31]NMR spin-lattice (T_1) relaxation times for the compounds observed in the ZDTP hydrolysis studies

Compound	T_1/s	Compound	T_1/s
Triphenyl phosphate	18.2	(6)	6.1
(1)	7.1	(7)	2.4
(3)	10.2	(8)	16.9
(4)	13.4	(9)	14.2
(5)	15.6	(10)	3.5

Thus, the signal intensities were proportional to their respective concentrations. In the case of ZDTP (1), it was found to be essential to use freshly prepared samples otherwise induction periods were observed presently arising from surface hydrolysis and the formation of coatings of zinc(II) oxide. All the hydrolysis were found to follow pseudo-first-order kinetics (Fig. 14.13); in the case of ZDTP (1) the plot was linear for only ca. two half-lives of the disappearance of substrate. During this period the only products to be observed were (3) and (6), i.e. before the formation of (8), (9), and (10), and the pH of the hydrolysis mixture decreased from 4.5 to 1.0. Thereafter, the plot for the hydrolysis of (1) showed an exponential increase presumably due to auto acid catalysis since no change occurred in the rate profile, even in the presence of large excess of water (30 equiv.).

The calculated pseudo-first-order rate constants (k_{obs}) for each species are presented in Table 14.5 and clearly establish that the rate of hydrolysis of the phosphorothioic acid (6) is very slow compared with that of its precursor the O,O-diethyl phosphorodithioate (3) which in turn is hydrolysed at a faster rate than ZDTP

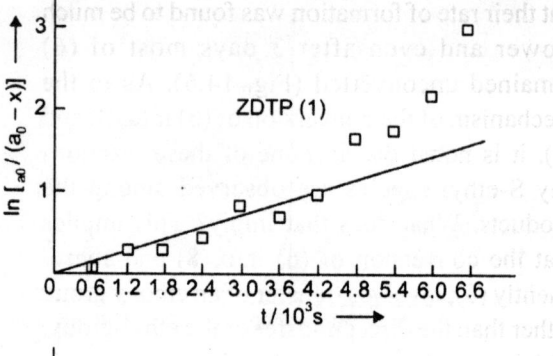

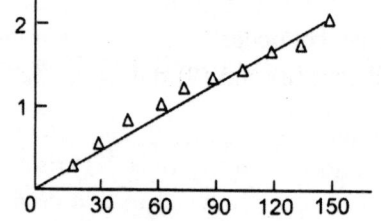

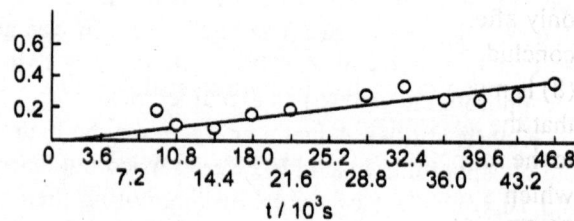

Fig. 14.13. Plots of pseudo-first-order decay of (1), (3), and (6) at 85 ± 1°C in DME with 10 equiv. of water.

(1). Obviously, this leads to a build-up in the concentration of (6) in the hydrolysis mixture (Fig. 10.1) and suggests that both monoethyl thiophosphate (8) and diethyl thiophosphate (9) originate from the esterification of (6) with (3) and/or ethanol which is a product of the hydrolysis (3). This assumption was verified when thiophosphoric acid (6) and O,O-diethyl S-hydrogen phosphorodithioate (3) were mixed in a 1:2 molar ratio in anhydrous DME and, upon being heated at 85°C for 15 minutes, were found to produce (8) and (9) together with the transesterification by-product (4) (Fig. 14.6). The same products could also be obtained from the esterification of (6) with ethanol under identical conditions

Table 14.5. Rate constant (k) for hydrolysis of (1), (3) and (6) under pseudo-first-order conditions (10 equiv. of water and 85 ± 1°C in DME)

Compound	$k_{obs}/10^{-4}$ s^{-1}
(1)	2.35
(3)	135.0
(6)	0.078

(8), (9) and (10) are formed only after the formation of (6)

but their rate of formation was found to be much slower and even after 3 days most of (6) remained unconverted (Fig. 14.6). As to the mechanism of the conversion of (6) into (8) and (9), it is noted that in none of these reactions any S-ethyl species are observed among the products. What does that imply? This implies that the conversion of (6) into (8) and subsequently (9), involves transfer of an ethoxy group rather than the direct transfer of the ethyl-group, which would be expected to lead to some S-ethylation that does not occur.

Further proof that (8) and (9) did not arise by the direct hydrolyses of (4) and (3) respectively, was obtained by monitoring the hydrolysis of (3) at room temperature to completion, whence (8) and (9) were observed only after the formation of (6). Thus, it can be concluded that the rate of esterification of (6) to (8) is much faster than its hydrolysis to (7) and that the subsequent hydrolysis of (8) gave rise to the formation of (10) as depicted in Fig. 14.9 which summarises the overall breakdown of ZDTP (1).

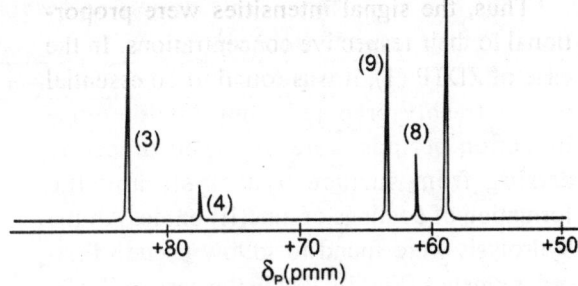

Fig. 14.14. ^{31}P NMR H-decoupled spectrum of the reaction between phosphorothioic O,O,O-acid (6) and (3) in anhydrous DME at $85 \pm 1°C$ after 15 min.

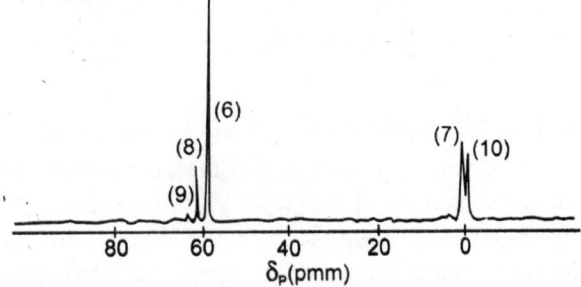

Fig. 14.15. ^{31}P NMR H-decoupled spectrum of the reaction of (6) with ethanol in anhydrous DME at $85 \pm 1°C$ after 3 days.

Finally, turning to the ultimate fate of the zinc in (1), it was note that hydrolysis is accompanied by the gradual formation of a colourless precipitate. It was assumed that the initially formed zinc complex (2) was transformed into insoluble zinc hydroxide, but the yield of precipitate was considerably higher than that expected (154% based on zinc hydroxide). An explanation for this ambiguity is that the zinc hydroxide undergoes further reactions with hydrogen sulphide and phosphoric acid formed during hydrolysis. This viewpoint is supported by the elemental analysis of a typical precipitate (Table 14.6) which showed that its composition is probably best formulated as a mixture of zinc hydroxide, zinc oxide, zinc sulphide, and zinc phosphates. Indeed, treatment of the precipitate with mineral acid resulted in evolution of hydrogen sulphide indicating the presence of a metal sulphide. In addition, ^{31}P NMR analysis of a solution of the precipitate in 2 mol dm^{-3} sodium hydroxide solution showed signals at +6.3 and +4.1 ppm which are identical with those for authentic samples of sodium phosphate and pyrophosphate, respectively. No NMR signals for sodium thiophosphate and/or pyrothiophosphate were observed. The yield of precipitate and soluble products increased and decreased, respectively, with time in keeping with the increase in concentration of phosphoric acid. The elemental ratios for the precipitate also changed with time, although it is important to note that the recovery of zinc from (1) in the precipitate was almost quantitative ($96.25 \pm 0.05\%$) regardless of its composition. This fact further reinforces the mechanism shown in Fig. 14.9 wherein attack of water occurs at the zinc centre, and in consequence does not give rise to any metal-containing soluble products.

Table 14.6. Elemental analysis of a precipitate from the hydrolysis of ZDTP (1)

Element	% weight	Elemental ratio
Zn	41.0	1
S	7.6	0.38
P	16.9	0.87
C	1.3	0.18
H	1.5	2.38
O	31.7	3.18

Further, to prove the point that the initial and rate determining step in the above hydrolysis reaction of zinc O,O-diethyl dithiophosphate, the corresponding cadmium (II) and nickel (II) dithiophosphates were subjected to hydrolysis. Comparison of the kinetic results showed that the order for rates of hydrolysis for the dithiophosphates for the metals was

$$Zn\ dtp > Cd\ dtp > Ni\ dtp$$

This is in keeping with the M–S bond strength.

Thus, you have seen that in the above example, where the products could not be isolated by the popular technique of thin layer chromatography (TlC), the research work has elegantly demonstrated that P–31 NMR spectroscopy could prove a wonderful tool in our hand to unravel the complexities of the reaction mechanism of reactions like hydrolysis of the zinc O,O-diethyl dithiophosphate.

14.4.7 Thermal Degradation of Zinc-O, O-Diethyl Dithiophosphate

As mentioned in the previous section Zinc dialkyl dithiophosphate (ZDTPs) have been widely used as commercial lubricant additives in the engine oils for their anti-wear action over half-a-century now. Despite a great deal of research, precisely how do the ZDTPs perform their anti-wear function is not clear as yet, although it is widely believed that they act by undergoing thermal degradation at higher temperature of the order of 170–190°C. So, Dewan (this author) reported investigation of their thermal degradation under such conditions i.e. at 190° in n-hexa-decane.

The thermal degradation of Zinc O, O-diethyl dithiophosphate was investigated at 190°C in n-hexadecane. The major products were identified as O, S, S-triethyl trithiophosphate, $(EtS)_2P(S)\ OEt$, O,O,S-triethyl dithiophosphate, EtS P(S) $(OEt)_2$, S,S,S-triethyl tetrathiophosphate, $(EtS)_3\ PS$, O,S,S-triethyl dithiophosphate, $(EtS)_3\ PS$, O,S,S,-triethyl dithiophosphate, $(EtS)_2\ P(O)\ OEt$, and O,O,S-triethyl thiophosphate, EtS P(O) $(OET)_2$. The degradation is suggested to involve thiono-thiolo isomerisation coupled with disproportionation of sulfur and oxygen linked to phosphorus.

The ZDTP readily underwent total decomposition in ca 45 min when heated at 190°C in dry n-hexadecane under nitrogen, giving a complicated mixture of products as indicated by the appearance of 7 new peaks in its [31]p NMR spectrum at 109.5, 95.8, 90.7, 69.5, 66.1, 53.7 and 27.6 pm as shown in Fig. 14.16. Since the peak at 96.5 ppm due to the diethyl ZDTP itself was absent, it was clear that the zinc dithiophosphate had undergone complete thermal decomposition to give rise to a number of phosphorus containing products.

Attempts to isolate the products by chromatography proved unsuccessful. The spectrum of the

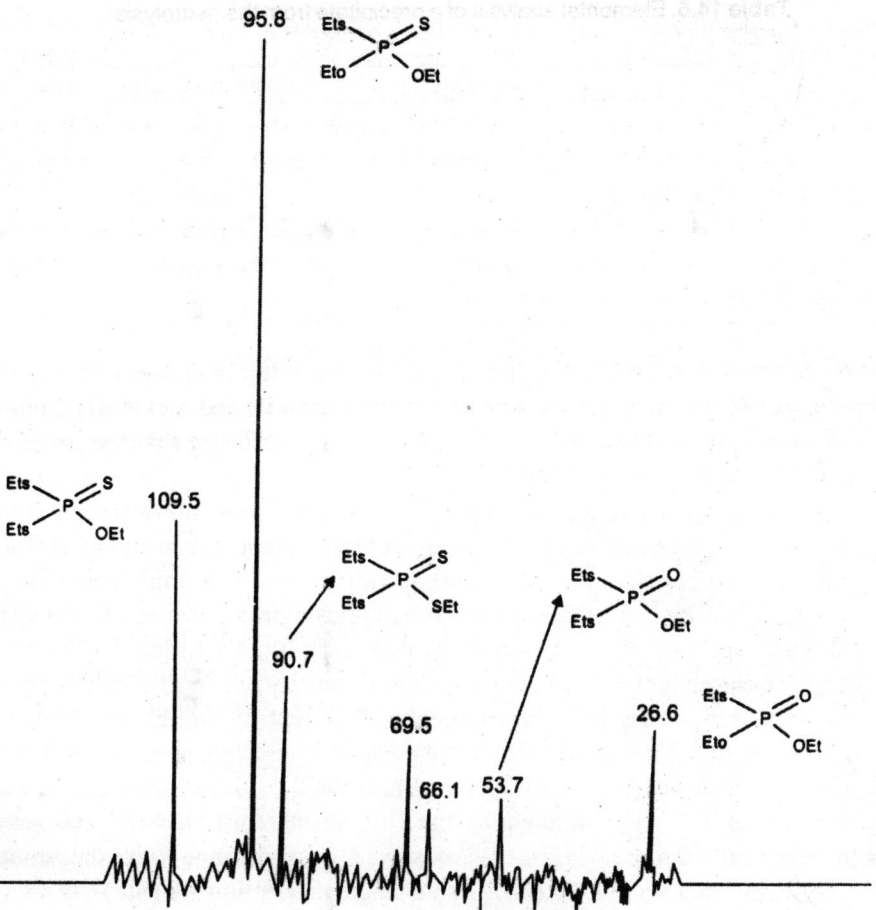

Fig. 14.16. ^{1}H-decoupled ^{31}P NMR spectrum of the thermal degradation products of zinc(II)-diethyldithiophosphate in the n-hexadecane after 45 min. at 190°C.

product mixture was very complicated, although it did show the presence of both P–O–CH as well as P–S–CH signals. However, Dewan used P–31 NMR spectroscopy for this purpose. Thus, the major products with ^{31}P chemical shifts at 109.5, 95.8, 90.7, 53.7 and 27.6 ppm were identified as O,S,S-triethyl trithiophosphate (EtS)$_2$, P(S) OEt, O,O,S-triethyl thiophosphate, (Ets) P(S) (OEt)$_2$, S,S,S-triethyl tetrathiophosphate (EtS)$_3$ P(S), O,S,S,-triethyl dithiophosphate (EtS)$_2$ P(O) (OEt) and O,O,S-triethyl thiophosphate, EtS P(O) (OEt)$_2$ respectively. Such types of products have been identified in the thermal depredation of zinc n-butyl dithiophosphate complexes. Based upon ^{31}p NMR analysis, these products were obtained in 19.8, 44.9, 10.8, 4.5 and 9.3% yield respectively. The identity of the remaining two (minor) peaks with shifts 69.5 (7.2%) and 66.1 ppm (3.6%) could not be known. However, neither was shown to correspond to O,O,O-triethyl thiophosphate, (EtO)$_3$ PS, an authentic sample of which resonated at 68.3 ppm. Identification of products was based on the "peak enhancement" of the ^{1}H-decoupled ^{31}P NMR signal on addition of an authentic samples to the reaction mixtures. The products identity was further confirmed by infra-red analysis which showed the presence of P–O–C (900–1300 cm^{-1}), P.S.C.

(500 cm^{-1}) and P=S (800–850 cm^{-1}) groups. Hydrogen sulfide and ethyl mercaptan were identified as the volatile products. A colorless solid was also formed which gave off hydrogen sulfide upon treatment with dilute HCl, indicating it to be mainly zinc sulfide.

Judging from the nature of the products formed, it seems highly likely that the mechanism of this fascinating degradation involves thiono-thiolo isomerization coupled with disproportionation as reported for some thiophosphoryl compounds.

In conclusion, it is clear that P–31 NMR spectroscopy has proved to be a wonderful tool in our hands to investigate this reaction involving complicated thermal decomposition as the products could not be isolated by TLC and also ^{1}H NMR was not successful.

14.4.8 Determination of Enantiomeric Excess of Chiral Alcohols

The enantiomeric excess of chiral alcohols can be obtained from the ratio of integrations of ^{31}P n.m.r. absorptions of diastereoisomeric O,O-dialkyl dithioates (3, $X = S$) derived therefrom.

Recently methods for determination of the enantiomeric excess (e.e.) of chiral alcohols, thiols, amino acid esters, and primary amines have been reported. The principle involved is the ^{31}P n.m.r. analysis of diastereoisomeric phosphorus derivatives of these compounds using PCl$_3$ (for alcohols) or MePXCl$_2$ ($X = O$ or S) as derivatizing agents. Consequently no auxiliary chiral compound is necessary in order to determine the e.e. by this method. In the case of phosphonates, derived from racemic alcohols, a mixture of a ($\pm$)-pair and two *meso*-isomers is formed, as is illustrated for *di-(s-buty)* phosphonate (Scheme). When a non-pseudochiral phosphorus atom is present, as in (3), only a ($\pm$) pair and one *meso*-isomer are expected. In general this stereochemical feature would be of advantage in e.e. determinations as only two ^{31}P n.m.r. signals will be present for racemic compounds. Phosphates (3, X = O, R = Bu^s) show only one absorption at – 0.16 p.p.m. (CDCl$_3$). It is remarkable that despite the high symmetry at phosphorus, ^{31}P n.m.r. non-equivalence for diastereoisomeric ($\pm$ and *meso*) O,O-di(s-butyl) hydrogen phosphorodithioate (Fig. 14.17) is observed. In accordance with expectation two singlets (50:50 ratio) for ($\pm$)- and *meso*-(4) ($\Delta\delta$ 6.6 Hz) and a single absorption for (S,S)-(4) are found.

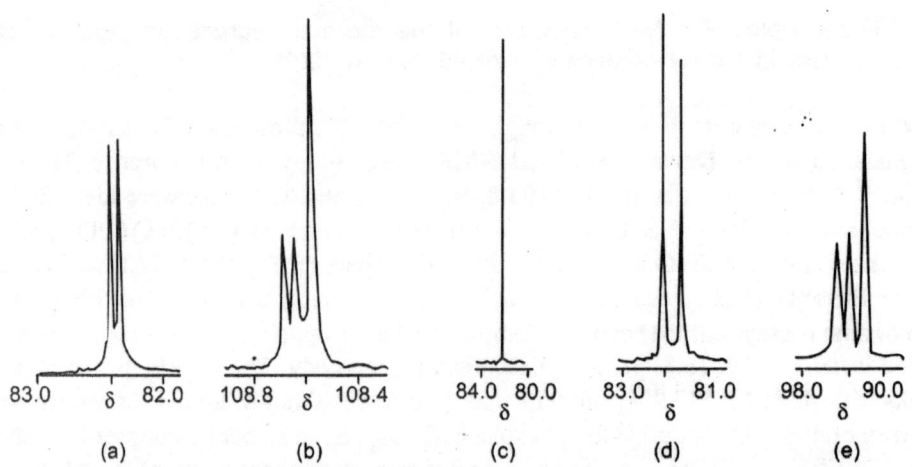

Fig. 14.17. ^{31}P n.m.r. spectra at 80.988 MHz [CDCl$_3$, 85% H$_3$PO$_4$ (d 0.0 ppm) as external standard]: (a) (4) derived from racemic s-butyl alcohol; (b) (–)-cinchonidine salt of racemic (4); (c) (7) derived from (–)-menthol; (d) (7) derived from racemic menthol; (e) (–)-cinchonidine salt os racemic (7).

Various chiral alcohols were converted into phosphorodithionic derivatives by stirring at 20°C a CDCl$_3$ solution of 2 equivalent of alcohol and 1 equivalent of O,O-diphenyldithioic-acid as a thiophosphorylating agent (Fig. 14.17). Fig. 14.17(d) shows the ^{31}P n.m.r. spectrum of derived from racemic menthol following this procedure. These results indicate that (5) can be used as an alternative reagent for determination of the e.e. of chiral alcohols, although chemical shift differences are generally smaller for the *meso-* and ($\pm$)-pair of these phosphorus derivatives. Furthermore it was possible to discriminate between the *meso-* and ($\pm$)-phosphorodithioic acids using chiral tertiary amines. The (–)-cinchonidine salts of (4) and (7) clearly give ^{31}P n.m.r. nonequivalence only for one of the phosphorodithioic isomers (Fig. 1). The low field ^{31}P n.m.r. absorption of acids (4) and (7) can therefore be assigned to the (RR, SS)-pair. These diastereoisomeric salts belong to dynamic diastereoisomeric systems and their n.m.r. nonequivalence critically depends on solvent, and amine structure and concentration. So far we have observed this phenomenon only using racemic phosphorodithioic acids with chiral tertiary amines in CDCl$_3$.

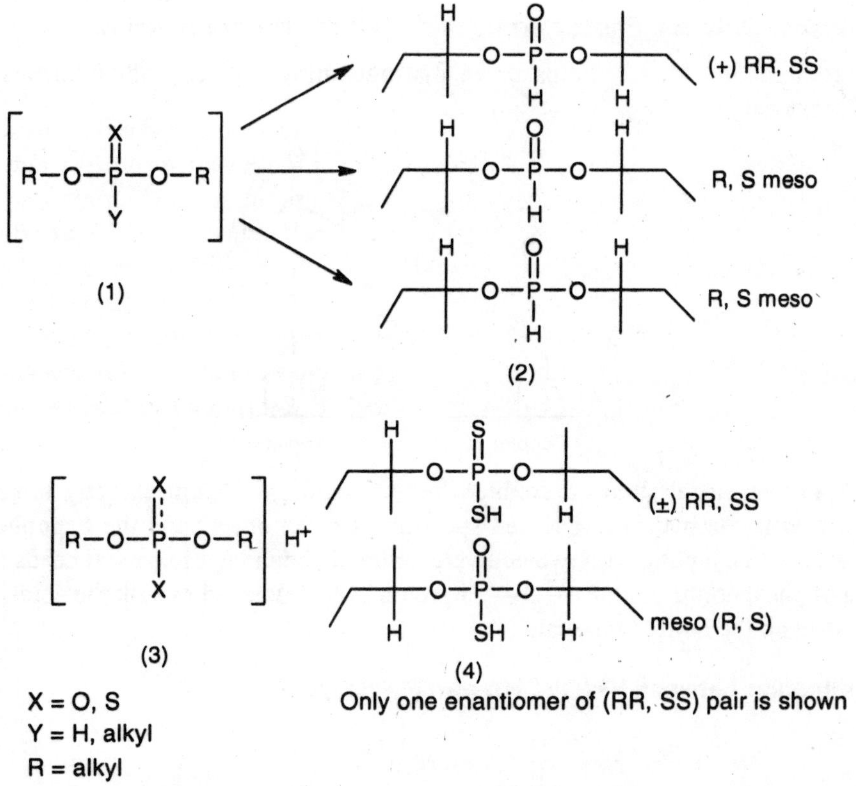

X = O, S
Y = H, alkyl
R = alkyl

Only one enantiomer of (RR, SS) pair is shown

Fig. 14.18 Only one enantiomer of (RR, SS) pair is shown.

These results demonstrated for the first time ^{31}P n.m.r. nonequivalence of diastereoisomeric salts of thiophosphates non-chiral at phosphorus. These observations might also be useful in elucidating the role of the prochiral phosphorus atom as a potential chiral binding site in phospholipids.

14.4.9 Distinction between Phosphorous and Hypophosphorous Acids

^{21}P NMR spectroscopy readily helps us in distinguishing between phosphorous (H_3PO_3) and hypophosphorous acid (H_3PO_2).

The phosphorous signal shows a doublet due to coupling with one directly linked hydrogen in phosphorous acid in the hydrogen-coupled spectrum. On the other hand the hypophosphorous acid shows a triplet due to coupling with two equivalent directly bound hydrogens. It needs to be noted that the coupling of phosphorous with P — O — H proton is not observed in both the acids because of fast proton exchange on the NMR time-scale.

14.4.10 Distinction between FP(O)(OH)$_2$ and F$_2$P(O)OH

The compound (I) shows a doublet in its P–31 spectrum (Fig. 14.18) due to coupling of P with the single fluorine (I = 1/2). Compound (II) shows a triplet due to coupling with the two fluorine atoms.

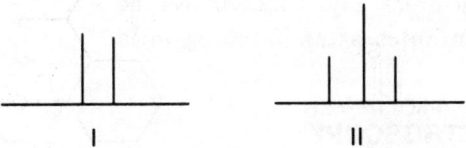

Fig. 14.19. ^{31}P NMR spectra of compounds (I) and (II).

14.4.11 Structure determination of P$_4$S$_3$

The structure of P_4S_3 is shown in Fig. 14.19. P–31 spectrum of this compound shows only two signals in the ratio 3:1 (A_3X system). That means there are two types of phosphorous nuclei in this molecule, three of one type and the single one of another type. This fits in with the proposed structure (Fig. 14.19).

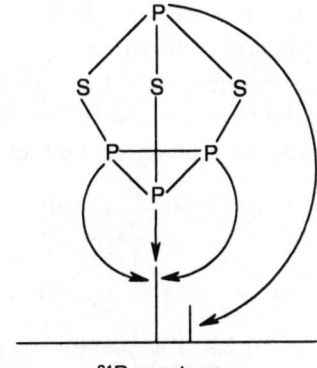

^{31}P spectrum

Fig. 14.20. The origin of two peaks in P$_4$S$_3$ in the P–31 spectrum.

14.4.12 ^{31}P NMR in Living Bodies

^{31}P NMR spectroscopy has been used for unravelling the mysteries of metabolism as well as to investigate the effects of and recovery from ischaemia (it means curtailment of supply of oxygen) at the metabolic level in a variety of tissues. Using this technique, partial and global mycardial ischaemia, ischaemic skeletal muscle and a model of kidney transplant have been investigated.

^{31}P NMR spectrum of the abdominal region of a live rat is shown in the Fig. 14.21. The three peaks β, α and γ are due to ATP. The next deshielded peak is due to PCr (Phosphocreatine) and Pi (the inorganic phosphate).

Further, ^{31}P NMR has been used in identifying and studying a disorder as recorded in Fig. 14.21 which shows the spectra obtained from the palmeris longus muscle, the muscle present in the forearm that is mainly responsible for clenching the fist. Fig. 14.21 shows the normal spectrum

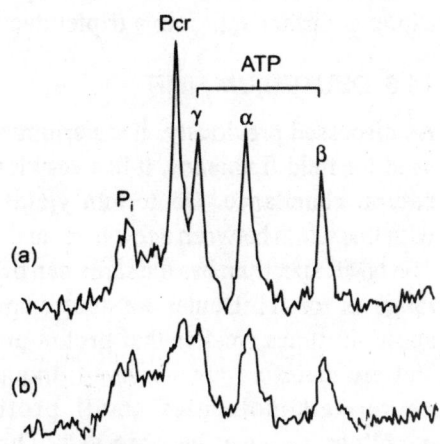

Fig. 14.21. ^{31}P spectra from the abdominal region of an intact live rat: (a) sensitive volume 40 mm diameter, (b) sensitive volume 20 mm diameter.

with ATP, PCr and Pi, in that order. Fig. 14.22 shows the spectrum obtained fifteen minutes after inducing mild ischaemia.

14.5 BORON-11 NMR SPECTROSCOPY

Boron-11 has spin of 3/2. Its natural abundance is 80.1%. Its receptivity is 0.133 compared to that of proton. The NMR spectra of *B-H* is of great importance in boron-containing compounds.

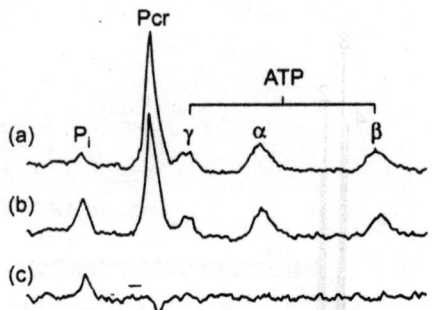

Fig. 14.22. ^{31}P spectra from human forearm: (a) normal resting condition, (b) 15 minutes after applying a tourniquet to the upper arm, (c) difference (a)–(b).

Structure of Diborane, B_2H_6

Diborane is known to occur in the following structure. The two BH_3 units are joined together such that there is no *B–B* bond, four terminal hydrogen lie in one plane and the remaining two join the two boron atoms and are therefore called bridging hydrogens and these lie in a plane perpendicular to the plane containing the two boron with four hydrogen atoms. In this example, we show here how proton and boron nmr spectra are of great help in confirming the structure of diborane.

B–11 spectrum is shown in the Fig. 14.23. The spectrum was taken of $^{11}B_2H_6$ which contained isotopically pure Boron–11 as the natural diborane also contains the normal ^{10}B with natural abundance of 19.6%. It is clear from the spectrum that the spectrum contains a triplet of triplets. The two borons are equivalent. Each boron is split by the two bridged hydrogens into a triplet and then each line of the triplet is further split into a triplet due to coupling with the two terminal hydrogens it is bonded to.

14.6 DEUTERIUM NMR

As discussed previously, ^{2}Deuterium NMR is usually used for field frequency. It has very low sensitivity at natural abundance. Deuterium yields broad signals with line width between a few hertz and a few kilohertz. The NMR spectrum has the same narrow chemical shift range as for ^1H. Deuterium-deuterium couplings are about 40 times smaller that proton-proton couplings and are therefore not observed, though, in partially deuterated molecules small proton-deuterium couplings $J_{H,D}$ can be observed. The major use of deuterium spectra is for determining the effectiveness of chemical deuteration as shown in Fig. 14.24 for effective specific deuteration of the methyl group of amphetamine sulfate-d$_3$.

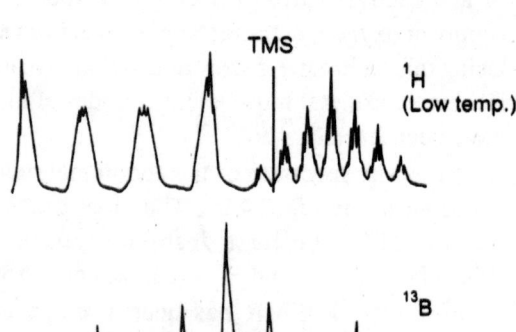

Fig. 14.23. (i) ^1H NMR and (ii) ^{11}B NMR of isotopically pure ^{11}B containing diborane.

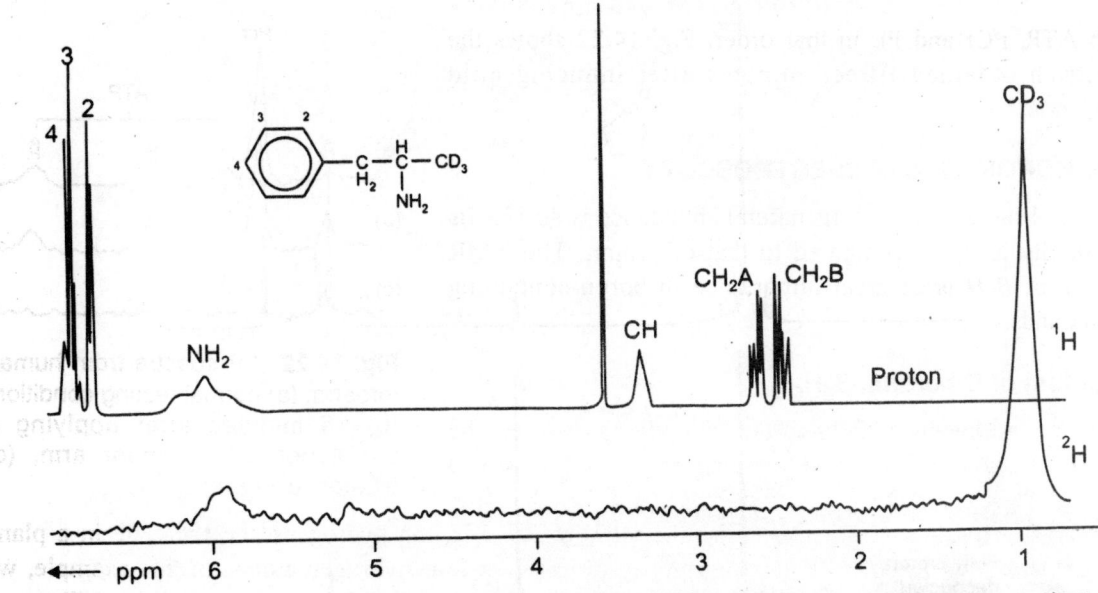

Fig. 14.24. Deuterium (and ^1H) spectra showing effective deuteration of the methyl group in amphetamine sulfate-d_3 in TFA-d (some deuteration of the NH$_2$ also occurs).

Similarly, Fig. 14.25 shows the ^2H NMR spectrum along with ^1H NMR spectrum of sec-butyl crotonate at 360.1 MHz. Fig. 14.26 shows the ^2H NMR as well as ^1H NMR spectra of another reaction for replacement of OH by Br in the mono-deuterated cyclopentane molecule.

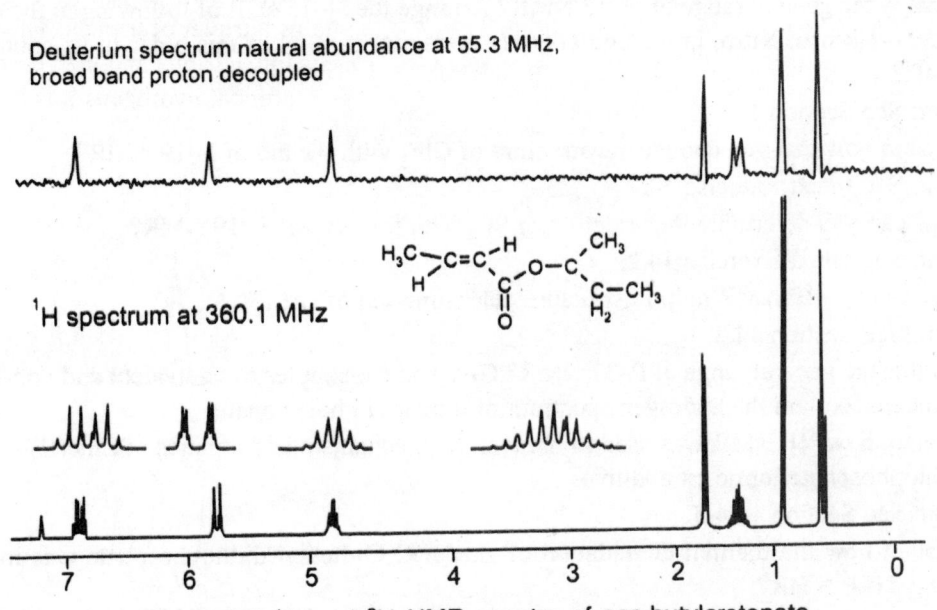

Fig. 14.25. ^1H and ^2H NMR spectra of sec-butylcrotonate.

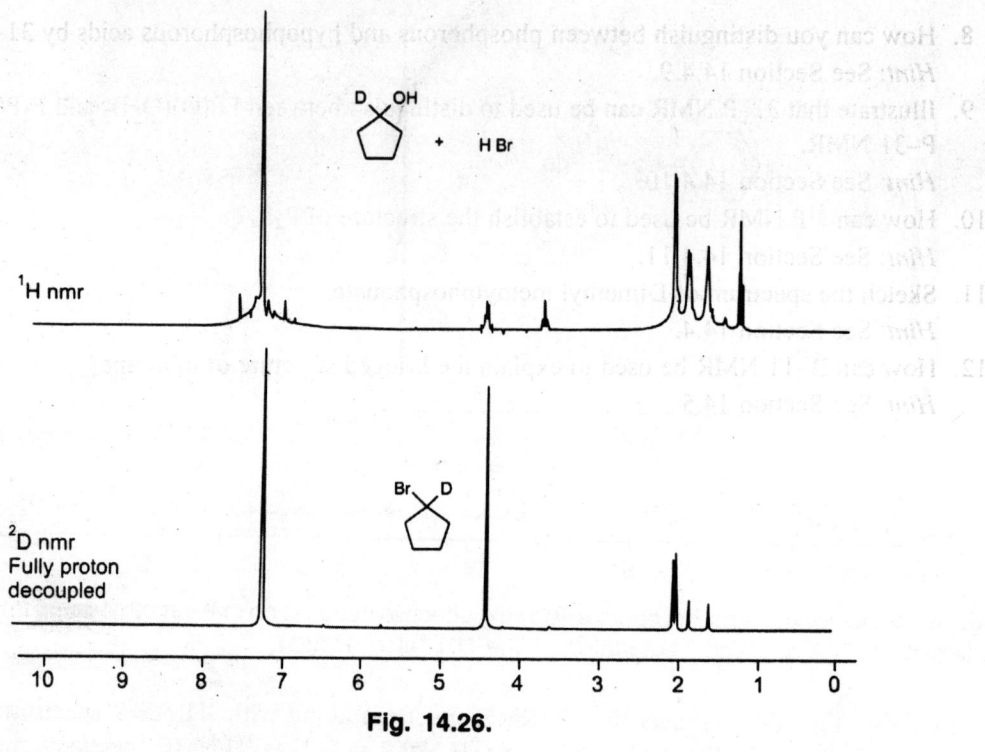

^{1}H nmr

^{2}D nmr
Fully proton
decoupled

Fig. 14.26.

PROBLEMS

1. What is the general range of N–15 NMR? Arrange the N–15 shift of following in the decreasing order—Nitroso, Nitro, imino and alkyl. Is there any parallel of this order in its counterparts in CMR?

   Hint: See Section 14.1.

2. Explain how can you deduce the structure of ClF_3 with the aid of F–19 NMR?

   Hint: See Intext Exercise 14.1.

3. How can you determine the structure of SF_4 with the help of F–19 NMR?

   Hint: See Intext Exercise 14.2.

4. How does F–19 NMR help in structure determination of BrF_5?

   Hint: See Section 14.3.

5. What is the general range of P–31 NMR? Give some examples of equivalent and non-equivalent P nuclei. Explain the hydrogen spectrum of dimethyl phosphonate.

6. Explain how ^{31}P NMR was used to unravel the mechanism and kinetics of Zinc(II)-O,O-diethyl dithiophosphate lubricant additives.

   Hint: See Section 14.4.5.

7. Explain how the thermal degradation of zinc(II)O,O-diethyl dithiophosphate was investigated using 31–P NMR?

   Hint: See Section 14.4.7.

8. How can you distinguish between phosphorous and hypophosphorous acids by 31–P NMR?
   Hint: See Section 14.4.9.
9. Illustrate that 31–P NMR can be used to distinguish between FP(O)(OH)$_2$ and F$_2$P(O)OH using P–31 NMR.
   Hint: See Section 14.4.10.
10. How can ^{31}P NMR be used to establish the structure of P$_4$S$_3$?
    Hint: See Section 14.4.11.
11. Sketch the spectrum of Dimethyl methylphosphonate.
    Hint: See Section 14.4.
12. How can B–11 NMR be used to explain the bridged structure of diborane?
    Hint: See Section 14.5.

15

Pulsed Gradient Field NMR (PFGNMR)

Pulsed gradient field NMR is concerned with the use of pulsed gradient fields (PGF). This is a technique of NMR spectroscopy which was originally developed for magnetic resonance imaging (MRI) that encodes spatial information along x, y and z axes instead of the chemical shift information in the FID. MRI would not have been possible without the development of this technique.

Let us first of all, become familiar with what is a gradient? A gradient is an additional magnetic field applied to the sample that is used to destroy homogeneity in a linear and designed way. Earlier, we learnt that in order to get a NMR spectrum of good quality, it is absolutely essential that we maintain homogeneous field throughout the sample solution in the NMR tube. Thus, when a gradient is applied along the z-axis to the NMR tube, it destroys homogeneity such that while the magnetic field strength Bo, is increased in the upper part of the NMR tube, it gets reduced in the lower part of the NMR tube, all in a linear approach. If Bo is the applied field. $Bg(z)$ is the magnetic field with the gradient applied, G_z is the strength of the gradient and Z is the position of the sample molecule along the z-axis, then the following relation exists between these:

$$Bg_{(z)} = Bo + G_z \times Z$$

Obviously, it can be concluded that the magnetic field strength is now a function of the position, a molecule holds in the NMR sample tube. Suppose we apply a 90° pulse to the sample solution in the NMR tube, the net magnetization vector now rotates in the $x'-y'$ plane. Of course, the rate of precession of this magnetization will depend upon the position of the molecule in the NMR tube. If we assume diffusion to be slow, that means the position of the molecule does not change. It we take zero of the z-axis at the centre of the sample, clearly the increased magnetization in the upper part of the NMR tube means faster precession of the magnetization vector compared to normal ($Bg > Bo$).

On the other hand, the rate of precession of the magnetization vector in the lower part of the sample gets reduced when compared to normal ($Bg < Bo$). What will be the result of these inhomogeneities in magnetic field around the sample? It may be a helix or twist form of the magnetization in the sample in the NMR tube. We can say that the magnetization will rotate as a function of z-coordinate throughout the sample solution in the upper part of the tube (where $Bg > Bo$), as all the protons undergo rotation in the counterclockwise direction at different rates as they are positioned at different vertical heights from the centre of the tube (where $Bz = Bo$, if we assume an on-resonance peak spins at the centre of the tube). This rotation becomes more and more pronounced as Z (position) from the zero or the centre increases. On the other hand, the spins below the centre of the tube where $Bg < Bo$, rotate in clockwise fashion. This is how a twisting of the magnetization occurs at the end of the gradient (Fig. 15.1).

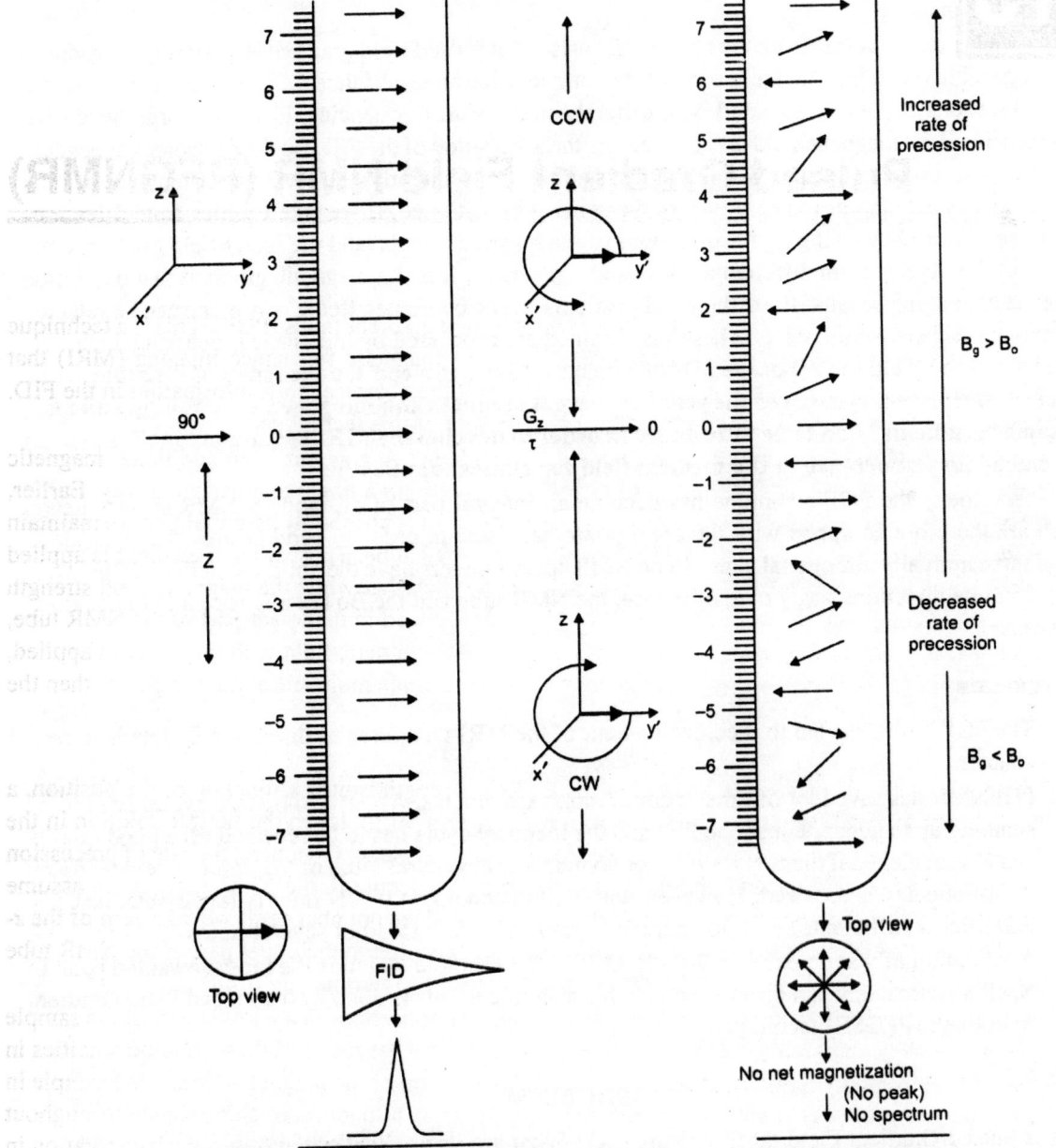

Fig. 15.1. Gradient along z-direction leads to destruction of signal.

What will happen if you now acquire the NMR spectrum at this point after the gradient? Will you get any peaks? No peaks will be obtained. Why? You can realise that all the spin vectors in the x'-y' plane point out in all possible directions such that they cancel out each other as shown in Fig. 15.1. There is no net observable magnetization vector at this particular point in time. This is how gradients are used to destroy the undesired peaks and artifacts in an NMR spectrum. The beauty of this method is that this technique accomplishes the task in just a single scan. Usually, the gradient time, τ is of the order of 1–2 ms.

In conclusion, it is clear from the above discussion that pulsed field gradients technology introduces inhomogeneities such that different parts of the sample solution experience different fields i.e. different spatial locations become associated with different precession frequencies. In other words, when the homogeneity of the magnetic field is "bent" during the acquisition of the FID, Bo field becomes dependent upon the position of molecules within the test sample. Consequently, the PMR spectrum acquires the form of a physical map or image of where the spins are positioned. If we take profiles from directions which are achieved by changing the directions of the magnetic fields, and the linear field gradients, the images of the objects from different angles can be recorded. It is the magnetic gradient that determine the plane of imaging because the orthogonal gradients can be combined freely, any plane can be selected for imaging. Subsequently, the profiles thus obtained are processed by the image processing technique in a computer to yield the 2D or the 3D MRI images. **Thus, you can see the irony of fate that while so many efforts were spent over the years to prevent magnetic inhomogeneities or the "gradients", the same "gradients" had to be introduced in order to develop the MRI technique that has proven of tremendous importance in the medical field for clinical applications.**

In fact, today the PGF technique has become an integral part of all modern NMR spectrometers which are therefore equipped with the appropriate hardware in order to bend/destroy the field along one of three mutually orthogonal axes. Some NMR spectrometers have the ability to deliver PF gradient in all the three directions – x, y or z, of course, the NMR tube and the Bo are aligned parallel i.e. along the z-axis.

Applications

1. The PGF NMR has led to the development of the MRI technique as discussed in details in next chapter.
2. PGFNMR has saved lot of time in correlation experiments. About 4–64 phase cycles have to be summed up to generate just one FID and the identical cycle has to be repeated till a good quality signal is achieved if the S/N ratio is not favourable. In general, time of the order of several hours to full one day is required. However, with PGF technology, if S/N ratio is favourable, just one FID scan is sufficient. So, it just requires a minute or so instead of several hours.
3. Annhilation of water peak in a 90% H_2O/10% D_2O sample which is the most unwanted peak in NMR spectroscopy can be achieved by this technique. This is done by the Pulsed Field Gradient Spin Echo (PFGSE) technique.

PROBLEM

What is Pulsed Gradient Field NMR (PFGNMR)? What are its applications?

16 | Magnetic Resonance Imaging (MRI)

16.1 INTRODUCTION

Magnetic resonance imaging, MRI is also known as Magnetic Resonance Tomography (MRT). Some also call it Nuclear Magnetic Resonance Tomography. As the word nuclear is associated in the public mind with ionizing radiation exposure, it is now referred to simply as MRI. This technique is used to image every part of our body. It is particularly useful for diagnosis of neurological conditions, disorders of muscles and joints as well as for evaluating turmoids and for detection of abnormalities in the host and blood vessels. A modern MRI scanner is shown in Fig. 16.1. MRI of brain is shown in Fig. 16.2.

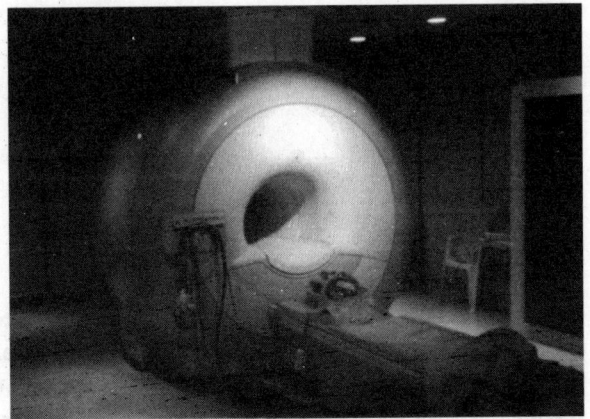

Fig. 16.1. MRI scanner.

16.2 WORKING OF MRI

16.2.1 Principle

Our body mainly (80% of total body atoms) contains water molecules. A water molecule contains two hydrogen atoms. In other words, our body is made up of untold billions of hydrogen atoms. As the hydrogen atoms keep spinning or precessing around their nuclear axis, imagine these billions of hydrogens spinning or precessing in every direction in our tissues. The MRI scanner has a horizontal tube running through the magnet from front to

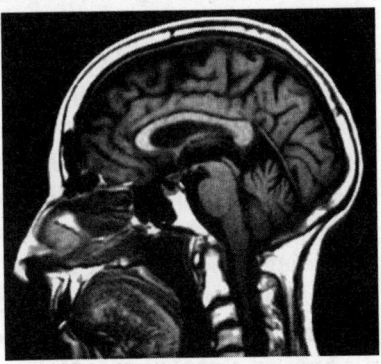

Fig. 16.2. MRI of brain.

back. This tube is called the bore of the magnet. **This bore is the equivalent of the NMR tube and the patient is equivalent to the sample.** Patient lying on the back is allowed to slide into the bore on a special table. Whether or not the patient goes in head first or feet first, and how far depends upon the type of examination to be done. Once, the body part to be scanned is in the exact centre or isocentre of the magnetic field, the scanning is started off.

The magnets in use are in the range 0.5 T–2.0 T (5,000 to 20,000 gauss) (1 T = 10,000 gauss). It should be noted that the Earth's magnetic field is equal to 0.5 gauss. This gives us a good understanding of the power of the magnetic field to which our body is subjected to in MRI scanners.

Anyway, inside the bore of the MRI magnet, the magnetic field runs straight down the centre of the tube in which we place the patient. So, a patient slides into the bore, **the billions of protons in his or her body align themselves with the direction of the applied field in the direction of the head or feet depending upon whether it is the head or the feet that goes first. The magnetic moments of vast majority of the protons cancel out each other. That is to say, for each one lined up towards the feet, that towards the head will cancel it up. In fact, it is just 1–2 protons out of every million protons** (Boltzman population excess) **that are not cancelled out.** And, it is these protons that do the wonder for us.

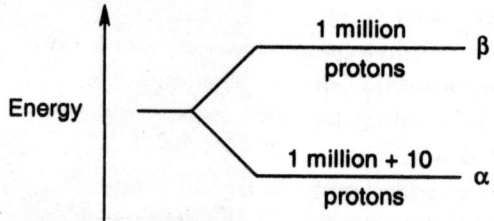

When a suitable radiofrequency is briefly turned on, it causes the water protons to absorb some energy as they get excited from α to the β-spin state. When this field is turned off, the excited protons (β spin state) relax and release this energy at a resonance radio frequency that is then detected by the scanner. It should be noted that the MRI machine system itself directs the *Rf* pulse towards the area (slice) of the body we want to examine. The specific Larmor frequency is calculated based on the particular tissue being examined or imaged and depending upon the strength of the main magnetic field Bo of the scanner. The radiofrequency pulses are applied via a coil. The MRI machines or scanners are equipped with different coils designed for different parts of the body such as head, necks, shoulders, wrists etc. These coils conform to the contour of the body part under imaging or at least reside very close to it during the examination.

As the protons in each active areas of the tissue sample are subjected to the same constant magnetic field, they will all produce the same frequency of radiation and hence give only one peak in the spectrum. This single peak shows the presence of protons. But there is no information regarding their location. This is obtained by adding a calibrated gradient field across the region of the sample with an increasing magnetic field as we move to the right across the sample. The resonance energy and the frequency of the emitted signal rises from left to right. Consequently, the emitted signal now contains different frequencies for the two proton concentration or density areas. This is how we are able to locate the position of protons (Fig. 16.3–16.4).

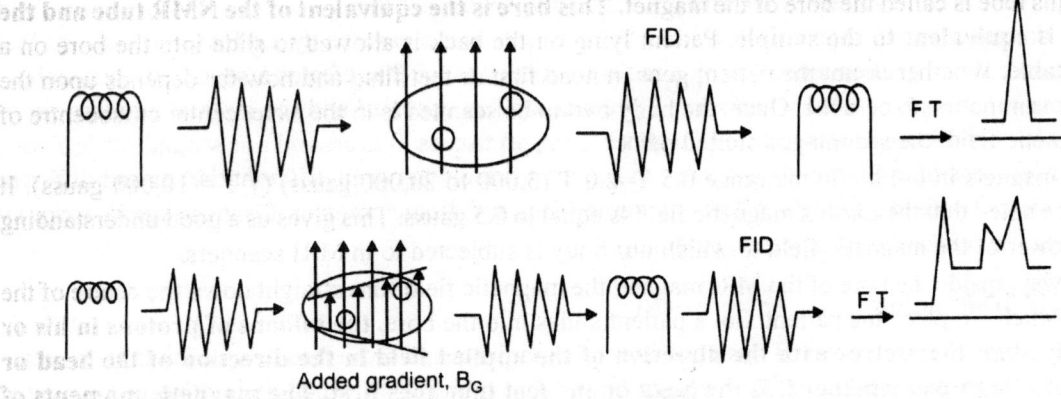

FID

FT

FID

FID

FT

Added gradient, B_G

Fig. 16.3. Locating the position of the hydrogens by gradient technique.

It should be noted at about the same time as the *Rf* pulse is turned on, the three gradient magnets (or coils) jump into action. These turn on and off very rapidly (producing the knocking sounds heard during an MR scan) such that they alter the main magnetic field, *Bo* at a very local level over a slice that is just a few millimeters thin. Further, you do not have to move for the MRI machine to get an image from a different direction. It is these gradient magnets of the scanner that do the job themselves.

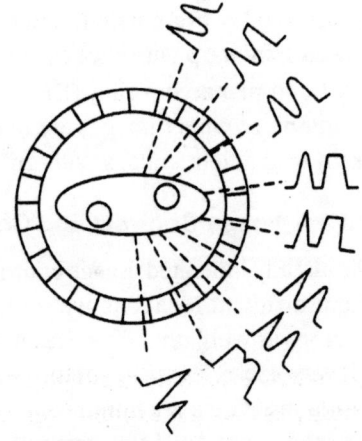

Fig. 16.4. Locating the position of protons.

Since the proton density varies with the type of tissue, a certain amount of contrast is achieved to image the organs and other tissue variations in the subject tissue. The bone of the skull does not have many protons, so, it shows up dark. Similarly, the sinus cavities also appear as dark.

As the protons in different tissues return to their equilibrium state at different rates, changing the parameters on the scanner, creates contrast between different types of body tissue. Contrast agents may be injected intravenously to enhance the appearance of blood vessels, tumors or inflammation. Contrast agents may also be directly injected into a joint in the case of arthrograms, MR images of the joints.

16.2.2 The FID, T_1 and T_2

After the absorption of energy when the radio frequency pulse is turned off, the transverse net magnetization vector component produces an oscillating magnetic field which indices a small current in the receiver coil, called the free induction decay (FID): In an idealized nuclear magnetic resonance experiment, the FID decays approximately exponentially with a time constant T_2. However, in practice small differences in the static magnetic field at different spatial locations (inhomogeneities) cause the Larmor frequency to vary across the body. This create destructive interference and shortens the FID. As noted earlier, in MRI, the static magnetic field is caused to vary across the body by a field gradient with the result that different spatial locations become associated with different precession frequencies.

It is the almost infinite variety of RF and gradient pulse sequences that gives MRI its versatility. Field gradient destroys the FID signal. But this can be recovered and measured by a refocusing gradient that creates a so-called "gradient echo" or by a radio frequency pulse that creates a so-called "spin-echo". The whole process is repeated when some T_1-relaxation has occurred and the thermal equilibrium of the spins has been more or less restored. In general, in soft tissues T_1 is around one second while T_2 and T_2^* are a few tens of milliseconds. As these values vary widely between different tissues and different external magnetic fields, this gives MRI its tremendous soft tissue contrast. Contrast agents work by shortening the relaxation parameters, especially T_1.

16.2.3 2D, 3D-Imaging

Many schemes have been devised that combine field gradients and radio frequency excitation to create an image. These are: the 2D or 3D reconstruction from projections, much as is done in Computed Tomography. Building the image point-by-point or line-by-line. Gradients in the RF field rather than the static field. These schemes are occasionally used in specialist applications. The majority of MR images today are created either by the Two-Dimensional Fourier Transform (2DFT) technique also called spin-warp with slice selection, or by the Three-Dimensional Fourier Transform (3DFT) technique.

Echo-planar imaging (EPI) is yet another scheme which is sometimes used, especially in brain scanning or where images are needed very rapidly. In this scheme, each RF excitation is followed by a train of gradient echoes with different spatial encoding.

16.2.4 Image Contrast and Contrast Enhancement

As already indicated, image contrast is created by differences in the strength of the NMR signal recovered from different locations within the sample. The contrast depends upon the relative density of excited protons as well, on differences in relaxation times T_1, T_2 and T_2^* of the protons after the pulse sequence. However, careful design of the imaging pulse sequence permits one contrast mechanism to be emphasized while the others are minimized. Thus, the ability to choose different contrast mechanisms as and when desired, gives MRI the tremendous flexibility. **T_1-weighting causes the nerve connections of white matter in the brain, to appear white, the congregations of neutrons of gray matter to appear gray, and the cerebrospinal fluid (CSF) to appear dark. Further the contrast of white matter, gray matter and cerebrospinal fluid can be reversed using T_2 or T_2^* imaging.** Furthermore, functional parameters like cerebral blood flow (CBF), cerebral blood volume (CBV) or blood oxygenation can affect T_1, T_2 and T_2^* parameters and hence can be encoded with suitable pulse sequences.

When it is not possible to generate enough image contrast to adequately show the anatomy or pathology of interest by adjusting the imaging parameters alone, a contrast agent may be administered which may be as simple as water (taken orally) for imaging the stomach and small bowel. In general, most contrast agents used in MRI are chosen for their specific magnetic properties. Most commonly, a paramagnetic contrast such as a gadolinium compound is given. The reason is the Gadolinium-enhanced tissues are fluids appear extremely bright on T_1-weighted images. Thus high sensitivity is achieved for detection of vascular tissues (e.g. tumors) and permits assessment of brain perfusion as in stroke.

Very recently, superparamagnetic contrast agents like iron oxide nanoparticles (Fig. 16.5) have been used which appear very dark on T_2^*-weighted images. These are used for liver imaging, because while normal liver tissue retains the agent, the abnormal areas like scars, tumors do not.

16.3 APPLICATIONS OF MRI

MRI scan is harmless to the patient. In clinical practice, MRI is used to distinguish pathologic tissue such as a brain tumor from normal tissue. It uses strong magnetic fields and non-ionizing radiation in the radio frequency range. In comparison, CT scans and traditional X-rays involve doses of ionizing radiation and hence increase the risk of malignancy, especially in a fetus. Although CT provides good spatial resolution which enables us to distinguish two structures an arbitrarily small distance from each other as separate. MRI provides comparable resolution with far better contrast resolution. It provides the ability to distinguish the differences between two arbitrarily similar but not identical tissues.

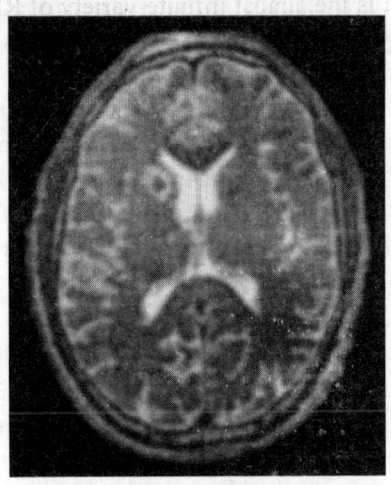

Fig. 16.5. T_2 weighting.

MRI is able to distinguish all groups one apart and is therefore ideally suited for map vision in our brain.

Although most MRI investigations used protons, other nuclei such as P–31, N–15, F–19 and Na–23 have also been extensively investigated in living systems. MRI is being used more for functional investigations rather than anatomical ones.

REFERENCES

1. P.C. Lauterbur, Image formation by Induced Local Interactions : Examples of Employing Nuclear Magnetic Resonance, Nature 242, 190–191, 1973.
2. L.F. Squire, R.A. Novelline, Squire Fundamentals of Radiology (5th ed.), Cambridge : Harvard University press. ISBN 0-674-93339-2.
3. C. Chen, D. Houtt, Biomedical Magnetic Resonance Technology. Medical Sciences, Taylor and Francis. ISBN 978-0852741184.
4. A Oppett., Imaging Systems for Medical Diagnostics : Fundamentals, Technical Solutions and Applications for Systems. Applying Ionizing Radiation, Nuclear Magnetic Resonance and Ultrasound, Wiley-VCH, ISBN 978-3895782268, 2006.

PROBLEM

What is MRI? Explain its principle and applications.

Infrared Spectroscopy
("Yoga" Spectroscopy or "Exercising" Spectroscopy or "Dancing" Spectroscopy)

17.1 INTRODUCTION

Infrared radiation corresponds to the region that lies in between the visible and microwave parts of the electromagnetic spectrum as shown in Fig. 17.1.

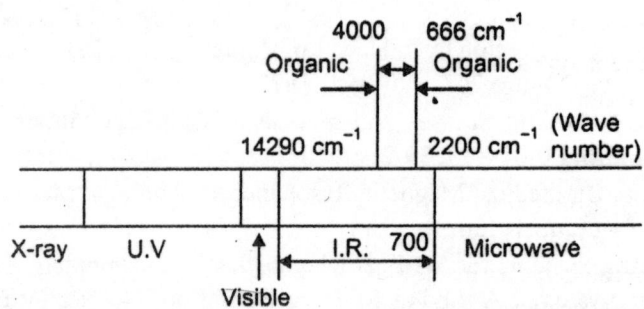

Fig. 17.1. The IR region (14290 cm⁻¹–200 cm⁻¹) organic IR (4000–666 cm⁻¹; 2.54 μ–15 μ).

Dewan (this author) has coined three more terms for the first time in the history of i.r. spectroscopy i.e. "Yoga Spectroscopy" or "Exercising Spectroscopy" or "Dancing Spectroscopy" for i.r. spectroscopy. As bonds display "Yoga" or Exercising or Dancing movements like we do i.e. stretching, compressing, rocking, scissoring, twisting or wagging, so the new terms are very much justified and should also be used as these would and fascinate the students towards this type of spectroscopy.

Infrared range: The complete infrared range is 14,290 to 200 cm⁻¹.

Near–1R range 14,290–4000 cm⁻¹ (0.75–2.5 μ).

Organic–1R range: This is the part of major interest to an organic chemist: 4000–666 cm⁻¹ (2.5 μ–15 μ). This is also called Medium IR region.

Far–1R range: 700 cm⁻¹–200 cm⁻¹.

Calibration of IR spectrum: This is done in wave numbers, $\bar{v}$ (2.5 µm to 25 µm)

$$\bar{v} = 1/\lambda$$

λ = v/c where v is the frequency and c is the velocity of light 3×10^8 cm/sec.

$\therefore$

$$\bar{v} = v/c$$

- The position of absorption in infrared spectrum generally done in wave number, $\bar{v}$ expressed in cm^{-1} as this is the reciprocal of wavelength, l.
- Wavelength λ, in micrometers, µ or µm: The calibration of the absorption can also be done in micrometer, µm, a unit of wavelength. µm = $1/cm^{-1} \times 10000$
- Why wave number expression is preferred?

The major reason for this is that wavenumber $(\bar{v})$ is directly proportional to energy. This enables us to compare the positions of absorptions of different bonds with their energy requirements as we will see later in terms of energy. Further, the wave numbers are larger values and easy to handle compared to wavelengths that are not easy to handle due to small differences in the values of functional groups.

- Relation between wave number $(\bar{v})$ and frequency v (cm)

$$\bar{v} = \frac{1}{\lambda \, (cm)} = \frac{v \, (cm)}{c \, (cm/sec)} = \frac{v}{3 \times 10^8} \, sec.$$

17.2 PRINCIPLE

In addition to the facile rotation of the groups about single bonds we talk about so often, molecules also experience many different types of motions, the vibrational motions. Such motions are obviously characteristic of their component atoms or bonds.

17.2.1 Diatomic molecules

According to classical approach, a diatomic molecule can have zero vibrational energy but wave mechanical approach predicts rather insists that in the molecule, the bond distance continually

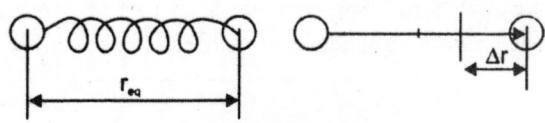

Vibrational motion

Fig. 17.2. Vibrational motion.

changes from an equilibrium value i.e. the bond always vibrates to some extent. In other words, the covalent bonds in molecules are not rigid sticks or rods, as seen in molecular model kits. Rather, they are more like stiff springs that can be stretched or bent (see Fig. 17.2). So, bond should be governed by Hooke's law.

A diatomic molecule XY can be imagined to be made up two masses X and Y connected by a spring. The bond X–Y has minimum internuclear distance r_{eq}, called bond length. The atoms in a bond are not stationary. They vibrate to a new distance, by a difference Δr. The force F between the two atoms will be given by Hooke's law:

$$F = Kr$$

where F is the force that tries to return the system to original position.

K is called Hook's law constant for spring-force constant for molecular system.

These atoms can not have zero vibrational energy. In other words, they can not be completely at rest with respect to each other.

The vibrations are quantized (Fig. 17.3). That is to say a molecule has many vibrational states, we can call them as v_0, v_1, v_2, v_3, v_4, v_5 etc. This can be understood like this. Consider a heteronuclear diatomic molecule such as HCl. This molecule has the vibrational states shown (Fig. 17.3).

Upon absorption of   red energy, the HCl molecule in the v_0 ground state stretches to go into the excited vibration state called v_1, (first excited stretching state). Supposing this bond has absorbed 10 kJ mole energy **(i.r. absorption provides energy in the range 8–   J)** for getting stretched into v_1 state. That mean   it will always require 10 kJ/mole energy to do that. This will not take up less than that amount to stretch to v_1 state i.e. 1 kJ or 2 kJ or 3 kJ to 9 kJ to 9.1 and even 9.9 kJ will not enable the HCl bond to stretch to v_1 level of stretching. Similarly, if the HCl bond requires 2 ×

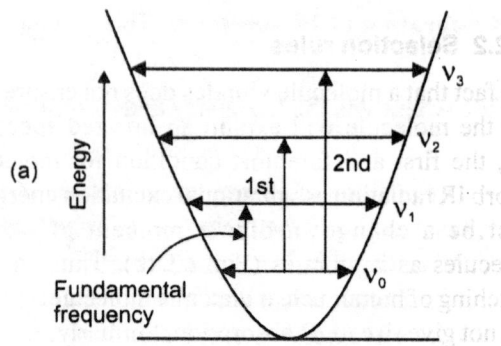

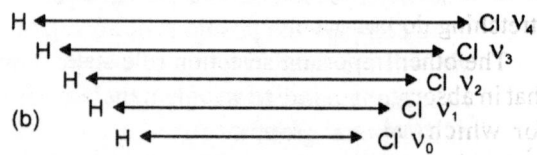

Fig. 17.3. (a) Fundamental frequency, (b) The quantized vibrational energy states for HCl symmetrical stretching.

10 kJ/mole to stretch to the level if v_2 state, it will not stretch to that level if it is provided with 11 to 19 or to even 19.9 kJ of energy. Bonds just do not stretch to any level. They do not stretch to just any level of your choice.or what we popularly quote in Hindi i.e. "Jitna Gur Utna Meetha" (you can sweeten a drink by adding as much sugar as you want). This is what is called the quantisation concept of vibrations. Not only stretching, symmetric or asymmetric but also all bending vibrations which we will study next are similarly quantised in nature.

Intext Exercise

1. With the help of a figure explain that the stretching vibrations in diatomic molecules such as H—Cl are quantised.

   Ans. As above (last paragraph) and give Fig. 17.3(b).

A quantum mechanical treatment based on Schrödinger equation of the molecular system gives the following equation for permitted energy states.

$$E_v = hv \left(v + \frac{1}{2}\right) \text{ joules (v in Hz)}$$

where v is integer 0, 1, 2, ... represented by vibrational quantum number of various states.

$E_v \rightarrow$ energy of Vth state

$h \rightarrow$ Planck's constant

$v \rightarrow$ fundamental vibrational frequency (cm^{-1})

As vibrational energy levels are not equally spaced levels and converge due to anharmonic oscillation, the deviation from the equation increases with increase in vibrational quantum number.

17.2.2 Selection rules

The fact that a molecule vibrates does not ensure in itself that the molecule will exhibit an infrared spectrum. In fact, the first and foremost condition for molecules to absorb IR radiation as vibrational excitation energy, there must be a change in dipole moment of molecules as it vibrates (Fig. 17.4b). Thus stretching of homonuclear diatomic molecule will not give rise to IR absorption. Similarly, $O=C=O$ stretching and is $CH_3-C\equiv C-CH_3$ stretching do not occur.

The other important selection rule states that in absorption of radiation only transition for which $\Delta v = +1$ can occur. As most molecules are in v_0 vibrational level at room temperature, most transitions will occur from v_0 to v_1 frequency. This energy is called Fundamental frequency (Fig. 17.3a).

Transitions between $v_0 \rightarrow v_2$ and $v_0 \rightarrow v_3$ i.e. 2 and 3 will not occur but due to the fact that most molecules are not perfect Harmonic oscillators, the rule breaks down and transitions do occur, known as 1st and 2nd overtones (intensity less than fundamental as shown in Fig. 17.2).

Classic approach further shows that the frequency for IR absorption is given as by the following Hooke's law expression:

$$\bar{v} = \frac{1}{2\pi c} \sqrt{\frac{K}{\mu}}$$

where $\bar{v}$ is called wave number (cm^{-1})

μ is the reduced mass:

$$\mu = \frac{1}{m_1} + \frac{1}{m_2} = \frac{m_1 m_2}{m_1 + m_2}$$

K is the force constant and has a value of 5×10^5 dynes/cm for single bonds (its magnitude for the double and tripple bonds is about twice or thrice this value respectively).

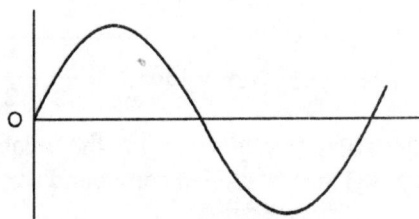

Fig. 17.4a. I.R. inactive stretching which do not involve a change in dipole moment.

The bending vibration of CO_2

Dipole moment

The vertical component of dipole

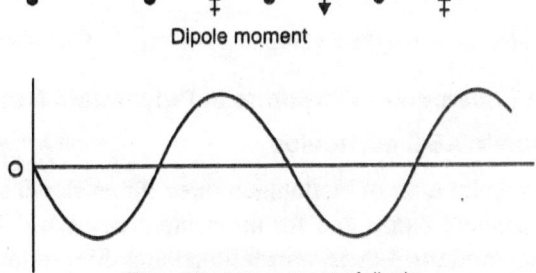

The asymmetric stretching vibration of CO_2

Dipole moment

The vertical component of dipole

Fig. 17.4b. Change in dipole moment is a must for a vibration to be i.r. active.

IR stretching frequencies can be roughly predicted by using harmonic oscillator model – the Hooke's law:

$$v = 1303\sqrt{K\left(\frac{1}{m_1} + \frac{1}{m_2}\right)}$$

where m_1 and m_2 are the relative atomic masses. K means force constant which assumes values of 5, 10 and 15 for single, double and triple bonds respectively.

This equation is particularly useful for predicting isotope shifts.

Thus, C–H stretching frequency:

$$\bar{v}_{CH} = 1303\sqrt{5\left(\frac{1}{12} + \frac{1}{1}\right)} = 3033 \text{ cm}^{-1}$$

Similarly, C–D stretching frequency:

$$\bar{v}_{CD} = 1303\sqrt{5\left(\frac{1}{12} + \frac{1}{2}\right)} = 2225 \text{ cm}^{-1}$$

Further, if the stretching frequency (n_0) in the unlabelled compound is known, then the respective stretching frequency (v_1) in the labelled compound can also be predicted:

$$v = v_0 = v_0\sqrt{\frac{\dfrac{1}{m_1} + \dfrac{1}{m_2'}}{\dfrac{1}{m_1} + \dfrac{1}{m_2}}}$$

m_1 and m_2 are the relative atomic masses of the involved atoms. m_2' is the atomic mass of the isotope. Thus:

$$v_{DO} = v_{HO}\sqrt{\frac{\dfrac{1}{16} + \dfrac{1}{2}}{\dfrac{1}{16} + \dfrac{1}{1}}} = 2539 \text{ cm}^{-1}$$

The actually observed value is 2540 cm^{-1}. This shows the power of the equation.

17.2.3 Fundamental Vibrations in Polyatomic Molecules

(i) Triatomic ABC molecules

Let us consider a set of N atoms in three-dimensional space. It has 3N degree of freedom. This is true for independent atoms and for molecules having an N atoms. For all non-linear molecules, external molecular motions – three translational and three-rotational account for six of these motions. Hence, this leaves 3N–6 vibrational modes. As a linear molecule has only two rotations, it has 3N–5 vibrational modes. Thus, a linear diatomic molecule has only one mode of vibration: N = 2, 3N – 5 = 6 – 5 = 1, this is bond stretching motion or vibration.

As per the 3N–6 vibrational modes formula, a bent triatomic molecule ABC has $(3 \times 3 - 6) =$ three modes of vibrations as shown in Fig. 17.5.

Further, it should be noted that, in general, a molecule has one bond stretching mode per bond. Of course, in rings and cages like systems, the stretching modes can not be described so simply.

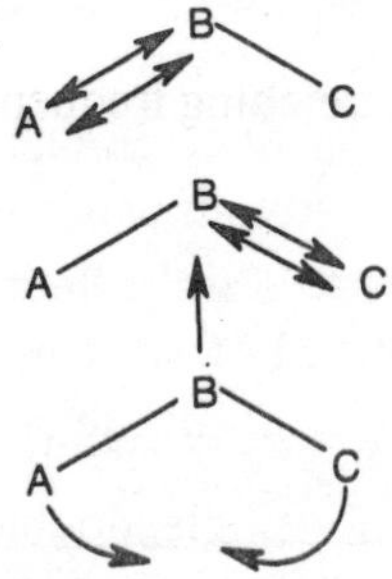

(ii) Triatomic molecules XY_2 Type

XY_2 molecule may have either a bent or linear structure.

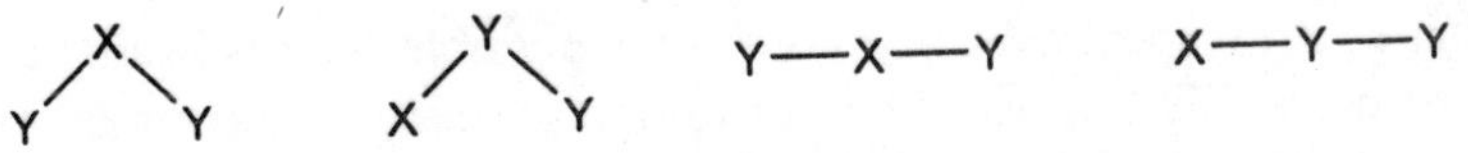

Fig. 17.5. Three modes of vibrations in a bent triatomic molecule, ABC.

A linear XY_2 (CO_2) molecule shows three normal modes of vibrations:

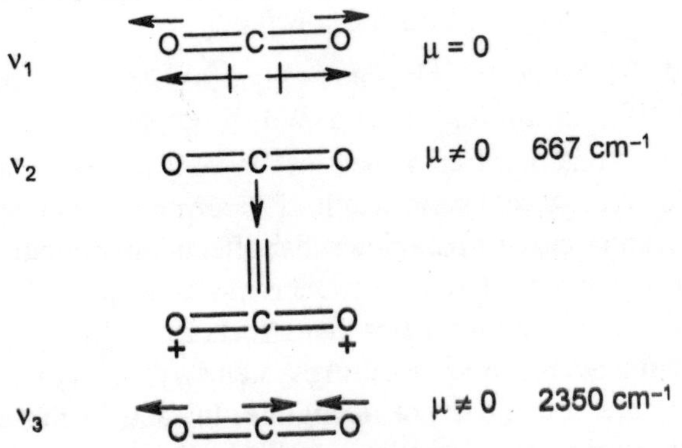

v_1 $\mu = 0$

v_2 $\mu \neq 0$ 667 cm^{-1}

v_3 $\mu \neq 0$ 2350 cm^{-1}

Intext Exercise

2. How many vibrational frequencies in the i.r. spectrum of carbon dioxide observed and why?

Ans. See the above discussion.

17.2.4 Infrared spectrum versus Raman spectrum

It needs to be noted that not all the fundamental vibrations as predicted by the formula 3n–6 non-linear molecules or 3n–5 for linear molecules are seen in i.r. spectrum. This is because some fundamental bands are too weak to be observed, some are so close that they coalesce but most important of all reasons is the failure of the vibrations not to cause a change in the dipole moment of the molecule.

In other words, when compared to vibrations active in Raman Spectrum we can say that those vibrations are i.r. active that do not have a centre of symmetry while they are Raman-inactive. When a molecule possesses a centre of symmetry, the vibrations symmetrical around that centre of symmetry are Raman-active but they are i.r.-active. That is what makes the Raman spectra and i.r.-spectra complementary to each other for structure determination of molecules. The i.r. spectra assume great importance for organic chemists as the organic molecules in general lack centre of symmetry which involve more change in dipole moment and give more intense i.r. spectra.

Intext Exercise

3. Why does Buckminster fullerence (C_{60}) show only four absorption bands in its infrared spectrum?

Ans. This reflects the highly symmetrical nature of C_{60} (Fig. 17.6a). Symmetric vibrations are infra-red inactive as these do not lead to a change in the dipole moment of the molecule.

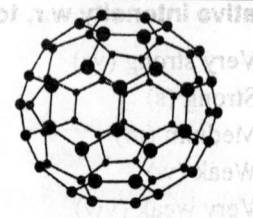

Fig. 17.6a. C_{60} fullerene.

17.2.5 Band Shapes and Intensity

Quantitative measures for peak intensities in i.r. spectroscopy is not readily possible. This is in contrast to the situation in UV-visible spectroscopy. That is why, the absorption intensity is expressed by subjective classifications: weak (w), medium (m), strong (s), and very strong (vs). What.

Intext Exercise

4. In contrast to UV and visible spectra it is not readily possible to give quantitative measures for absorption peak intensities in infrared spectra. Why?

Hint: The major reason is that in infrared spectroscopy, the monochromator slot width is of the order of magnitude identical to the band width of absorption bands in routine measurements. Thus, the slit width is an important parameter that affects the measured optical density as the light passing through the sample is non-monochromatic. In fact, the non-monochromaticity also governs the band shape. Another factor that affects band shape is the speed of the scanner (or sluggish response of detection and recording systems), particularly so for those parts where absorption of light by the solvent is not negligible. In fact, in those parts of the spectrum wherein the solvent transmission is less than ~ 35%, the light energy that reaches the detection system is not sufficient for reliable working. Under these conditions, the recording system becomes erratic such that the spectra obtained are difficult to interpret.

As the first and foremost condition for a vibration to be i.r.-active is that it must lead to a change in dipole moment of the molecule, that is to say that a band in the i.r. spectrum will be obtained only if the vibration causes the change in molecular dipole moment (Fig. 17.6b), it is clear that the intensity of the band will be dependent upon the magnitude of the change caused in the dipole moment. Greater the change in molecular dipole moment, greater the intensity of the band (as in $C=O$), smaller the change in molecular dipole moment, weaker the band (as in cis $C=C$). The bands observed in the i.r. spectrum are usually classified as being strong, medium, weak or very weak. This is usually done by taking the most intense peak as of 100% intensity.

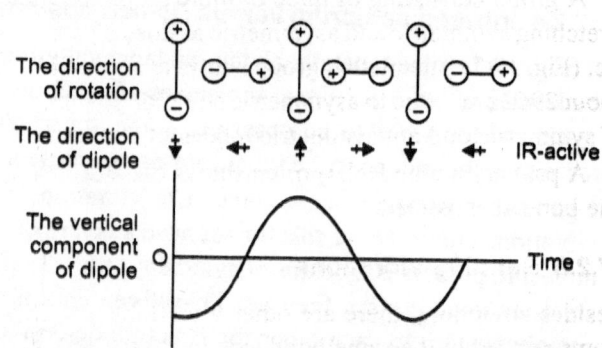

Fig. 17.6b. The vertical component of dipole of HCl molecule as a function of time.

Relative intensity w.r. to base peak taken as 100%

Very strong (vs)	80%
Strong (s)	80–60%
Medium (m)	60–50%
Weak (w)	50–30%
Very weak (vw)	< 30%

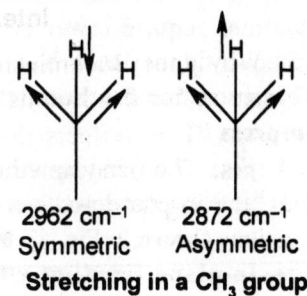

2962 cm^{-1} 2872 cm^{-1}
Symmetric   Asymmetric

Stretching in a CH$_3$ group

17.2.6 IR bands are broad due to rotational coupling

It needs to be noticed that the i.r. bands are broad rather than sharp discrete lines. This is because of rotational coupling i.e. a single vibrational energy change is accompanied by a number of rotational energy changes. Even though the rotational frequencies of the molecule as a whole are i.r.-inactive, they usually couple with the stretching and bending vibrations. Consequently the i.r. peaks are broad and have fine structure.

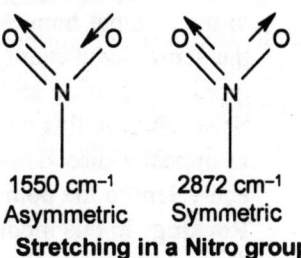

1550 cm^{-1} 2872 cm^{-1}
Asymmetric   Symmetric

Stretching in a Nitro group

17.2.7 Stretching and bending vibrations

Stretching and bending vibrations are the simplest types of vibrational motion that cause infrared absorptions.

H—C
Stretching

Bending

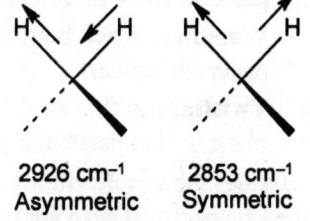

2926 cm^{-1} 2853 cm^{-1}
Asymmetric   Symmetric

Stretching in a CH$_2$ group

Fig. 17.7. Some stretching vibrations.

Stretching is of two types as can be readily imagined. Symmetric when the atoms stretch in the same direction. Asymmetric when the atoms stretch in opposite directions. Asymmetric stretching vibrations require more energy and so occur at higher frequencies compared to symmetric stretching vibrations.

A group consisting of three or more atoms in which two atoms are identical, shows two modes of stretching symmetric and asymmetric as does a heteronuclear diatomic molecule: CH$_3$, CH$_2$, anhydrides etc. (Fig. 17.7) The methyl group shows at about 2872 cm^{-1} due to symmetric stretching and another at about 2962 cm^{-1} due to asymmetric stretching. Similarly, the anhydride functional group shows because of symmetric and antisymmetric modes of stretching C = O region.

A primary amine RNH$_2$ often shows two absorption due to N–H stretching, a 2° amine shows only one bond as expected.

17.2.8 Bending Vibrations

Besides stretching, there are other vibrations called bending vibrations (or deformations). While the atoms remain in the same bond axis in stretching vibrations, the atoms in bending vibrations may not remain in the same bond axis. Although unlike in stretching vibrations, the distance between atoms remains fixed, the positions of the atoms may change with regards to the original bond axis. Bending vibrations require lower energy to occur and consequently they absorb at lower frequency. **It is easier to bend a bond than to stretch or compress it!**

Types: The bending vibrations are of two types: the in-plane and out-of-plane bending vibrations shown in Fig. 17.8.

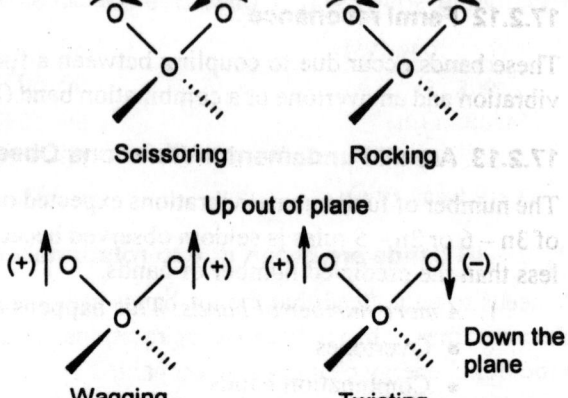

Fig. 17.8. Bending vibrations.

- **In-plane bending vibrations:** In such vibrations, although the bonds bend w.r. to the original bond axis, they remain in the same nodal plane. These are of two types – scissoring and rocking.
- **Scissoring:** In this mode, the atoms move in opposite directions, the motion being equivalent to the points of a pair of scissors. Hence, the name.
- **Rocking:** In this mode both the atoms show rocking movement on one side or the other.
- **Out-of-plane (OOP) vibrations:** In these bending vibrations, the atoms bend out of the nodal plane in two modes called wagging and twisting.

   Wagging: When both the involved atoms either go up the plane or down out of the plane of the paper, in concert.

   Twisting: In this mode, while one atom goes up the plane, the other atom goes down out of the plane at that particular point in time.

Besides the simple vibrations of stretching and bending, some other vibrations are often also noticed in the i.r. spectra. These are overtones, combination bands, difference bands, fermi resonance etc.

17.2.9 Overtones

These are the vibrations that occur at twice, thrice etc. the value of fundamental vibrations, that is to say these are the vibrations which occur at $n\bar{v}_0$ where n is an integer and can have values 2, 3, 4 etc.

$$\text{Overtones} = n\bar{v}_0 = 2v_0, 3v_0, 4v_0 \text{ etc.}$$

Thus, if fundamental vibration occurs at 600 cm^{-1}, the first overtone $(2v_0)$ will occur at $(2 \times 600) = 1200$ cm^{-1}, the second $(3v_0)$ at 1800 cm^{-1} etc.

These can prove very useful as diagnostic bands, say for example in aromatic compounds.

17.2.10 Combination bands

These are the bands that result due to combination or coupling of fundamental frequencies. For example $\bar{v}_1 + \bar{v}_2$ may couple or combine to give a new frequency band called combination band:

$$v_{comb} = \bar{v}_1 + \bar{v}_2$$

17.2.11 Difference bands

Sometimes, bands are seen to occur at a frequency that is the difference of the two bands, hence the name:

$$\bar{v}_{diff} = \bar{v}_1 + \bar{v}_2$$

17.2.12 Fermi resonance

These bands occur due to coupling between a fundamental vibration and an overtone or a combination band (Fig. 17.9):

$$\bar{v}_0 = 2\bar{v}_0 + \bar{v}_{\text{Fermi resonance}}$$
Fundamental Overtone

$$\bar{v}_0 + (\bar{v}_1 + \bar{v}_2) = \bar{v}_{\text{Fermi resonance}}$$
Fundamental Combination

Fig. 17.9. Fermi resonance.

17.2.13 Are all Fundamental Vibrations Observed?

The number of fundamental vibrations expected on the basis of $3n - 6$ or $2n - 5$ rules is seldom observed because of the following reasons. In fact, it can be more or less than the predicted number of bands.

1. *A more number of bands:* This happens due to:
   - Overtones
   - Combination bands
2. *Lesser number of bands*: A reduced number of bands occurs due to following reasons:
   - When a vibration does not involve a change in dipole moment.
   - When the fundamental bands fall outside the region 4000–667 cm^{-1}.
   - When the bands are too weak to be observable.
   - When the vibrations occur very close to each other such that they coalesce.
   - In highly symmetrical molecules several absorptions of the same frequency give rise to a degenerate band.

17.3 FACTORS THAT AFFECT FREQUENCY OF A VIBRATION

We have already learnt that the frequency of a vibration can be calculated by using the Hooke's law:

$$\bar{v}_0 = \frac{1}{2\pi c}\sqrt{\frac{k}{\mu}} \qquad k = \text{force constant}; \quad \mu = \frac{1}{m_1} + \frac{1}{m_2} \text{ (reduced mass)}$$

As can be seen from the formula $\bar{v}$ depends upon both the force constant as well as reduced mass, μ.

(i) Force constant factor

Thus, it is expected that stronger the bond, higher the k, higher the frequency. As tripple bonds are stronger than double, which, in turn, are stronger than single bonds between the same two atoms, therefore the increasing order of frequencies should be observed. Indeed, it is so

$$C \equiv C \qquad\qquad C = C \qquad\qquad C - C$$

$\longleftarrow$
Increasing K and $\bar{v}$

2150 cm^- 1650 cm^{-1} 1200 cm^{-1}

(ii) Reduced mass factor

The reduced mass is expected to increase if the atoms bonded to carbon increases in mass. Consequently, the frequency of vibration will decrease. This can be seen from comparison of the following:

$$C - H \qquad\qquad C - C \qquad\qquad C - O$$

3000 cm^{-1} 1200 cm^{-1} 1100 cm^{-1}

$$\text{C – Cl} \atop 750 \text{ cm}^{-1} \qquad \text{C – Br} \atop 600 \text{ cm}^{-1} \qquad \text{C – I} \atop 500 \text{ cm}^{-1}$$

Increasing μ   →   Increasing μ   →

Decreasing ν   →   Decreasing ν   →

Another example is:

Increasing μ   →

$$\text{C = O} \atop 1700 \text{ cm}^{-1} \qquad \text{C = S} \atop 1350 \text{ cm}^{-1}$$

Decreasing ν   →

Intext Exercise

5. Although the atomic mass of fluorine is higher than that of carbon, the F–H stretching occurs at 4138 cm^{-1} compared to C–H stretching at 3040 cm^{-1}.

   Ans. Obviously, here, the reduced mass factor is not being dominant. In fact, it is the force constant, K factor which is in operation. The F–H force constant is greater than that of the C–H bond.

6. What will be the C–D stretching frequency if that of C–H stretching is 2900 cm^{-1}.

   Ans. We know

   $$\frac{\nu_{C-H}}{\nu_{C-D}} = \sqrt{2}$$

   or

   $$\frac{\nu_{C-D}}{\nu_{C-H}} = \frac{1}{\sqrt{2}}$$

   or

   $$\nu_{C-D} = \nu_{C-H} \times \frac{1}{\sqrt{2}}$$

   $$= 2900 \times \frac{1}{\sqrt{2}}$$

   $$= 2900 \times \frac{1}{1.414}$$

   $$= 2060 \text{ cm}^{-1}$$

17.4 INSTRUMENTATION

These are of two types, Double Beam IR spectrum and FTIR spectrometer.

17.5 MODERN DOUBLE BEAM IR SPECTROMETER

It consists of five main parts and is shown in Fig. 17.10.

1. **Radiation source:** Nernst filament (made up of oxides of Zr, Th, Ce + binder) that is heated at 1000–1800°C or Globar – small rod of SiC. Radiation from the source is divided into two parallel

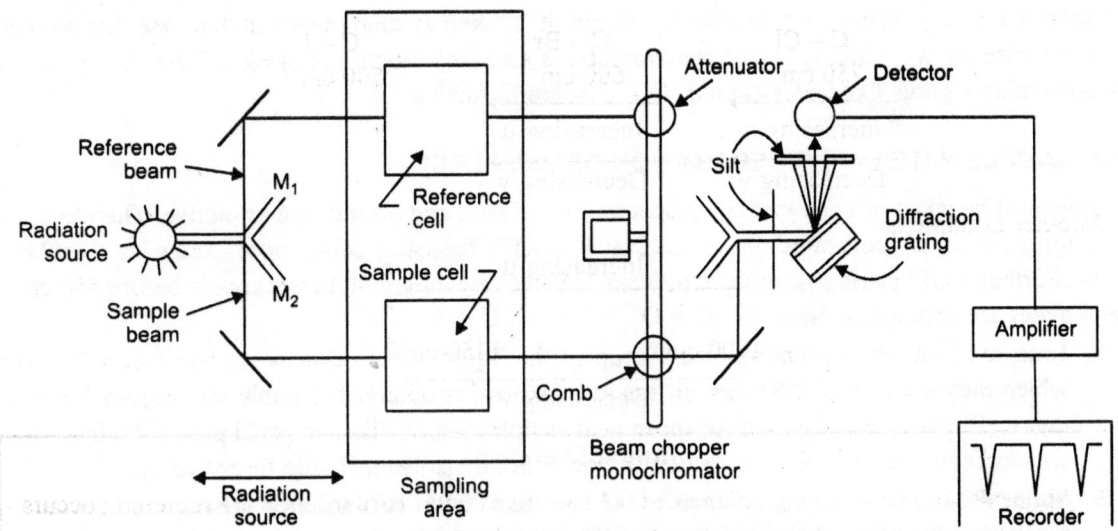

Fig. 17.10. Modern double beam IR spectrometer.

beams – called reference and sample beam by means of mirrors M_1, M_2 respectively of equal intensity radiation.

2. **Sampling area:** Reference and sample beam enter into the reference sampling area pass through the reference and sample cells respectively.

3. **Photometer:** The reference beam passes through the attenuator and the sample beam through the comb. In the photometer zone, the two beams are combined into a single beam of alternating segments. The attenuator is driven in and out of the reference beam in response to the signal created at the detector by the sample beam. So, when the sample beam is absorbed by the sample, the attenuator is driven into the reference beam until its intensity matches that of the sample beam.

4. **Monochromator:** The monochromator is a rapidly rotating beam chopper. It passes the two beams alternatively to a diffraction grating that rotates slowly which changes the frequency of rotation reaching the thermocouple detector.

5. **Detector (thermocouple):** The sensitive fast thermocouple detects the ratio between the intensities of the reference and sample beam so that it is able to determine frequencies have been absorbed by the sample and those that are unaffected by the light passing through the sample.

6. **Recorder:** The signals from the detector are electronically amplified by the amplifier. Afterwards the recorder records the resulting spectrum of the sample on a special graph paper. Double beam IR spectrometer are said to record a spectrum in the frequency domain i.e. the spectrum is recorded as the frequency of i.r. radiation changes by rotation of the diffraction grating. The i.r. spectrum is a plot of frequency ν (cm^{-1}) against the per cent transmittance ($Is/Ir \times 100$) where Is is the intensity of sample beam and Ir that of the reference beam.

You might be wondering about the interference, the bands of the solvent will cause in an i.r. spectrum. Well, do not worry as the instrument is well taught to subtract the spectrum of the solvent from that of the sample solution. In case, the sample is a liquid, it is taken as such (neat). In that case this problem does not arise anyway. Similarly, the spectrometer is also well taught not to record the absorptions of the atmospheric gases like water-vapour, CO_2 that are i.r.-active.

17.6 SAMPLE HANDLING (PREPARATION OF SAMPLES)

Sample must be taken in a cell that is transparent in i.r. Glass and plastics are i.r.-active. Therefore, the cells are made up of ionic substances like. NaCl or KBr, the latter being more expensive than NaCl plates. Further, NaCl starts absorbing at 650 cm^{-1}. Since few important bands appear before 650 cm^{-1}, NaCl plates are commonly used.

A. **Liquids:** Neat or in solution. One 1 drop of the liquid is placed between NaCl or KBr plates which means a film of 0.01 mm or less in thickness, is obtained. Sample size required is 1–10 mg. AgCl plates may be used for those neat samples which dissolve NaCl plates. Further, there should be no water as NaCl dissolves in water. So, the solvent should be anhydrous.

B. **Solids solutions:** 1–10 mg volumes of 0.1 to 1 ml of 0.05–10% solution are required for readily available cells of 0.1–1 mm thickness. CCl$_4$ is used which, of course, absorbs strongly at about 785 cm^{-1}. CS$_2$ may also be used. CS$_2$ absorbs below 1333 cm^{-1}, while CCl$_4$ is relatively free of absorption at > 1333 cm^{-1}. Solute and solvent combinations to that react must be avoided.

C. **Solids:** Sample + KBr under pressure give pellets called KBr pellets. But as KBr absorbs moisture, the interference will be seen. If good pellets are obtained, no interference is seen.

Nujol mull sample + mineral → placed between NaCl or KBr pellets. Nujol absorbs at 2924, 1462, 1377 cm^{-1} (disadvantages!).

Sample + solvent (CCl$_4$/CS$_2$): Non-polar solvents are better as polar solvents may show H-bonding. Fig. 17.10b shows the i.r. spectra of Nujol, KBr and CCl$_4$.

17.7 FOURIER TRANSFORM INFRARED (FTIR) SPECTROMETER

The FTIR instruments have a number of advantages over the double-beam dispersive IR instruments. An FTIR is shown in Fig. 17.11a. In such instruments, the optical pathway used to record the spectrum of the sample, actually produces what is called an **interferrogram** that is a plot of intensity of all bonds against time. In other words, it is a **time-domain** rather than the routine **frequency domain** i.r. spectrum. Fourier transformation of these interferrograms then converts these from time-domain into the routine frequency domain i.r. spectra. It is similar to what you learnt in the chapter on NMR spectroscopy.

An interferrogram is obtained in less than a second. In order to increase the S/N ratio, dozens of interferrograms of a sample are taken and then accumulated. This is done by a computer. Thus, the i.r. spectrum is obtained in about half-a-minute. Therefore, FTIR saves our time. They are not only fast but also more sensitive.

Further, while a dispersive double-beam i.r. instrument records only one peak at a time,.in a successive pattern, FTIR instrument records all peaks all at once.

The FTIR is based upon coupling of a Michelson interferometer with a highly sensitive infrared detector. No monochromator is used in the Michelson interferometer as infrared radiation having a large number of frequencies is allowed to strike the sample. The idea is to catch all frequencies absorbed

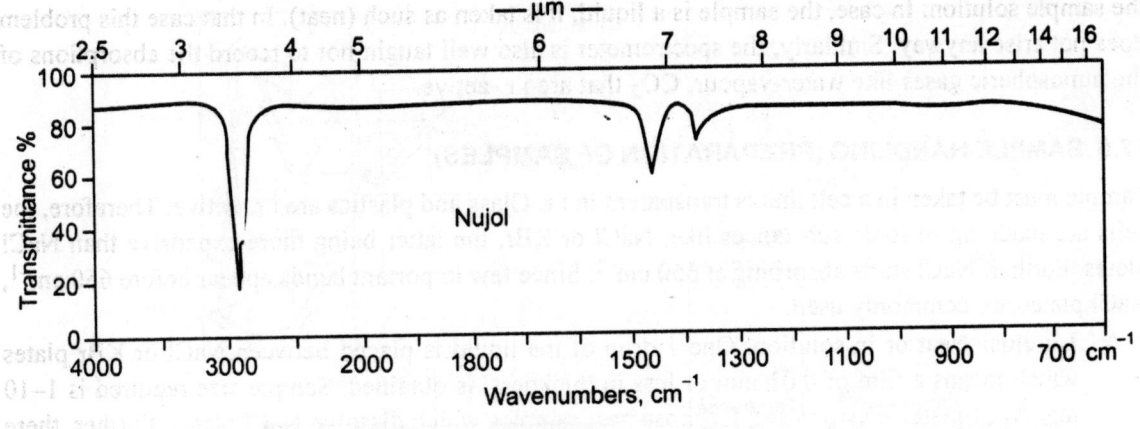

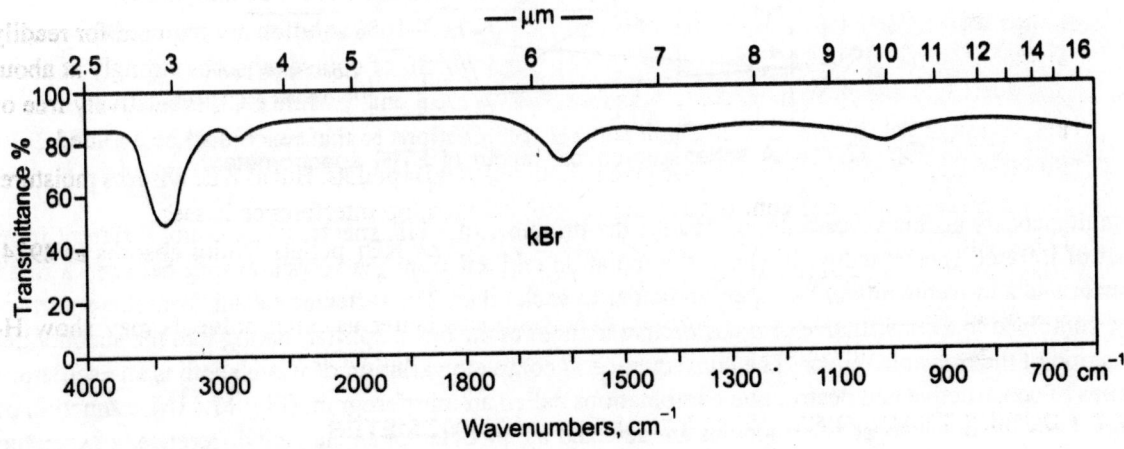

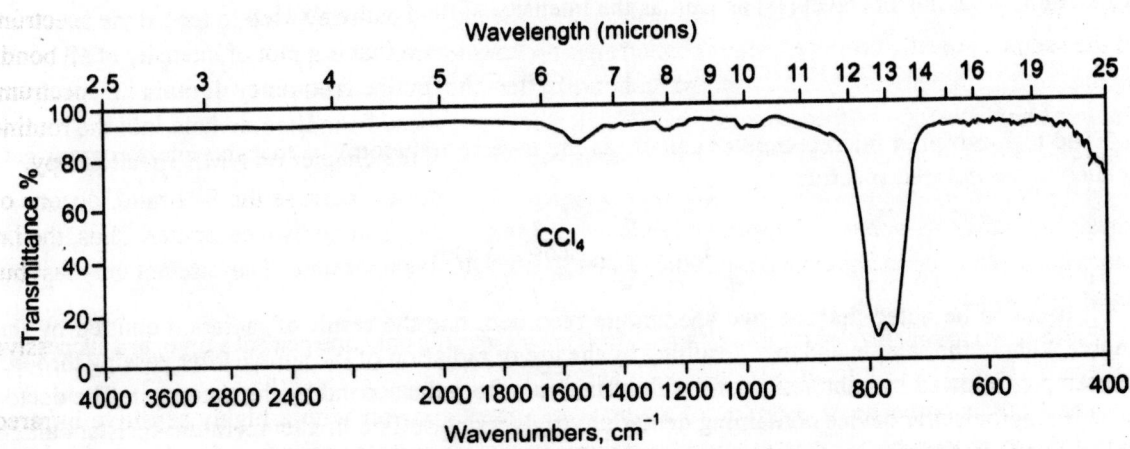

Fig. 17.10b. IR spectra of Nujol, KBr and CCl₄.

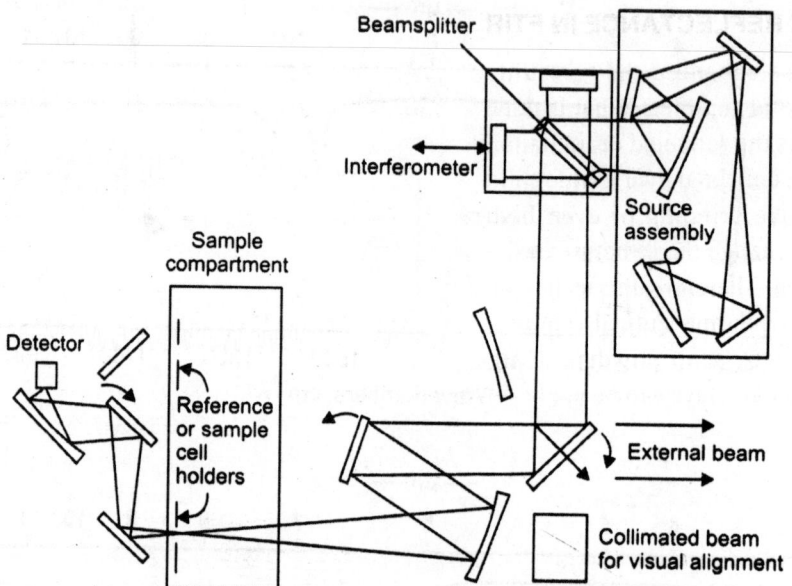

Fig. 17.11a. A schematic optical layout of FTIR spectrometer.

simultaneously as this saves time, of course, the principle of FTIR spectroscopy is not different from that of infrared spectroscopy. In short, the radiation emitted from the source is split between a fixed mirror and a movable mirror held perpendicular to each other. The reflected beams from these mirrors are combined in a constructive or a destructive manner at the beam splitter, taking into the account the position of the movable mirror. The consequence of complete variation of wavelength is an oscillatory series of constructive and destructive combinations called an interferogram (Fig. 17.11b), a function of time. Only the nonabsorbed frequencies are detected by the detector as the path difference between the two beams is altered. The cosine fourier transform relates the intensity of the obtained interferogram as a function of the mirror travel (I_x) as well as the intensity of the frequency (I_v).

$$I_{(x)} = \int_{-\infty}^{\infty} I_{(v)} \cos(2\pi vx)dv$$

The high-powered microcomputer calculates the inverse transform so that the interferogram gets related to the infrared spectrum.

$$I_{(v)} = \int_{-\infty}^{\infty} I_{(x)} \cos(2\pi vx)dv$$

It needs to be noted that the two spectra are recorded, one the result of radiation emitted by the source without the sample and that, resulting by the use of radiation of the source after passing through the sample followed by subtraction of the first spectrum from the second by the computer. The dector used is a pyroelectric device containing deuterium triglycerine sulfate in a temperature-resistant alkali halide window. Mercury-cadmium-telluride (MCT) detectors have of course, increased the sensitivity of the FTIR instruments.

17.7A DIFFUSE REFLECTANCE IN FTIR

This technique has enhanced the versatility of the FTIR for solid samples. What is done in this technique is the reflected i.r. radiation from the sample is collected over a wide solid angle. No extensive grinding or even high pressure that can change the structure of the sample are required. Therefore, this technique is widely used for pharmaceutical samples, drugs, food products, soap powders. Even inorganic samples like clays can be analysed in next form.

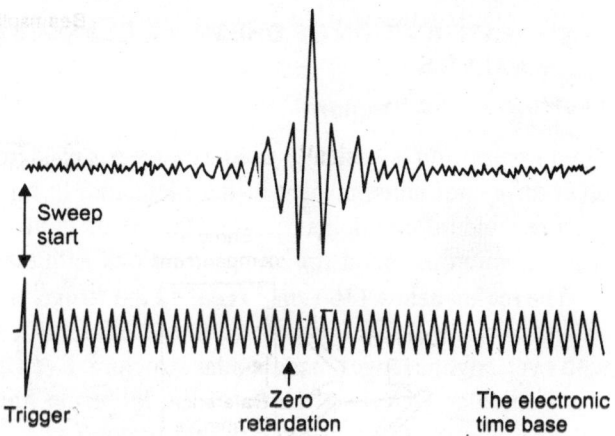

Fig. 17.11b. An interferogram of polychromatic source.

Advantages

1. These instruments are fast and record the spectrum of a sample within merely a period of thirty seconds.

2. They are very sensitive and give a good S/N ratio and high resolution.

3. These yield spectra in which there is uniformity in wave number all over whereas variation is often noticed in the spectra recorded by dispersive i.r. spectrometers.

4. The i.r. spectra of solid polymeric substances with intractable nature can be obtained. Thus, a high melting, hard and insoluble copolymer of phenylene oxide and styrene has been examined. When this substance is rubbed with an amery paper, the deposited powder can be examined to give a good i.r. spectrum by diffuse reflectance method.

5. The radiation power throughput of the interferometer is significantly larger (about forty times) than for the dispersive instrument. Furthermore, excellent spectra from very small samples can be obtained. An FTIR unit can therefore be used in conjunction with HPLC or GC.

6. As with computer-aided spectrometer, spectra of pure samples or solvents, already stored in the computer can be subtracted from the mixtures.

7. Several manufacturers offer GC-FTIR instruments with which a vapour phase spectrum can be obtained with nanogram amounts of a compound eluting from a capillary GC column.

8. Furthermore, the vapour phase spectra resemble those obtained at high dilution in a non-polar solvent. Obviously, the concentration-dependent peaks are shifted to higher frequency in comparison to those obtained from concentrated solution, thin films, or the solid state.

9. Still further, flexibility in spectral print out is also available. Spectra linear in either ν or λ can be obtained for the same data set.

10. They are cheaper than classical monochromator IR instruments. All modern IR spectrometers are FTIR instruments.

11. On top of it all, FTIR instruments can have very high resolution (≤ 0.001 cm^{-1}).

17.8 IDENTIFICATION OF CHEMICAL CLASSES (FUNCTIONAL GROUPS) BY INFRARED ANALYSIS

The Organic I.R. Region

The i.r. spectrum is basically used as a means of identifying the types of functional groups as well as other structural units, present in the molecule. In this context, the region 4000–1500 cm^{-1} gives the most reliable information as most of the bonds in this region arise due to specific bond vibrations like X–H and multiple-bond stretching vibrations with reasonable certainty.

The region below 1500 cm^{-1} is called the "fingerprint region". This is because it contains a complex pattern of bands that is entirely reproducible for any type of compound. However, it varies significantly with even slight changes in molecular structure. Even though it is not possible to assign each absorption to a particular vibrational mode of the molecule, this region, while acting as a valuable source of information, acts like a **"finger-print"** region.

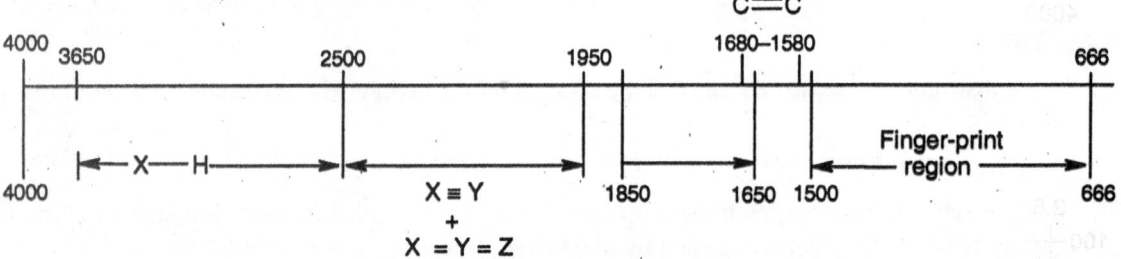

The infra-red region: 3650–1500 (X–H and multiple bond stretching region and 1500–666 (the finger-print region (not to scale).

We would show herein the application of infrared spectroscopy to different chemical classes or functional groups.

17.8.1 Alkanes

- **C–H stretching occurs around 3000 cm^{-1}**: C–H stretching absorption always occurs at frequencies less than 3000 cm^{-1}. Two strong bands each for CH_3 and CH_2 occur in the region 3000–2840 cm^{-1}. CH_2 shows a characteristic bending absorption at approximately 1465 cm^{-1} due to CH_2 scissoring plus CH_3 asymmetric bending.
- CH_3 groups shows a diagnostic bending absorption at about 1375 cm^{-1} due to symmetric bending.
- The long chain bending i.e. the motion linked with four or more CH_2 groups appears at ~ 720 cm^{-1}. The i.r. spectrum of n-decane and cyclooctane are shown in Fig. 17.12a and b respectively.

17.8.2 Alkene

Diagnostic peaks are as follows:

- C–H stretching occurs at more than 3000 cm^{-1}, generally in the range 3095–3020 cm^{-1} = C–H bending (out-of-plane) appears in the region 1000–650 cm^{-1}.
- C = C stretching occurs at 1660–1580 cm^{-1} in non-conjugated alkenes. In conjugated alkenes, this appears at lower frequencies.

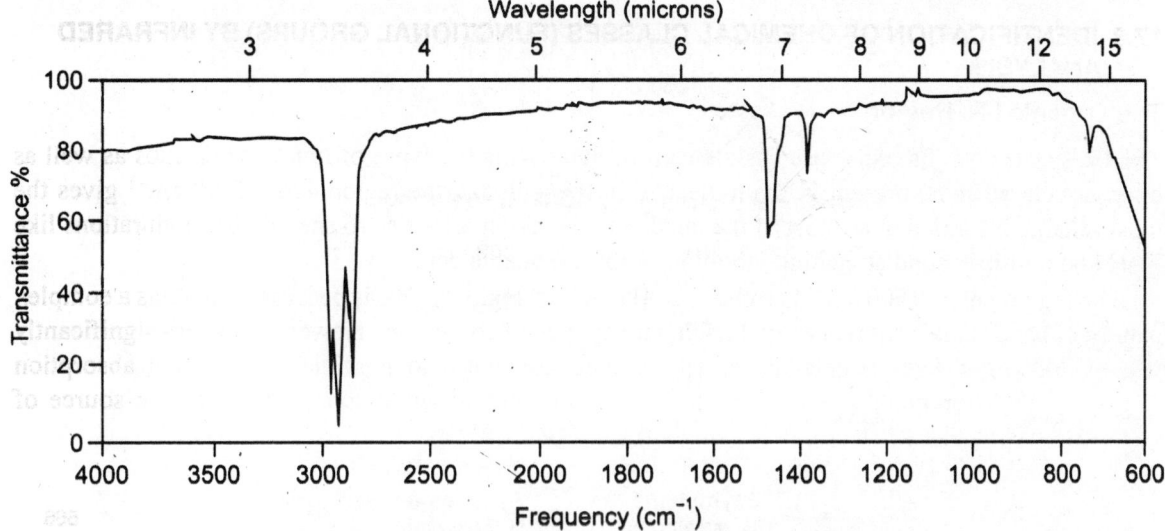

Fig. 17.12a. IR spectrum of n-Decane $CH_3(CH_2)_8CH_3$ (NaCl).

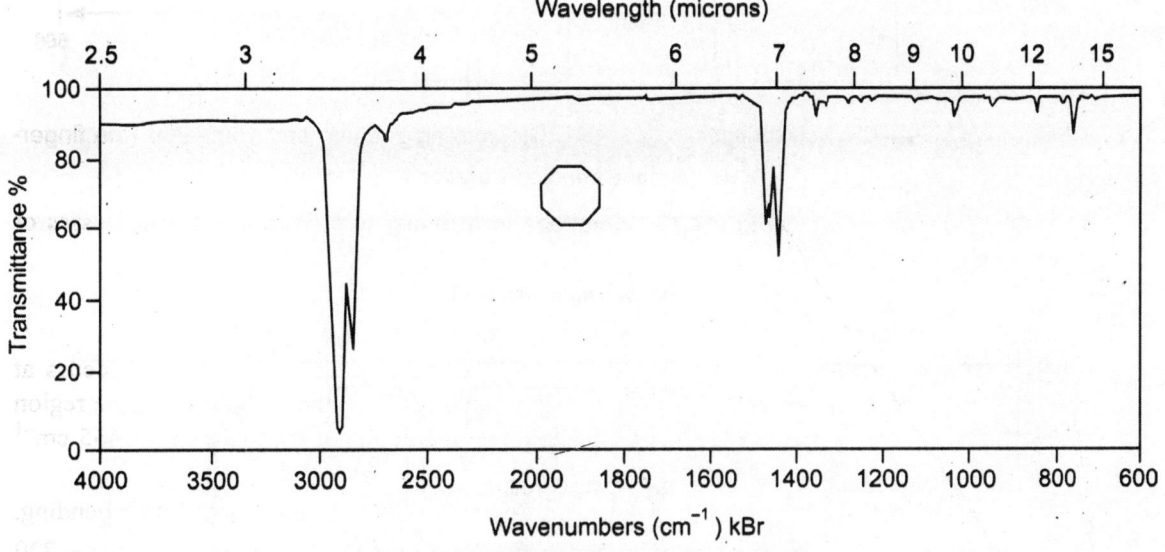

Fig. 17.12b. IR spectrum of cyclooctane.

The i.r. spectrum of trans-Stilbene is shown in Fig. 17.14a. It does not show C=C stretching as this absorption does not lead to a change in dipole moment, trans-stilbene being a symmetrical molecule. IR spectrum of cyclohexene is shown in Fig. 17.14b.

Substitution pattern of alkenes via C – H bending: Those peaks that appear in the region 1000–650 cm^{-1} serve as diagnostic peak for ascertaining the substitution pattern of alkenes (Fig. 17.15a).

Two strong bonds at 990 cm^{-1} and 910 cm^{-1} indicate a monosubstituted alkene. A vinyl group also shows an overtone at 1820 cm^{-1}.

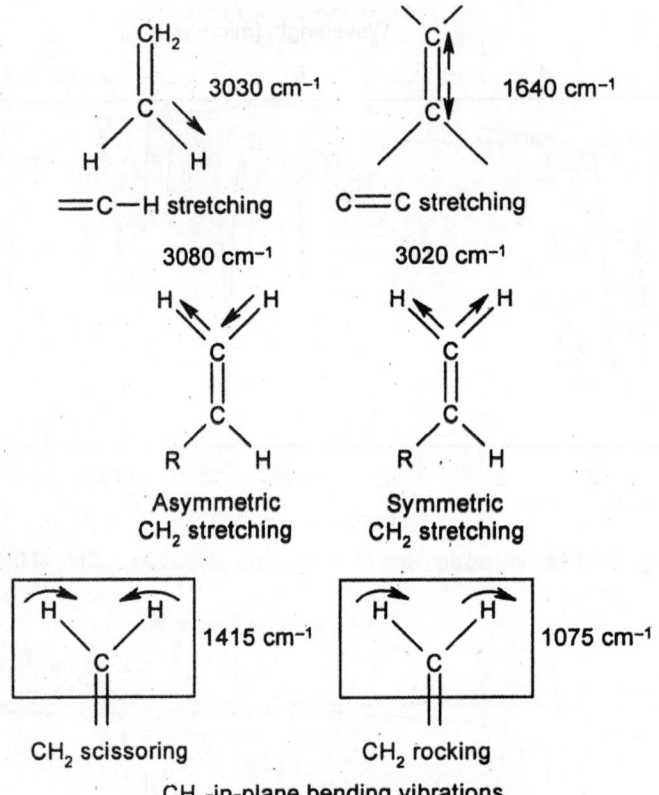

=C—H stretching   C=C stretching

Asymmetric CH₂ stretching   Symmetric CH₂ stretching

CH₂ scissoring   CH₂ rocking

CH_2-in-plane bending vibrations

Fig. 17.13. Vibrations in alkenes.

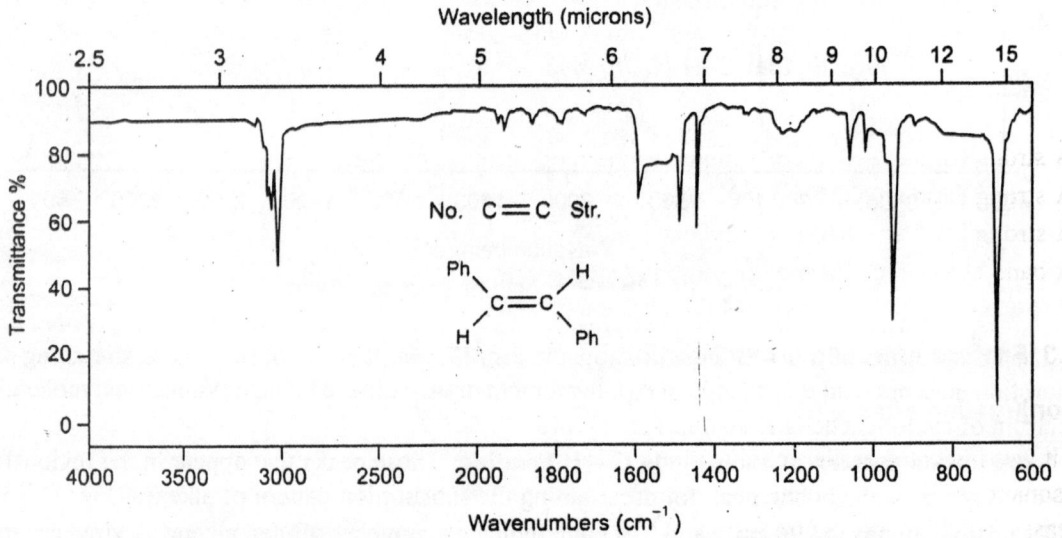

Fig. 17.14a. I.R. spectrum of trans-Stilbene. No C=C stretch.

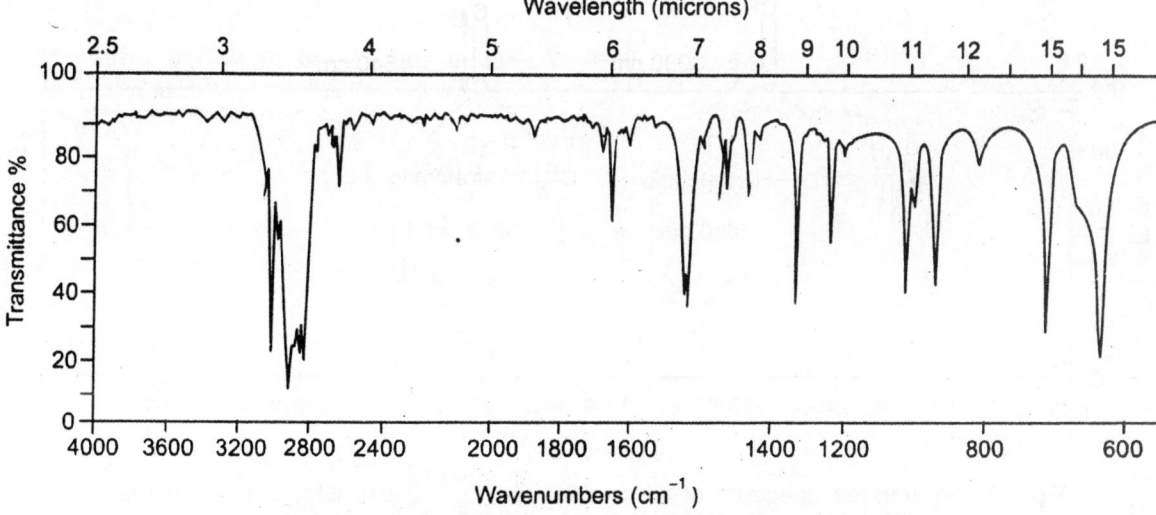

Fig. 17.14b. Infrared spectrum of Cyclohexene neat (KBr).

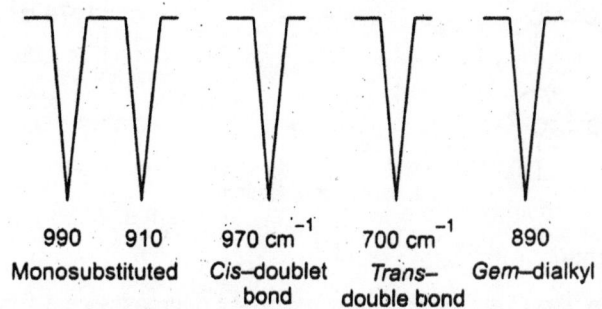

990	910	970 cm⁻¹	700 cm⁻¹	890
Monosubstituted		*Cis*–doublet bond	*Trans*– double bond	*Gem*–dialkyl

Fig. 17.15a. C–H (OOP) and substitution pattern in alkenes.

A strong band at ~ 970 cm^{-1} indicates the trans substitution pattern.

A strong band at 700 cm^{-1} indicates the cis-substitution pattern.

A strong band at ~ 890 cm^{-1} indicates a gem-dialkyl substituted olefinic bond.

A band at 815 cm^{-1} of medium intensity indicates a trisubstituted double band.

17.8.3 Factors Affecting C = C Stretching Vibration

1. Conjugation effects

Like it was indicated earlier, conjugation lowers the C = C stretching frequency. Why? This is because of resonance. The C = C character becomes C ⎯⎯ C (1.5 bonds). Obviously, the force constant K decreases which lowers the frequency of vibration. For example, the vinyl double bond in styrene gives an absorption at 1630 cm^{-1} and that in crotonaldehyde at 1632 cm^{-1} (see Fig. 17.15b).

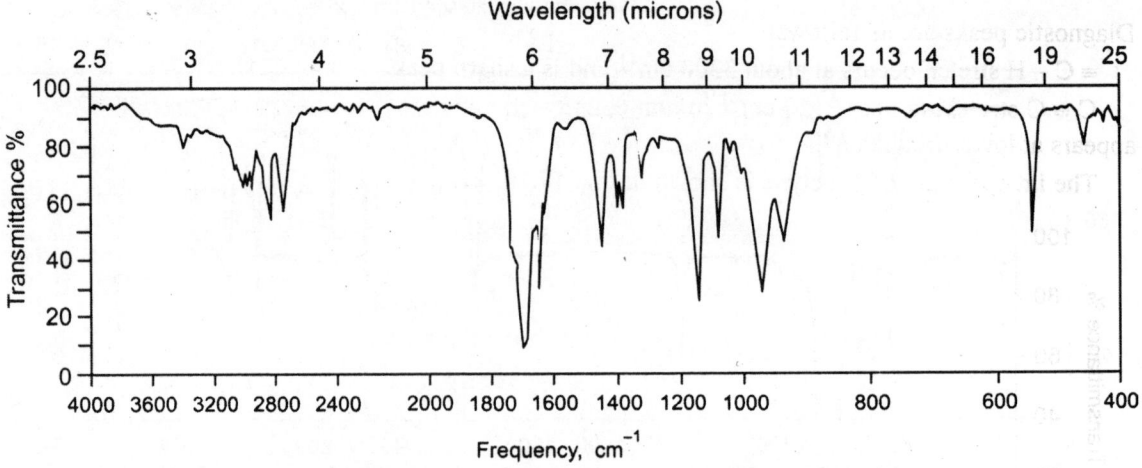

Fig. 17.15b. Infrared spectrum of crotonaldehyde, neat (KBr), CH_3–CH $=$ CHCHO.

Effect of conjugation

2. Effects due to ring size

With decrease in ring size, the C $=$ C stretching frequency decreases as a function of the decrease in internal angle:

1650 cm⁻¹   1646 cm⁻¹   1611 cm⁻¹   1566 cm⁻¹

The peak shifts to the right due to strain. An exception is cyclopropene that shows C $=$ C at 1656 cm⁻¹, due to ring strain.

When a double bond present exo to the ring, then the trend is reversed. The C $=$ C decreases with ring size.

1780 cm⁻¹   1678 cm⁻¹   1657 cm⁻¹   1651 cm⁻¹

17.8.4 Alkynes

Diagnostic peaks are as follows:

$\equiv C - H$ stretch occurs at about 3300 cm^{-1} and is a sharp peak.

$C \equiv C$ stretching near 2120 cm^{-1} in non-conjugated alkynes. Of course, in conjugated alkynes, it appears at lower frequency.

The i.r. spectrum of 1–octyne is shown in Fig. 17.16.

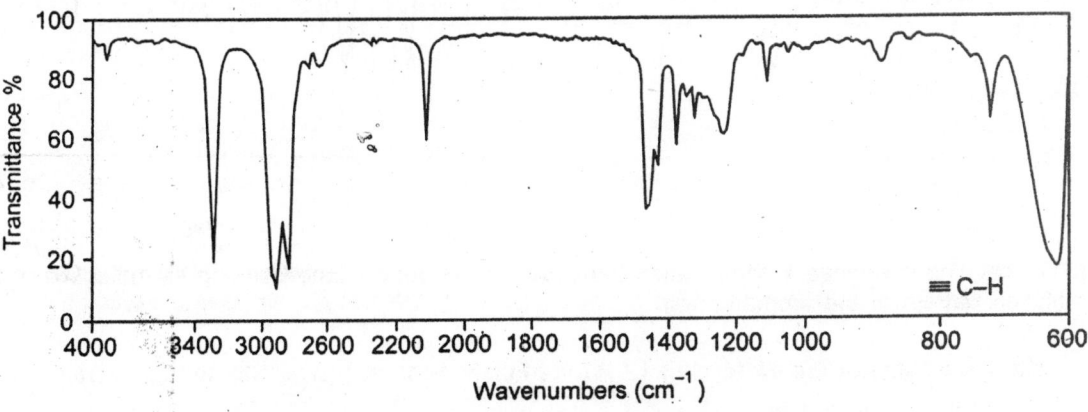

Fig. 17.16. IR spectrum of 1-octyne (thin film).

17.8.5 Aromatic Compounds

The diagnostic peaks are as under:

- $C - H$ stretch appears at frequencies greater than 3000 cm^{-1} as a shoulder on the stronger alkane C–H stretching peaks.
- Overtone plus combination bands appear in the region 2000–1667 cm^{-1} (Fig. 17.17). These indicate the substitution pattern of the ring.

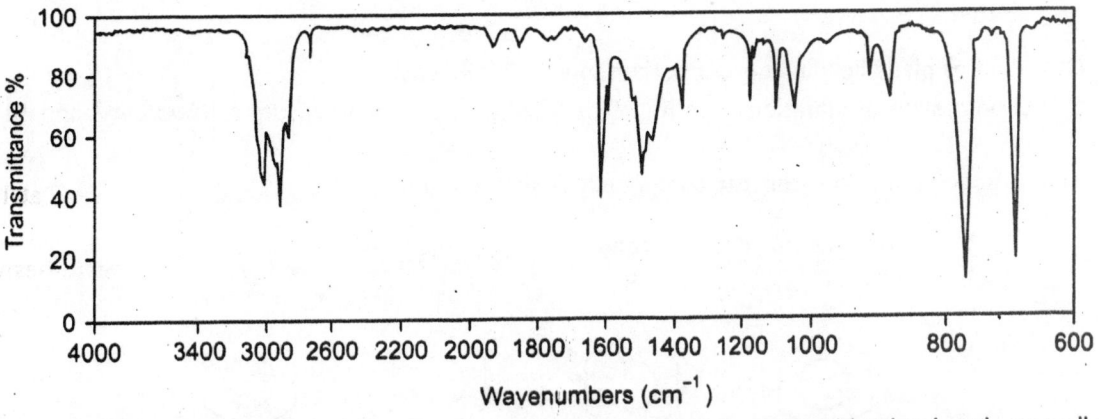

Fig. 17.17. IR spectrum of m-xylene (thin film) showing overtones and combination bonds as well as peaks at 780 and 690 cm^{-1} for a substitution pattern.

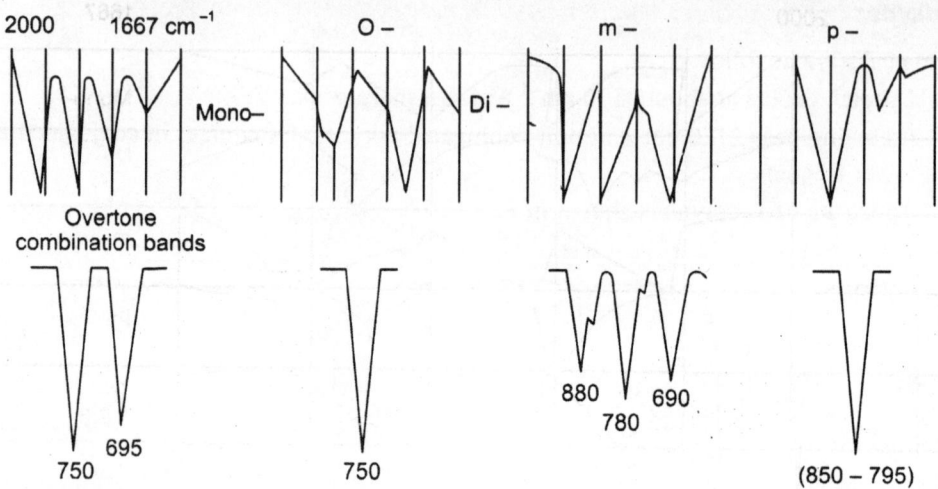

Fig. 17.18a. The overtones + combination bands and C–H out-of-plane bending as indicative of the substitution pattern of the aromatic ring.

Knowing substitution pattern via C–H out of plane bending please refer to Fig. 17.18a to learn about this.

1. **Mono substitution ring:** A strong band due to 5H at 690 cm^{-1} indicates mono substitution pattern. Further in case this is not present in the spectrum, it implies absence of a monosubstituted ring. Another strong band at 750 cm^{-1} is also observed.

2. **Ortho-disubstituted ring:** A band of strong intensity at ~ 750 cm^{-1} (770–735) indicates ortho-disubstitution pattern.

3. **Meta-disubstituted ring:** Two bands at ~ 690 cm^{-1} (725–680) and ~ 780 cm^{-1} (810–750) and third band at 880 cm^{-1} medium intensity confirm meta-disubstituted pattern.

4. **Para-disubstituted ring:** A strong band in the range 795 to 860 cm^{-1} confirms p-disubstituted pattern.

C – H out of plane bending appear in the range 900–690 cm^{-1}.

C = C ring (skeletal vibrations, see Fig. 17.19) stretching in pairs occurs at 1600 cm^{-1} and 1475 cm^{-1}.

The i.r. spectra of some aromatic compounds is shown in Fig. 17.18.

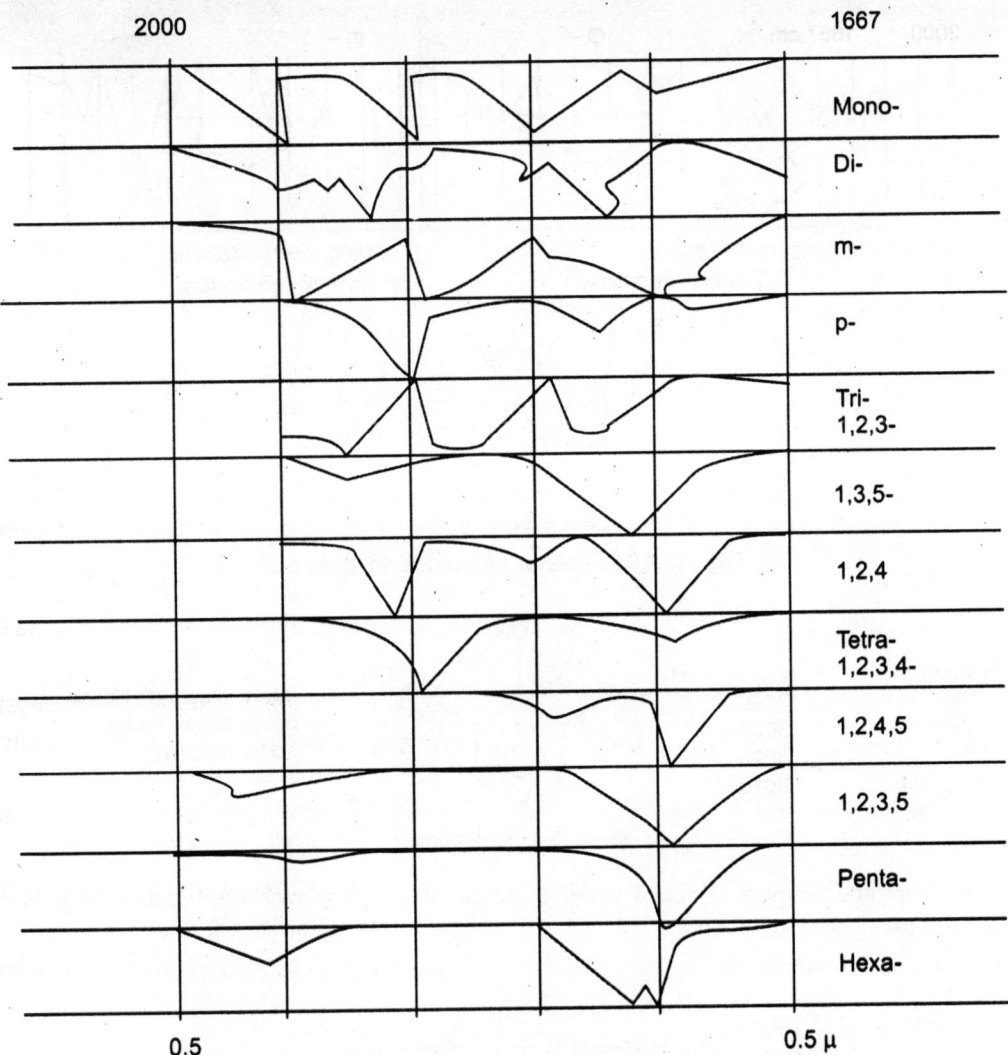

2000   1667

Mono-

Di-

m-

p-

Tri-
1,2,3-

1,3,5-

1,2,4

Tetra-
1,2,3,4-

1,2,4,5

1,2,3,5

Penta-

Hexa-

0.5   0.5 μ

Fig. 17.18b. Overtone bands in substituted benzenes.

17.8.6 Alcohols and Phenols

The diagnostic peaks are as follows:

As these compounds undergo H-bonding, the i.r. spectra vary with the physical state of the sample. O–H (broad) occurs at 3400–3200 cm^{-1}. When the H-bonding is eliminated by dilution with a non-polar solvent such as CCl_4, O–H free stretching appears at ~ 3600 cm^{-1}. In 1° alcohol, 2° and 3° alcohols, this occurs respectively at 3640, 3630 and 3620 cm^{-1}. In phenols, the free OH occurs at 3610 cm^{-1}.

Compounds which cannot show H-bonding despite the presence of X–H and Y units show free O–H stretching. For instance 2,6–di–tertbutyl phenol.

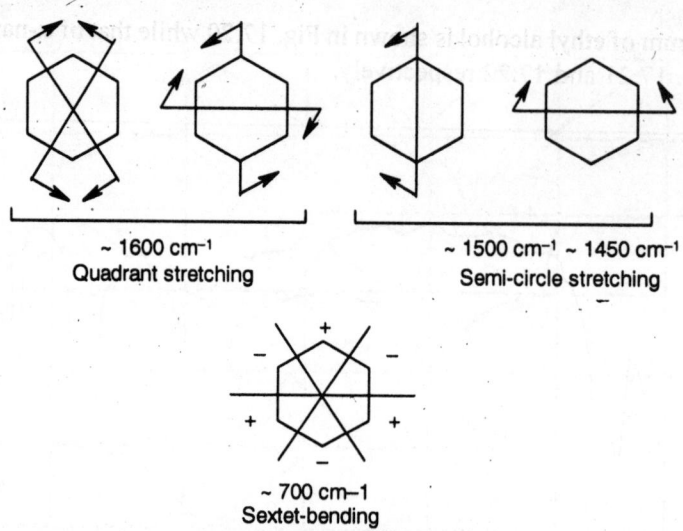

$\sim 1600\ \text{cm}^{-1}$
Quadrant stretching

$\sim 1500\ \text{cm}^{-1}$ $\sim 1450\ \text{cm}^{-1}$
Semi-circle stretching

$\sim 700\ \text{cm}{-}1$
Sextet-bending

Fig. 17.19. Skeletal vibrations in benzene.

Alcohol	ν_{CO}
1°	3640
2°	3630
3°	3620
Phenol	3610

Intermolecular H bonding
not possible due to
steric factors

Free O–H stretching

Further, there are compounds like 3–ethyl–3–pentanol which show both free as well as H–bonded O–H stretchings:

- C–O–H in-plane bending occurs at 1440–1220 cm^{-1} as a broad (weak) band, often buried under CH$_3$ bending bands which appear at 1375 cm^{-1}.
- C–O stretching occurs at 1250–1000 cm^{-1}. This is used to distinguish 1°, 2° and 3° alcohols.

Alcohol	C–O stretching cm^{-1}
Primary alcohol	1050
Secondary alcohol	1100
Tertiary alcohol	1150
Phenols	1220

- OH OOp: These appear at 770–650 cm^{-1}.

The i.r. spectrum of ethyl alcohol is shown in Fig. 17.20 while that of α-naphthol and β-naphthol appear in Fig. 17.21 and 17.22 respectively.

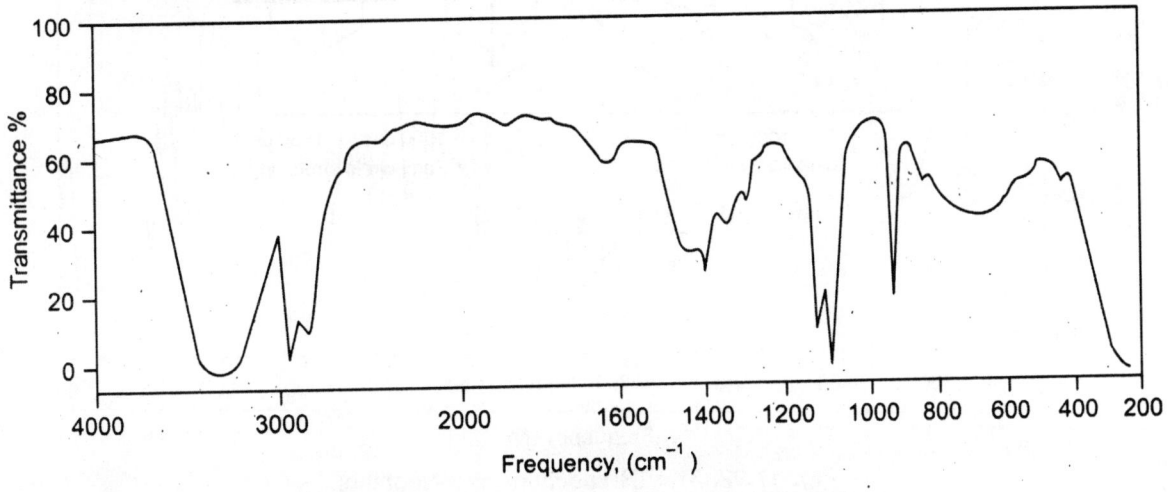

Fig. 17.20. The IR spectrum of ethyl alcohol.

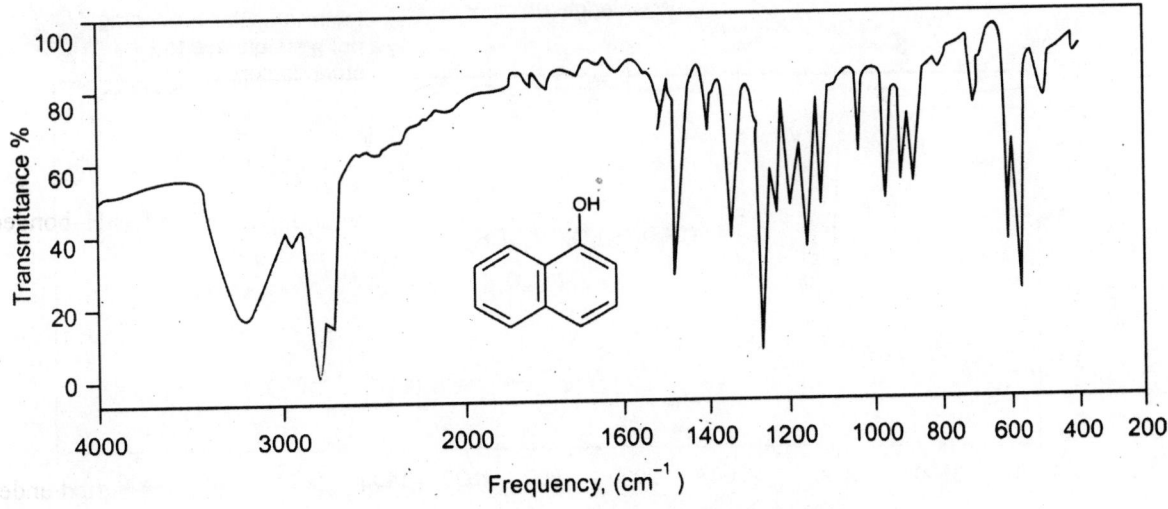

Fig. 17.21. The IR spectrum of α-Naphthol.

17.8.7 Ethers

The i.r. spectrum of Di-n-amyl ether is shown in Fig. 17.23.

The diagnostic band is the C–O stretching at 1300–1000 cm^{-1}. This coupled with the absence of C=O and O–H bands indicates that the observed C–O stretching is not due to other oxy compounds like alcohols, esters, etc. In dialkyl ethers the asymmetric a single strong C–O–C stretching is noticed at ~ 1120 cm^{-1}, the symmetric stretching being i.r. inactive. On the other hand, the unsymmetrical aryl alkyl

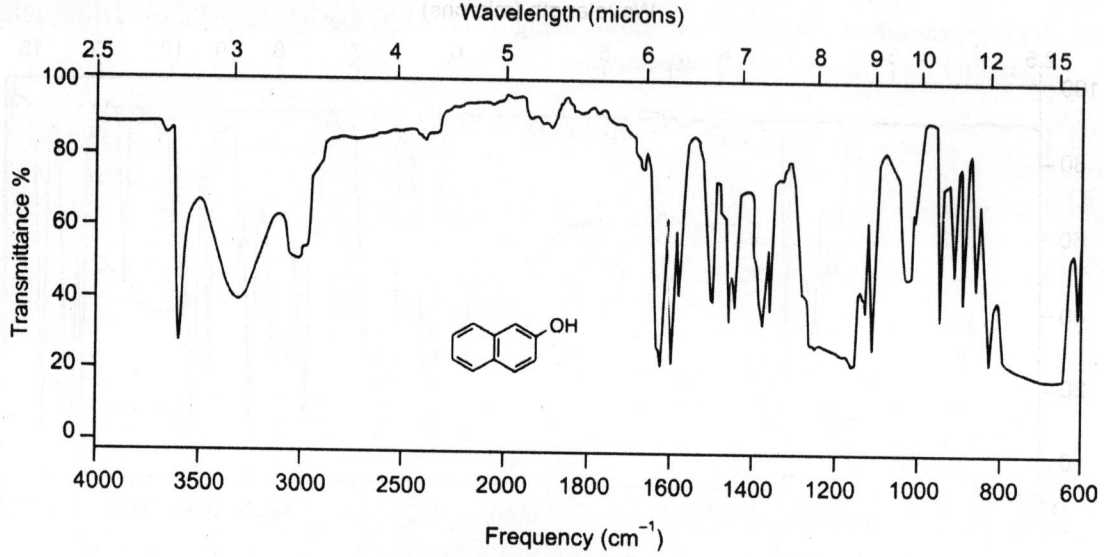

Fig. 17.22. The IR spectrum of β-Naphthol.

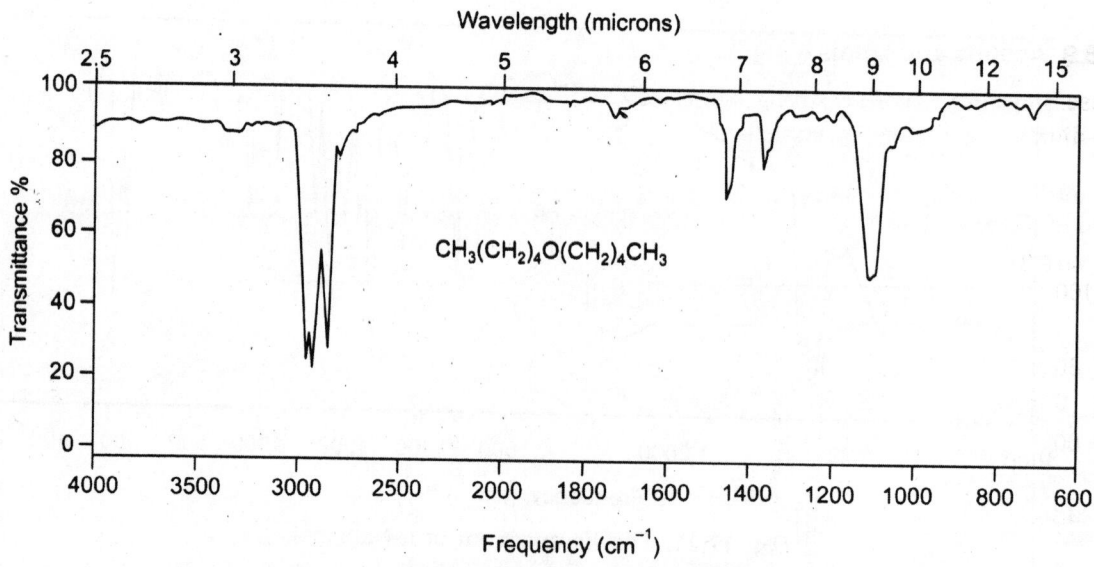

Fig. 17.23. Infrared spectrum of Di-n-amyl ether.

ethers show two strong bands due to C–O–C stretching at 1250 cm^{-1} (asymmetric) and symmetric one at 1040 cm^{-1}. The i.r. spectrum of anisole is recorded in Fig. 17.24a.

17.8.8 Epoxides

Epoxides give a weak ring stretching at 1280–1230 cm^{-1}.

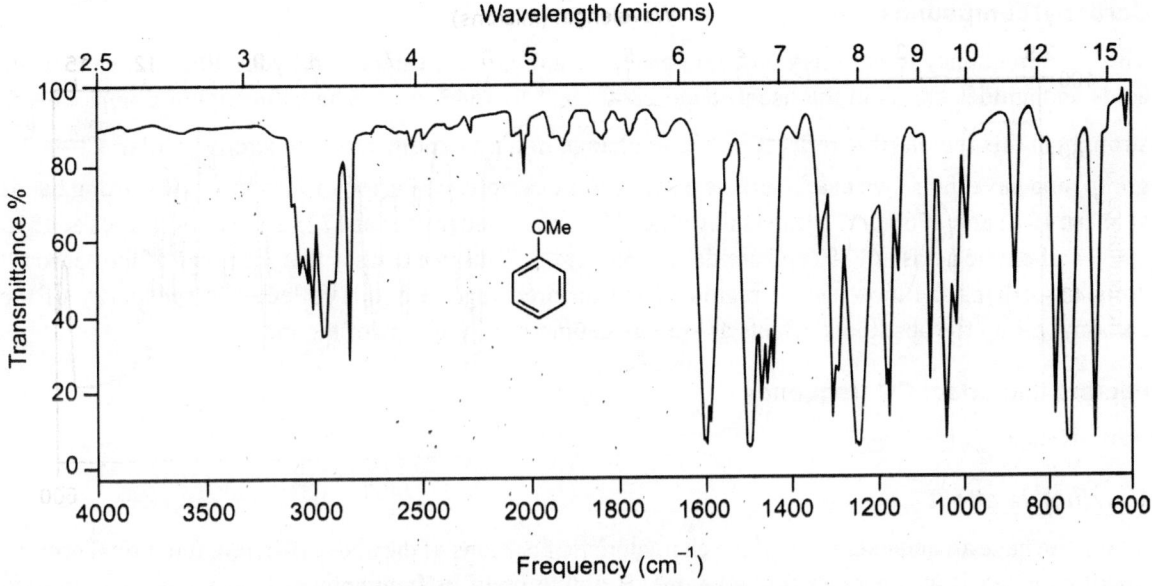

Fig. 17.24a. IR spectrum of anisole.

17.8.9 Acetals and ketals

These show four or five strong bands at 1200–1020 cm^{-1}. See Fig. 17.24b for i.r. spectrum of 2,2–dimethoxypropane, a simple ketal.

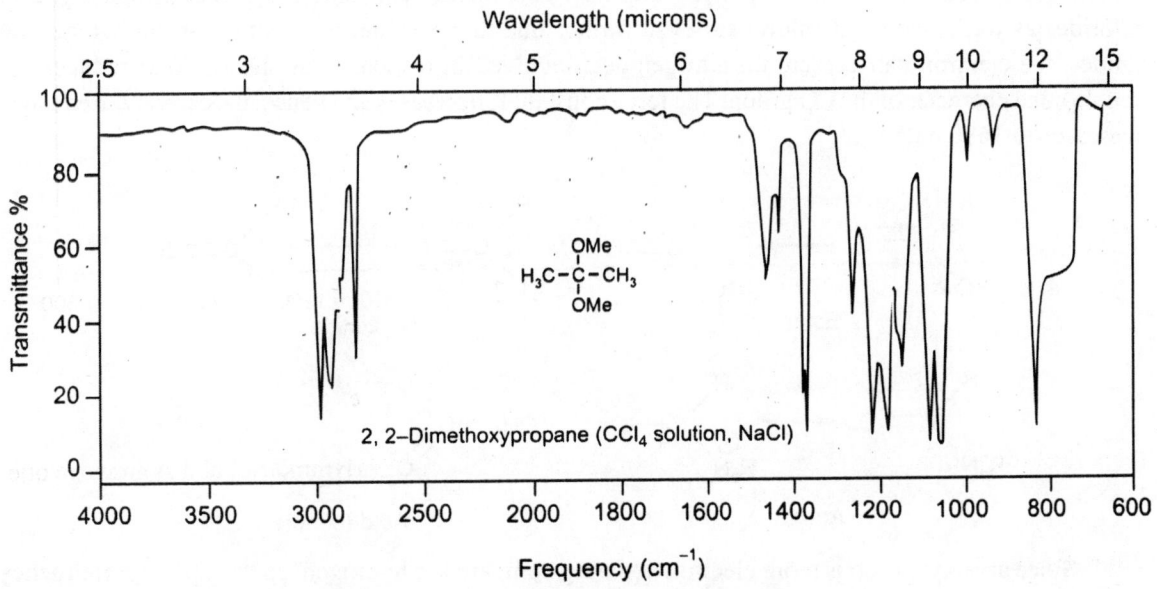

Fig. 17.24b. IR spectrum of 2,2–Dimethoxypropane.

Carbonyl compounds

The C=O frequency in various functional groups – anhydrides, esters, aldehydes, ketones, carboxylic acids and amides etc. is in the usual range 1850 cm^{-1} to 1545 cm^{-1}. These functional groups absorb strongly in this region (that reflects immense change in dipole moment in the strongly polar $\overset{+\delta}{C}=\overset{\delta-}{O}$ group) and have their own characteristic pattern. For example, while anhydrides show two strong bands at about 1810 and 1760 cm^{-1}, testers absorb at 1735 cm^{-1}, aldehydes at 1725 cm^{-1} and ketones at 1715 cm^{-1}, carboxylic acids at 1710 and amides at 1690 cm^{-1}. Thus, we can say that the range of the carbonyl group is perhaps the most useful region of the infrared region as this reflects the sensitivity of the carbonyl group to substituent effects as well as geometry of the type of the molecule.

Factors that affect CO frequency

Various factors affect v_{CO}.

1. Inductive effect

In order to have an understanding of the characteristic positions of the above different functional groups, it will be better if we consider first a ketone. Building upon its frequency as base value, we can then discuss the effect of varying the substituents electron withdrawing and electron releasing conjugation, resonance, ring strain and hydrogen bonding – various factors affecting CO frequency.

The base value for a ketone such as acetone is observed to be 1715 cm^{-1}. If an alkyl substituent is replaced by an electron withdrawing group (EWG), such as an OR, transforming the ketone into an ester, the carbonyl frequency rises to 1735 cm^{-1}. This is as per expectation since withdrawl of electrons from oxygen to carbon gives a triple bond character to the C=O bond. As the force constant K increases, the stretching frequency of the carbonyl group now gets raised. This is exactly what happens in acid chlorides as well. The C=O value rises even further due to electronegative nature of the halogen. In amides, the electron pair present on nitrogen gets involved in resonance as shown. That reduces the double bond character of the CO group. The force constant K decreases and hence, the carbonyl frequency decreases to 1690 cm^{-1}.

Since an alkyl group is more electron donating compared to hydrogen, so the carbonyl frequency of ketones is relatively lower than aldehydes which absorb at 1725 cm^{-1}.

2. Effects of H-bonding

As for carboxylic acids are concerned, the oxygen of OH group is electron withdrawing which should raise the carbonyl frequency but the observed value is rather smaller than 1715 cm^{-1}. This is due to hydrogen bonding that converts carboxylic acids into dimers. As the C=O gets stretched, the force constant is lowered, so that it absorbs at 1680 cm^{-1} in methyl salicylate (oil of wintergreen) whose i.r. spectrum of methyl salicylate is recorded in Fig. 17.24c.

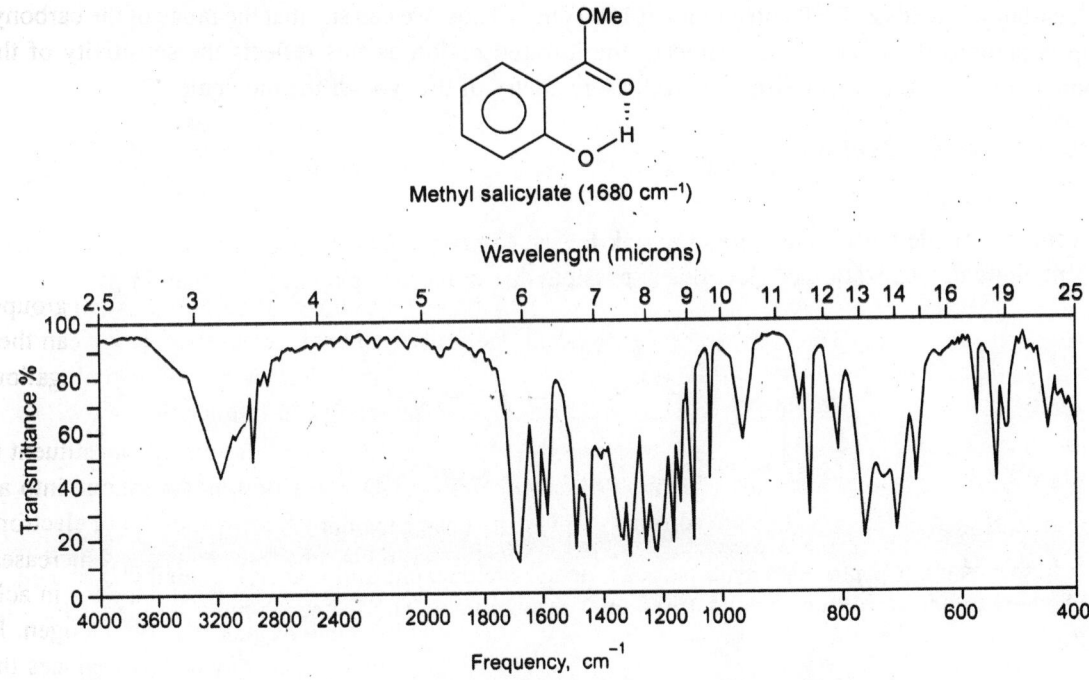

Methyl salicylate (1680 cm^{-1})

Fig. 17.24c. Infrared spectrum of methyl salicylate, neat (KBr).

3. Effect of conjugation

When a C=O group is present in conjugation with a C=C, the C=O stretching frequency is lowered down because of delocalization of π electrons which reduces the double bond character of the C=O group. A reduction in the force constant lowers the carbonyl frequency as anticipated. It has been observed that, in general, the decrease is about 30 cm^{-1} (0.1 μ). Greater the number of C=C attached to the carbonyl group in conjugation, larger is the decrease. For example, in acetophenone, the C=O frequency appears at 1685 cm^{-1}. Introduction of a yet another C=C in conjugation with the C=O leads to a further decrease as anticipated albeit by about 15 cm^{-1} (0.05 m).

Conjugation effect

4. Steric effects

When the conjugation effect is prevented by say a reduction in the coplanarity of the unsaturated system, two carbonyl frequencies are observed instead of just one. For instance, α, β unsaturated ketones like benzal acetone exists as s-trans as well as s-cis isomers. This molecule shows two bands at 1674 cm^{-1} and 1699 cm^{-1}, due respectively to the s-trans and s-cis carbonyl groups. In s-trans, there is no steric hindrance while the reverse is true in the s-cis form.

s-trans   s-trans

Benzalacetone

Similarly, while the ketone I shows a peak for the C=O at higher position than the ketone II. As is evident, more delocalization of electrons is possible due to more coplanarity in I than in II.

I. More coplanar   II. Less coplanar

A further example is provided by its pair of 1–acetyl cyclohexene and 1–acetyl–2–methyl cyclohexene which show bonds at 1686 cm^{-1} and 1693 cm^{-1} respectively. The former is more co-planar than the latter.

1–acetyl cyclohexene
(1686 cm^{-1})

1–acetyl–2–methyl cyclohexene
(1693 cm^{-1})

5. Field effect or the α-substitution effects

Replacement of a α-hydrogen to the carbonyl carbon by a halogen raises the C=O bond frequency. This happens as a result of the electron-withdrawing ability of the halogen such that the non-bonded electron pairs of the carbonyl oxygen are shifted into the carbonyl double bond, thereby increasing its double bond character. As the force constant is increased, the frequency is raised. In such a situation, it is but natural, to expect two C=O frequencies from these types of ketones. Thus, α-chloro acetophenone exhibits two bonds in its infrared spectrum. This happens because in one form, the chloride is present on the same side as the C=O group while in the other form, the chlorine is rotated on the other side of the CO group.

6. Ring strain effect

Ring strain leads to an increase in carbonyl frequency (see Fig. 17.24d). More the strain, higher the frequency as is reflected in the following series i.e. as the bond angle around the CO decreases, v_{CO} increases.

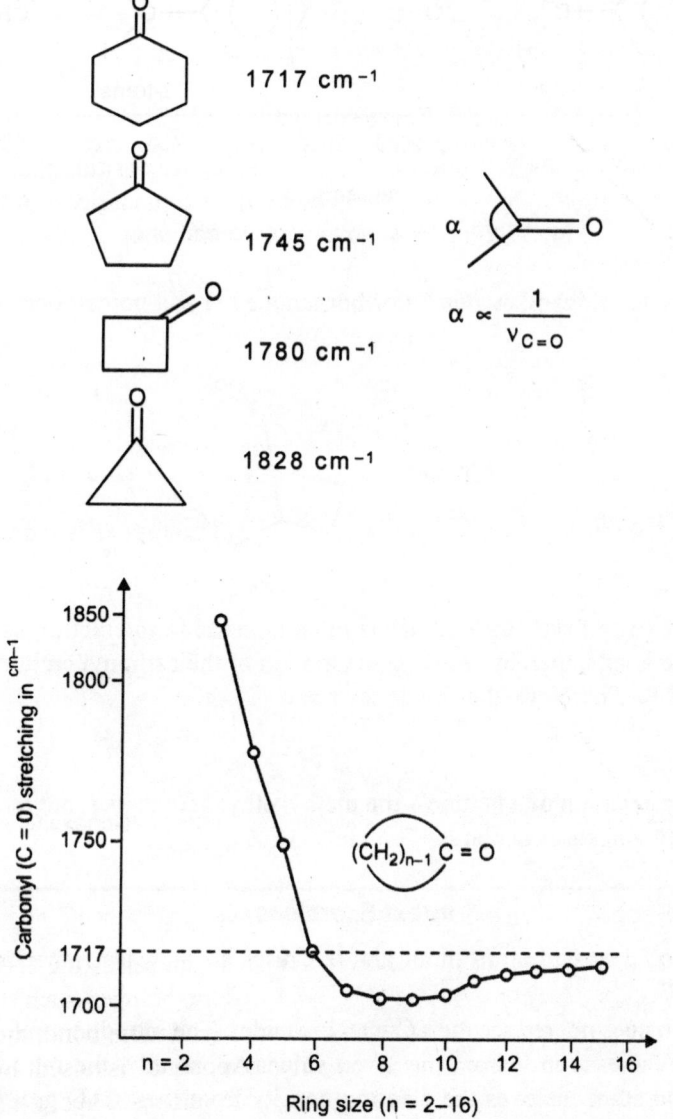

1717 cm^{-1}

1745 cm^{-1}

1780 cm^{-1}

1828 cm^{-1}

$\alpha \propto \dfrac{1}{v_{C=O}}$

$(CH_2)_{n-1} C = O$

Carbonyl (C = O) stretching in cm^{-1}

Ring size (n = 2–16)

Fig. 17.24d. C=O frequency versus ring size in cycloalkanones.

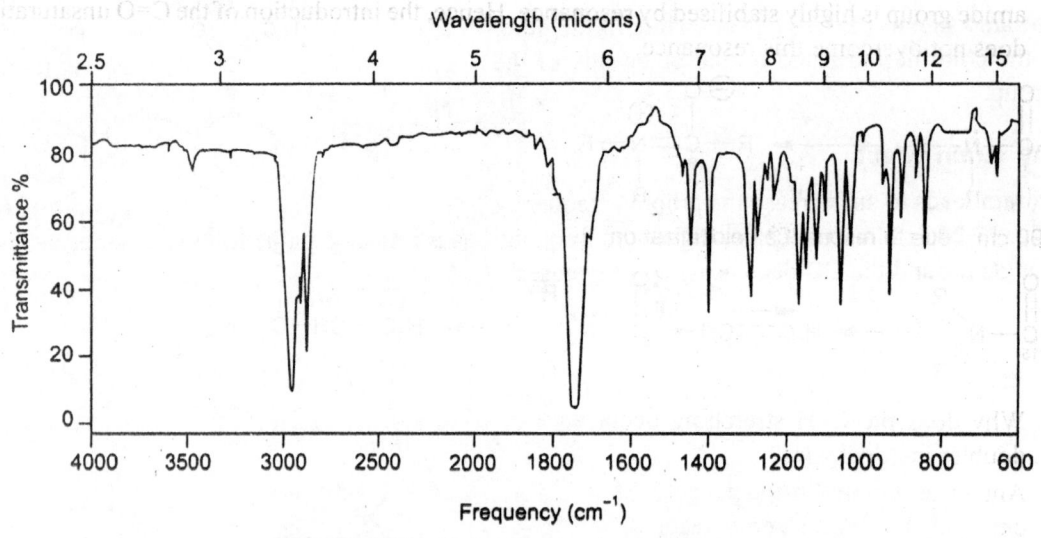

Fig. 17.24e. IR spectrum of norcamphor.

More strained bicyclic bridged ketones 7 nor bornanone (1) and norcamphor (2) absorb at higher values (Fig. 17.24e).

(1)   1800 cm⁻¹

(2)   O 1748 cm⁻¹

A decrease in bond angle from 109°–28′ leads to an increase in interaction between the C=O and the neighbouring single bonds, thereby resisting the motion of the carbonyl carbon. That increases the value of force constant K. Therefore, the frequency rises.

7. Effect of solvent

This is illustrated by observation of a ketone – the methyl ethyl ketone in about ten percent solution of methyl alcohol in which it absorbs at about 1706 cm⁻¹.

Intext Exercises

4. Introduction of α, β unsaturation in an amide causes an increase rather than a decrease in frequency. Why?

   Ans. Conjugation does not reduce the >C=O ν in amides. The introduction of α,β-unsaturation rather causes an increase in ν from the given value. Apparently, the introduction of the sp² hybridised carbon atom removes the electron density from the >C=O group, strengthens the bond instead of interacting by resonance as in the other >C=O examples. In fact, the parent amide group is highly stabilised by resonance. Hence, the introduction of the C=O unsaturation does not overcome this resonance.

$$R-\underset{\underset{R}{|}}{\overset{\overset{O}{\|}}{C}}-\underset{1}{\ddot{N}}-R \quad\longleftrightarrow\quad R-\underset{\underset{R}{|}}{\overset{\overset{\ominus O}{|}}{C}}=\underset{9}{\overset{\oplus}{N}}-R$$

1690 cm^{-1} due to resonance delocalization

$$R-\overset{\overset{O}{\|}}{\underset{15}{C}}-N\overset{R}{\underset{R}{\diagup}} \quad\longrightarrow\quad H_2C=CH\longleftarrow\overset{\overset{:O}{\|}}{\underset{23}{C}}-\ddot{N}\overset{R}{\underset{R}{\diagup}} \quad\longleftrightarrow\quad H_2\overset{\oplus}{C}-CH-\underset{32}{\overset{\overset{\ominus}{\overset{O}{|}}}{C}}-N\overset{R}{\underset{R}{\diagup}}$$

5. Why does the C–H stretching occur as a doublet in Aldehydes?

Ans. The doublet in the range 2830–2695 cm^{-1} occurs due to Fermi resonance. The fundamental C–H vibration i.e. C–H in plane bonding at 1390 cm^{-1} couples with the first overtone (1390 × 2) at 2780 cm^{-1}. These two close molecular vibrational frequencies resonate or rather exchange energy.

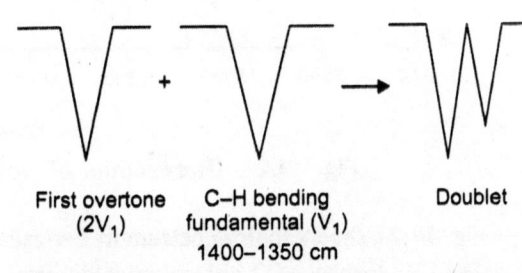

First overtone (2V$_1$) C–H bending fundamental (V$_1$) 1400–1350 cm Doublet

Fig. 17.25. Fermi resonance in action in aldehydes

17.8.11 Aldehydes

The diagnostic peaks are as follows:

- C–H stretching occurs a doublet of weak bands at 2830–2695 cm^{-1}, due to Fermi resonance, a phenomenon explained earlier (see Fig. 17.25). In some cases, the higher frequency peak in the doublet is obscured by the C–H aliphatic peak.
- C=O stretching occurs at 1740–1725 cm^{-1} for aliphatic aldehydes. In aromatic aldehydes, this goes down to 1700–1660 cm^{-1} due to conjugation. More the conjugation, still lower the frequency:

$$Ph-\underset{|}{C}=\underset{|}{C}-\overset{\overset{O}{\|}}{C}-H \qquad 1680 \text{ cm}^{-1}$$

$$R-\overset{\overset{O}{\|}}{C}-H \qquad 1740\text{–}1725 \text{ cm}^{-1}$$

$$-\underset{|}{C}=\underset{|}{C}-\overset{\overset{O}{\|}}{C}-H \qquad 1700\text{–}1680 \text{ cm}^{-1}$$

$$Pr-\overset{\overset{O}{\|}}{C}-H \qquad 1700\text{–}1660 \text{ cm}^{-1}$$

- C–H OOP occurs at 975–780 cm^{-1}.

Fig. 17.26 shows i.r. spectrum of iso-valeraldehyde.

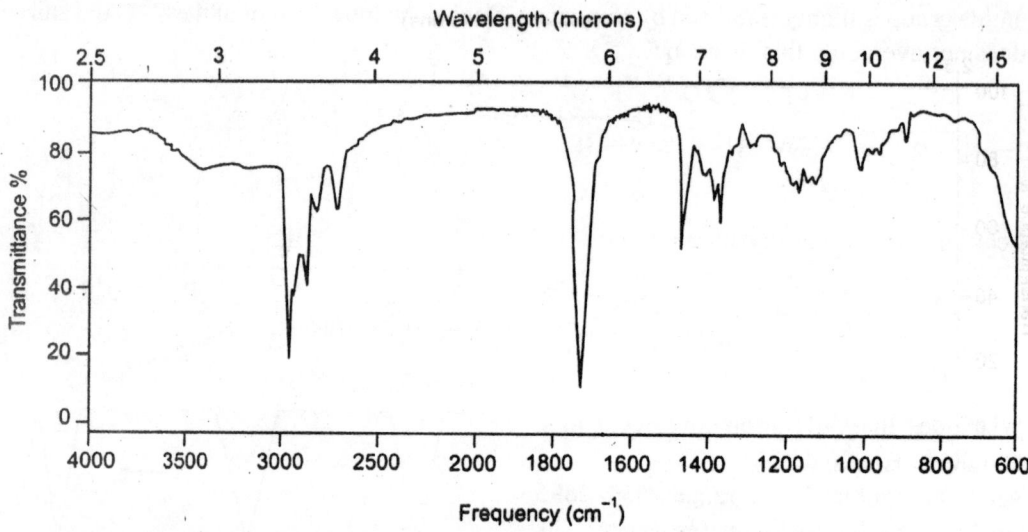

Fig. 17.26. IR spectrum of Isovaleraldehyde, $(CH_3)_2CHCH_2CHO$.

Fig. 17.27 shows their spectrum of benzaldehyde.

The I.R. spectra of O-chlorobenzaldehyde, cinnamaldehyde are shown in Fig. 17.28, 17.29 and 17.30 respectively.

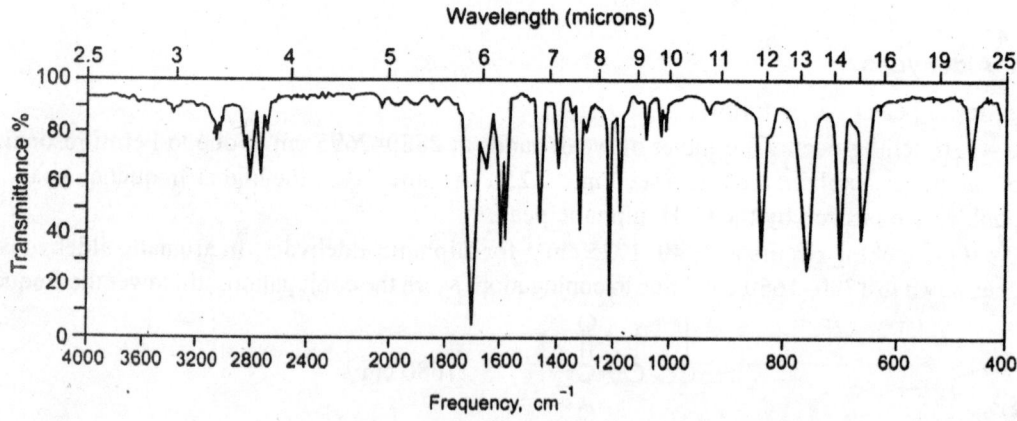

Fig. 17.27. Infrared spectrum of Benzaldehyde, neat (KBr).

17.8.12 Ketones

The diagnostic hands are:

- The C=O stretching in aliphatic ketones (non-conjugated) occurs in the region 1720–1708 cm⁻¹ but conjugation with C=C decreases it to 1700–1675 cm⁻¹.

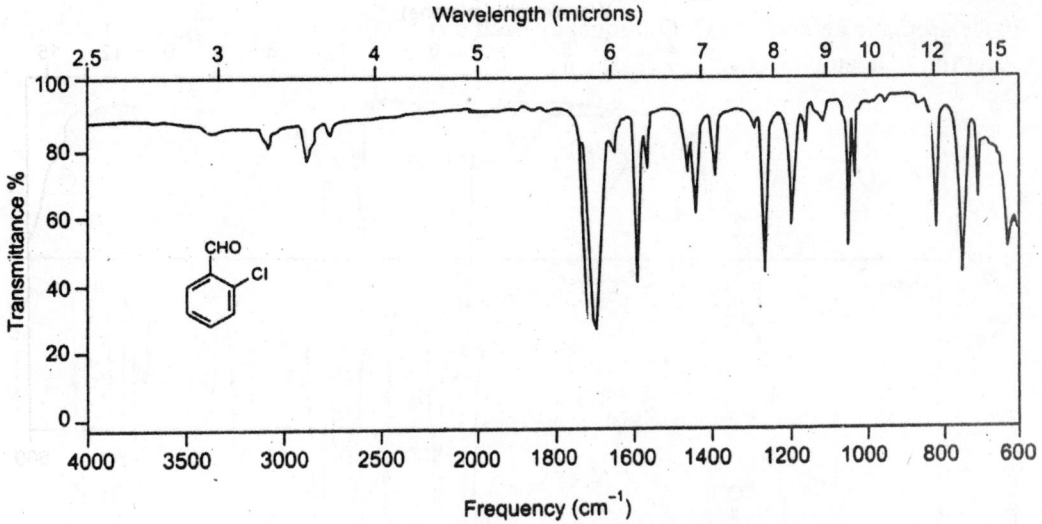

Fig. 17.28. IR spectrum of O-chlorobenzaldehyde (NaCl).

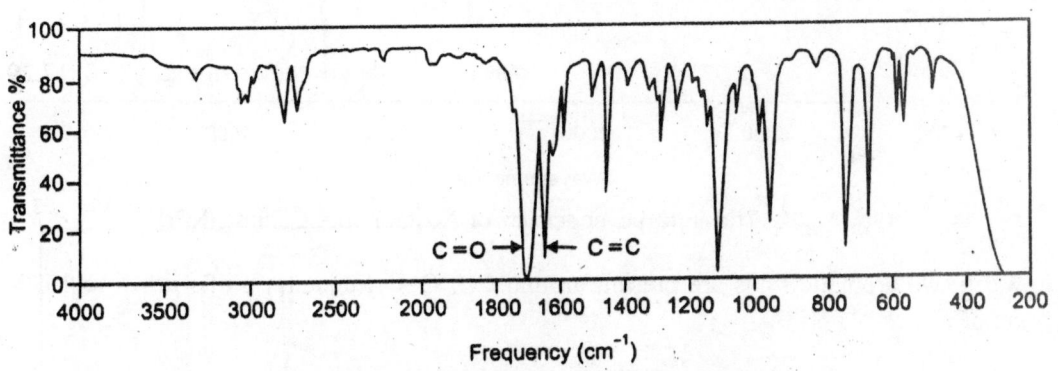

Fig. 17.29. IR spectrum of Cinnamaldehyde.

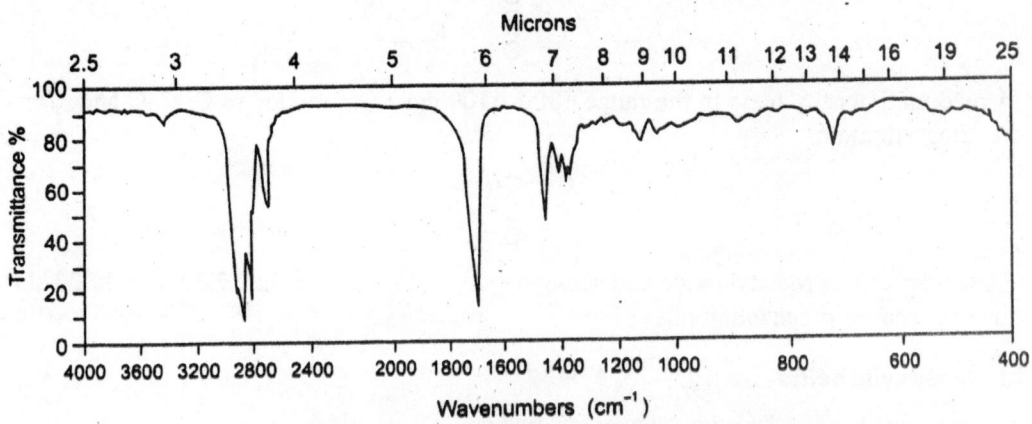

Fig. 17.30. Infrared spectrum of nonanal (thin film).

- In the aromatic ketones the C=O frequency occurs at 1700–1680 cm^{-1}. Fig. 17.31 shows the i.r. spectrum of acetophenone.

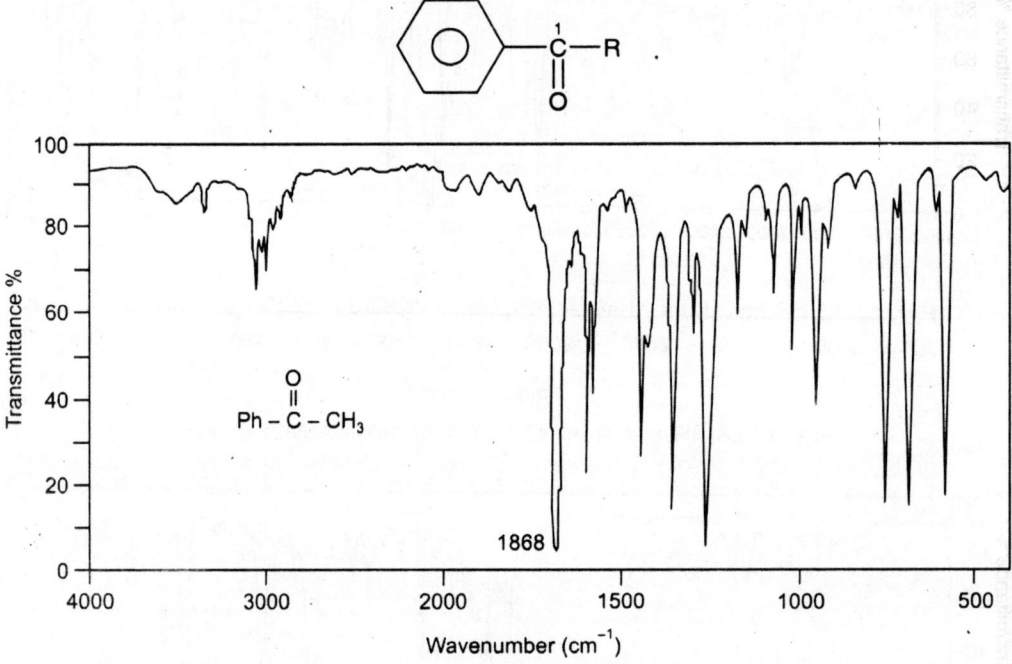

Fig. 17.31. The infrared spectrum of Acetophenone, neat (KBr).

- When two aromatic rings are present around CO, C=O frequency shifts down to 1670–1600 cm^{-1}.

- A medium intensity band in the range 1300–1100 cm^{-1} occurs due to C–C–C and C—C—C bending vibrations.

The i.r. spectra of Mesityl oxide and acetophenone are shown in Fig. 17.32. Fig. 17.33 shows the i.r. spectrum of p-benzoquinone.

17.8.13 Carboxylic acids

The diagnostic bands of carboxylic acids are as under:

- A very broad band in solid or liquid phase in the range 3400–2400 cm^{-1} due to O–H stretching.

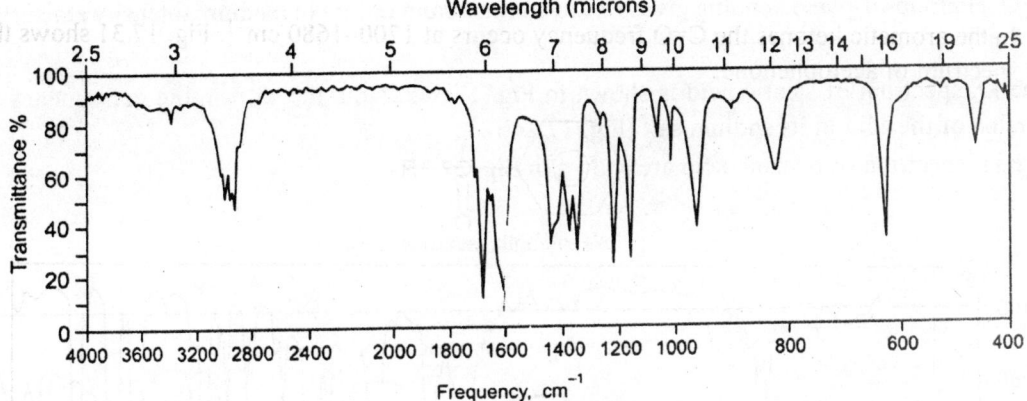

Fig. 17.32. IR spectrum of Mesityl oxide $CH_3COCH = C(CH_3)_2$ (neat, KBr).

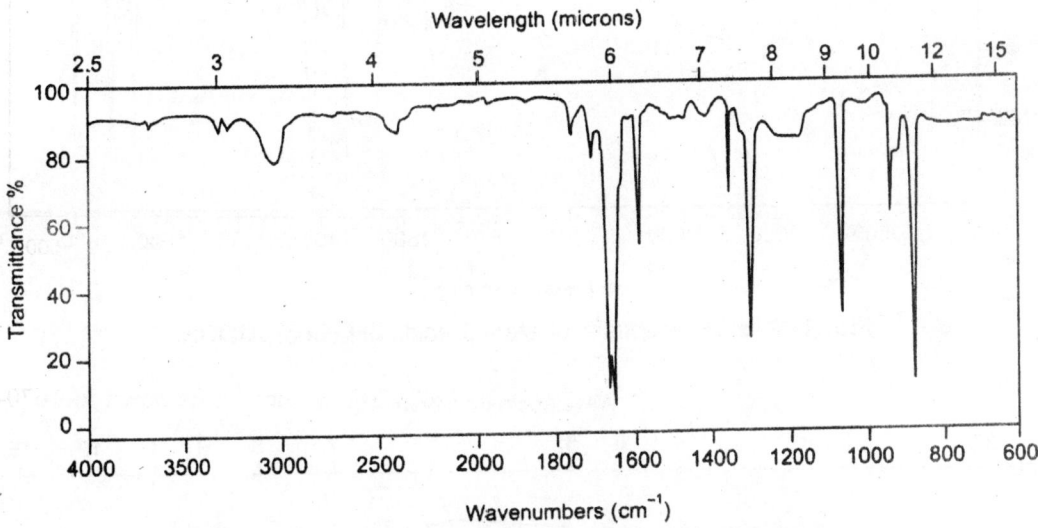

Fig. 17.33. Infrared spectrum of p-benzoquinone (NaCl).

Usually this band overlaps with the C–H stretching bands (3100–2800 cm^{-1}). This O–H is due to existence of acids mainly in the dimeric form. This O–H band, however, appears at an increased frequency at 3520 cm^{-1} when the acids are examined in vapour phase wherein the acids mainly exist in the monomer form. So, we may call this as the free O–H stretching.

- The carbonyl stretching broad band appears in the region 1730–1680 cm^{-1}. This band is even broader and more intense than those of the ketones and aldehydes. However, the band shifts to 1760–1730 cm^{-1} upon dilution of the acid with a non-polar solvent when acids exist mainly in monomeric form.

- The O–H in-plane bending and C–O stretching bands at 1450 cm^{-1} and 1300 cm^{-1} are the other diagnostic peaks.

- A medium intensity band at 1320–1210 cm^{-1} due to C–O stretching.

- O–H group-of-plane bending gives rise to a broad band of low to medium intensity at nearly 930 cm^{-1}.

The i.r. spectrum of stearic acid is shown in Fig. 17.34a. Note the shift in the cofrequency upon conversion of the acid in its sodium salt (Fig. 17.34b).

The i.r. spectrum of benzoic acid are shown in Fig. 17.35.

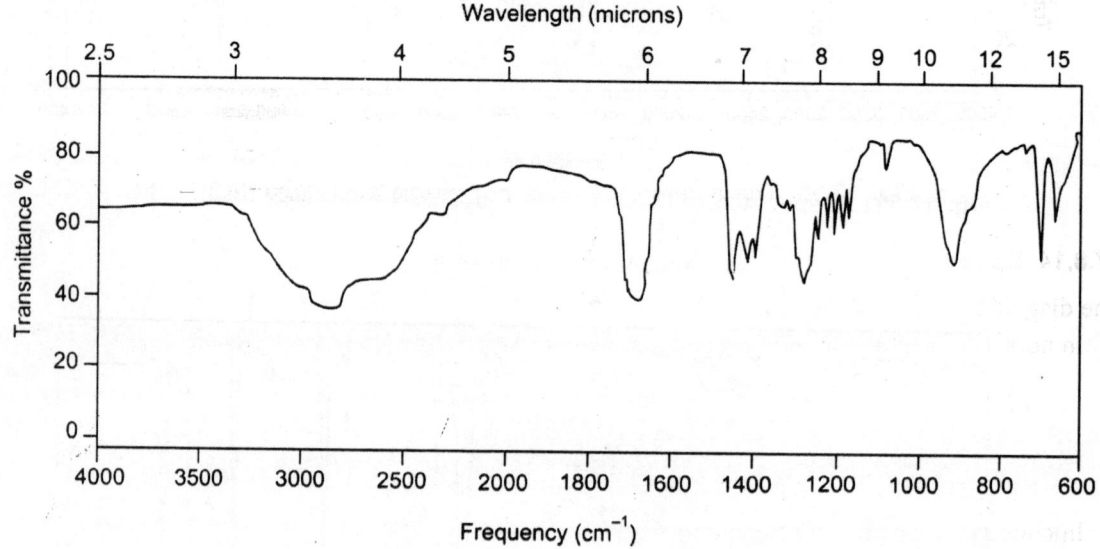

Fig. 17.34a. IR spectrum of stearic acid, CH$_3$(CH$_2$)$_{16}$COOH.

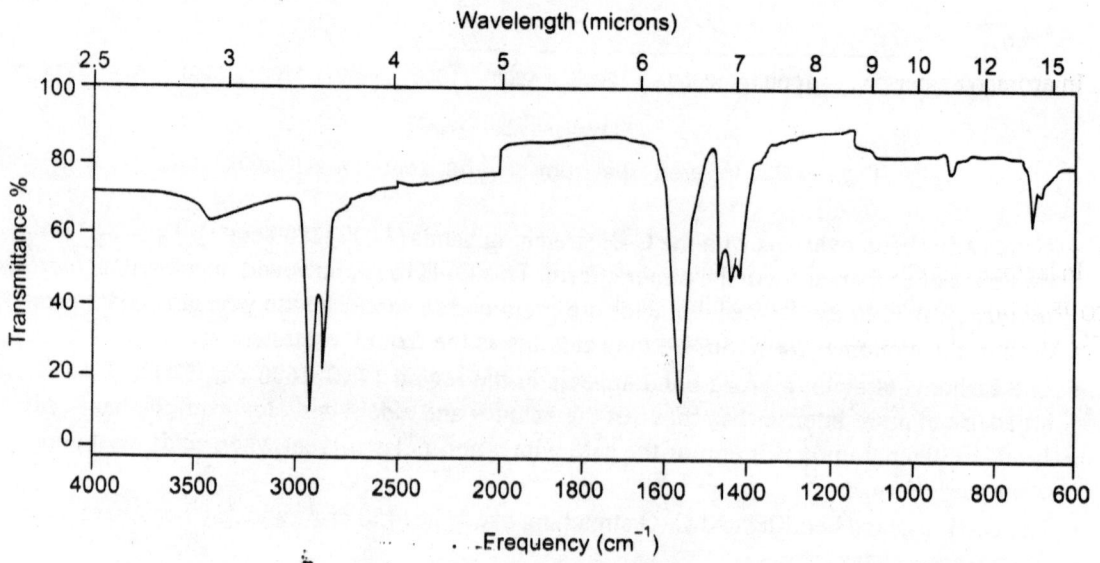

Fig. 17.34b. IR spectrum of sodium salt of stearic acid, CH$_3$(CH$_2$)$_{16}$COONa.

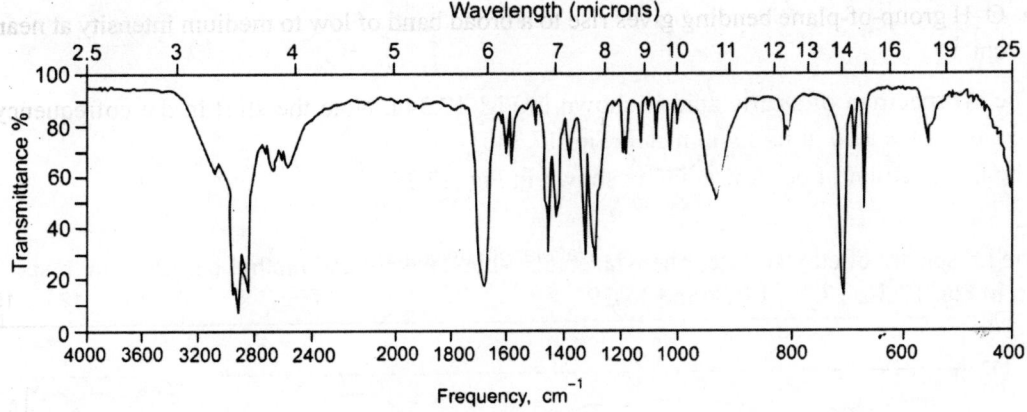

Wavelength (microns)

Fig. 17.35. The infrared spectrum of Benzoic acid, Nujol (KBr).

17.8.14 Esters

The diagnostic bands of esters are:

In normal aliphatic esters (non-conjugated) C=O stretching absorbs at 1750–1735 cm^{-1}.

$$R—\underset{\underset{O}{\|}}{C}—OR$$

1750–1735 cm^{-1} (stretching)

In conjugated esters C=O frequency shifts to 1740–1750 cm^{-1}.

$$—\underset{|}{C}{=}\underset{|}{C}—\underset{\underset{O}{\|}}{C}—O—R$$

1740–1715 cm^{-1} (stretching)

In aromatic esters, v_{CO} appears at 1740–1715 cm^{-1}.

$$Ar—\underset{\underset{O}{\|}}{C}—O—R$$

1740–1715 cm^{-1} (stretching)

In lactones (cyclic esters) $v_{C=O}$, increases with the decreasing ring size. For six-membered (δ-lactones) v_{CO} is similar to that in straight-chain unconjugated esters. However, with decreasing ring size, the C=O vibrations increase to higher frequencies.

1750–1735 cm^{-1} δ-valero lactone   γ-butyro lactone   1750 cm^{-1}
                   1755 cm^{-1} 1770 cm^{-1}

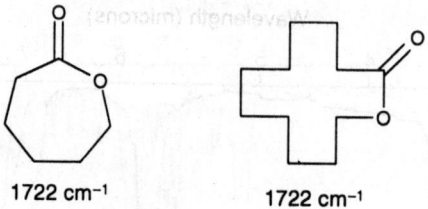

1722 cm⁻¹   1722 cm⁻¹

The i.r. spectra of ethylacetate, phenylacetate, n-butylacetate and methyl benzoate are respectively shown in Fig. 17.36, 17.37, 17.38 and 17.39.

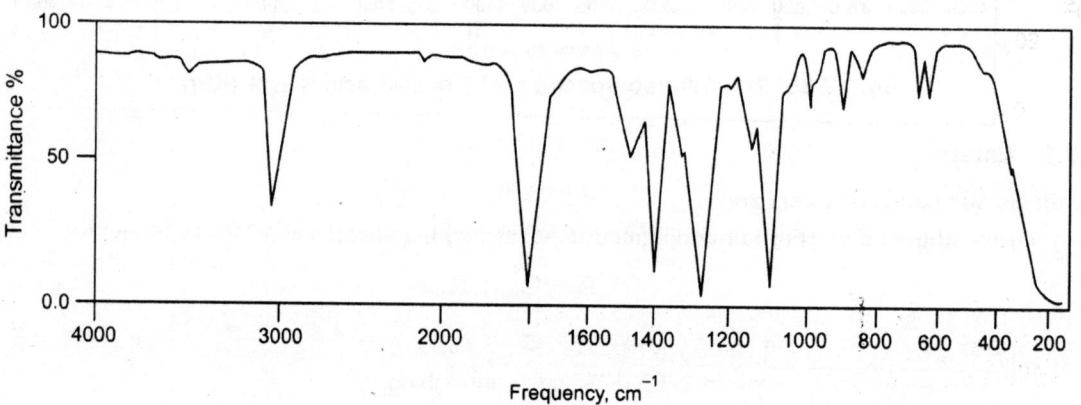

Fig. 17.36. The infrared spectrum of ethylacetate, $CH_3COOC_2H_5$, neat.

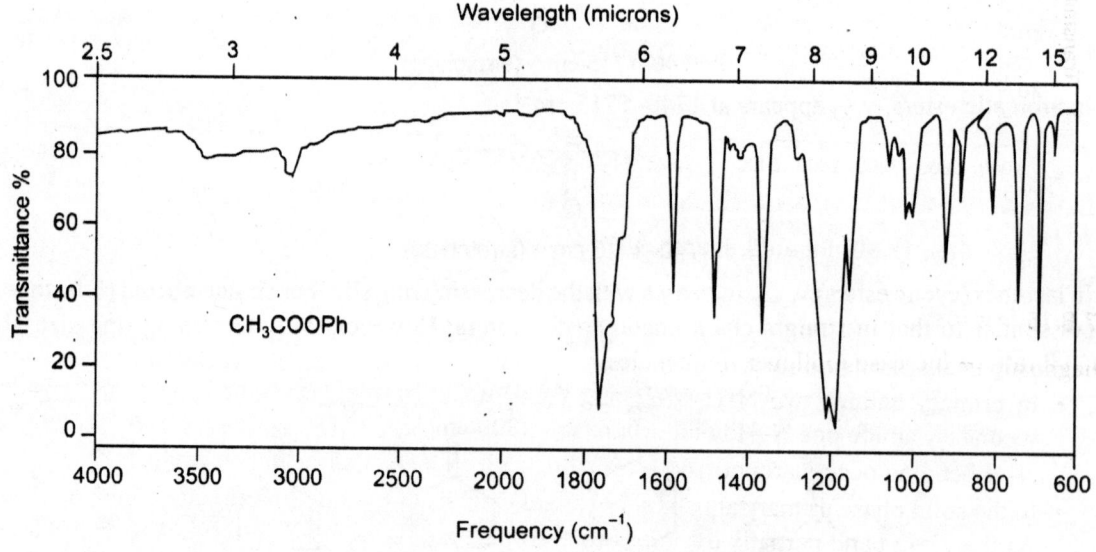

Fig. 17.37. IR spectrum of phenylacetate.

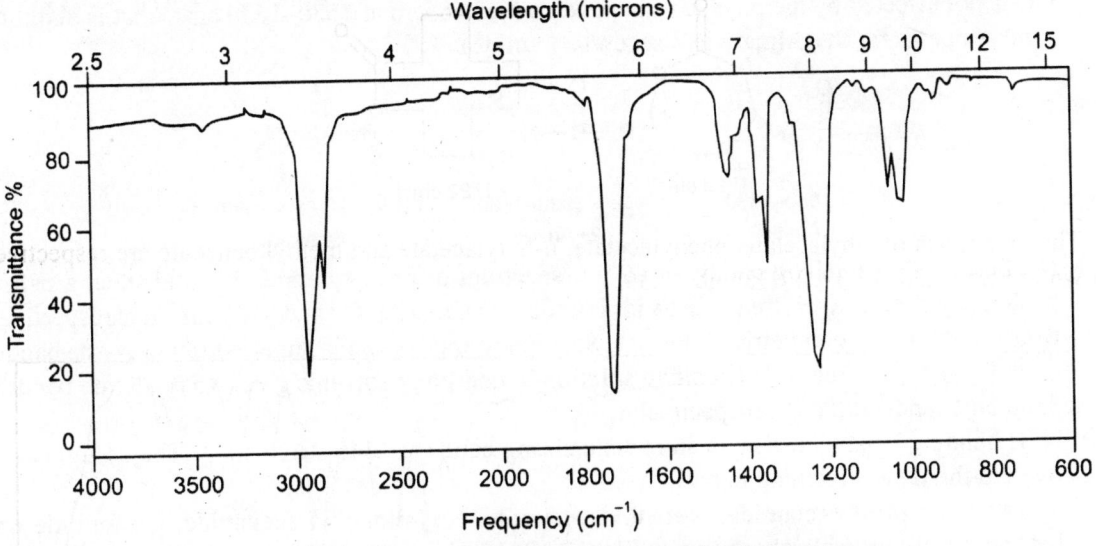

Fig. 17.38. IR spectrum of n-Butylacetate (KBr).

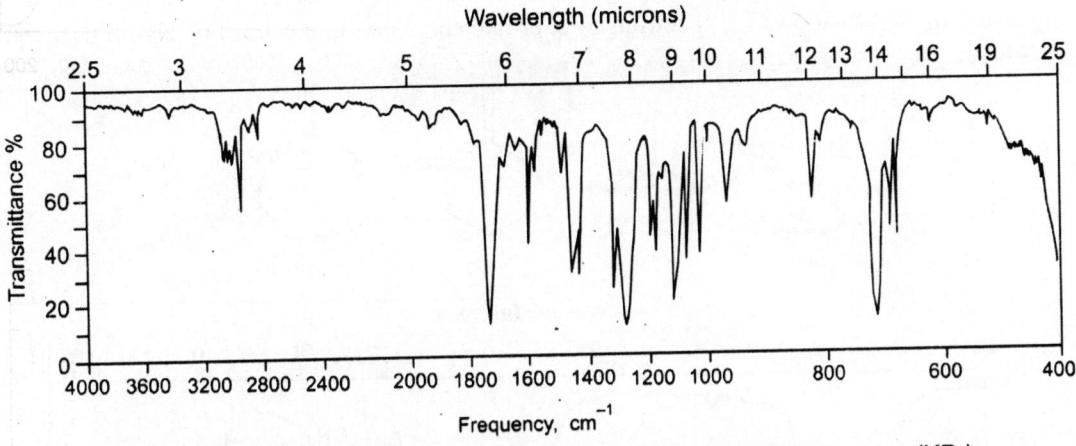

Fig. 17.39. Infrared spectrum of methyl benzoate, PhCOOCH$_3$, neat (KBr).

17.8.15 Amides

Diagnostic peaks are as follows:

- In primary amides two N–H stretching bands occur at about 3350 and 3180 cm^{-1} while in secondary amide one N–H bond occurs at ~ 3800 cm^{-1}.

  N–H bending occurs around 1640–1550 cm^{-1} for primary and secondary amides.

- In the solid phase primary amides show broad C=O band **(Amide I band)** at 1680 to 1630 cm^{-1}. As this C=O band partially overlaps due to N–H bending which in the region 1640–1620 cm^{-1} **(Amide II band)**, the C=O + N–H bands appear as a doublet. In secondary amide, the CO appears as a strong band at 1680–1640 cm^{-1}. As tertiary amides cannot form hydrogen bonding,

CO is not affected by the physical state and so they absorb at 1680–1630 cm^{-1} that is about the same range as for the primary and secondary amides.

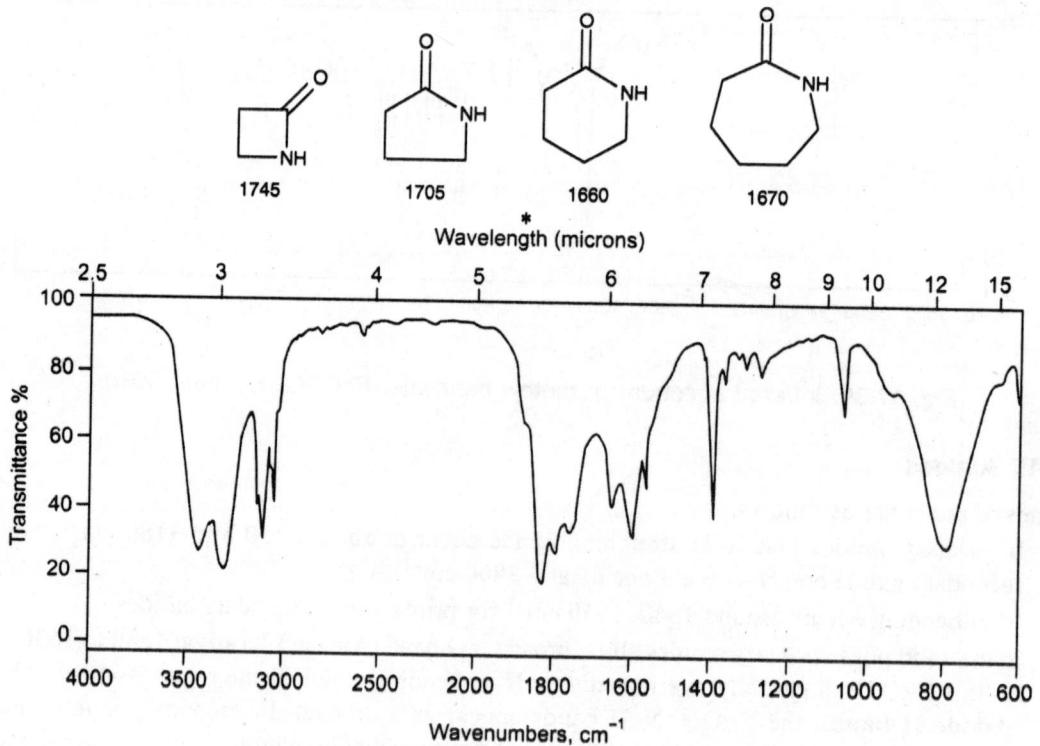

ν_{CO} = 1680–1630
1° Amide

ν_{CO} = 1680–1630
2° Amide

ν_{CO} = 1680–1630
3° Amide

- N–H and C–N stretching bands: In the i.r. spectrum of primary amide in solid state, a pair of moderately intense N–H stretching bands is noticed at about 3350^{-1} and 3180 cm^{-1} due respectively to asymmetric and symmetric vibrations. Secondary amides and lactams exhibit only one band at ~ 3000 cm^{-1}. The free N–H (in dilute solution in non-polar solvents give two moderate bands at 3500 cm^{-1} and 3400 cm^{-1} respectively.
- N–H bending bands, i amide in solid state strong bands at 1640–1620 cm^{-1}. They often nearly overlap the C=O stretching bands.

The i.r. spectra of acetamide, N-methylacetamide, N,N-dimethyl acetamide, acetamilide and benzamide are respectively shown in Fig. 17.40, 17.41, 17.42, 17.43 and 17.44

Cyclic amides display a rise in CO frequency due to ring strain, of course, the frequency rising with the ring size. Fig 17.44b shows i.r. spectrum of caprolactam. The i.r. spectrum of Nylon is shown in Fig. 17.44c.

1745

1705

1660

1670

Wavelength (microns)

Fig. 17.40. IR spectrum of acetamide (thin film).

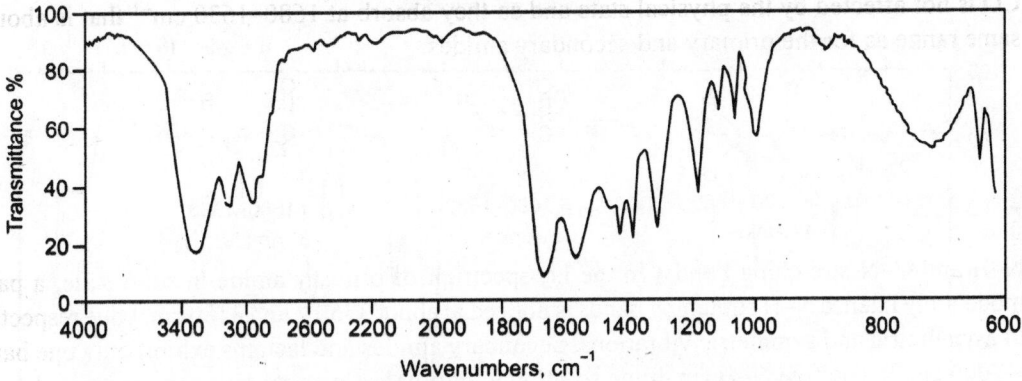

Fig. 17.41. IR spectrum of N-methylacetamide (melt).

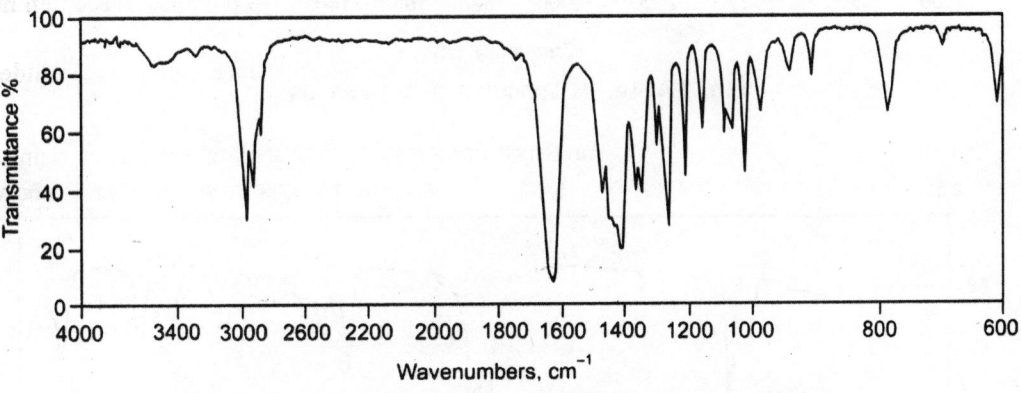

Fig. 17.42. IR spectrum of N,N-diethylacetamide (thin film).

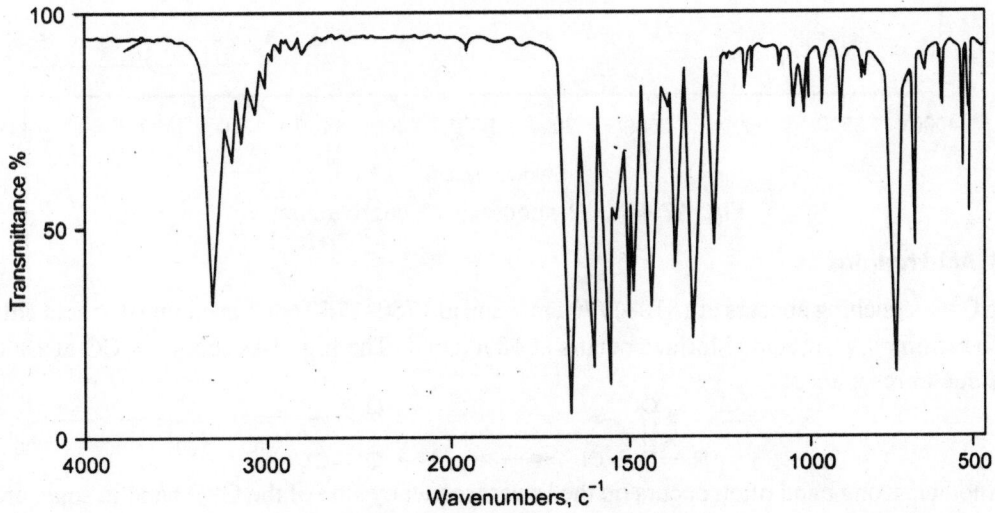

Fig. 17.43. IR spectrum of acetanilide.

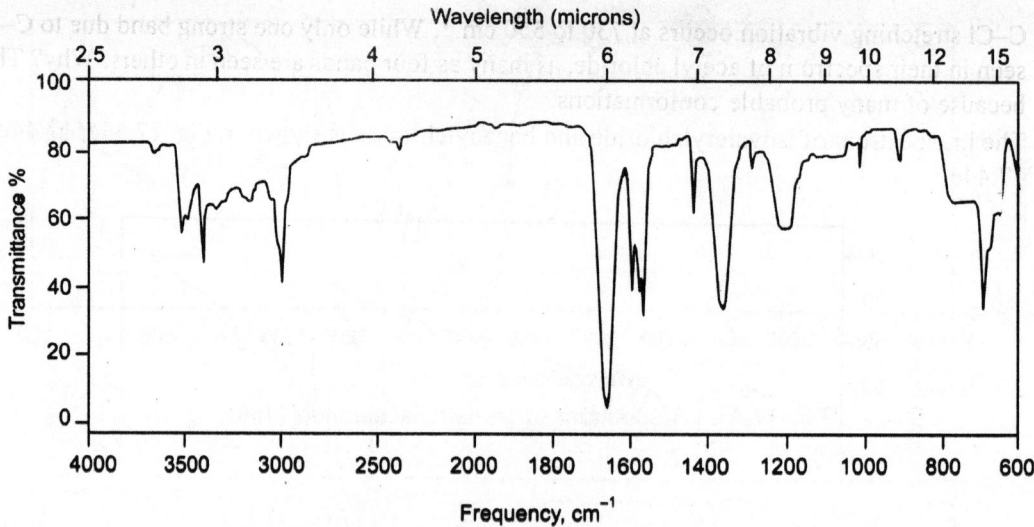

Fig. 17.44a. IR spectrum of benzamide.

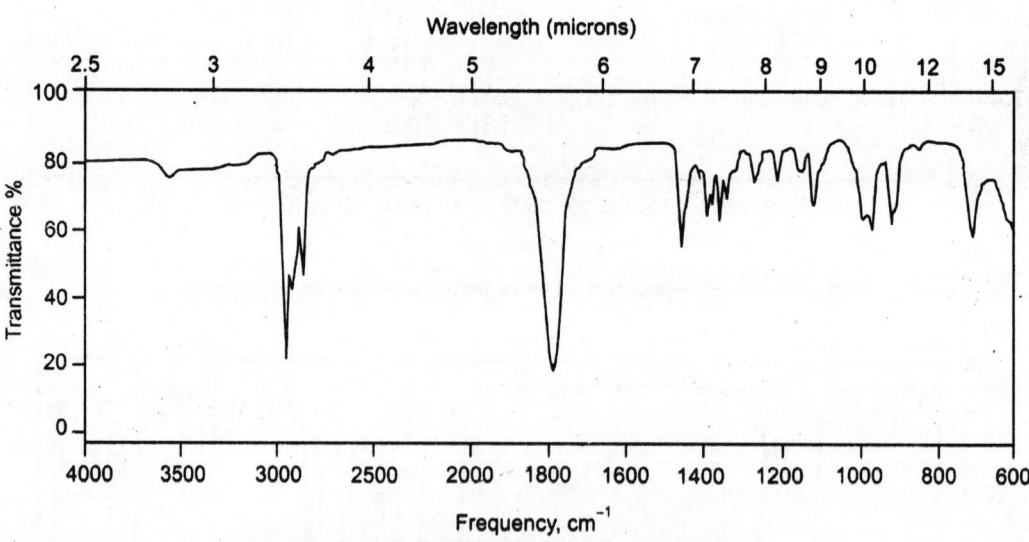

Fig. 17.44b. IR spectrum of caprolactum.

17.8.16 Acid halides

A strong C=O stretching appears at 1810–1770 cm^{-1} and at 1780–1760 cm^{-1} in conjugated acid chlorides.

- The strong v_{CO} of acid chlorides occurs at 1800 cm^{-1}. The high frequency for CO at 1800 cm^{-1} is due to resonance:

$$R—\overset{\overset{\displaystyle O}{\|}}{C}—\ddot{Cl} \longleftrightarrow R—\overset{\overset{\displaystyle O^-}{|}}{C}=\overset{\oplus}{Cl}$$

Another strong band often occurs on the lower frequency side of the C=O band in some aromatic acids. Consequently the $v_{C=O}$ appears as a doublet. This is due to fermi resonance.

- C–Cl stretching vibration occurs at 730 to 550 cm^{-1}. While only one strong band due to C–Cl is seen in their spectrum of acetyl chloride, as many as four bands are seen in others. Why? This is because of many probable conformations.

  The i.r. spectrum of isovalerylchloride and benzoylchloride is shown in Fig. 17.44c, 17.44d and 17.44e.

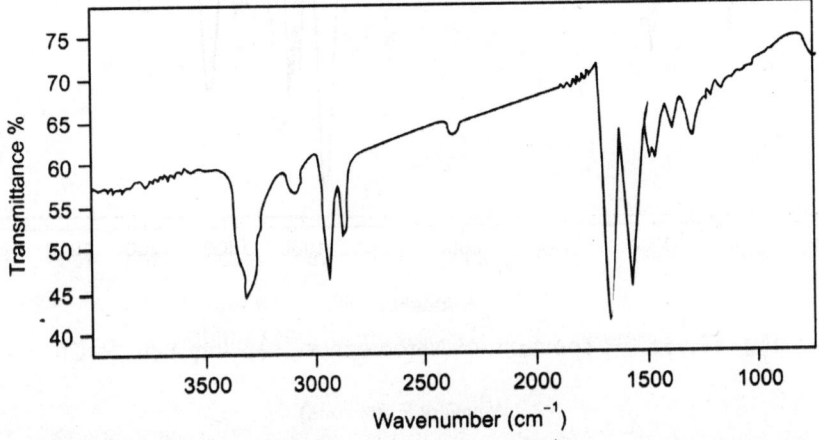

Fig. 17.44c. . Infrared spectrum of nylon, $-\left[\!\!\begin{array}{c} C-(CH_2)_5-NH \\ \parallel \\ O \end{array}\!\!\right]_n$ showing the N–H and C=O bands clearly.

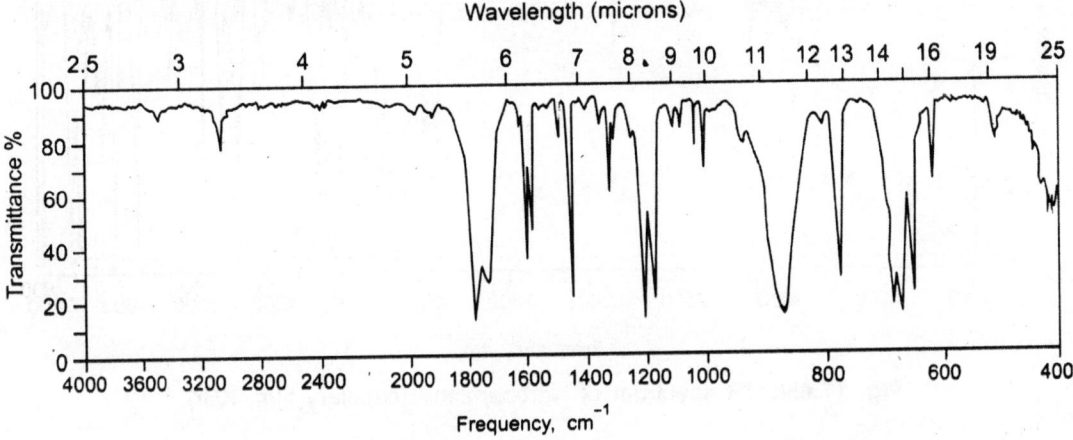

Fig. 17.44d. Infrared spectrum of benzoyl chloride, neat (KBr).

17.8.17 Nitro Compounds

- The aliphatic nitro compounds – assymetric stretching (strong) occurs at 1600–1530 cm^{-1} (Fig. 17.45a) while the symmetric stretching occurs at 1390–1300 cm^{-1}. These bands occur at lower frequencies in aromatic nitro compounds, assymetric stretch 1550–1490 cm^{-1} symmetric stretch 1355–1315 cm^{-1} due to conjugation. The i.r. of nitrobenzene is shown in Fig. 17.45b.

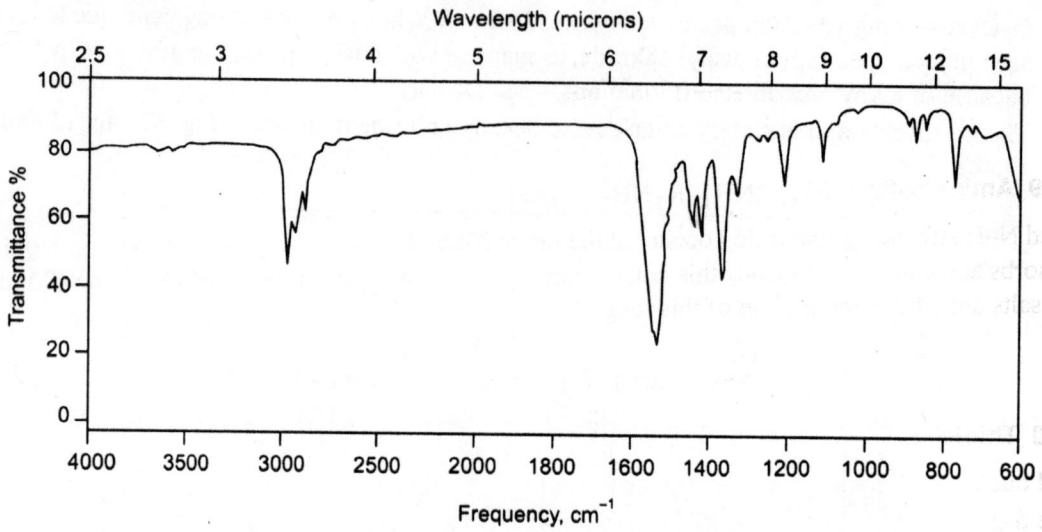

Fig. 17.45a. IR spectrum of Nitropropane (capillary film, NaCl)

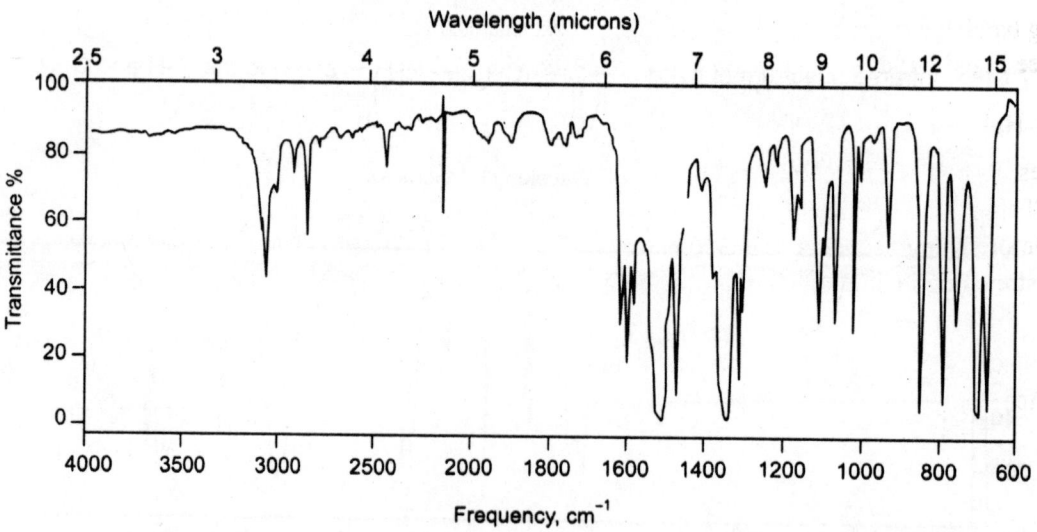

Fig. 17.45b. IR spectrum of Nitrobenzene (capillary film, KBr).

17.8.18 Carboxylate salts

$$R—C—O^-—Na^+$$
$$\underset{O}{\overset{||}{}}$$

These show an asymmetric stretching band at 1600 cm^{-1}. The symmetric stretching is seen at 1400 cm^{-1}. It is because of resonance that the frequency of C=O absorption is lowered. IR spectrum of sodium stearate is shown in Fig. 17.34b, while that of stearic acid in Fig. 17.34a.

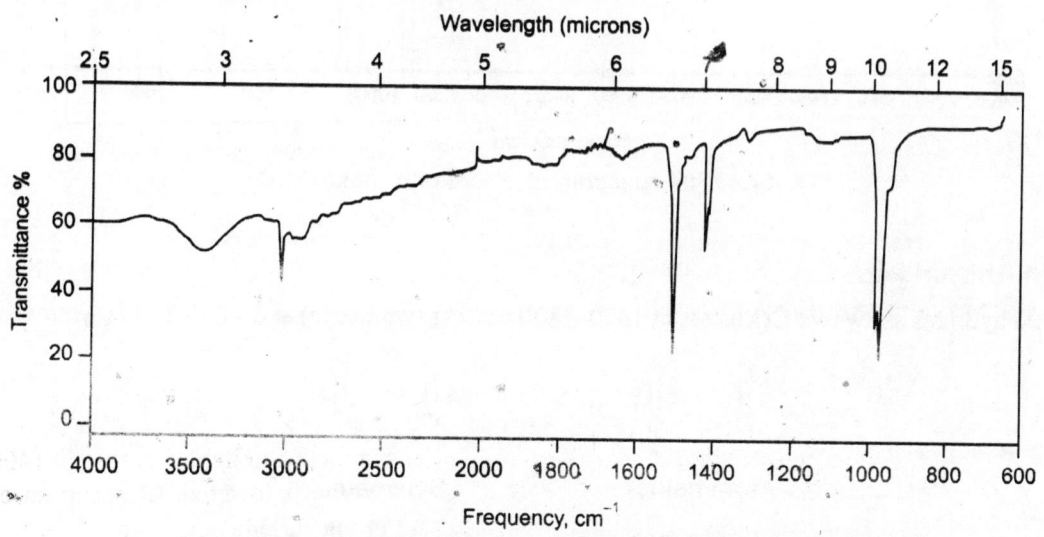

17.8.19 Amine salts $(NH_4^+, RNH_3^+, R_2NH_2^+, R_3NH^+)$

A broad N–H stretching absorption occurs in the range 3300–2600 cm^{-1} (Fig. 17.45b) The ammonium ion absorbs at the higher frequency this range while the 3° amine salt absorbs to the right. The 1° and 2° amine salts absorbs in the middle of this range.

$$\overset{\oplus}{(NH_4)} \quad 3300 \text{——} 2600 \text{ (amine salts)}$$

17.8.20 Thiols

A band due to N–H bending occurs in the range 1610–1500 cm^{-1}.

The S–H stretching occurs at ~ 2250 cm^{-1}.

17.8.21 Sulfoxides

A strong band due to S=O stretching occurs at about 1050 cm^{-1}. The C–S stretching occurs at 800–600 cm^{-1} (see Fig. 17.45d).

17.8.22 Halides

Fluorides, R–F: C–F stretching in aliphatic fluorides 1400–1000 cm^{-1}.

C–Cl stretching in range 785–540 cm^{-1} (Fig. 17.46).
C–Br stretching occurs at 650–510 cm^{-1}.
C–I stretching in aliphatic iodides occurs at 600–485 cm^{-1}.

Fig. 17.45c. The IR spectrum of tetramethyl ammonium chloride (KBr).

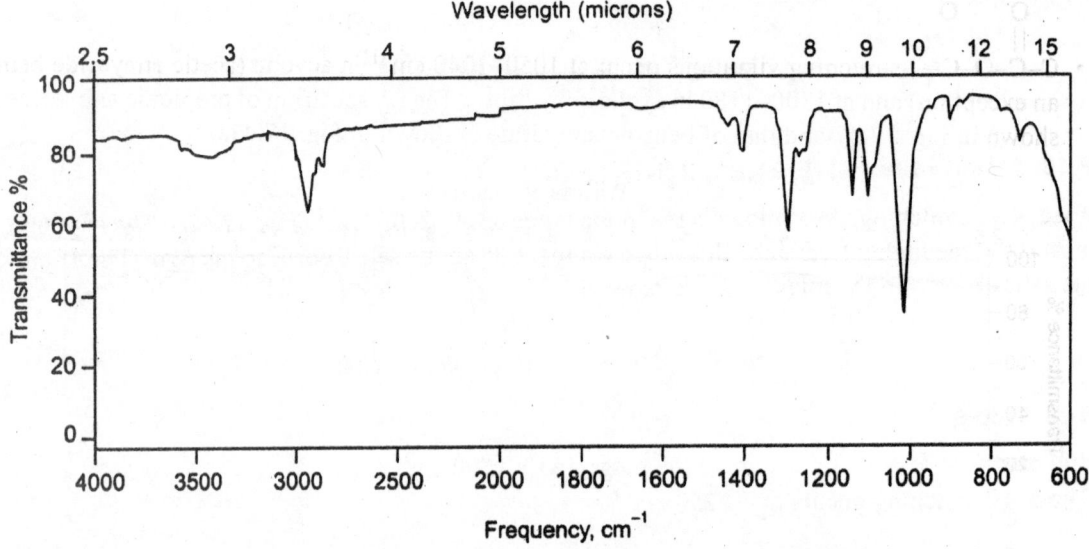

Fig. 17.45d. IR spectrum of tetramethyline sulfoxide.

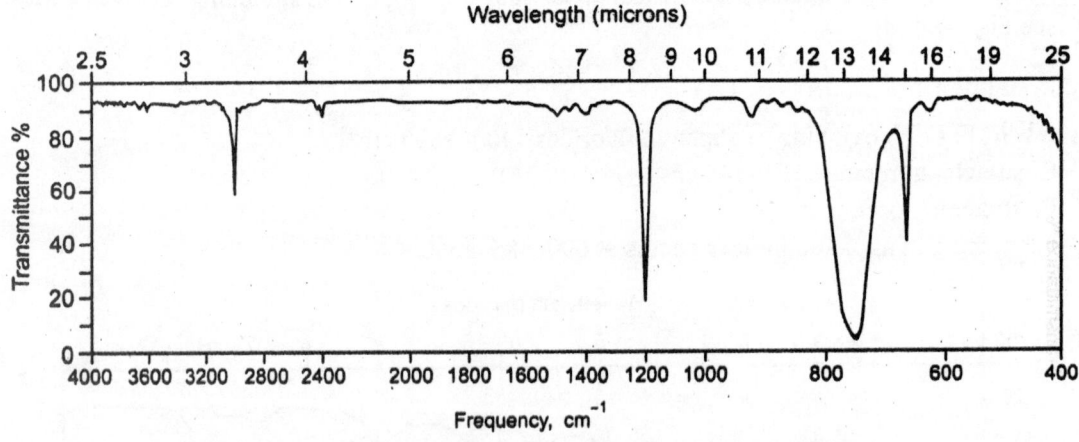

Fig. 17.46. IR spectrum of chloroform, neat (KBr).

17.8.23 Anhydrides

- Anhydrides show two CO bands at 1830–1800 cm^{-1} (asymmetric) and 1775–1740 (symmetric).

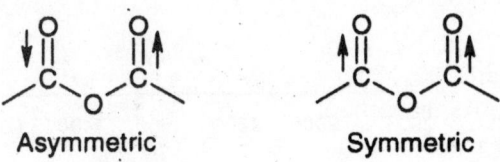

- C–O stretching appears at 1300–900 cm^{-1}.

- C–C–O–C–C stretching vibrations occur at 1050–1040 cm^{-1} in acyclic (acetic anhydride being an exception) and at 1300–1180 in cyclic anhydrides. The i.r. spectrum of propionic anhydride is shown in Fig. 17.47 and that of benzoic anhydride is shown in Fig. 17.47a.

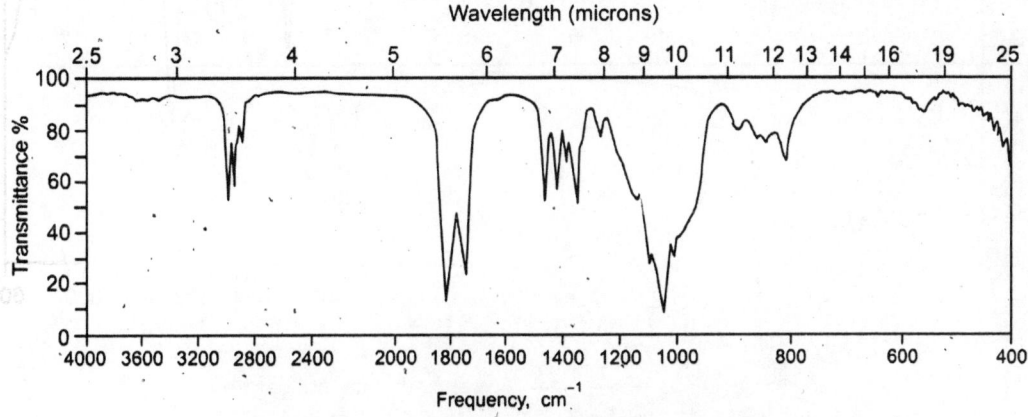

Fig. 17.47. IR spectrum of propionic anhydride.

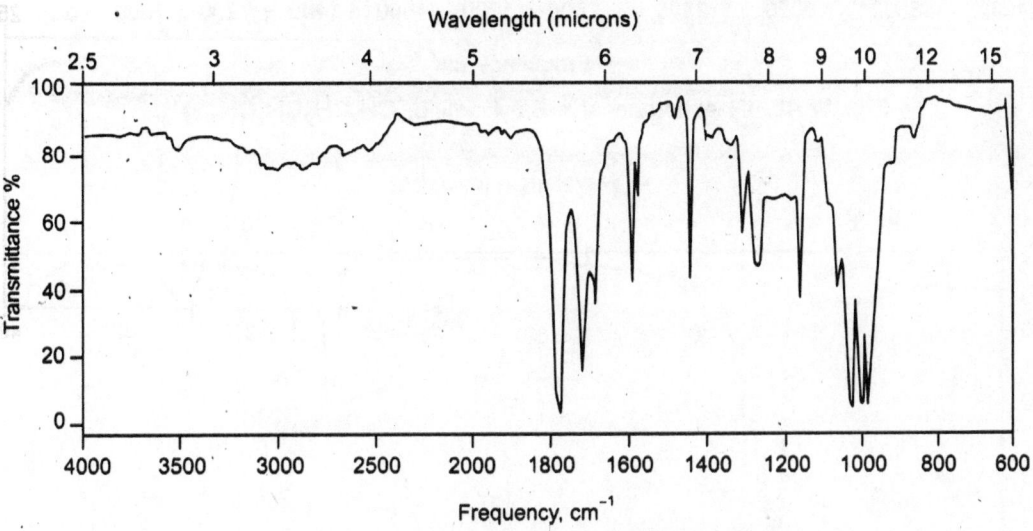

Fig. 17.47a. IR spectrum of Benzoic anhydride.

17.8.24 Amines

- N–H stretching occurs at 3500–3300 cm^{-1}. While primary amines exhibit two bands, secondary amines show one band. As the tertiary amines do not have a hydrogen, so they do not show a band in N–H stretching region.
- A broad band due to N–H bending in primary amine is seen at 1640–1560 cm^{-1}. 2° amines show this band at about 1500 cm^{-1}.

- Out of plane N–H bending occurs at about 800 cm^{-1}.
- C–N stretching occurs in the range 1350–1000 cm^{-1}.

The i.r. spectrum of a 1°, 2° and 3° amines are shown in Fig. 17.48 to 17.50. Figs. 17.51–17.53 show i.r. spectrum of p-Toluidine.

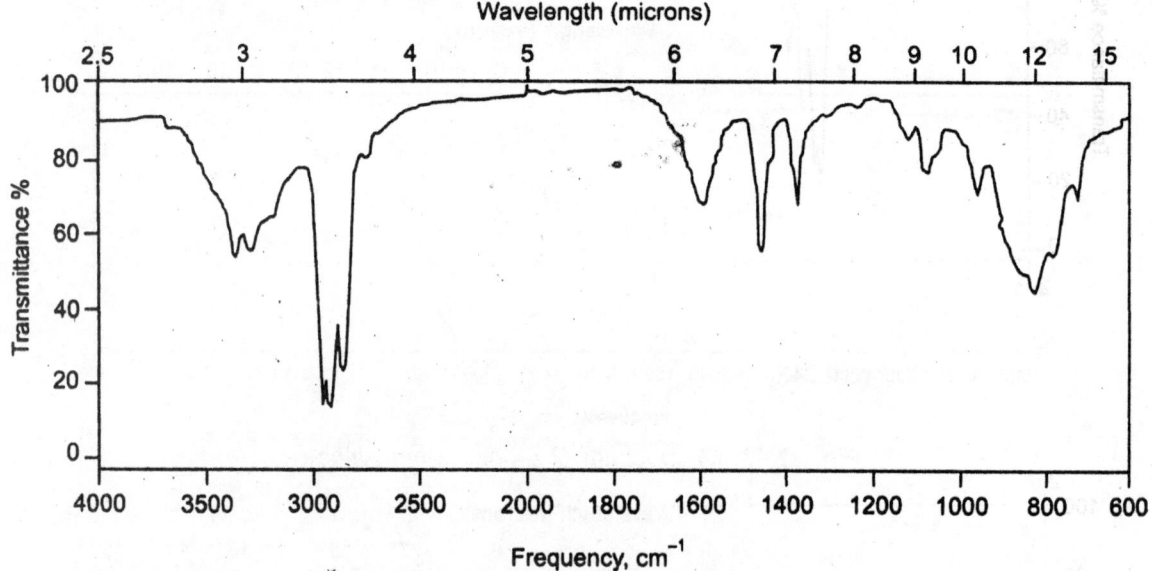

Fig. 17.48. IR spectrum of n-Butyl amine, $CH_3CH_2CH_2CH_2NH_2$.

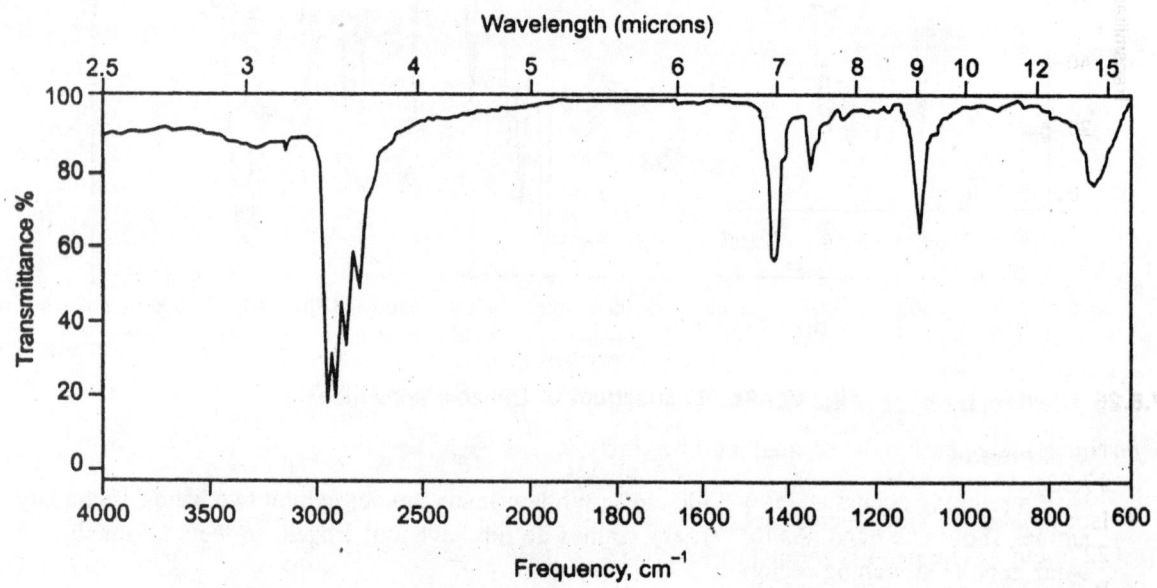

Fig. 17.49. IR spectrum of Di-n-butylamine.

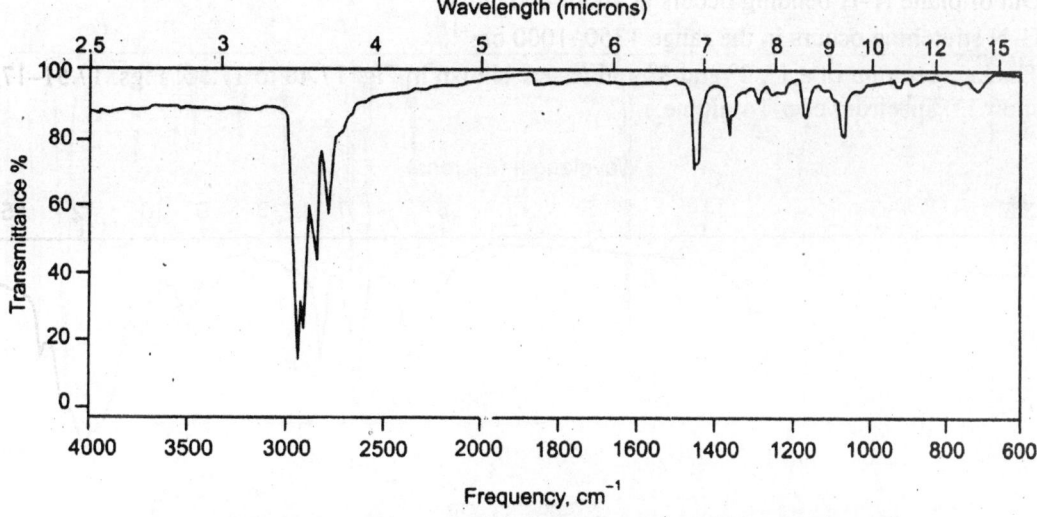

Fig. 17.50. IR spectrum of Tri-n-butylamine, $(CH_3CH_2CH_2CH_2)_3N$.

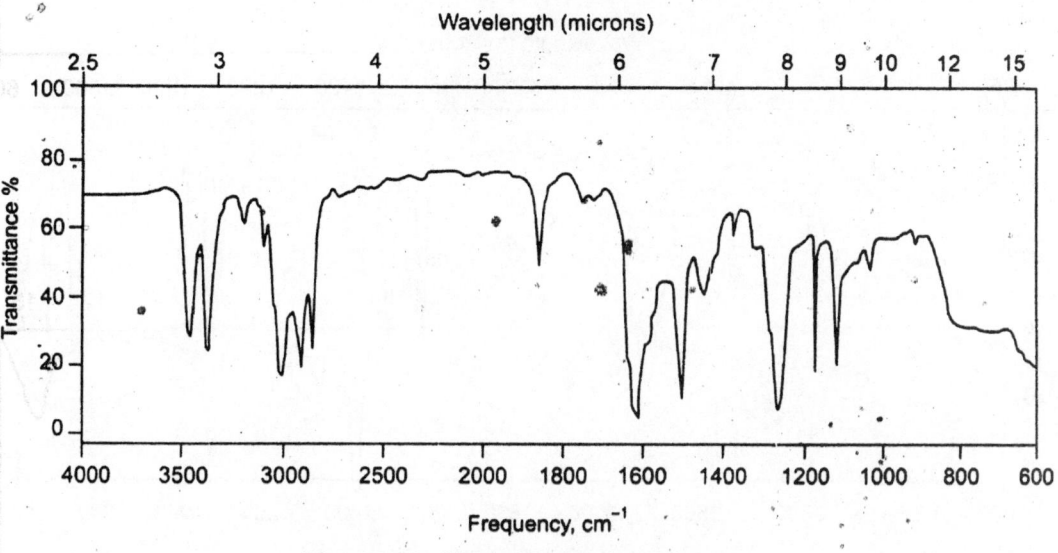

Fig. 17.51. IR spectrum of p-Toluidine.

17.8.25 Nitriles, Isocyanates, Isothiocyanates and Imines

- Nitriles is a sharp band of medium intensity, due to $-C\equiv N$ stretching occurs at 2250 cm^{-1} (Fig. 17.52)
- Isocyanates: In isocyanates gives a broad, intense band due to R–N=C=O stretching occurs at 2270 cm^{-1}. The band is frequently split or is accompanied by shoulders (Fig. 17.53).
- R–N=C=S stretch in it gives one or two bands which are broad centering near 2125 cm^{-1}.
- Oximes and imines show due to $-C = N -$ stretching in a band at 1690–1640 cm^{-1}.

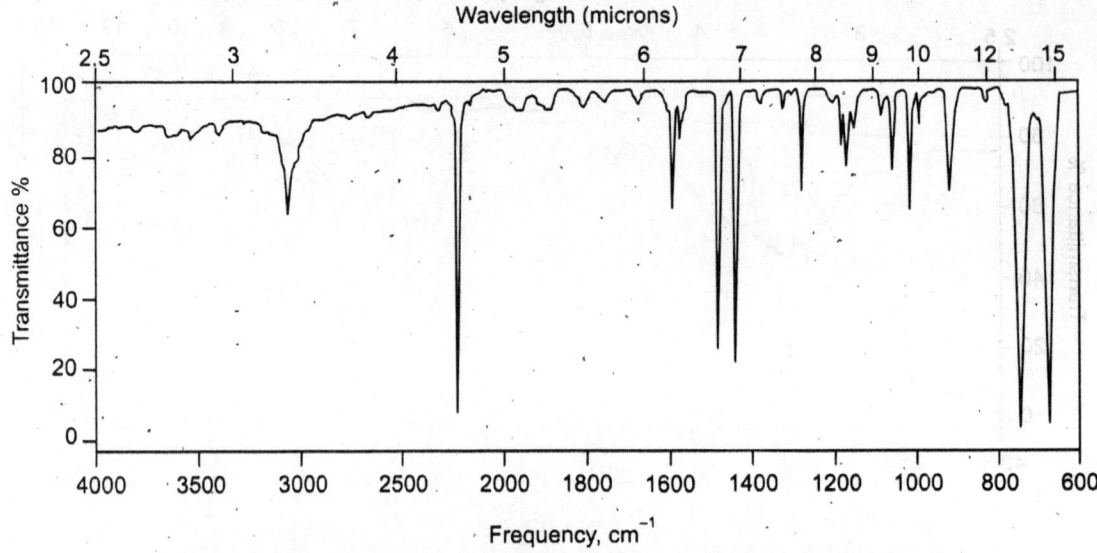

Fig. 17.52. IR spectrum of Benzonitrile (capillary film, NaCl).

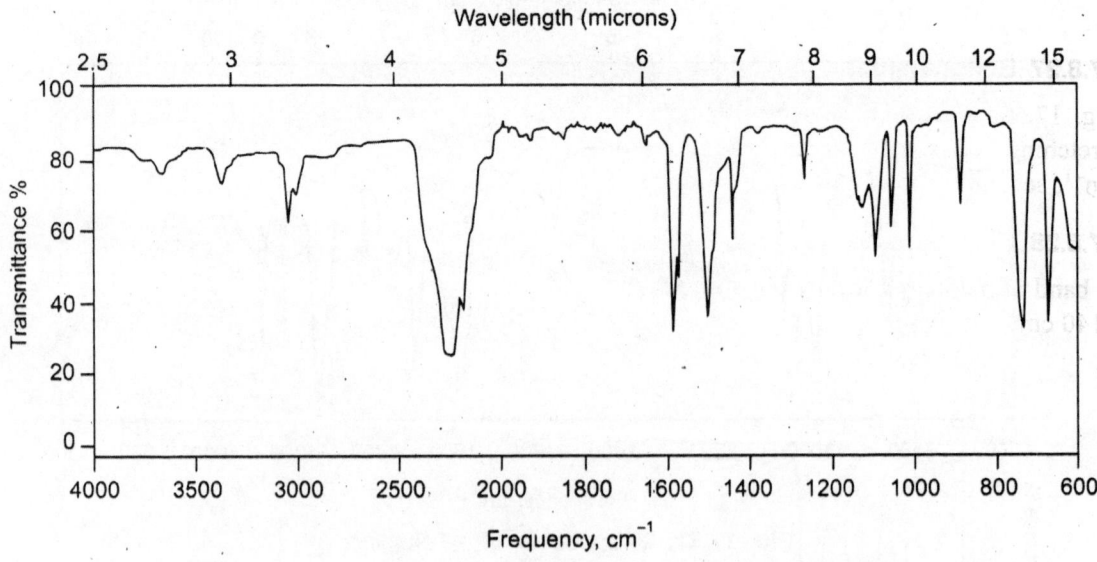

Fig. 17.53. IR spectrum of phenyl isocyanate, Ph–N=C=O.

17.8.26 Amino Acids

These occur as Zwitter (dipolar) ions and show bonds originating from $COO^{\ominus}$ group (asymmetric stretching at ~ 1600 cm^{-1} and symmetric stretching at ~ 1400 cm^{-1}) and $NH_3^{\oplus}$ stretching bands that overlap CH bands at 3000 cm^{-1}; overtones sometimes seen at 2600–1900 cm^{-1} and asymmetric bending at ~ 1600 cm^{-1} and symmetric bending at about 1500 cm^{-1}. Fig. 17.54 shows i.r. spectrum of L-isoleucine.

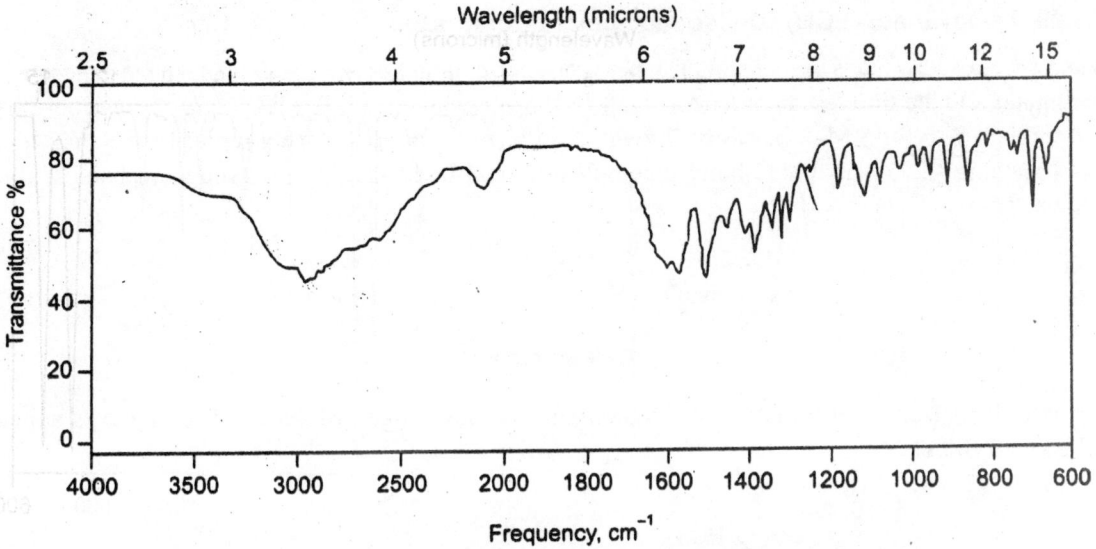

Fig. 17.54. IR spectrum of isoleucine, $(CH_3)_2CHCH_2CH-COO^-$
$\overset{|}{\underset{NH_3^{\oplus}}{}}$

17.8.27 Sulfonamides

Fig. 17.55a shows i.r. spectrum of benzenesulfonamide, $PhSO_2NH$ (Mujol, KBr). S=O symmetric stretching occurs at 1140 cm^{-1}, S=O asymmetric stretch at 1325 cm^{-1}. Primary N–H at 3350, 3250 cm^{-1}; secondary N–H at 3250 cm^{-1}; bending at 1500 cm^{-1}.

17.8.28 Thiocyanates

A band of medium intensity but stronger than that in isocyanates due to S–C=N stretching appears at 2140 cm^{-1}.

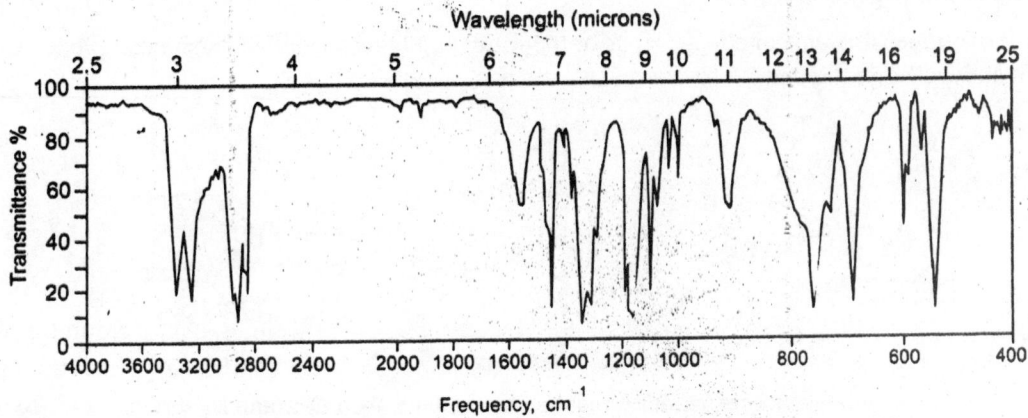

Fig. 17.55a. IR spectrum of benzenesulfonamide (KBr).

17.8.29 Thiocyanato (SCN) and Isothiocyanato Complexes

The i.r. spectroscopy helps us to distinguish between such complexes readily. One of the most thoroughly investigated and the simplest ambidentate ligand is the thiocyanate ion. The NCS^- group may coordinate to M through S to form M–S bonds or through N to form M–N bonds or through N and S. While the C–N stretching ≤ 2050 cm^{-1} in N-bonded complexes, the S-bonded complexes show this band at about 2100 cm^{-1}.

M–SCN $\qquad\qquad$ M–NCS

Thiocyanato $\qquad\qquad$ Iso-Thiocyanato

$\sim$ 2100 cm^{-1} $\qquad\qquad$ $\leq$ 2050 cm^{-1}

C–N stretching

It is further interesting to note that CN stretching in the bridged M–NCS–M^1 complexes appears well above 2100 cm^{-1}.

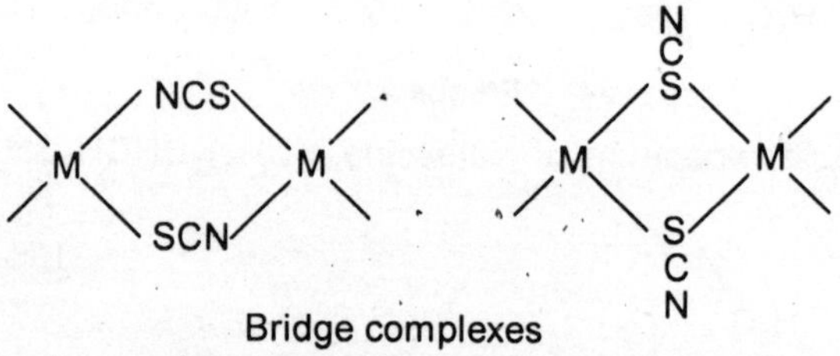

Bridge complexes

CN stretching > 2100 cm^{-1}

- ν_{CS} in   N bonded compplexes 860–780 cm^{-1}
  S bonded complexes 720–690 cm^{-1}
- δ_{NCS} in   N bonded complexes – sharp near 480 cm^{-1}
  In S bonded complexes – low intensity $\sim$ 42 (several bands)

Further $\nu_{M-IV} > \nu_{M-S}$ in far IR region.

Complexes of β-Diketones

Many β-diketones form metal chelate rings of the following types; acetylacetonate complexes are well known and well investigated:

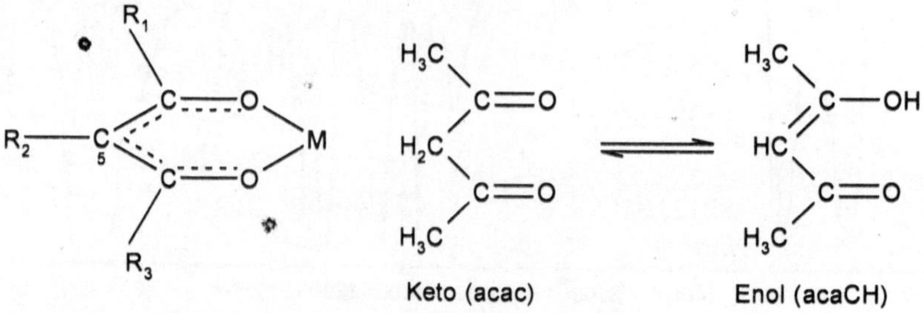

Keto (acac) $\qquad\qquad$ Enol (acaCH)

Acetylacetone (ac aCH) most common, $R_1 = R_3 = CH_3$ and $R_2 = H$

IR spectra of M (acac)$_2$ and M(acac)$_3$ type complexes have been reported extensively.

Examples of Complexes of Neutral Acetylacetone

(i) In some compounds, the keto form of acetyl–acetone forms a chelate ring in which n_{CO} is found to appear at 1700 cm^{-1}.

$$\gamma_{CO} = 1700 \text{ cm}^{-1}$$

In Mn (acaCH)$_2$ Br$_2$ – enol form (unidentate ligand) n_{CO} and n_{CC} occur at 1627 cm^{-1} and 1564 cm^{-1} respectively.

$v_{C \cdots O}$ 1627 cm^{-1}

$v_{C \cdots C}$ 1564 cm^{-1}

(ii) Carbon bonded Acetyl acetonato organometallic compounds are also known which can be readily distinguished by i.r. spectroscopy. In [Pt(acac)$_2$Cl$_2$]^2 one of the acac is C bonded.

	O–bonded	*C–bonded*
$v_{C=O}$	–	1652, 1626
$v_{C \cdots O}$	1563, 1380	–
$v_{C \cdots C}$	1538, 1288	–
v_{C-H}	–	1350, 1193
v_{C-H}	1212, 817	1193, 852
v_{Pt-O}	650, 478	–
v_{Pt-C}	–	567

As can be seen from the above examples, the v_{M-O} of acac complexes are most interesting because they provide us direct information regarding M–O bond strength.

17.9 SPURIOUS BANDS IN IR SPECTRA

While interpreting IR spectra care needs to be taken as sometimes spurious bonds are noticed in infrared spectra. These may originate from the following sources:

(i) Water even when present in traces in solvents like $CHCl_3$ and CCl_4 shows bands at ~ 3700 and 3600 cm^{-1} and a broad one at ~ 1650 cm^{-1} (see Fig. 17.55b).

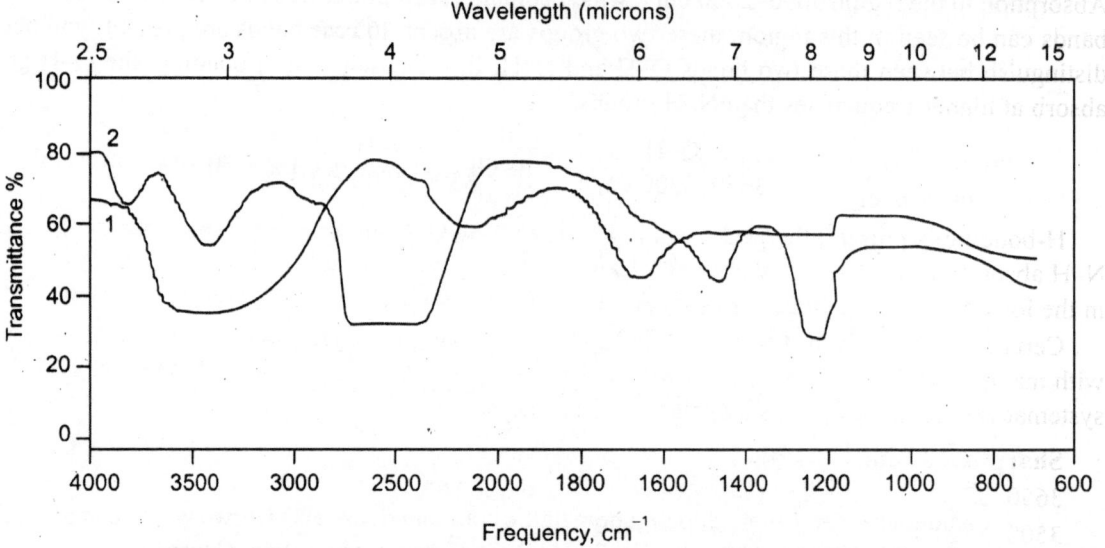

Fig. 17.55b. IR spectra of water (1) and deuterium oxide (2).

(ii) Water vapour shows many sharp peaks in the range 2000–1280 cm^{-1}. In fact, when these vapours are present in relatively high amounts, the detection system stops working momentarily giving rise to a shoulder while scanning is being carried out through a steep flank of a strong band as in case of carbonyl absorption bands in the stretching region.

(iii) Another source is dissolved CO_2. This generates a band at 2325 cm^{-1}. Sometimes spurious bands are seen due to protonated amines which are formed as a result of formation of H_2CO_3 from CO_2 and water. When the instrument (double beam) is not adequately balanced, the dissolved CO_2 contributes three peaks at 2630, 2335 and 667 cm^{-1}.

(iv) A band at 1725 cm^{-1} is due to phthalates, the plasticisers present in commercial polymeric materials but that enter the test samples somehow. Sometimes, a band appears at 1755 cm^{-1} due to phthalic anhydride that is formed upon reactions on phthalates.

Phthalates   Phthalic anhydride
1725 cm^{-1} 1755 cm^{-1}

(v) CCl_4 liquid shows a peak at 788 cm^{-1}, when it is present on the outer wall of the cell. CCl_4 vapour evaporating from a leaky cell exhibits a band at 788 cm^{-1}.

(vi) Silicones are also encountered as a common impurity and show a band at ~ 1265 cm^{-1}, and another at 1100–1000 cm^{-1}.

17.10 INTERPRETING AN I.R. SPECTRUM

As soon as you have an i.r. spectrum in your hand, you should look into the spectrum in the following sequence:

1. X–H Stretching Region, 3650–2500 cm⁻¹

Absorption in the region 3650–2500 cm^{-1} which contains absorptions due to O–H or N–H bonds. If no bands can be seen in this region, these two groups are absent. In case bands are present, you need to distinguish between these two bonds O–H and N–H. In the absence of H-bonding, the O–H groups absorb at higher frequencies than N–H groups:

$$\begin{array}{cc} \text{O–H} & \text{N–H} \\ 3650\text{–}3200 \text{ cm}^{-1} & 3500\text{–}3300 \text{ cm}^{-1} \end{array}$$

H-bonding is present, the peaks would be broad. The O–H group gives more broad peaks and the N–H absorptions are usually sharp and of lower intensity compared to N–H bands. Thus, sharp peaks in the lower part of the range are usually attributable to N–H bonds.

Certain OH (notably the OH of carboxylic acids) and NH absorptions exhibit very broad absorptions with maxima on the low frequency side of the C–H bands i.e. below 3000 cm^{-1} (see Fig. 17.56). The systematization that follows is a useful guide to interpretation.

Sharp bands cm⁻¹

3650–3500	O–H free or with a single H-bridge
3500–3400	O–H or N–H
3400–3100	N–H (most likely); 1° amines and 1° amides show two (sometimes more) peaks. 2° amines and 2° amides — only one peak

Broad bands cm⁻¹

3400–3200	O–H (most likely) due to polymeric association
3300–2500 (very broad)	O–H of RCOOH; Amine salts (NH_3^+, NH_2^+, NH^+) often show broad absorptions in this range; C–H

Once you have the indications from the above analysis about the presence of OH or NH compounds, you need to do the following examination in other parts of the spectrum:

- For alcohols and phenols, look for a strong C–O stretching at 1200–1000 cm^{-1} and in fact, this is among the strongest bands seen in the finger print region.
- For carboxylic acids, look for a strong C=O stretching at 1725–1650 cm^{-1}.
- For amides try to notice a strong C=O stretching band at 1700–1630 cm^{-1}.
- For primary amines you will notice a band at 1650–1580 cm^{-1} due to NH$_2$ deformation. Remember 1° and 2° amides show a similar band called amide II band.

2. Absorptions in the range 1850–1660 cm⁻¹

Now go to the region 1850–1540 cm^{-1} to look for strong bands due to carbonyl stretching. In case you detect a strong band, then if COOH group is present, you will have to read this in conjunction with OH stretching discussed in point. Similarly, you need to confirm the presence of amide group in combination with the N–H peaks of medium intensity at about 3400 cm^{-1}.

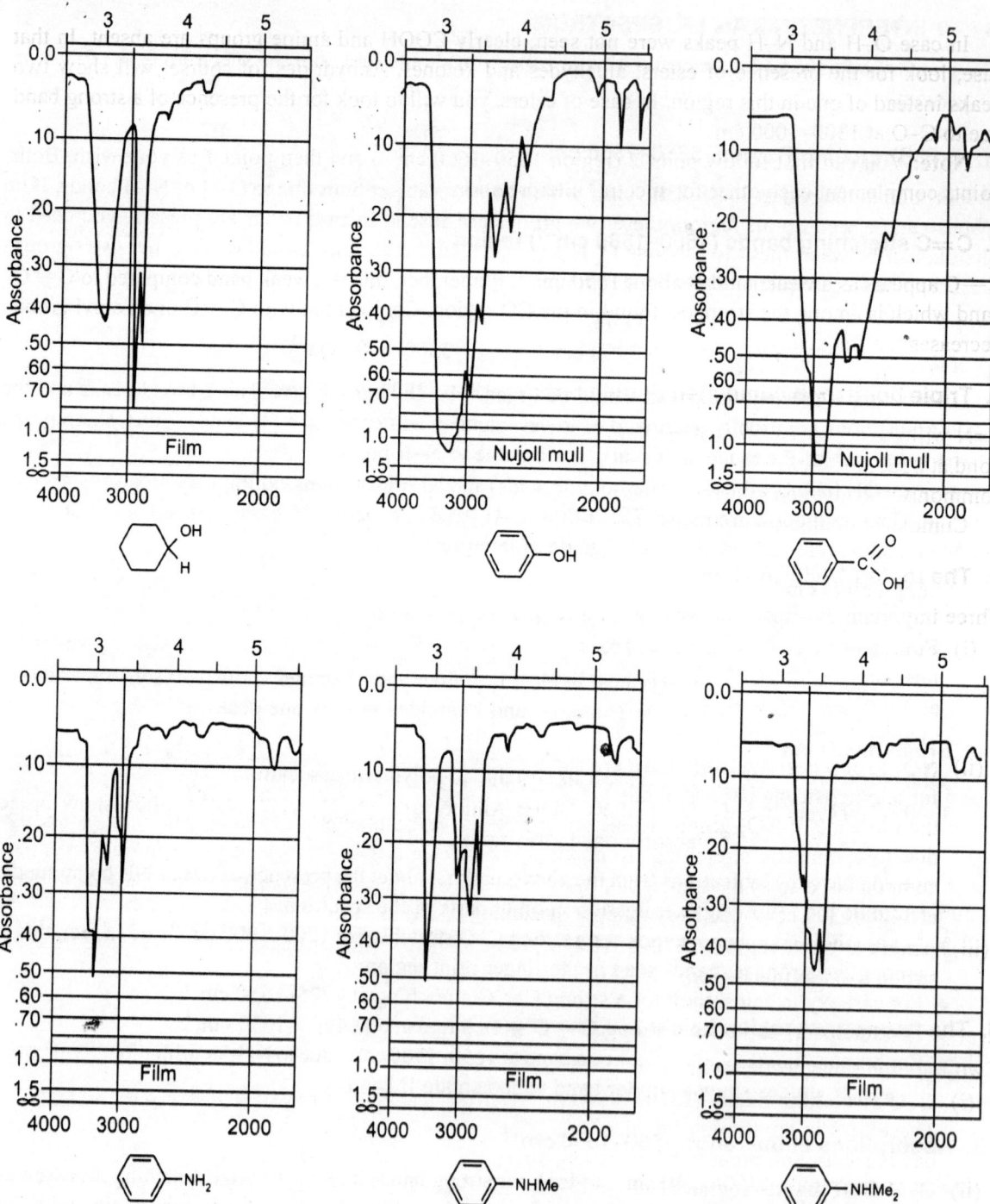

Fig. 17.56. IR spectra of some OH_2, NH_2, $> NH$ containing compounds emphasising their X–H bands (X = O or N).

In case O–H and N–H peaks were not seen, clearly COOH and amine groups are absent. In that case, look for the presence of esters, aldehydes and ketones. Anhydrides, of course, will show two peaks instead of one in this region. In case of esters, you will to look for the presence of a strong band due to C–O at 1300–1000 cm^{-1}.

Note: You can first follow point 2 (region 1850–1660 cm^{-1}) and then point 1 as your wish. Both points complement each other for spectral interpretation.

3. C=C stretching bands (1660–1580 cm^{-1}) region

C=C appears as a weak band at about 1650 cm^{-1}. Remember, this is a weak band compared to C=O band which is among the strongest found in the CO region. Conjugation with C=C or an amyl group decreases the frequency.

4. Triple bond (and cumulated double bond) region (2500–1950 cm^{-1})

C≡N will show a sharp band of medium intensity at 2260–2215 cm^{-1}. C≡C will appear a sharp weak bond at 2260–2100 cm^{-1} N = C = O will show up at 2275–2240 cm^{-1}. It should be noted that other less commonly encountered systems of the type X = Y = Z also absorb in this region.

Cumulated double bonds, C = C = C will appear in this region 1970–1950 cm^{-1}.

5. The region 1600–1450 cm^{-1}

Three important diagnostic absorptions are as follows:

(i) **Four bands, aromatic, 1600, 1580, 1500 and 1450 cm^{-1}:** If there are four bands of variable intensity at ~ 1600, 1580, 1500 and 1450 cm^{-1}, then aromatic ring is indicated. In fact, the bands at 1600 and 1500 cm^{-1} are the most constant in position and often, these are the only ones visible.

(ii) **NO$_2$ group region (1565–1510 cm^{-1}):** If you notice a strong band in this region, you must look for another strong band at about 1350 cm^{-1}. The presence of both these strong bands indicates the presence of NO$_2$ group. The first band is due to asymmetric stretching, while the second is due to symmetric stretching. Remember, carboxylate ions that are isoelectronic with nitro compounds, display the similar bands at 1610–1550 cm^{-1} due to asymmetric stretching and another at 1420–1300 cm^{-1} due to symmetric stretching.

(iii) **Amide II band region, 1570–1510 cm^{-1}:** The amide II band of secondary amides appears as a strong band in this region.

6. The finger-print region below 1500 cm^{-1}

Two important diagnostic groups are:

(i) **C–O stretching bands (1310–1000 cm^{-1}):** These are often **strongest** bands below 1500 cm^{-1}. These help in confirming the alcohols, phenols and ester groups. In case, the O–H and C=O bands are absent, proceed to recognise esters.

(ii) **C–H OOP bands region (1000–600 cm^{-1}):** These bands help us in detecting the presence of unsaturation or aromatic rings. In fact, the position of these bands gives excellent information about the substitution pattern in an ethylene or benzene derivative.

For monosubstituted benzene: Two strong peaks at 770–730 and 710–690.

Disubstituted benzenes:
ortho – one peak –(770–735 cm^{-1}) strong
meta – three peakls – (900–860) medium, (810–750) strong, (725–680) medium
para – one band – 860–800 cm^{-1} (strong)
For monosubstituted ethylenes such as vinyl group
Two bands – 995–985(s) and 915–905 cm^{-1}(s)
For 1,2–disubstituted ethylenes
cis – one peak – 730–665 cm^{-1} (strong)
trans – one peak – 980–960 cm^{-1} (strong)

7. C–H stretching bands region

- If C ≡ C stretching is confirmed at 2260–2100 cm^{-1}, a peak at ~ 3000 cm^{-1} due to acetylenic C–H will be noticed.
- Peaks in the region 3100–3000 cm^{-1} will confirm the presence of olefinic C–H and or aromatic (C–H).
- Saturated C–H will be seen at 3000–2850 cm^{-1}. The strongest absorption of Nujol is seen here.
- A pair of peaks (doublet) present at 2820 and 2720 cm^{-1} (due to Fermi resonance) will confirm the presence of CHO, the aldehyde group if a strong peak in the C = O stretching region is noticed at 1740–1660 cm^{-1}. It is advisable not to analyse the C–H stretching band region at ~ 3000 cm^{-1} in the beginning.

The interpretation sequence is shown in Fig. 17.57.

Entry

1. 3650–2500 cm^{-1} (X–H region)
  ↓
2. 1850–1660 cm^{-1} (CO region)
  ↓
3. 1680–1580 cm^{-1} (C = C region)
  ↓
4. 2500–1950 cm^{-1} (C * C, C = C = C, N = C = O region)
  ↓
5. 1600–1450 cm^{-1} (fourbands) Ar, NO$_2$, Amide II region)
  ↓
6. Below 1500 cm^{-1} (finger print region)
  ↓
7. 3100–2820 cm^{-1} (C–H stretching region)

Exit

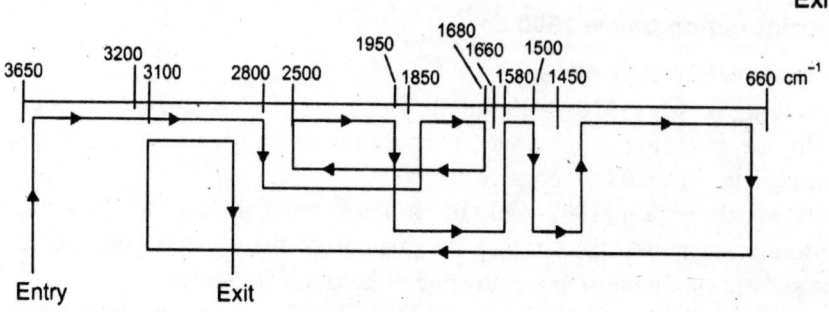

Fig. 17.57. Region-wise path to be followed for complete i.r. spectral interpretation.

17.11 HANDY-DANDY CHART FOR INFRARED SPECTRAL ANALYSIS IN LABORATORY

Sr. No.	Molecule type	ν (mode)		

1. **Alkanes**

2960	C–H	St. Asymm (3000–2840) –CH_2– Scissoring	2925
			2850
			1470
			1250

Rocking [720]

2870	C–H Sym.	
1460	C–H i.p. asym. bending	CH_3
1380	C–H i.p. sym. bending	

2. **Alkenes**

3080	asy. C–H str. (= C–H)
2975	C–H str. stm.
~ 1420	i.p. (scissoring)
~ 900	op 1070 (rocking) = CH_2.
1640	C = C, conjugation moves it to lower frequencies

(= CH_2)

cis disub.	730–675	op (cis–di) (about 700 cm^{-1})
trans disub.	965	op
tri substd	840– 800	op

3. **Alkynes**

3300 ≡ C–H	
2260–2150	C ≡ C

4. **Aromatic**
   Diagnostic for const. pattern

3070	C–H st. (differentiation between C = C–H or Ar (C–H difficult)
2000–1650	Overtones + combination bends of i.p. and op bending (characteristic of sub. pattern)

1600	quadrant st.	
1580		Skeletal with C = C within the ring (vs. C = C for alkenes - 1650)
1500	semi circle st.	
1450		

1300–1000	C–H i.p. (many) - rarely useful due to overlapping of other absorptions
880–671	C–H op bending
750–710	(o, p monosubstituted benz) - 2 bands
750	o disubstituted (4 and H)
830	p disubstituted (2 and H system) (800–850 range)
880, 780, 690	m - disubstituted (1 adj. H system, 2 adj. H system)

5. **Alcohols**
   ROH

3650–3590	(OH non bonded)
3400–3200	(OH bonded)
1410–1260	O–H bending (i.p.)
1260–1040	O–O str.
770–650	O–H bending (op)

6. **Ethers**

1300–1000	C–O–C

7. **Aldehydes**
	2900–2700	C–H stretch, doublet
	1740–1720	C = O stretch
	1705–1680	Conjugated C = C
	1715–1695	Aryl aldehyde
	975–980	C–H oop

8. **Ketones**
	1725–1705	Dialkyl ketone
	1685–1665	α,β-unsaturated
	1700–1680	Aromatic
	1325–1215	C COC skeletal (alkyl)
	1225–1075	C COC skeletal (aryl)

9. **Acids**
   RCOOH
	Free 3520	(vap. phase) (O–H)
	3000–2500	(H-bonded, dimer)
	2700–2500	(ragged bands) overtones + OH i.p. bending (1420) + C–O st coupling (1300–1200)
	1760 > CO	Monomer
	1710 > CO	Dimer $\left(\text{⬡–COOH }1685\right)$, (1650–1500, 1420–1300) (RCOŌ)
	1420	(OH ip)
	1300–1200	(C–O)

10. **Esters**
	1750–1735	(CO str.)
	1300–1050	(2 bands, C–O) asy, sym bending

11. **Lactones**
	1820–1760

$\left(\square{=}O\right)$ (ring C=O 1770)   (ring C=O 1735)   (30–35 cm^{-1} less for α, β, unsaturation)

1820   1770   1735

12. **Anhydrides**
	1850–1800	2 bands Asy C = O
	1790–1740	Sym C = O
	1300–900	$\left(-\overset{O}{\underset{}{C}}-O-\overset{O}{\underset{}{C}}-\right)$
	1050–1040	(C–O)

13. **Acid halides**
	1815–1790	(CO)

14. **Amino acids**
	1650–1550	2 bands 3220–2640 $\overset{\oplus}{N}H_3$ asy. stretching
	1440–1360	2220–2000 $\overset{\oplus}{N}H_3$ asy. bending

15. **Amino acid**
    HCl
	3350–2380	OH + NH$_3$ sy.
	1735–1700	CO – only one
	1620–1585	$\overset{\oplus}{N}H_3$ asymmetric bending
	1555–1485	$\overset{\oplus}{N}H_3$ symmetric bending

	1220–1190	C — C — O stretching $\overset{\|}{O}$
16. **Nitro (NO_2)**	1565–1515	Asymm. NO_2
	1385–1335	Symm. NO_2
	870	C–N bending
	610	C–N–O bending
17. **Nitrites**	1686–1655	N = O st. trans isomer
O–N=O	1630–1600	N = O st. cis isomer
	3350–3200	N = O st. overtones
	690–615	O–N = O bending in cis isomer
	630–560	O–N = O bending in trans isomer
18. **Amides**	3500–3400	N–H non-bonded – 2 bands R $CONH_2$ (Asym. + Sym.)
	3325–3125	N–H (multiple bands) trans 1° amide (dimer + polymers)
	1695–1675	C = O + N–H i.p. 2 bands (amide I) (amide II)
	1400	C–N–H (NH ip + C–N st.) amide III
	700	N–H op (amide V)
	700	O CN bending (amide IV) 700 640
19. **Amines**	3500–3300	(2 bands NH asym., sym.) 1° amides 1 band for 2° amine
RNH_2	1600–1575	N–H ip
	1260–1000	C–N (aliphatic)
	1340–1240	C–N (aromatic)
	1350–1280	2° aromatic
	1360–1310	3° aromatic
	909–667	NH bending (multiple bands) 1°
	750–700	Aliphatic 2° amines

17.12 APPLICATIONS OF INFRARED SPECTROSCOPY IN PHARMACEUTICAL SCIENCES AND ORGANIC CHEMISTRY

1. Identification of functional groups and structure determination

We have already learnt in details how i.r. can be used to identify the various functional groups. Different functional groups show their characteristic vibrations and so, they can be easily identified. Thus C=C and C=N absorb in the region 1650–1550 cm^{-1} while carbonyl group at 1800–1650 cm^{-1} (stretching).

2. Detection of impurities (purity of a known compound)

If a compound under investigation contains additional peaks than the characteristic peaks of the known compound, it is clear that the compound is not pure. As an example, cyclohexanol usually contains an impurity cyclohexanone which shows itself as a strong band in the region of the carbonyl group.

3. Identification of known compounds

In case of doubt about the identity of a known compound, its i.r. spectrum can be compared with the reference spectrum of the most suspected compounds. If the i.r. spectra of this compound overlaps peak-by-peak, that can be clearly checked by using a light-box, the two compounds unquestionably are identical.

4. Monitoring of progress of a reaction

It is often possible to monitor the progress of a reaction as a reactant with a characteristic functional group gets converted into a product having a different functional group. Thus, if a ketone is being reduced in the reaction to give an alcohol, then with time, i.r. analysis will show that the peak due to C=O gets diminished and finally disappears, while that due to O–H appears and intensities.

5. Elucidation of reaction mechanism

This is done by taking samples out of the reaction vessel after short regular intervals and recording their i.r. spectra. Characteristic peaks of the suspected functional groups can be recognised, thus enabling us to propose a most appropriate mechanism.

6. Chromatographic separations

IR analysis can be very helpful in ensuring complete separation by say column chromatography. The portions that contain no impurities as indicated by the absence of the additional peaks in their i.r. spectra can be collected and separated apart. Mixed samples as indicated by the presence of additional peaks in their spectra can be discarded.

7. Quantitative analysis

This is done by finding out the relative intensities of absorption bands and measuring optical density of the absorption band of the pure component and comparing them with the standard working curves obtained by plotting optical density versus percent content. As an example, o–, m– and p–xylenes present in a mixture can be quantitatively estimated like this:

• This estimation is possible as ortho, meta and p-xylenes show bands at different positions for the C–H oop bending at 740, 880 and 830 cm^{-1} respectively. So, what is done is that we prepare mixtures of known composition of these three isomeric xylenes and draw their working curves by plotting optical density versus content of isomers for the three bands at 740, 800 and 830 (see Fig. 17.58). Finally, all you have to do is to know the optical density values for the commercial xylene samples and read the percentage composition from the working curves directly (see Fig. 17.58).

8. Investigation of optical isomerism

Although the solution i.r. spectra of racemates and enantiomers are identical, their i.r. spectra taken in the solid state form are different.

9. Investigation of rotational isomerism

While the CH_2 rocking in-plane vibrations in trans (staggered) 1,2–dichloroethane appears at 1291 cm^{-1}, the gauche (skew) isomer absorbs at 1235 cm^{-1}. With increase in temperature, the gauche conformer becomes dominant over the trans rotational conformer (Fig. 17.60).

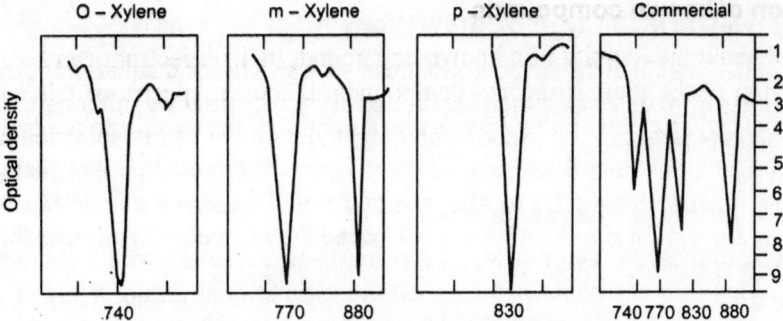

Fig. 17.58. Significant regions of the i.r. spectra for quantitative estimation of the three isomeric xylenes and the commercial sample.

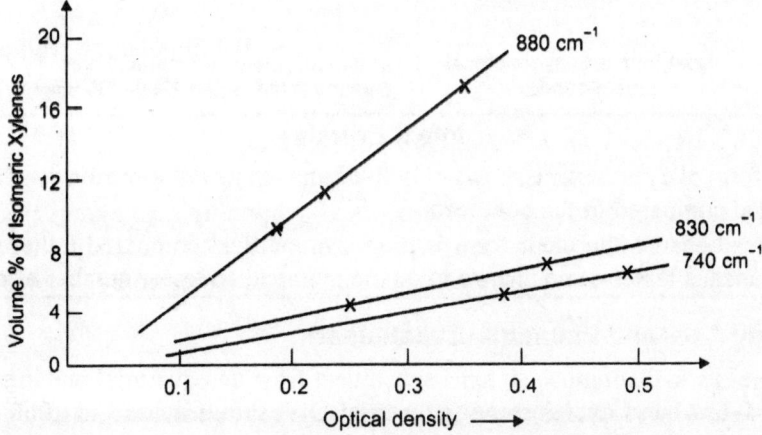

Fig. 17.59. Optical density versus percentage of the isomeric xylenes in a commercial sample.

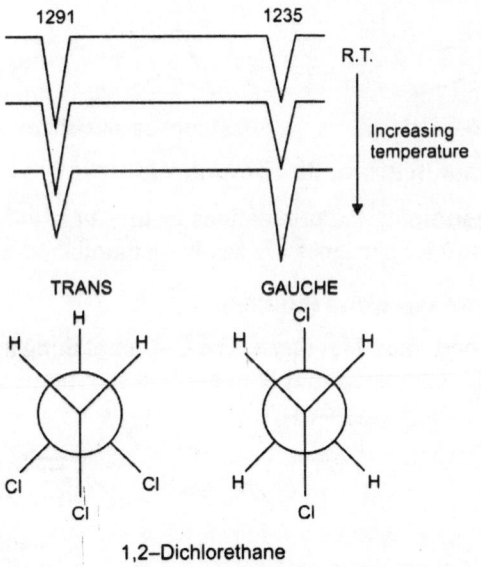

Fig. 17.60a.

10. Estimating relative stability of conformations

Alicyclic compounds exist in different conformations such as axial and equatorial. Analysis by infrared spectroscopy enables us to determine their relative stability. For instance, although, the chair as well as the boat conformations are expected to show forty eight vibrational bands, selection rules allow far less in the chair form than in the boat form on grounds of symmetry/dipole moment changes. Thus, while a total of eighteen C–C stretching, CH_2 rocking and twisting vibrations are to be expected from the boat form, only five are forcast for the chair form. And indeed the i.r. spectrum of chair form shows just five bands in the expected region – 1350–700 cm^{-1}.

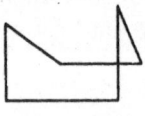

Boat form less symmetrical   Chair form more symmetrical only
more bands   5 bands in the region 1350–700 cm^{-1}

Intext Exercise

6. The chair form of cyclohexane shows only five bands in its i.r. spectrum even though 48 peaks are expected compared to the boat form.

   Ans. This is because the chair form is more symmetrical compared to the boat form. More symmetry means lesser or no change in dipole moment, so lesser number of bands are seen.

---

11. Investigating Axial and Equatorial Substituents

IR analysis enables us to distinguish an axial substituent from an equatorial one in cyclohexane. Thus, while the trans–4–tert-butyl cyclohexane (equatorial OH) shows a band at 1060 cm^{-1} due to C–O stretching, the cis (axial O–H) absorbs at 951 cm^{-1}.

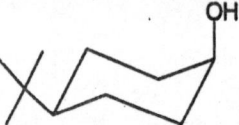

951 cm^{-1} axial OH   1060 cm^{-1} equatorial OH   C–O stretching

12. Elucidating orientations in aromatic compounds

The C–H oop help us in determining the orientations or the substitution pattern on benzene ring. The ortho, meta and para disubstituted benzenes are easily distinguished as we have already learnt.

13. Distinguishing between cis-trans isomers

Let us consider cis–2–pente and trans 2–pentene. The C=C stretching in the symmetrically disubstituted trans–2–pentene is very weak compared to that in the less symmetrically disubstituted cis–2–pentene.

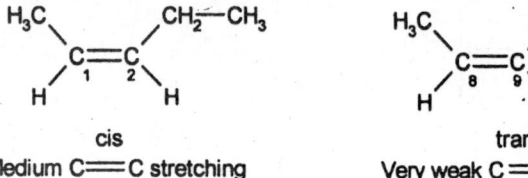

cis   trans
Medium C=C stretching   Very weak C=C stretching

Similarly, C=C stretching is not observed in trans–2–butene while it is observed in the cis isomer.

C=C stretching missing   C=C stretching present

14. Keto-enol tautomerism

Unlike simple ketones or 2,4–diketones, 1,3–diketones also called β-diketones, show a complicated i.r. spectrum because they exist in keto-enol tautomerism. The enol form is the major one because of hydrogen-bonding.

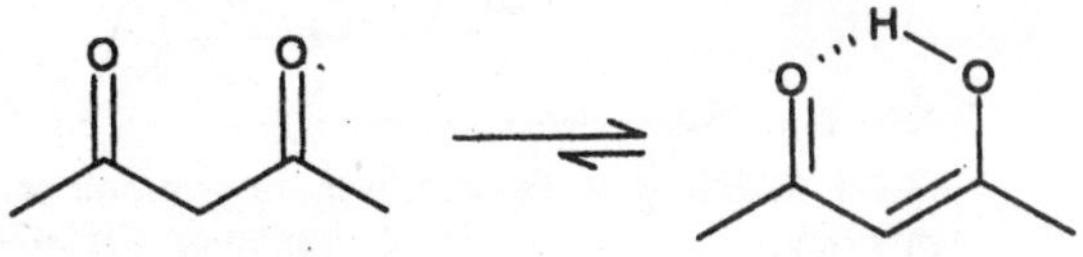

Keto   Enol

Acetylacetone

| General 1730–1695 | Two C=O bands Symmetric 1723 cm^{-1} Asymmetric 1706 cm^{-1} | ~ 1622 cm^{-1} (C=O H-bonded) 3200–2400 cm^{-1} | General 1640–1570 cm^{-1} (O–H H-bonded broad) |

Thus, the keto tautomer shows a doublet for CO because of symmetric and asymmetric stretching. The C=O moves down to a lower frequency in the enol tautomer at 1622 cm^{-1}, due to a couple of effects, the intramolecular H-bonding as well as resonance that makes it some one even a half bond. Further O–H stretching appears at 3200–2400 cm^{-1}.

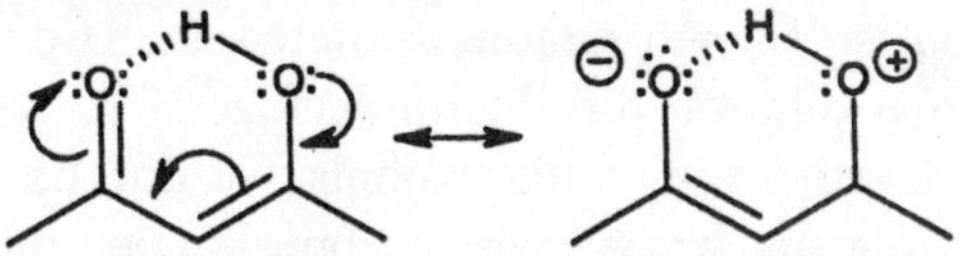

Resonance in Enol tautomer
consequence C=O ⟶ C⁚⁚O

As the % composition of the two tautomers depends upon nature of the solvent, therefore, it is but natural that the relative intensities of the bands from these tautomers would vary as we noticed this in the chapter on NMR.

It should be noted that unlike β-diketones β-keto esters, in general, do not enolize or enolize to a very weak extent. Thus, ethyl acetoacetate shows a doublet for C=O stretching because of existence keto (major) and ester CO. The O–H seen in enolic form in b-diketones is not seen in b-diketones as the enol form is only a very minor one.

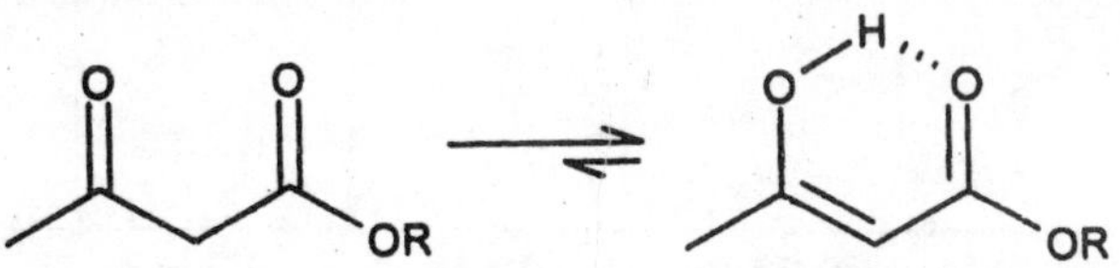

Ethylacetoacetate

General	Keto		Enol	General
R	R=Et		R=Et	R ≠ Et
	C=O doublet			
	1733			
1740	1710		1645 cm^{-1}	1650
1720				

15. Hydrogen bonding

Like we saw in the chapter on NMR, i.r. can also be used to indicate the existence of hydrogen bonding in a given compound. H-bonding occurs in a molecule possessing X–H and Y groups where both X and Y can be F, O or N. So X–H bond is lengthened and force constant is reduced. Hence ν stretching is lowered.

$$X—H + Y \longrightarrow X—H \cdots Y$$

COH, CONH$_2$,   H-bonding

OH, NH$_2$

In fact, both the X—H and H....Y stretching frequencies are lowered. Obviously, stronger the H-bonding, lower will be the O—H stretching. So, the O—H stretching frequency can be taken as a measure of the strength of the H-bond. Further, the shape and intensity of the band also depends upon the extent of H-bonding. Absorption bands due to H-bonding, in general, become broad as well as intense. Thus, O—H in alcohols appears at 3400–3300 cm^{-1} while the non-H-bonded (free) OH stretching appears at 3650–3590 cm^{-1}.

We have also seen the effect of H-bonding on β-diketones and β-ketoesters.

Whether the H-bonding is intermolecular, or intermolecular? This can also be investigated by i.r. analysis of the diluted samples. When a sample is diluted, the H-bonds are broken down between different molecules. Thus, upon dilution the intermolecular H-bonding decreases and free X—H stretching appears. Hence if we are dealing with alcohols, we find the H-bonded O—H stretching at 3400–3300 cm^{-1} decreases in intensity and finally disappears upon dilution, while the free O—H at 3650–3590 cm^{-1}, appears as a sharp band and increases in intensity (Fig. 17.60b). On the other hand, i.r. analysis shows that the H-bonded X—H stretching remains unaffected upon diluting the test sample in case of intramolecular H-bonding e.g. in methyl salicylate ("oil of wintergreen").

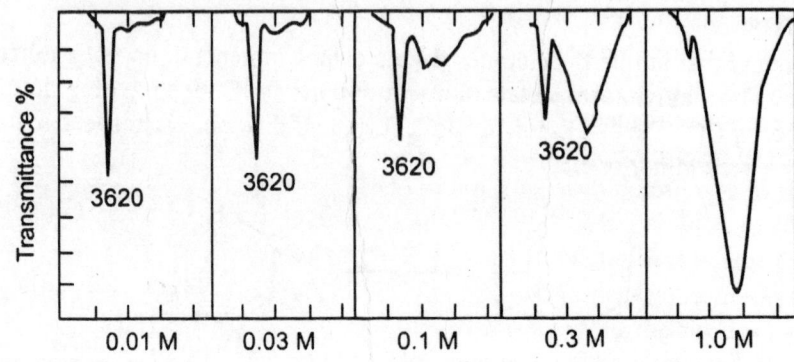

Fig. 17.60b. Effect of dilution on intermolecular H-bonding in ethyl alcohol.

16. Degree of Polymerization

By measuring at a specific frequency over time, changes in the character or quantity of a particular bond can be measured. Modern research instruments can take infrared measurements across the whole range of interest as frequently as 32 times a second. This can be done while making simultaneous measurements using other techniques. Thus it makes the observations of chemical reactions and processes quicker and more accurate.

17. Quality of Tea Leaves

Techniques have been developed to assess the quality of tea-leaves by using infrared spectroscopy. Thus, highly trained experts, also called 'noses' can be used more sparingly, at a significant cost saving.

18. In Semiconductor Electronics

Infrared spectroscopy is useful in inorganic chemistry, in the field of semiconductor microelectronics. For example, infrared spectroscopy can be applied to semiconductors like silicon, gallium arsenide, gallium nitride, zinc selenide, amorphous silicon, silicon nitride, etc.

17.13 INFRARED SPECTROMICROSCOPY : INFRARED SPECTRUM AND FORENSICS (INFRARED MICROSCOPY)

Many of the materials encountered at crime scenes are too small to be analysed by means of standard instrumentation, even at infrared wavelengths. But it is now possible to do that by infrared spectromicroscopy.

It is less well known as to how forensic science has benefitted from infrared radiation. Many of the materials encountered at crime scenes are too small to be analysed using standard instrumentation even at infrared wavelengths. But, "infrared spectromicroscopy" has led to significant advantage in forensic science.

In addition to simple material and chemical samples, the technique lends itself nicely to the study of more complex system. Crime scenes offer many examples of composite vibrationally active samples, including blood smears on surfaces, mixed tissue and body fluids.

Infrared spectroscopy reveals the molecular fingerprint of the compounds in a given sample. Such fingerprints are invaluable for identifying particular molecules, their structure and their chemical reactions.

Little wonder then that infrared spectroscopy has assumed a significant role in forensics, today. Indeed, the technique has become one of the work horses of the standard forensics laboratory. It has proved a highly effective technique for analysing samples from crime scene, such as blood, fabrics and soil particles. Infrared spectroscopy enables crime investigators to compare a sample with a known compound in order to determine whether they share any chemical or physical properties. In fact, the future applications of synchroton-based infrared spectromicroscopy to forensics are virtually limitless. Infrared spectromicroscopy is ideal for examining the minute traces of blood found at crime scenes because of its high spatial resolution and high sensitivity characteristics.

In an infrared microscopy instrument shown in Fig. 17.61, i.r. rays arising either from a thermal source or a synchroton beam are allowed to enter the Michelson interferometer from the right. Afterwards, the modulated light leaves the interferometer to enter an infrared microscope where it is focussed onto a test sample. The outgoing components of light that are not absorbed are focussed onto an infrared detector. If desired, visible images of the test sample can also be recorded at the same time. The infrared spectrum can be mapped with micron precision as the sample is positioned on a computer-controlled microstage.

Microscopes extend the use of i.r. to samples of the order of 10 μm. Use of a microscope provides us the ability to align the small sample in the i.r. beam and also for focussing the energy.

The use of i.r. in forensics is especially useful as it is non-destructive.

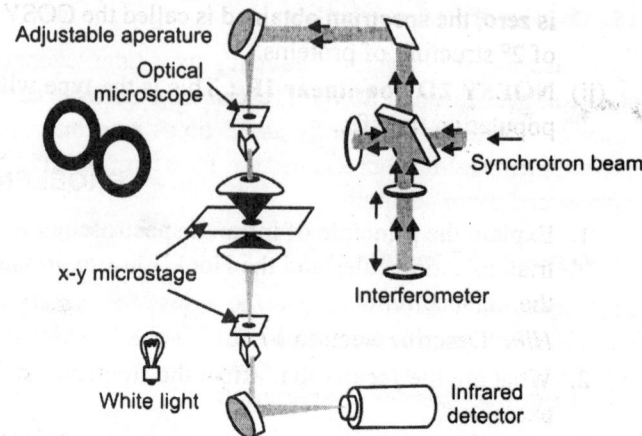

Fig. 17.61. An infrared spectromicroscopy where it is focussed onto a sample.

17.14 TWO-DIMENSIONAL FT INFRARED SPECTROSCOPY

Two-dimensional infrared correlation spectroscopy analysis involves the application of 2D correlation analysis on FT infrared spectra.

Nonlinear two-dimensional infrared spectroscopy : This technique allows the observation of coupling between different vibrational modes. This is also used to monitor molecular dynamics on a picosecond time scale. Although, it is still a largely unexplored technique but has high potential for fundamental research. In fact, this technique is the infrared version of correlation spectroscopy. This is the result of the development of femtosecond infrared laser pulses. In this experiment first a set of pump pulses are applied to the sample. A waiting time allows the system to relax. This period lasts over zero to several picoseconds. The duration can be controlled with a resolution of tens of femtoseconds. A probe pulse is now applied. A signal is emitted from the sample. The resultant infrared spectrum is a two-dimensional correlation plot of the frequency ω_1 that was excited by the initial pump pulses and the frequency ω_3 excited by the probe pulse after the waiting time.

As in 2DNMR spectroscopy, this 2D IR technique spreads the spectrum in two dimensions. Cross peaks that contain information on the coupling between different modes. Further, this also involves the excitation to overtones which result in excited state absorption peaks. These peaks are noticed below the diagonal and cross peaks.

Types

The 2D nonlinear IR spectra are of two types being analogous to COSY and NOESY techniques of 2D NMR :

(i) **COSY 2D nonlinear IR :** If the waiting period t_2 in the pulse sequence used above

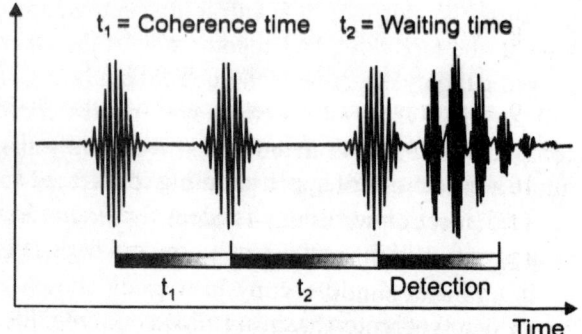

Fig. 17.62 Pulse sequence in 2D FT IR spectrum.

is zero, the spectrum obtained is called the COSY 2D non-linear IR. This finds use in elucidating of $2°$ structure of proteins.

(ii) **NOESY 2D non-linear IR :** This is the type with finite waiting time, t_2 that allows vibrational population transfer.

PROBLEMS

1. Explain the principle of infrared spectroscopy including fundamental vibrations in diatomic and triatomic molecules and the Hook's law expression? Are all fundamental vibrations observed in the i.r. spectrum?

   Hint: Describe Section 17.2.

2. What are the factors that affect the frequency of a vibration in infrared spectrum? Explain with examples?

3. With the help of a diagram explain that stretching vibrations in molecules such as HCl are quantized?

   Hint: See Fig. 3 and its discussion in Section 2.

4. Explain the following terms:
   (i) Stretching vibrations with types
   (ii) Bending vibrations with types
   (iii) Overtones
   (iv) Combination bands
   (v) Difference bands
   (vi) Fermi resonance

5. Why does Buckminster fullerene (C_{60}) show just four absorption bands in its i.r. spectrum?

   Hint: See Intext Exercise 3 (Section 2).

6. Although the atomic mass of fluorine is higher than that of carbon, the F–H stretching occurs at 4138 cm^{-1} compared to O–H stretching at 3040 cm^{-1}.

   Hint: See Intext Exercise 4 (Section 3)

7. How many vibrational absorptions are expected to be observed in the i.r. spectrum of carbon dioxide?

   Hint: See Intext Exercise 2 (Section 2).

8. Why do the following groups show two types of stretching? Explain with the help of figures.
   CH_3, CH_2, NO_2, anhydride and RNH_2.

9. Explain the construction and working of a double beam infrared spectrometer. What is an FTIR spectrometer? What are its advantages?

10. Discuss the sample handling (preparation of the sample) in infrared spectroscopy in brief.

11. How can we use C–H out-of-plane bending to determine substitution pattern of an alkene?

12. What are the factors that affect C=C stretching in acyclic and cyclic alkenes having endo and exo double bonds?

13. What are overtones and combination bonds and how do they help us in determining the substitution pattern on a benzene nucleus?

14. How can we distinguish among hexane, 1–hexene and 1–hexyne on the basis of i.r. spectroscopy?

15. Discuss with suitable examples, the effects of inductive effect, resonance and ring size in C=O stretching frequencies?

16. Discuss the following factors that affect $v_{C=O}$: field effect, steric factors, and ring-strain effect.

17. Introduction of α,β-unsaturation in an amide causes an increase rather than a decrease in $v_{C=O}$. Why?

    Hint: See Intext Exercise 4 (Section 8.11).

18. How will you distinguish between the following pairs by infrared analysis?
    (a) Aldehydes (RCHO) from ketones (RCOR)
    (b) RCOOH and RCOOR
    (c) Primary amines and secondary amines
    (d) Cyclohexanone and cyclobutanone
    (e) Cis 2–butene and trans 2–butene

19. How can you distinguish between the following pairs by infrared spectroscopy?
    (a) $PhCH_2NH_2$ and $PhCONH_2$

    (b) and

    (c) and

20. How can you distinguish between intramolecular and intermolecular hydrogen bonding by infrared spectroscopy?

21. How can you distinguish between:
    (a) Organic thiocyanates and isothiocyanates
    (b) Thiocyanato and isothiocyanato complexes
    (c) β-keto (acac) and enolic acetylacetonato (acaCH) complexes and carbon-bonded acetylacetato and complexes. Hint: See the discussions on these topics within sections 8.25, 8.26 and 8.27.

22. How does infrared spectroscopy help us in investigating keto-enol tautomerism in β-diketones and β-ketoesters?

    Hint: See the discussion on this topic in keto-enol tautomerism in section 9.14.

23. The chair form of cyclohexane shows only five bands in its i.r. spectrum even though the number of peaks expected is forty eight. Why?

    Hint: See Intext Exercise 6 (Section 9.10).

24. Can we distinguish between axial and equatorial substituents in cyclohexane? Explain by taking the example of trans–4–tert-butylcyclohexan and its cis isomer.

Hint: Based upon C–O stretching, it can be done (Section 9.11)

axial O–H in trans = 951 cm^{-1}

equatorial O–H in cis = 1060 cm^{-1}

25. The dehydration of 1,2–dimethyl cyclohexanol, cis or trans yields three alkenes. Propose their structures and suggest how can you disginguish among these by infrared spectroscopy.

Hint:

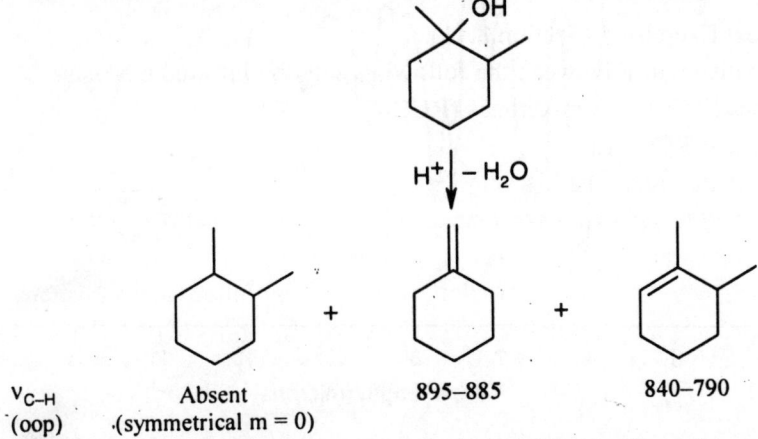

v_{C-H} Absent   895–885   840–790
(oop)   (symmetrical m = 0)

26. The i.r. spectrum of a pure liquid, with MF $C_4H_{10}O$ is given. Deduce the probable structure of this compound.

Hint: $CH_3CH_2CH_2CH_2OH$ (n-butanol).

27. Deduce from the following i.r. spectrum (film) the structure of the probable compound.

Hint: Anisaldehyde.

28. What is 2D FTIR spectroscopy?

29. Assign the bands observed in the i.r. spectrum of the following three compounds to the appropriate vibrational modes.

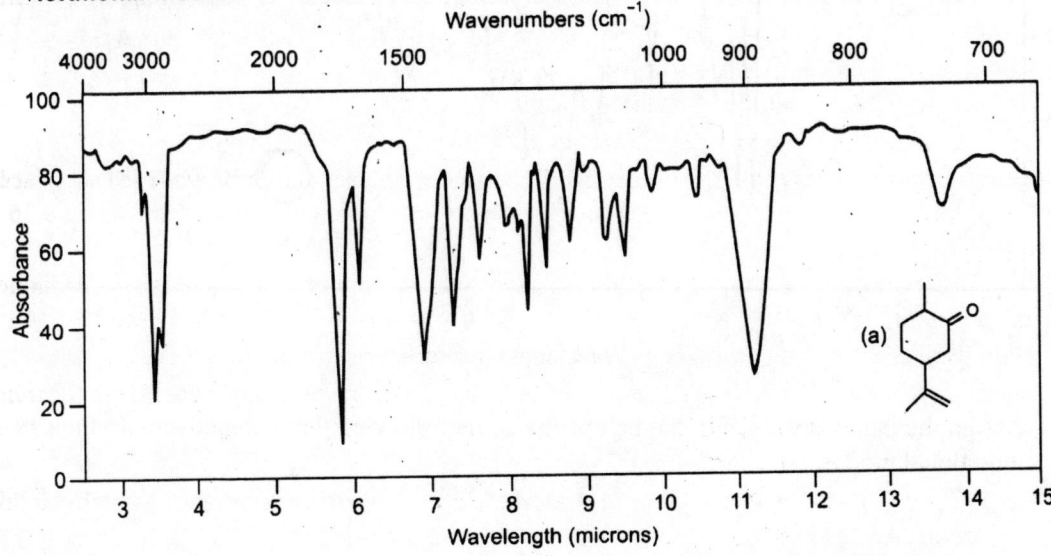

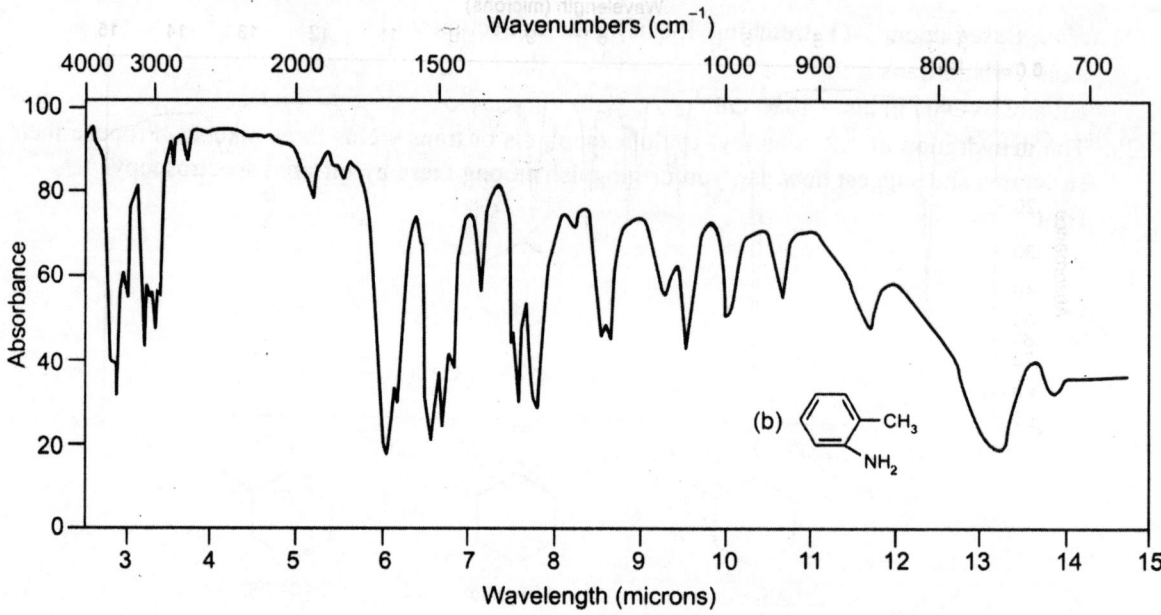

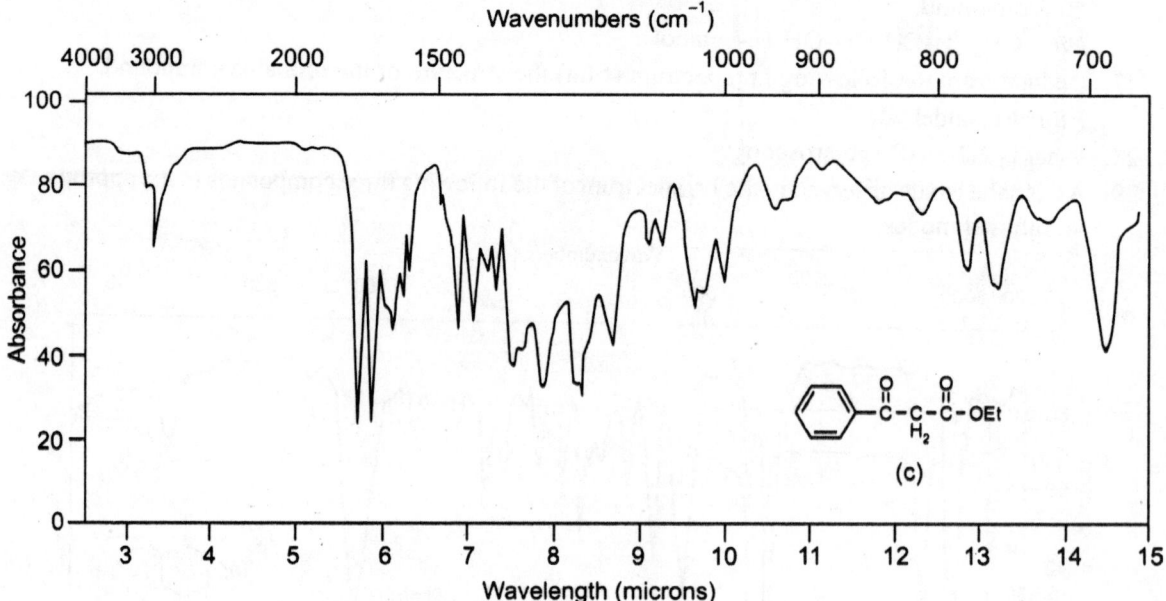

30. Assign the bands observed in the i.r. spectra of the following three compounds to their possible vibrational modes.

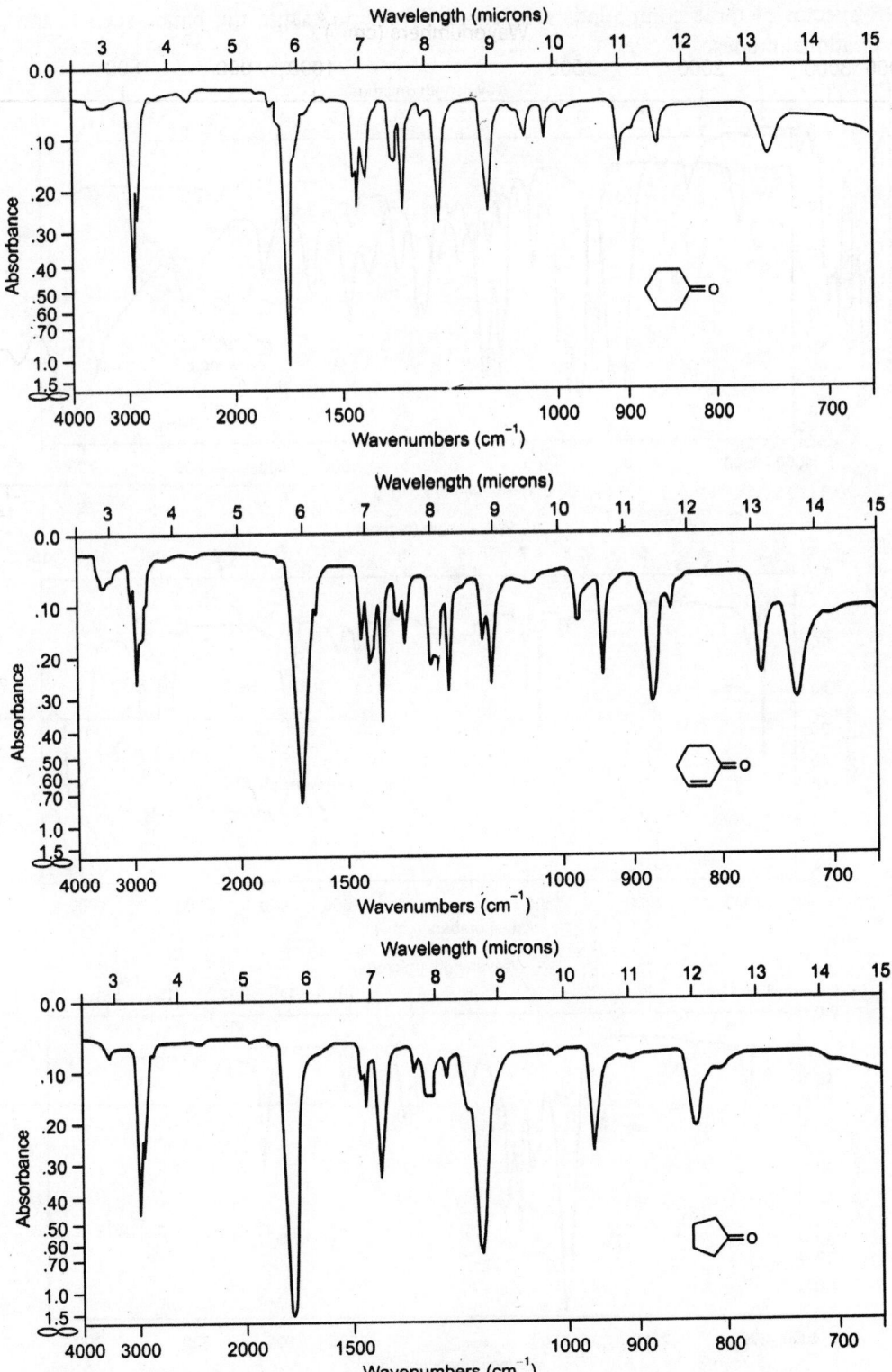

31. IR spectra of three compounds are recorded herein. Assign the bands seen to the possible vibrational modes.

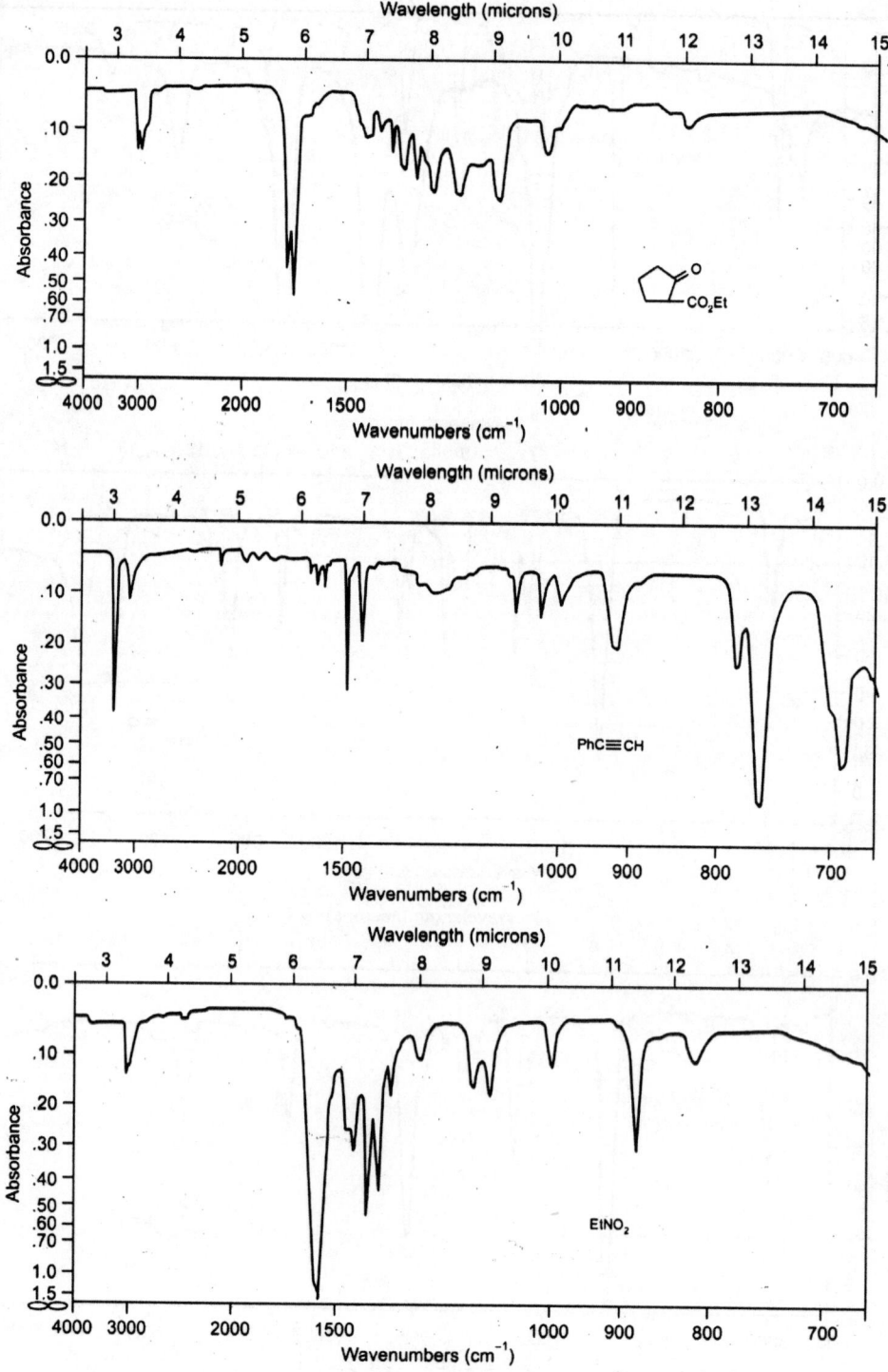

32. The IR spectra of acetone and isopropyl alcohol are shown below. Relate the bands observed to their vibrational modes.

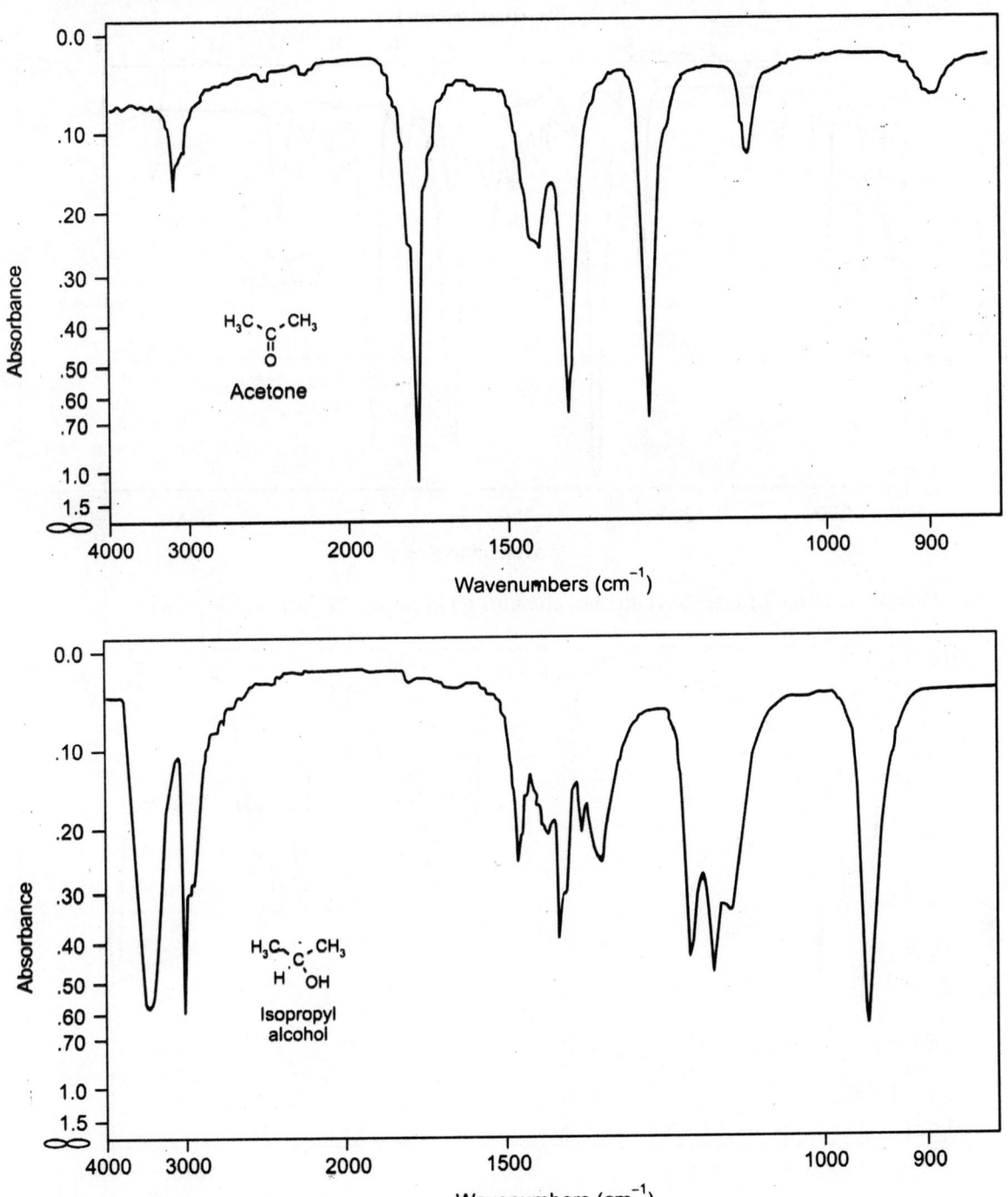

33. This IR spectrum of Acetone contains an impurity. What could be that?

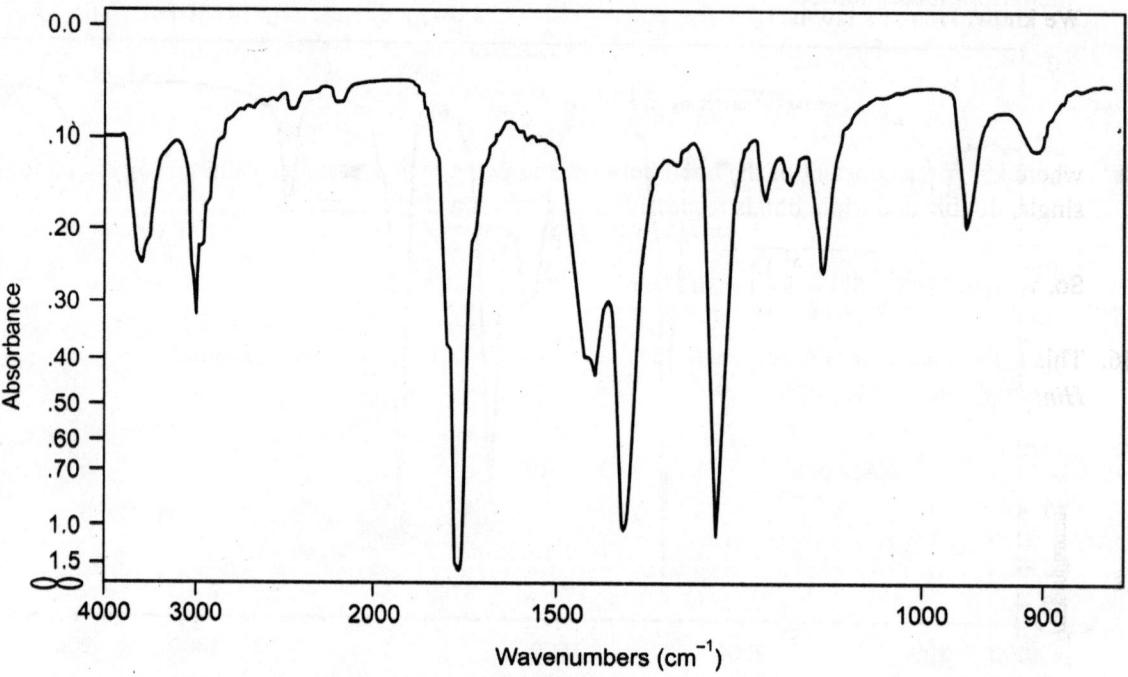

34. This IR spectrum of Isopropyl alcohol contains an impurity. What could be that?

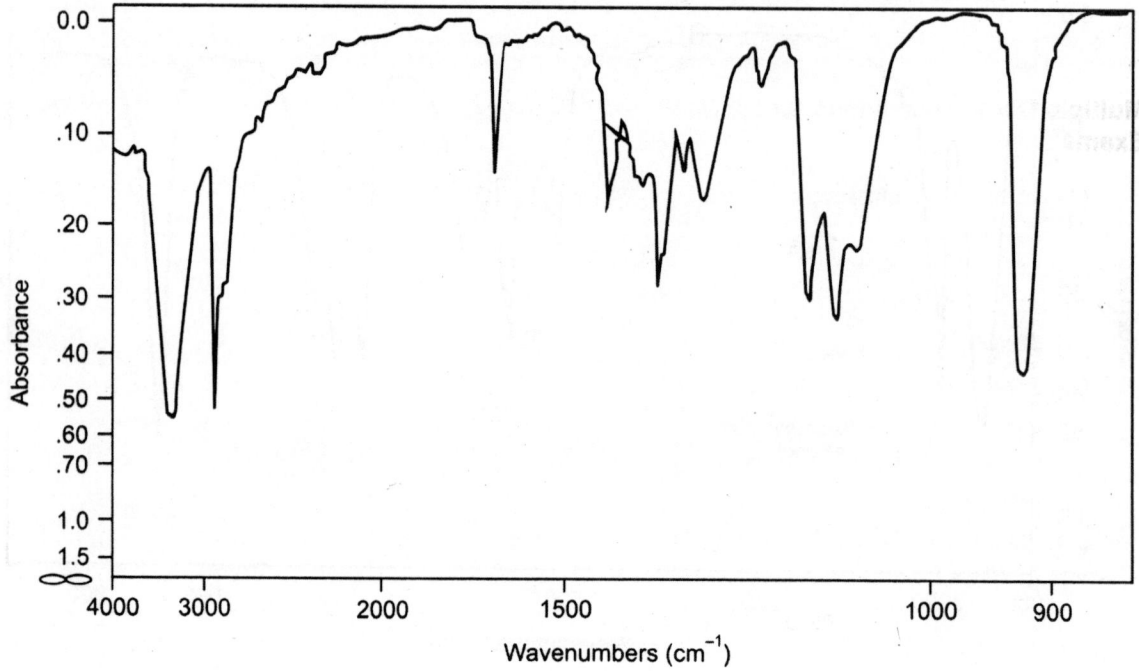

35. Predict, using Hooke's law the v_{C-H}.

We know, Hooke's law is:

$$v_{stretching} = 1303 \sqrt{k\left(\frac{1}{m_1} + \frac{1}{m_2}\right)}$$

where k = force constant of the bond between the two atoms. k assumes values of 5, 10, 15 for single, double and triple bonds respectively. As this is a single bond, C–H, k = 5.

So, $v_{C-H} = 1303 \sqrt{5\left(\frac{1}{12} + \frac{1}{1}\right)} = 3033$ cm^{-1}

36. This is the spectrum of 4-octyne. It does not show C≡C stretching. Why? Explain.

Hint: See selection rules, Section 1.

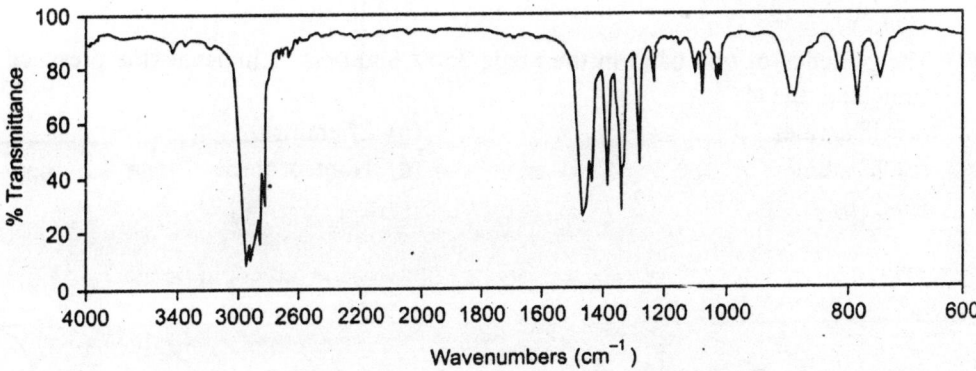

Multiple Choice Questions for NET, GAIT, GPAT, SLAT, GRE, CSE, HCS etc. Competitive Exams

(1) Infrared spectroscopy for organic compounds involves electromagnetic waves with wave number:

    (a) 4000–800 cm^{-1} (b) 4000–667 cm^{-1}

    (c) 5000–800 cm^{-1} (d) 5000–667 cm^{-1}

    Hint: (2).

(2) Infrared region lies between:

    (a) Ultraviolet and radiowaves   (b) Visible and radiowaves

    (c) Visible and microwaves   (d) UV and visible waves

    Hint: (3).

(3) Oct–4–ene shows C = C frequency in the range:

    (a) 1680–1600 cm^{-1} (very weak)   (b) 1680–1600 cm^{-1} (strong)

    (c) 1680–1600 cm^{-1} (medium)   (d) No peak in this region

    Hint: (4).

(4) C_{60} fullerene shows lesser number of peaks in the infrared spectrum because:
    (a) It is asymmetric in nature   (b) It contains sp^3, sp^2 and sp carbons
    (c) It contains a graphite like structure   (d) It has a symmetrical structure

(5) Anhydrides show two hands at 1820 cm^{-1} and at 1750 cm^{-1}. It shows that:
    (a) The two CO groups are non-equivalent .
    (b) The CO peak is split into a doublet due to Fermi resonance
    (c) One peak is due to CO group, while the other is due to COO group
    (d) None of these
    Hint: (d).

(6) The presence of two bands in the range 3500–3300 cm^{-1} indicates the presence of N–H stretching due to:
    (a) $1°$ amines   (b) $2°$ amines
    (c) $3°$ amines   (d) None of these
    Hint: (a).

(7) The presence of one band in the range 3500–3300 cm^{-1}, indicates the presence of N–H stretching due to:
    (a) $1°$ amines   (b) $2°$ amines
    (c) $3°$ amines   (d) None of these
    Hint: (b).

18

Mass Spectrometry ("Plus-Minus" or "Addition-Subtraction" Spectrometry)

This is an analytical technique that is used for determining molecular mass of a sample compound as well as for generating structural information about the compound. The molecular mass is determined to an accuracy of about 0.01% for the large biomolecules. That means an accuracy of within 4 Daltons (Da) or atomic mass units (amu) error for a molecule having molecular mass of 40000 Da. Further, this technique tells us about the whole structure of the compound. In fact, this technique provides us some necessary whole structural information that can not be obtained from any other spectrum. The information about molecular mass is obtained from the highest peak seen in the mass spectrum which is a plot of ion abundance (intensity) versus m/e values. In mass spectrometry the test sample is converted into a molecular cation radical, $M^{\ddagger}$ by loss of one electron. This ion then fragments into charged species which give rise to their own peaks in the mass spectrum as per their mass (m/e) values. Structural information is obtained by subtracting an m/e value from a higher m/e value or by adding some value to the lower m/e value to see if it gives rise to the higher m/e value as you will see later on. That is why, the author has coined two new terms for mass spectroscopy – "Plus-Minus" or "Addition-Subtraction" spectroscopy. Because all you got to do while interpreting the m/e for the peaks in a mass spectrum is to do the plus-minus or the addition-subtraction arithmetic calculations in order to recognise the fragments generated. Therefore, these terms are very rightly justified and should also be used as these will popularise this important branch of spectroscopy among the students. Another beauty of the technique is that is requires only very minute quantities of the test sample available in just picograms.

18.1 PRINCIPLE

In this type of spectroscopy, no electromagnetic radiation is used for excitation. Hence, the preferred term spectrometry over spectroscopy. Instead, the molecules are bombarded with high energy (70 eV) electron beam to knock off electrons from the molecules. As a result, the molecules are converted into ions, the positively charged radical ions:

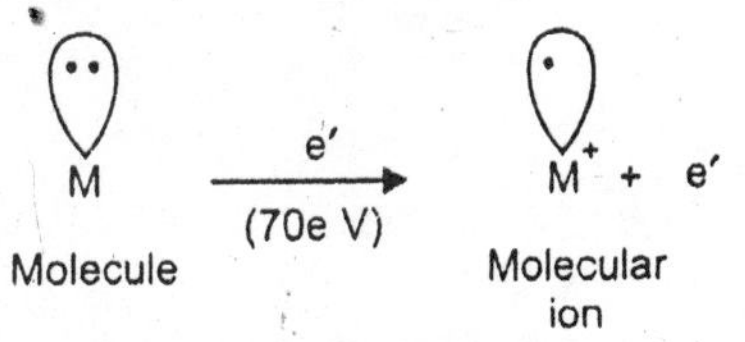

Fig. 18.1.

These ions are then accelerated by positive potential (also called accelerating potential) in general. Because the ions are positively charged, so they get repelled and consequently travel with great speed along a straight path. Now a magnetic or an electric field is applied with the help of repeller plates to these accelerated ions so that they travel in a curved path instead of moving in a straight path. Consequently, these ions get separated depending upon their mass-to-charge (m/z) ratio. This happens due to the fact that the mass (m) and charge (z) of the accelerated (V being accelerating potential) radical cations formed in the ionizer force it to follow a curved flight path (with r being its radius of curvature) in a magnetic field (H) as per the equation:

$$\frac{m}{z} = \frac{H^2 r^2}{2V}$$

Changing the strength of the magnetic field determines which ion travels the radius r to where the detector is positioned because the radius of curvature depends on their respective masses. Every time a separated ion is detected, the signal is sent to a data system in the computer whereby the m/z ratios are stored together along with their relative abundance and this is called a (m/z) mass spectrum.

Thus the detector detects r. And this allows us to calculate the mass (m/z) of the ion when z is known. Even as multiply charged species can be produced in the gaseous phase, z is mainly equal to +1.

18.2 MASS SPECTROMETER

A schematic mass spectrometer is shown in Fig. 18.2. This consists of three parts - the ionization source (chamber), the analyzer and the detector.

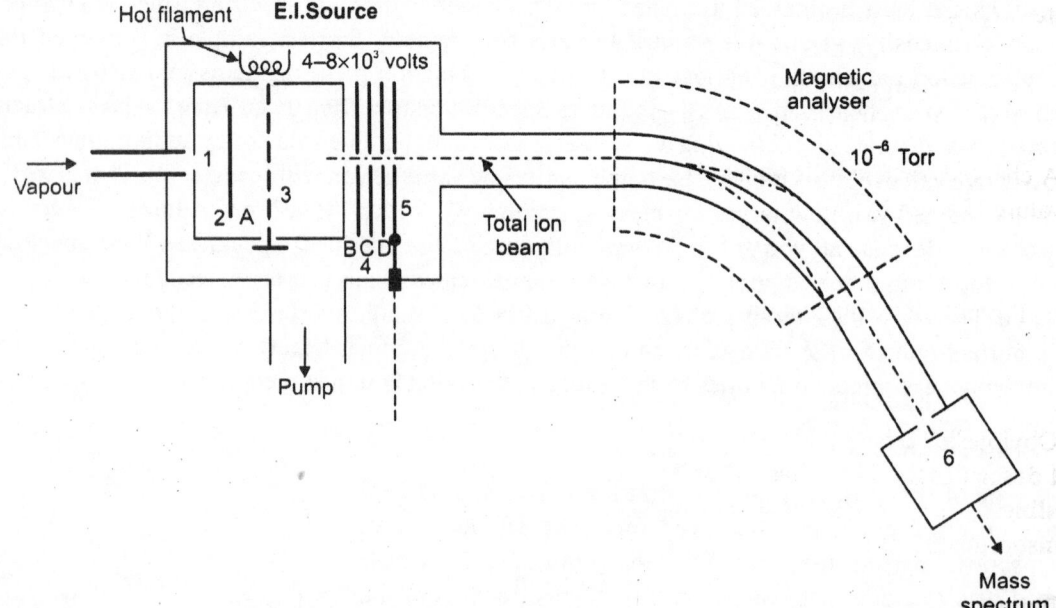

Fig. 18.2. A schematic mass spectrometer: (1) sample inlet, (2) ion-repeller plate, (3) ionizing electron beam, (4) plates for accelerating and focussing ion beam, (5) total ion monitor plate, (6) ion detector—usually an ion multiplier.

1. Ionization source (chamber)

This is the chamber in which ionization of the test molecules occurs. The sample is introduced from a reservoir into the ionization chamber via a sample inlet. The ionization chamber is maintained at a pressure (10^{-6} to 10^{-5} torr) lower than that of the reservoir so that the sample molecules are drawn into it easily. Further, this vacuum gives ions a reasonable chance to travel from one end to the other without encountering any hindrance from air molecules. Thus, a stream of molecules is let into the source without any problem when the sample is gas or liquid. For a non-volatile solid sample, a direct probe technique is used for this purpose. The sample is placed on the tip of the probe and heated. It is then with the help of a vacuum lock, allowed to enter the chamber.

2. Mass Analyzer

This is a curved tube that is maintained under high vacuum through which the ion beam passes from the ion source to the collector.

The major function of a mass analyzer is two-fold, one to resolve ions having identical m/z ratio from all other ions and second to focus the individual ion beams of discrete mass onto a detector or into a second ionization chamber or into a collision cell.

The energetics of electron removal: For most of organic compounds, the ionization potential required lies between 8 and 15 eV but the electron beam has to be powered with 50–70 eV to generate the ions. The kinetic energy of an accelerated ion is given by:

$$\frac{1}{2} mv^2 = eV$$

where m = mass of ion
v = velocity of ion
e = charge of ion
V = Potential difference of ion-accelerating plates

A charged particle follows a curved flight path in the presence of a magnetic field whose radius of curvature is given by:

$$r = \frac{mV}{eH}$$

From these two equations, we get:

$$\frac{m}{e} = \frac{H^2 r^2}{2V}$$

Obviously, higher radius of curvature is associated with higher m/e value. **Hence, it is this equation that describes the behaviour of an ion in terms of its m/e for detection in the mass analyzer. It is possible to vary V with H as constant so as to bring each m/e species to the same focus (Nier-Johnson geometry).**

3. Detector

If the molecular ion or any of its fragments have lifetimes of at least 10^{-6} s, they are able to reach the detector. Detector is a counter. It generates an electronic signal when struck by an ion. As the current is directly related to the number of particles striking it, the detector records the abundance of each m/z particle. Timing mechanisms that integrate the signals with the scanning voltages enable the instrument to report which m/z strikes the detector.

The Mass Spectrum

As indicated earlier, the mass spectrum is a graph of ion abundance against m/e ratio. It has the following features (Fig. 18.2):

(i) **Base peak:** The tallest peak in the mass spectrum corresponds to the most abundant ion formed in the ionization chamber. This is called the base peak. This is a very important peak in the spectrum because the relative abundances of all the other peaks are reported as percentages of the abundance of this base peak.

(ii) **Molecular ion:** The highly energetic beam of electrons transforms some of the sample molecules to positive ions in the ionization chamber. As an ion is formed by the removal of an electron from a molecule, its weight is the actual molecular weight of the original molecule. We call this ion as the molecular ion, M^+. In fact, the molecular ion is a radical cation. This is because it contains an unpaired electron and a positive charge. The peak due to this ion called the molecular ion peak is usually the heaviest peak in the spectrum. However, we also need to take note of the existence of isotopes as well. Thus, hydrogen occurs mainly as ^1H and the isotope ^2H (0.02%). Similarly, carbon is mainly C–12 but also contains about 1.1% of the heavier isotope C–13. So, it is but natural that the heavier isotopes would also give ions which will contribute peaks in the mass spectra. The relative abundances of the isotopic peaks as expected are proportional to their abundances of the isotope.

(iii) Further, we also see the M+1 and M+2 peaks in the spectrum. Ions which have lifetimes of 10^{-6} sec. get accelerated in the ionization chamber even before they have an opportunity to disintegrate so that these get detected. However, some unstable ions do get disintegrated into fragments on their way to the analyzer. These fragment ions have considerably lower energy than normal ions. Why? This is because some of the energy that the ion receives is carried away as it gets the uncharged portion of the original ion accelerated. Consequently, the fragment ion follows an abnormal flight path to the detector and is detected at an m/e ratio that is dependent both on its mass and that of the original ion from which it formed. The peaks contributed by these ions are called **metastable ion peaks**. These peaks are usually broad peaks and appear

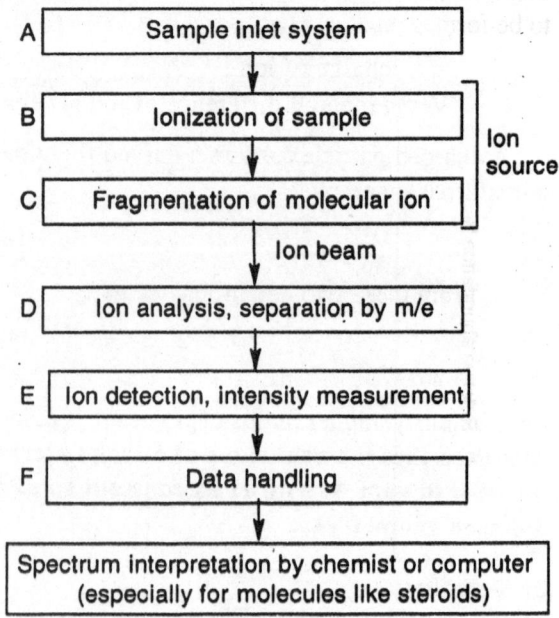

Fig. 18.3a. Mass spectral analysis involves six steps A to G.

at nonintegral values of m/e, often. The position of the metastable ion peak to the mass of the original ion is predicted by the equation:

$$m* = \frac{(m_2)^2}{m_1}$$

for $m_1^+ \longrightarrow m_2^+ + \text{fragment}$

$m*$ is the apparent mass of the metastable ion m_1 is the mass of the original ion from which gave rise to the fragment and m_2 is the mass of the new fragment ion.

18.3 RECOGNITION OF MOLECULAR ION M⁺ PEAK

The peak with the highest m/e value in the mass spectrum obtained on a low-resolution mass spectrometer represents the mass of the $M^{+\cdot}$ ion. When EI ionization technique is used, often the molecular ion $(M^{+\cdot})$ peak may either be very weak or absent altogether, as already discussed. Therefore, you have to be very cautious while recognizing such a peak. In case of doubt, if you lower the energy of the electron beam, the intensity of the $M^{+\cdot}$ increases as the molecular ion will have lower energy to fragment. The best solution to this problem will be to do the ionization via C.I. mode wherein in place of $M^{+\cdot}$ peak, $[MH]^{+\cdot}$ peak is obtained as we learnt earlier in the discussion of this method. Thus, it is better to obtain both the EI and the CI spectra in routine. Of course, the $[M-H]^+$ peak may also be seen in the CI spectrum as a result of the hydride abstraction.

These peaks can arise from the isotopic $[M+1]^+$ and $[M+2]^+$ ions as shown in Fig. 18.4 for 2–butanone. Carbon exists in mainly two isotopes – C–12 (98.89%) and C–13 (1.11%), hydrogen as H–1 (99.98%) and H–2 (D, 0.01%), oxygen as O–16 (99.76%) and O–17 (0.04%) and O–18 (0.20%). Thus, not only the normal molecular ions $(M^{+\cdot})$ but those arising from their isotopes are also expected to be formed and detected as $[M+1]^+$ and $[M+2]^+$. Clearly, the peak at m/z 72 is due to the compound

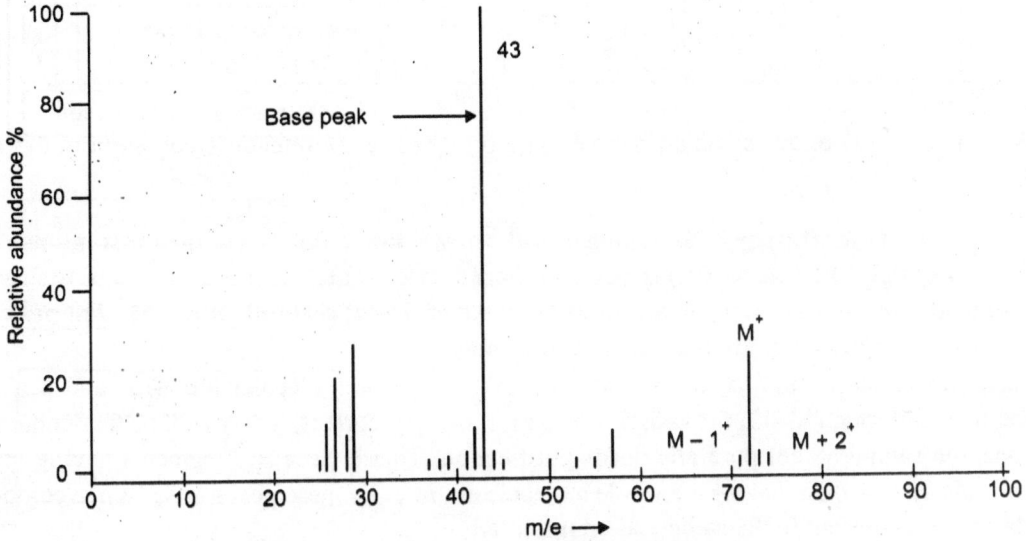

Fig. 18.3b. Mass spectrum of 2–butanone.

containing all normal (major) isotopes of C, H and O i.e. $^{12}C_4{}^1H_8{}^{16}O$. Evidently, the molecule containing one C–13 atom i.e. $^{13}C^{12}C_3{}^{13}H_8{}^6O$ having additional mass of one unit, will contribute a peak at $[M+1]^{\ddagger}$ that is at 73. Of course, the two other probable molecules can also contribute to $[M+1]^{\ddagger}$ peak i.e. $^{12}C_4{}^2H^1H_7O_{16}$ and $^{12}C_4{}^1H_8{}^{17}O$.

How to be sure about the $M^{\ddagger}$ ion peak when many peaks are observed in the highest m/z region? In general, when heteroatoms – Cl, Br and/or S are absent, of the following four patterns, one out of the four common patterns (Fig. 18.3c) is likely to be present. As for pattern (i) is concerned, clearly the two peaks correspond to $M^{\ddagger}$ and $[M+1]^{\ddagger}$ ions, the $[M+1]^{\ddagger}$ peak is the one having lower intensity as per the relative abundance of the isotope involved. The pattern number (ii) exhibits three peaks due to $M^{\ddagger}$, $[M+1]^{\ddagger}$ and $[M+2]^{\ddagger}$ when an additional peak enters such a pattern, then it is due to the $[M-1]^{\ddagger}$ ion, of course one of the peaks could be due to $[M+3]^{\ddagger}$ ion, of course that is rarely seen. When five peaks are observable as in pattern (iv), clearly, as the $[M+3]^{\ddagger}$ peak is rare, so we will ignore this and we will consider the four starting from lowest m/z value as $[M-2]^{+}$, $[M-1]^{+}$, $[M^{\ddagger}]$ and $[M+2]^{\ddagger}$ peaks. Obviously the $[M-1]^{\ddagger}$ is more intense than $M^{\ddagger}$ peak in the pattern (iv) but the $M^{\ddagger}$ peak is more intense than the $[M+1]^{\ddagger}$ or the $[M+2]^{\ddagger}$ peaks.

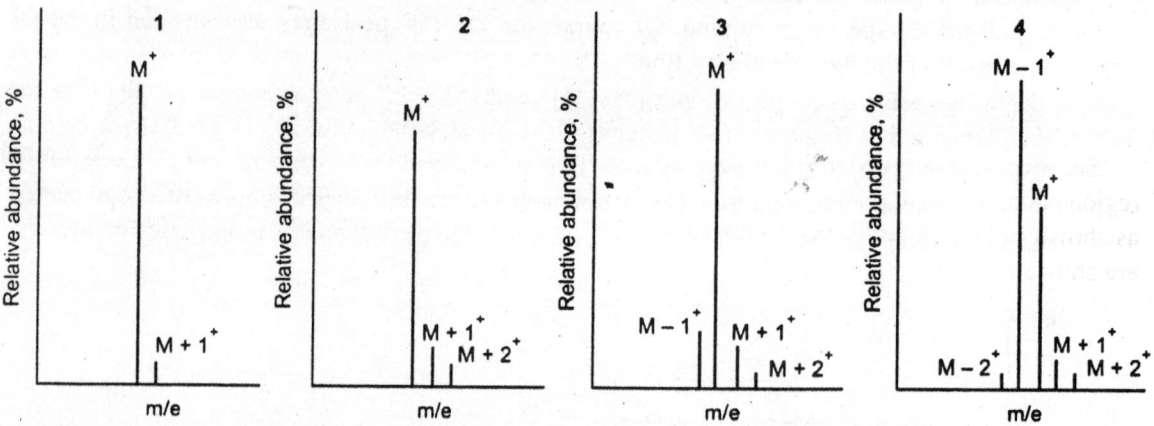

Fig. 18.3c. Four (1–4) of the common patterns in the highest peak (mass) region seen in the mass spectra.

Further, a notable strategy in assigning a peak to $M^{\ddagger}$ ion is that when the most intense peak (the one at the highest value of m/z) is odd-numbered, two situations may arise: one the sample contains an odd number of nitrogen atoms or the peak is almost certainly not a $M^{\ddagger}$ ion peak. For an even number of nitrogen atoms, $M^{\ddagger}$ has even mass.

Furthermore, in case the highest m/z value is assigned to the molecular ion $M^{\ddagger}$, and peaks are observed at M–3 through M–13, the assignment is most likely incorrect, it may well be that under these conditions, the sample is not pure and needs purification. This is because fragments having masses between 3 and 13 less than that for the whole molecule are rare. Or these peaks arise from a compound with a larger mass present in the sample as an impurity.

When S, Cl or Br are present, then the ratio M/M + 2 can be used to confirm that:

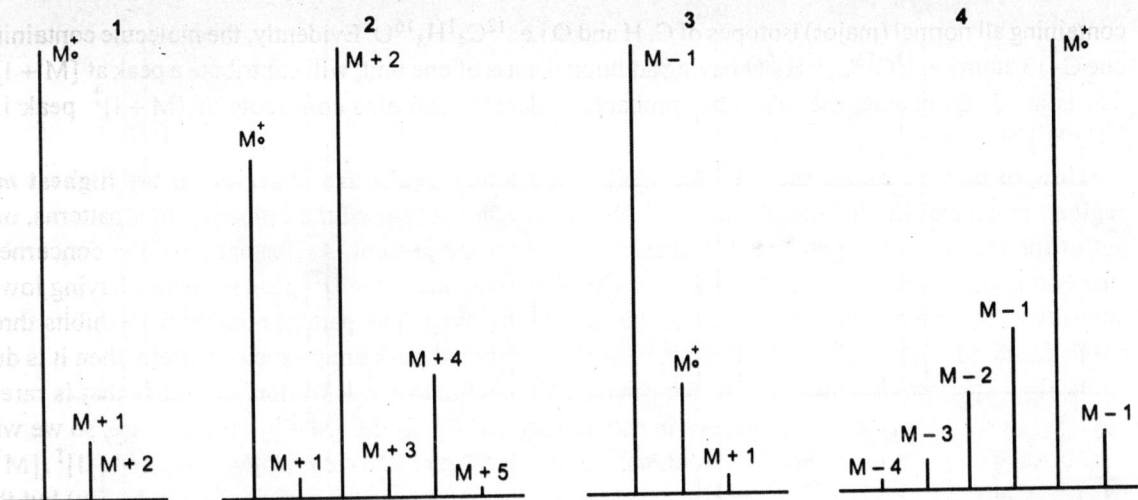

Fig. 18.3d. Highest mass spectra regions for: (1) phenylacetylene, (2) 1–bromo–2–chlorobenzene, (3) 2–styrylpyridine, (4) biphenyl.

	S $^{32}S/^{34}S$	Cl $^{35}Cl/^{37}Cl$	Br $^{79}Br/^{81}Br$
M/M + 2	24/I	3/I	1/I

So, a comparison of the intensities of the peaks separated by two mass units in the highest m/z region not only aids in identifying the M^{+} ion but also confirms the presence of these three heteroatoms as shown in Fig. 18.3e. Relative isotope populations for some combinations of chlorine and bromine are shown in Fig. 18.3f.

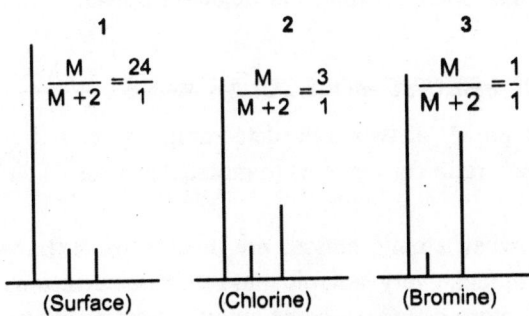

Fig. 18.3e. Comparison of M/M + 2 ratio for the highest mass region of compounds possessing (1) sulfur, (2) chlorine, (3) bromine.

Nitrogen rule: According to this rule if a molecule contains an even number of nitrogen atoms, its molecular ion will appear at an even mass value; if it contains an odd number of nitrogen atoms, it will form a molecular ion with an odd mass. The basis for the nitrogen rule is that although nitrogen has an even mass, it has an odd numbered valence. As a result, an extra hydrogen atom is included as a part of the molecule, giving it an odd mass.

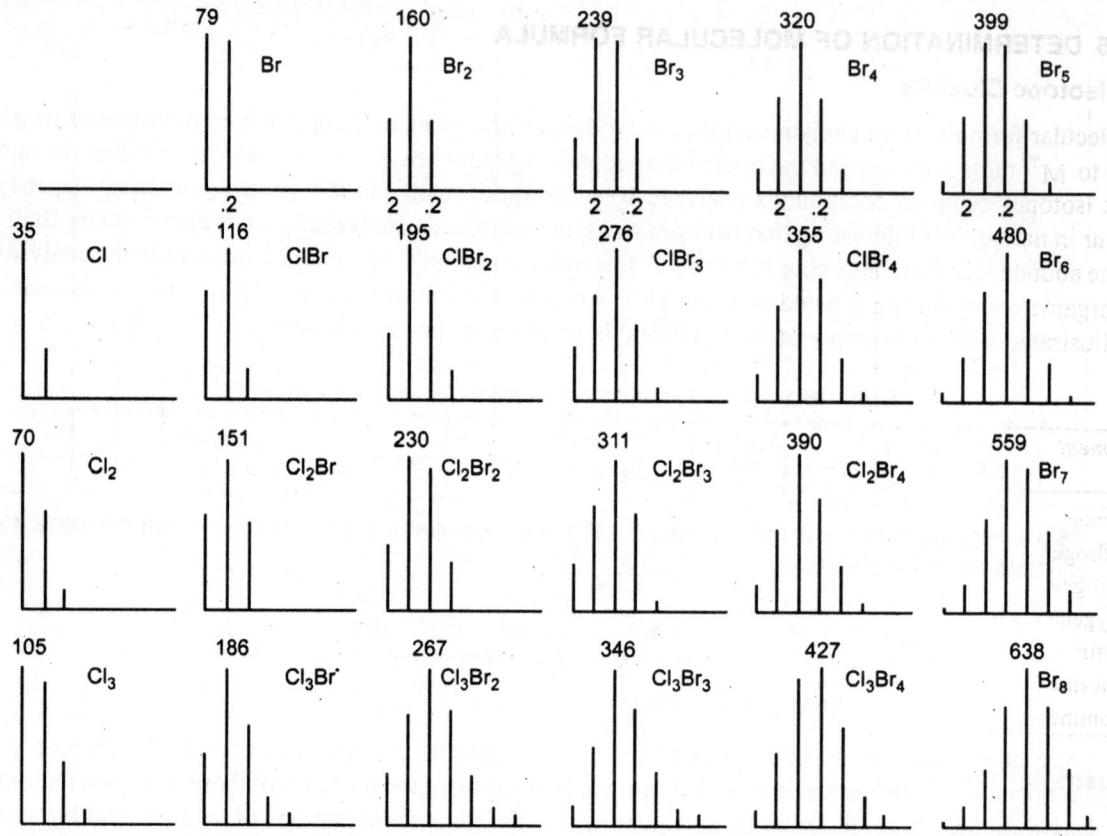

Fig. 18.3f. Some possible combinations of chlorine and bromine in highest mass regions with a difference of two atomic mass units between the adjacent peaks.

18.4 DETERMINATION OF PRECISE MOLECULAR MASS

When the analyte molecular ion M^+ arrives at the detector intact i.e. without undergoing fragmentation, molecular ion peak whose m/e ratio corresponds to molecular mass of the original molecule is seen at mass in the m/z spectrum.

It should be noted that when atomic masses are determined even with sufficient precision, the molecular mass is not true. In fact, every isotopic mass is characterized by a small "mass defect". This is because the mass of each atom differs by some amount from a whole mass number. This is called nuclear packing fraction. High-resolution mass spectrometers take this into account and so give the precise molecular masses which help us in knowing the exact structure of the compound. The accuracy is 0.005% compared to $\pm$ (0.1–1%) by chemical method.

Further, as mass spectral patterns are reproducible, there is a library of published mass spectra for various categories of functional groups. Thus, mass of the investigated sample can be deduced on the basis of fragmentation pattern. Instrument computers generally contain spectral libraries which can be searched for matches.

18.5 DETERMINATION OF MOLECULAR FORMULA

By Isotope Clusters

Molecular formula of an analyte sample can be determined by examining relative intensities of peaks due to M^+ molecular ion and the related ions containing more heavy isotopes. This is based on the fact that isotopes occur in compounds analyzed by mass spectrometry in the same abundances that they occur in nature. It is interesting that isotopes occur in compounds analyzed by mass spectrometry in the same abundances that they occur in nature. A few of the commonly encountered isotopes in the analyses of organic compounds are listed in Table 18.1. An example of how they can aid in peak identification is illustrated with an example of methyl bromide whose m/e spectrum is shown in Fig. 18.5.

Table 18.1. Isotope abundance (relative) of common elements

Element	Isotope	Relative abundance	Isotope	Relative abundance	Isotope	Relative abundance
Carbon	^{12}C	100	^{13}C	1.11	–	–
Hydrogen	^1H	100	^2H	.016	–	–
Nitrogen	^{14}N	100	^{15}N	.38	–	–
Oxygen	^{16}O	100	^{17}O	.04	^{18}O	0.20
Sulfur	^{32}S	100	^{33}S	.78	^{34}S	4.40
Chlorine	^{35}Cl	100	–	–	^{37}Cl	32.5
Bromine	^{79}Br	100	–	–	^{81}Br	98.0

Illustration

Example 1 : Methylbromide : Methylbromide, CH_3Br which contains the common isotope of bromine with mass 79, shows a M^+ peak at m/z 94 (Fig. 18.4). Let us now imagine that the molecule contains a heavy isotope Br–81. Therefore, it should show another peak at m/z 96 ($M + 2$) and with a relative abundance of 98% compared to 100% for the peak at m/e 94. This is because the isotopes occur in the same abundances as they occur in nature. And

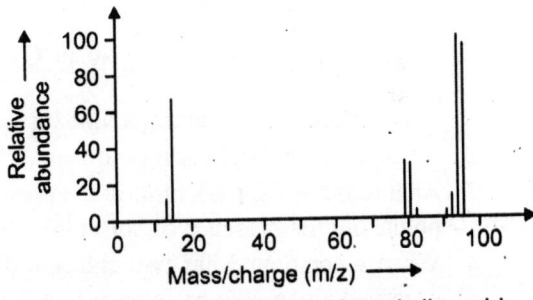

Fig. 18.4a. m/z spectrum of methylbromide.

indeed the mass spectrum shown in Fig. 18.4a, exhibits two peaks at m/z 94 and m/z 96 in the relative ratio of 1.020 (100/98).

CH_3–Br	Observed	Natural abundance
$79BrCH_3$ m/z 94	100	100
$81BrCH_3$ m/z 96	98	98

Thus, it is evident that the m/z spectrum is due to methyl bromide, CH_3Br. This is how isotopic peak ratio helps us in identifying the M^+ ion and in deducing the molecular formula. An $M + 1$ peak appears at m/e 95 with a relative abundance of 6.1.

The ratio of relative abundances of peaks containing ^{79}Br (m/z 94) and its isotope ^{81}Br (1.0204) (m/z 96) confirms the presence of bromine in the compounds as it is equal to the ratio of their natural abundances (100/98) = 1.0204.

$$
\begin{array}{l}
\text{Br} \!-\!\!\!-\!\!\!- \text{CH}_3 \\
\quad\text{m/z = 15} \\
\text{(79)BrCH}_3 \text{ m/z = 94} \\
\text{(81)BrCH}_3 \text{ m/z = 96}
\end{array}
$$

Example 2 : Ethane containing most common isotopes of C and H has molecular mass of 30, as per its molecular formula C_2H_6. Its m/z peak at m/z 30. Let us now imagine one carbon atom is a heavy isotope C–13. So the m/z spectrum should contain a peak at m/z 31 and its relative intensity would be 1.08% because in mass spectra, the isotopes occur in the same abundances as they occur in nature. As ethane molecule contains two carbons, therefore, we will see a peak at m/z 31 with a relative abundance of 2.16%. This is indeed so.

Similarly, let us imagine a H atom of ethane being replaced by a deutrium atom $_1^2H$ (D), the molecule should show an additional peak at M + 1 value i.e. 30 + 1 = 31. What would be its intensity like? Because the natural abundance of deuterium is just 0.016% of that of a H atom, the intensity of the peak at m/e 31 should be 0.016 multiplied by six i.e. 0.096% of that of molecular ion (M^+) peak. Further as the molecule may contain one C–13, the total intensity of M + 1 peaks should be (0.096 + 2.16%) = 2.26% to that of molecular ion peak, M^+.

Molecular formula by comparison of intensities of M^+, M + 1 and M + 2 peaks (isotopic ratio):

1. Number of carbon atoms in the analyte sample can be obtained from the relative heights say h of M^+ and h + 1 of (M + 1) ions respectively. This is given by the formula :

$$
\text{No. of C atoms} = \frac{100(h + 1)}{1.1\,h}
$$

This is because the natural abundance of C–13 relative to C–12 is 1.1%.

2. An odd molecular weight points out at the presence of odd number of nitrogen atoms.

3. An intense M + 2 peak hints at the presence of chlorine and bromine. A less intense M + 2 peak points out the presence of sulfur.

4. When a compound has two chlorine or bromine atoms, M + 4 peak, a very clear cut peak is observed along with an intense M + 2 peak.

5. When two molecules have about the identical molecular mass, the relative intensities of the M + 1 and M + 2 peaks would clearly prove them different.

6. In order to deduce molecular formula of the sample analyte, it is necessary to know the accurate mass of M^+, the molecular ion. Tables or calculations can be used based on Beynon and Williams work. For an illustration consider the M^+ peak at m/e 100 in a m/z spectrum. This can correspond to the following elemental compositions.

M^+	Mass (accurate)
$C_3H_6N_3O$	100.0511
$C_4H_8N_2O$	100.0637
$C_5H_{10}NO$	100.0762
C_7H_{16}	100.1251

In the accurate mass was found to be 100.0760, the precise M.F. would be $C_5H_{10}NO$.

For all combinations of common elements having M.F. upto mass of 500, relative values of M + 1 and M + 2 ion peaks are available in the tables.

18.6 DOUBLE FOCUSSING HIGH RESOLUTION MASS SPECTROMETERS

Ordinary mass spectrometers are a single focussing instrument type. They are also called low-resolution mass spectrometers as they are unable to discriminate between small differences in mass. The double beam mass spectrometers have high resolution power so that they can discriminate between small mass differences. They can measure mass of an ion upto an accuracy of ± 0.0001 amu. Therefore, it becomes possible to distinguish between ions having same nominal or integral mass but differing in their exact masses. A double focussing mass spectrometer uses an electric and a magnetic sector to work to such a high resolution is shown in Fig. 18.4b.

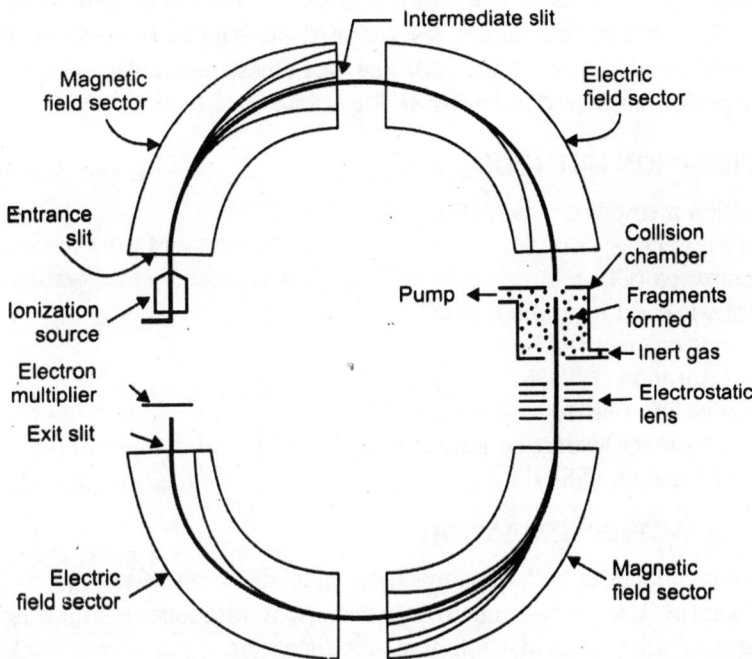

Fig. 18.4b. A schematic high resolution mass spectrometer with a collision cell.

Resolution (R)

This is the power of a mass spectrometer that is a measure of its ability to resolve or separate two ions of any defined mass difference, resolution is given by:

$$R = \frac{M}{\Delta M}$$

where M is the mass of the particle and ΔM represents the difference (M_2-M) in mass between the particle having mass M and another with next higher mass M_2. When the two masses are separated by a ten percent valley the resoluting power of the mass spectrometer for two masses say 100.000 and 100.005, will be:

$$R = \frac{100.000}{100.005 - 100.000} = \frac{100}{0.005} = 20000$$

Such instruments are called high resolution instruments. Low resolution instruments have much lower resolving power, say up to 2000. A low resolution instrument with R = 100 can resolve an ion with m/e 100.000 from another with mass, m/e 101. Thus, it is better to use high resolution instruments for accurate mass measure-

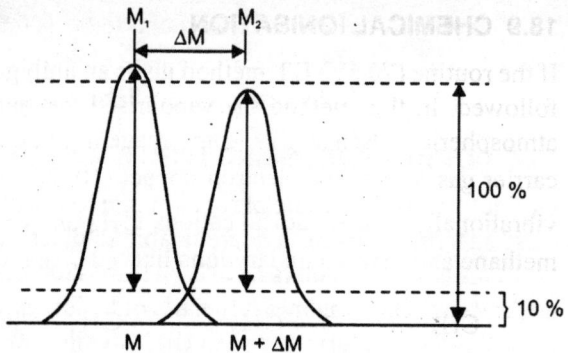

Fig. 18.4c. Valley resolution (ten percent) in a mass spectrum.

ments. Low resolution instruments separate unit masses. R typically ranges from 100 to 500000 (5 lakh). It is important to note that determining resolution, the two adjacent peaks of approximately equal intensity are chosen so that the height of the valley between these peaks is equal to nearly ten percent of the intensity of the peaks considered as shown in Fig. 18.4c.

18.7 SAMPLE IONIZATION METHODS

A number of ionisation methods are available :
1. Electron Impact (EI)
2. Chemical Ionisation (CI)
3. Field Desorption (Field Ionisation) (FD/FI)
4. Fast Atom Bombardment (FAB)
5. Electrospray Ionisation (ESI)
6. Nanospray Ionisation (NSI)
7. Matrix Assisted Laser Desorption Ionisation (MALDI)
8. Thermospray Ionisation (TSP)

18.8 ELECTRON IMPACT (EI) IONISATION

We have already become familiar with this ionisation method that operates at 70 eV. The first method, EI ionisation method is a "hard" ionisation. This is because it introduces a large amount of energy into molecules. Consequently, the molecular ion does not appear or contributes a weaker smaller peak in the m/z spectrum. So, there was a need for "soft" methods. The chemical ionisation is one such method which is next described.

Characteristics of EI technique

1. Relatively easy to obtain EI spectra.
2. Compounds that are air- and moisture-sensitive can also be analysed.
3. EI mode can be used in GC/MS systems as well as with direct inlet methods.
4. EI is a sensitive technique.
5. EI is restricted to thermally stable compounds having low molecular masses up to about 2000 Da.
6. EI is a hard technique as sometimes M^{+} peaks are not observed.

18.9 CHEMICAL IONISATION

If the routine (70 eV) E.I. method gives an ambiguous molecular ion, the chemical ionisation method is followed. In this method the vapourised test sample is introduced into the ionisation chamber near atmospheric presence with some reagent gas like methane taken in excess. The latter is also called carrier gas. Under the electron impact (10–20 eV), the gas having excess energy gets ionised to give vibrationally excited radical cations $C\overset{+\cdot}{H}_4$ and CH_3^+. These methane-derived ions react with the excess methane and give secondary ions like CH_5^+ and $C_2H_5^+$:

$$CH_4 + e \xrightarrow[\text{(i)}]{-2e} C\overset{+\cdot}{H}_4 \xrightarrow[\text{(ii)}]{H^+} \overset{+}{C}H_3 \text{ (1}^\circ \text{ ions)}$$

(iii) $C\overset{+\cdot}{H}_4 + CH_4 \rightarrow C\overset{\cdot}{H}_5 + \overset{\cdot}{C}H_3$ (2° ion)

(iv) $C\overset{+}{H}_3 + CH_4 \rightarrow C_2H_5^+ + H_2$ (2° ion)

The sample (RH) now reacts with secondary ions in acid-base type reaction (not electrons) to give (M–1) ions eventually.

(v) $RH + C\overset{+}{H}_5 \rightarrow RH_2^+ + CH_4$

RH_2^+ with mass 1 amu greater than the $M^{\ddagger}$ ion are called **quasi-molecular ions.**

(vi) $\underset{\text{(base)}}{RH} + \underset{\text{(acid)}}{C_2H_5} \rightarrow \underset{\text{(M + 1)}}{RH_2^+} + C_2H_4$

$RH_2^+ \rightarrow R^+ + H_2$

The C.I. source along with EI source is shown in Fig. 18.5. The reagent gases and ions are shown in Table 18.2.

Note: The students can avoid showing reactions (i), (ii), (iii) and (v) and can only write reaction (vi) or (v) to convey the point to the paper evaluator in exam. This will suffice for the sake of examination.

Example 1 : Proline : Like we noted in the beginning, in case molecular ion peak is not observed In E.I., CI method is of help. This

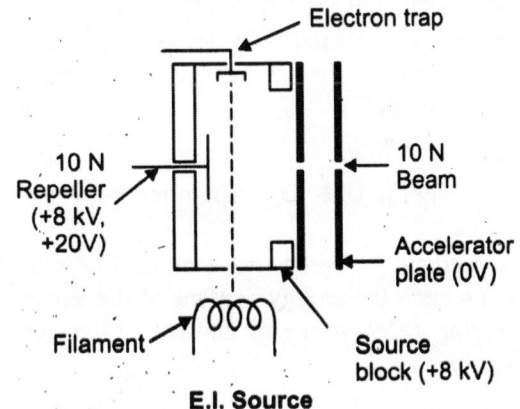

E.I. Source

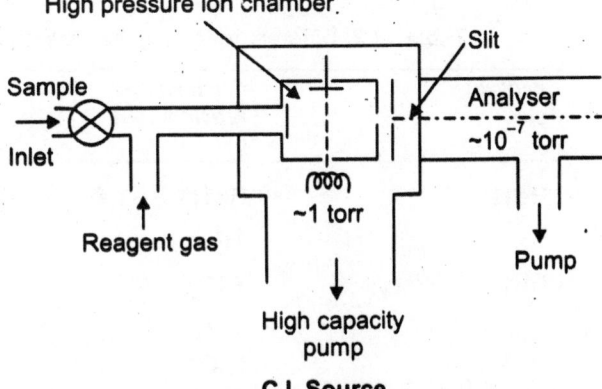

C.I. Source

Fig. 18.5. The C.I. source.

is proven by the example of proline where the $M^{\ddagger}$ peak that should have been observed at m/e 115 is missing in EI based m/z spectrum but can be noticed (as a base peak rather!) in the CI based m/z spectrum in Fig. 18.5.

Example 2 : *n*-Butyl propionate : This is shown in Fig. 18.7. It is clear from Fig. 7 and Fig. 8 that the **fragmentation pattern is reduced under *CI* significantly compared to that under *EI*.** However, the two are complementary.

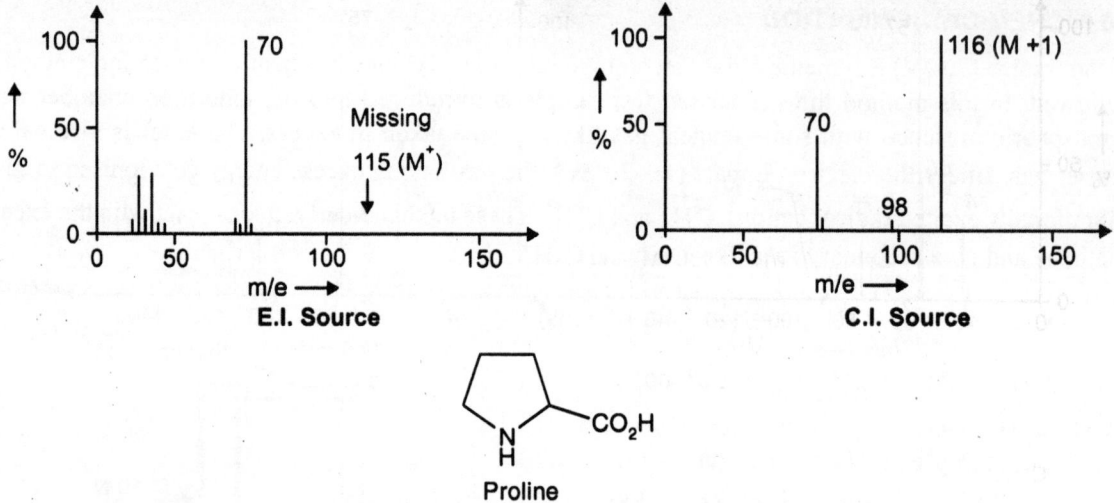

Proline

Fig. 18.6. The difference between EI (70 eV) and C.I. (10–20 eV) methods.

It needs to be noted that a number of reagent gases shown in Table 18.2 are used. The choice depends upon the energy content of the secondary ions derived from these gases. For example, the decreasing order of energy content of the derived secondary ions in cases of CH_4, isoobutane and ammonia is :

$$CH_5^+ > C_4H_9^+ > NH_4^+$$

Table 18.2. Different reagent gases with their characteristics for chemical ionization

Reagent gas	Predominant reactant ions	Proton[a] affinity (kcal/mole)	Hydride affinity (kcal/mole)
He/H	He/H$^+$	42	–
H$_2$	H$_3^+$	101	299
CH$_4$	CH$_5^+$	127	272
	C$_2$H$_5^+$	159	272
H$_2$O	H$_3$O$^+$	164	–
CH$_3$CH$_2$CH$_3$	C$_3$H$_7^+$	182	249
(CH$_3$)$_3$CH (isobutane)	C$_4$H$_9^+$	195	232
NH$_3$	NH$_4^+$, (NH$_3$)$_2$H$^+$, (NH$_3$)$_3$H$^+$	207	–
(CH$_3$)$_2$NH	(CH$_3$)$_2$NH$_2^+$, [(CH$_3$)$_2$NH]$_2$H$^+$, C$_3$H$_8$N$^+$	222	–
(CH$_3$)$_3$N	(CH$_3$)$_3$NH$^+$	226	–

[a] Increasing magnitude of proton affinity implies decreasing strength of a Bronsted acid and consequently decreasing effectiveness in effecting fragmentation.

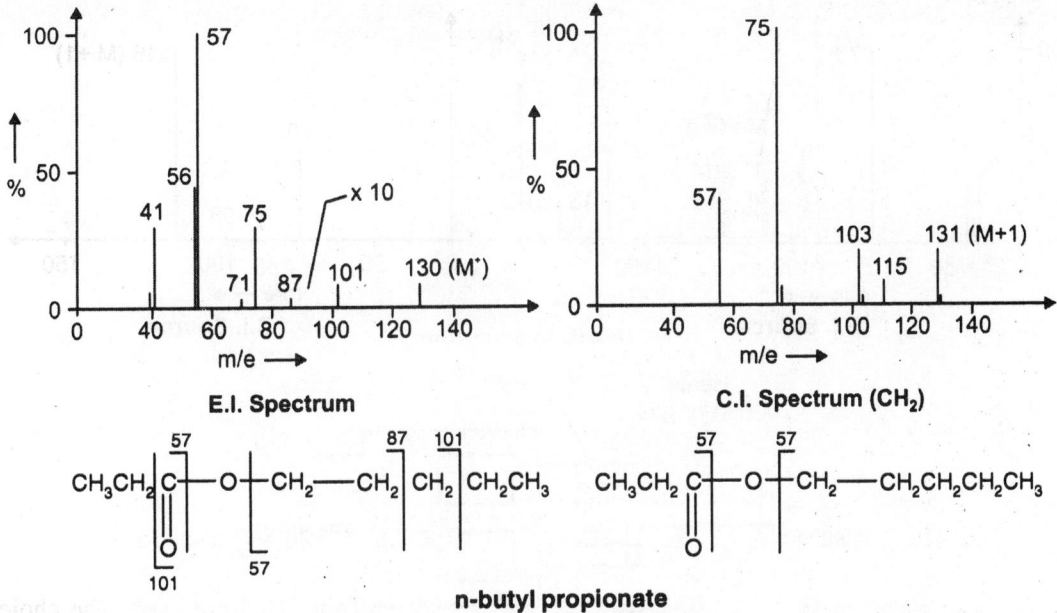

Fig. 18.7. Differences in fragmentation patterns under EI (70 eV) and CI (10–20 eV) methods.

18.10 FIELD DESORPTION

Those compounds that are either involatile or thermally unstable can not be analysed by the electron impact or the chemical ionisation techniques. For such compounds another technique called Field Desorption (FD) or Desorption Ionisation (DI) is used. In this technique the sample is placed on the anode of a pair of electrodes. An intense electric field is passed between the pair of electrodes. The sample that was absorbed now gets desorbed and both molecular ions are generated. [M + H]$^+$ i.e. M + 1 is the prominent ion peak in the spectrum. The FI source is shown in Fig. 18.8a.

Thus, while EI method fails to give a peak at m/e 284 for molecular ion of Xanthosine, the FD (FI) ionisation technique does give the M‡ peak at m/e 284 (see Fig. 18.8b).

This technique works well for polymers upto 1000 Da but is unsuccessful with polymers having molecular mass less than 10,000 Da. For such molecules the FAB technique is a popular one.

18.11 FAST ATOM BOMBARDMENT (FAB)

This is used for larger polar molecules like peptides having molecular weights less than 10,000 Da that are different to get into gaseous phase. Bombardment of the sample dissolved in a highly viscous matrix like glycerol is done by fast moving neutral atoms of xenon or argon:

$$Xe^{\ddagger} + Xe \rightarrow Xe + Xe^{\ddagger}$$

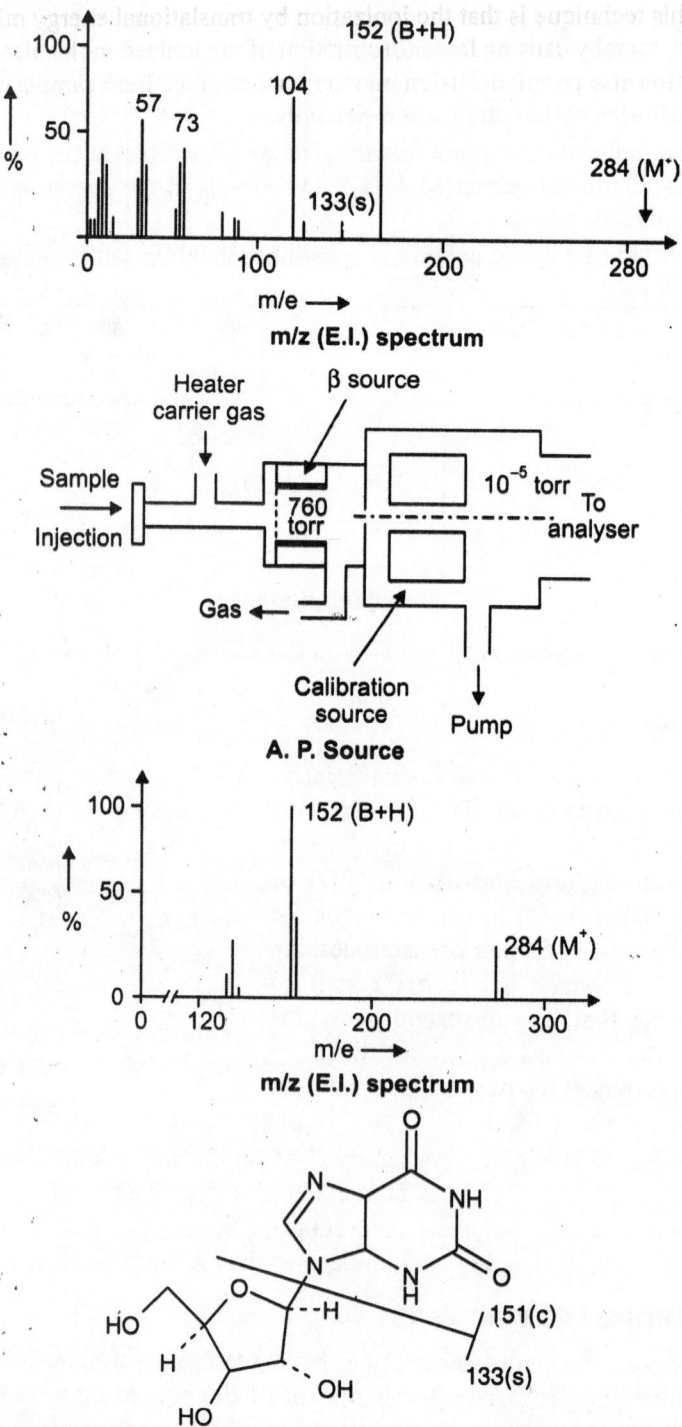

Fig. 18.8b. The FI spectrum of xanthosine FI versus EI method.

The main basis of this technique is that the ionization by translational energy minimizes the extent of vibrational excitation, thereby causing lesser destruction of the ionized molecules. Further, the polar solvents catalyse ionization also permit diffusion into the surface of the fresh sample material. **However, FAB requires 20–30 minutes rather than a few seconds.**

In FAB, RH_2^+ (quasi-molecular ions) are intense. The drawback is that the matrix (glycerol) also forms ions and so gives additional peaks $(M + H]^+$, $[M + Na]^+$ in the spectrum. Nevertheless, the fragment ions give conspicuous peaks.

Example: FAB spectrum of a cyclic peptide, a quasi-phosphonium salt is shown in Fig. 18.9.

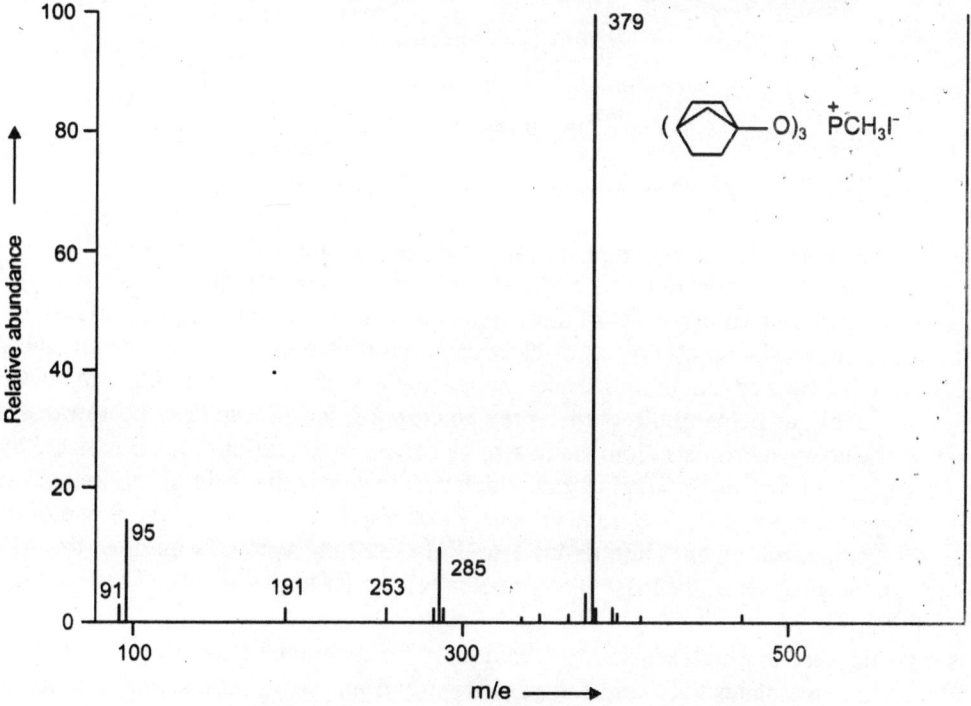

Fig. 18.9. FAB-MS of a quasiphosphonium salt.

18.12 ELECTROSPRAY IONISATION (ESI)

Electrospray Ionisation (ESI) is an **Atmospheric Pressure Ionisation (API)** technique well-suited to the analysis of polar molecules, 100 DA – 1,000,000 DA like water soluble biomolecules such as peptides, carbohydrates etc. ESI yields a mass spectrum in which the prominent peaks arising from molecular ions having a different number of attached charges. Thus, a molecular ion having molecular mass of 12,000 Da and charge 10 would be equivalent to a molecular ion having molecular mass ten times less (12000 ÷ 10) i.e. 1200 Da. That means a mass spectrometer with a modest resolution can be used. ESI ionization source is shown in Fig. 18.10.

The sample is dissolved in a polar, volatile solvent. It is pumped through a narrow stainless steel capillary (75–100 micrometers i.d.) at a high flow rate of 1 mL/min to 1 mL/min. A high voltage of 3 or 4 kV is applied to the tip of the capillary, situated within the ionisation source of mass spectrometer.

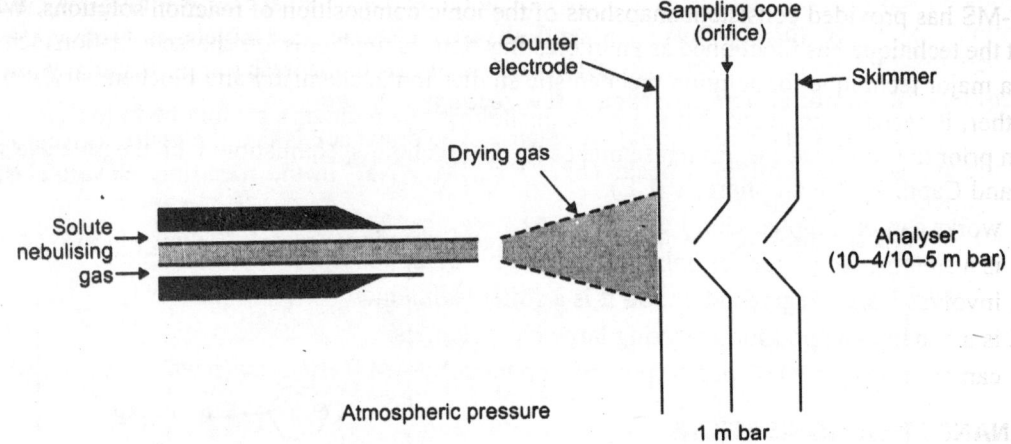

Fig. 18.10 The standard electrospray ionisation source.

Consequently, the sample emerging from the tip is dispersed into a fine aerosol of highly charged droplets. The droplets formed get reduced in size due to evaporation until they reach the Rayleigh limit (that occurs when surface charge density of the droplet becomes equal to the liquid surface tension). At this point the droplet breaks up as a result of electrostatic forces, thereby producing smaller droplets. This process is aided by a co-axially introduced nebulising gas (nitrogen), flowing around the outside of the capillary. This gas helps to direct the spray emerging from the capillary tip towards the mass spectrometer. The charged droplets diminish in size by solvent evaporation. This is assisted by a warm flow of nitrogen gas known as the **drying gas** which passes across the front of the ionisation source. Eventually charged **sample ions**, free from solvent get released from the droplets. Some of these pass through an orifice (**sampling cone**) into an **intermediate vacuum** region. From there through a small aperture they go the analyser of the mass spectrometer held under **high vacuum**. The process is shown in Fig. 18.11.

ESI is a gentle, fast and high sensitivity technique. This technique may allow even short-lived or loosely bounded intermediates to be transferred efficiently from the reaction solution to the gas phase. In fact, it has proven to be a very important method for the analysis of biological molecules in that they can be extracted from solution, ionized and transferred to the gas phase for mass spectral analysis.

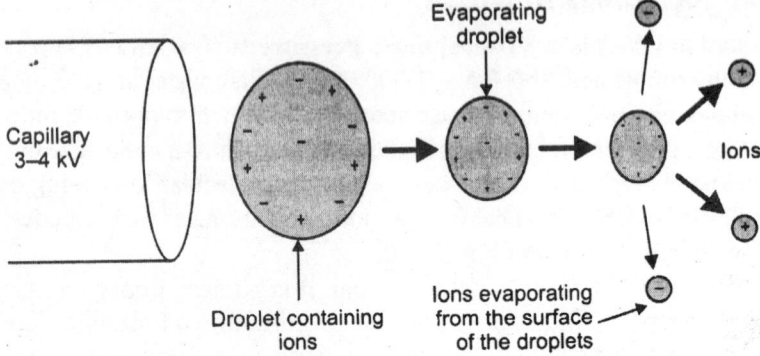

Fig. 18.11. ESI, the electrospray ionisation process.

ESI-MS has provided consistent snapshots of the ionic composition of reaction solutions. We can say that the technique has functioned as an interesting "ion-fishing" plus ion characterization technique and as a major technique for solution mechanistic studies in the chemistry and biochemistry.

Further, it needs to be noted that the prerequisite that a peptide or a protein be in ionized state in solution prior to transfer to the gas phase makes the ESI technique compatible with the reversed-phase HPLC and Capillary Electrophoresis (CE).

ESI works can be coupled with LC/MS.

ESI is a suitable technique for polar and even ionic compounds like metal complex.

ESI involves lesser fragmentation. So it is a softer technique.

ESI is a suitable method for analyzing large bio-polymers.

ESI can generate $[M + H]^+$ peaks (positive ion mode) or $[M - H]^+$ peak (negative ion mode).

18.13 NANOSPRAY IONISATION

This is a low flow rate version of electrospray ionisation. A small volume (1–4 microL) of the sample dissolved in a suitable volatile solvent (at a concentration of ca. 1–10 pmol/microL) is transferred into a miniature sample vial. A high voltage of (ca. 700–2000 V) is applied to the specially manufactured gold-plated vial. This results in sample ionisation and spraying. The flow rate of source and solvent is very low (30–1000 nL/min). Hence far less sample is consumed than with the standard electrospray ionisation technique. Further a small volume of sample lasts for several minutes. This enables multiple experiments to be performed. A common application : protein digest mixture is analysed to generate a list of molecular masses for the components present. Then each component is further analysed by tandem mass spectrometric (MS-MS) amino acid sequencing techniques.

In positive ionisation mode, a trace of formic acid is often added to aid protonation of the sample molecules. Proteins and peptides are usually analysed under positive ionisation conditions. In negative ionisation mode a trace of ammonia solution or a volatile amine is added to aid deprotonation of the sample molecules. Saccharides and oligonucleotides are analysed under negative ionisation conditions.

In ESI technique, samples (M) with molecular masses up to ca. 1200 Da give rise to singly charged ions usually protonated molecular-related ions, $(M + H^+)$ in positive ionisation mode, and deprotonated molecular ions $(M - H)^-$ in negative ionisation mode.

Example: The m/z spectrum of the pentapeptide leucine enkephalin, YGGFI whose molecular formula is $C_{28}H_{37}N_5O_7$ and the calculated monoisotropic molecular weight through ESI procedure is 555.2692 Da.. The mass spectrum is shown in Fig. 18.12a. As can be seen, the m/z spectrum shows dominant ions at m/z 556.1. These are consistent with the expected protonated molecular ions, $(M + H^+)$. These molecular ions are expected as the sample was analysed under positive ionisation conditions. As m/z ions are singly charged, so the m/z value is consistent with the molecular mass, because the value of z (number of charges) equals 1. So, the measured molecular weight comes to 555.1 Da which is close to the calculated mass.

Other ions with lower intensity (ca. 25% of the m/e 556.1 ions) at m/e 557.2 are also seen. These peaks represent the molecule in which one ^{12}C atom has been replaced by a ^{13}C atom because carbon has a naturally occurring isotope one atomic mass unit (Da) higher. Further, the intensity of these isotopic ions relates to the relative abundance of the naturally occurring isotope multiplied by the total number of carbon atoms in the molecule. Furthermore, the fact that the ^{13}C ions are one Da higher on the m/e scale compared to the ^{12}C ions means that z = 1. So, the sample ions are singly charged. In case

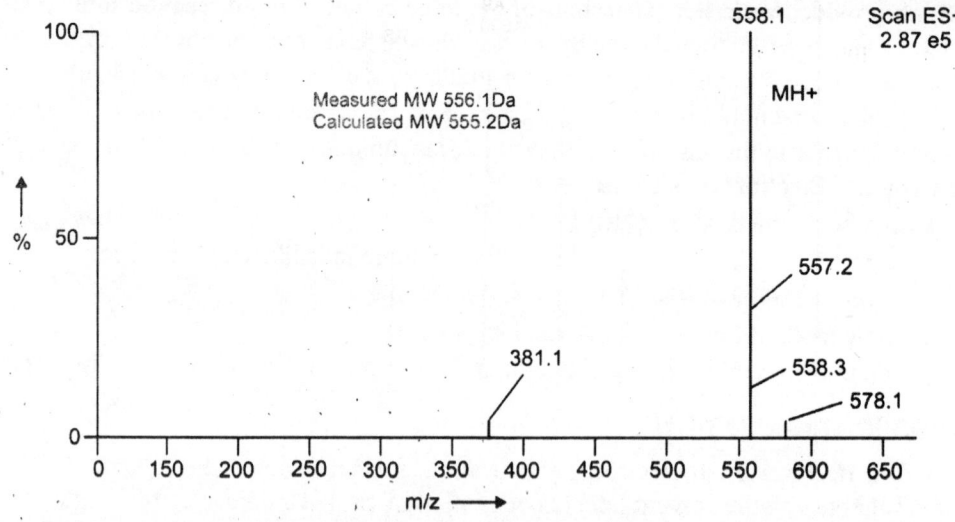

Fig. 18.12a. Mass spectrum (positive ESI-MS) of leucine enkaphalin, YGGFL.

the sample ions were doubly charged, then the m/e values would differ by just 0.5 Da as the number of charges were two.

Further, the mass spectrum peaks at m/z 578.1, some 23 Da higher than the expected molecular mass which means these are the sodium adduct ions $(M + Na)^+$. Such adduct ions are quite common in electrospray ionisation.

Unlike E-1 method, ESI is a "soft" ionisation method as the sample is ionised by the addition or removal of a proton so that very little extra energy remains behind to cause fragmentation of the formed sample ions.

Further, samples with molecular weights higher than ca. 1200 Da form multiply charged molecular-related ions $(M + nH)^{n+}$ in positive ionisation mode and $(M − nH)^{n−}$ in negative ionisation mode. Proteins have many suitable sites for protonation. In fact, all of the backbone amide nitrogen atoms could be protonated theoretically speaking..

Example : Mass spectrum (positive ionisation) of protein hen egg white lysozyme shown in Fig. 18.12b.

As can be seen, the mass spectrum shows a Gaussian-type distribution of multiply charged ions ranging from m/z 1101.5 to 2044.6. In fact, each peak represents the intact protein molecule carrying a different number of charges – protons. The individual peaks in the multiply charged series become closer together at lower m/z values. As the molecular weight is the same for all of the peaks, peaks with more charges appear at lower m/z values compared to those with fewer charges.

The m/z values in these cases are equal to:

$$m/z = (MW + nH^+)/n$$

wherein

m/z = the mass-to-charge ratio marked on the abscissa of the spectrum;

n = the integer number of charges on the ions;

H = the mass of a proton equal to 1.008 Da.

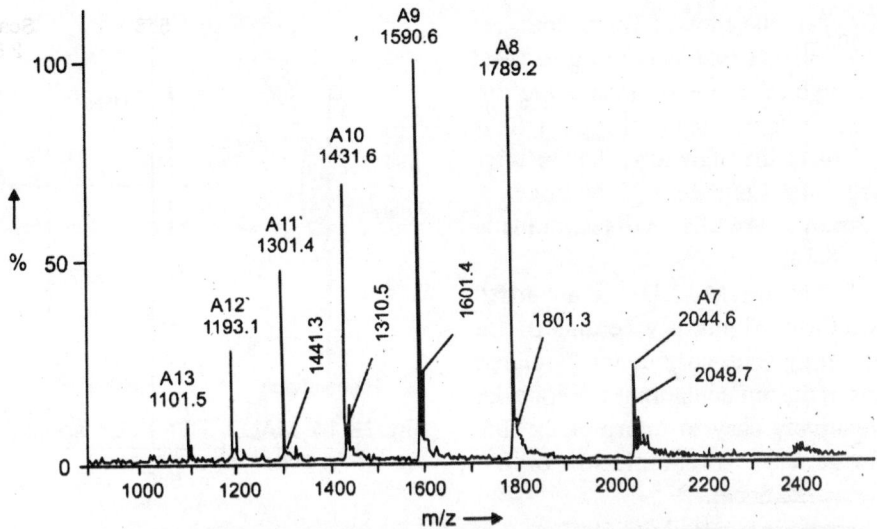

Fig. 18.12b. Positive ESI-MS spectrum of the protein hen egg white lysozyme.

18.14 MATRIX ASSISTED LASER DESORPTION IONISATION (MALDI)

MALDI is used for thermolabile, non-volatile organic compounds which have high molecular mass and is very successful for the analysis of proteins, peptides, glycoproteins, oligosaccharides and oligonucleotides and ionic metal complexes. Modern instruments are capable of measuring masses to within 0.01% of the molecular mass of the sample of at least upto ca. 40,000 Da. Nicotinic acid and sinnapinic acid are used as a matrix.

Basis: MALDI is based on the bombardment of sample molecules commonly with a laser, a pulsed nitrogen laser of wavelength 337 nm light which causes sample ionisation. The sample has to be pre-mixed with a highly absorbing matrix compound for the most consistent and reliable results. Only a low concentration of sample to matrix works best. The matrix transforms the laser energy into excitation energy for the sample. This leads to sputtering of analyte and matrix ions from the surface of the mixture such that energy transfer is efficient. Also the analyte molecules are spared excessive direct energy that may otherwise cause decomposition. The MALDI technique can be represented by the Fig 18.13.

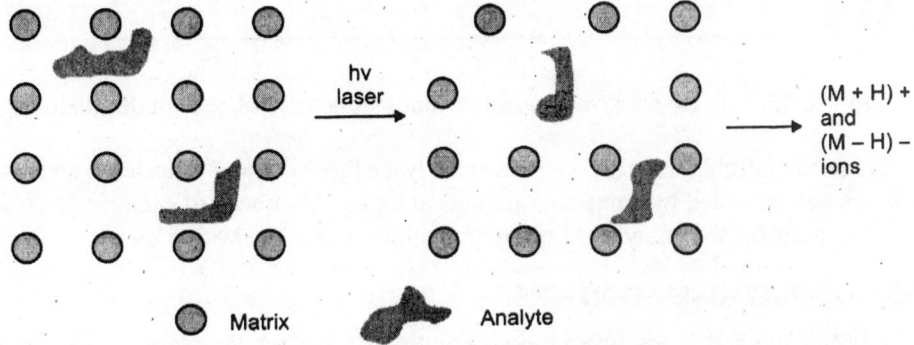

Fig. 18.13. A schematic matrix assisted laser desorption ionisation (MALDI).

In MALDI, it is the time-of-flight analyser that is used to separate ions according to their mass (m)-to-charge (z) ratios by measuring the time it takes for ions to travel through a field free region known as the flight tube. The heavier ions are more slow than the lighter ones. A schematic diagram of MALDI-TOF technique is shown in Fig. 18.14.

Unlike EI method MALDI is a "soft" ionisation method. It mainly leads to the generation of singly charged molecular-related ions regardless of the molecular mass. Hence the spectra are relatively easy to interpret. In this technique, in general, fragmentation of the sample ions does not occur.

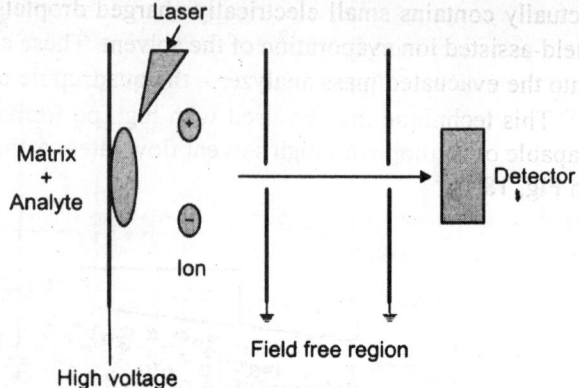

Fig. 18.14. MALDI-TOF mass spectrometry (linear mode) (a schematic diagram).

The protonated molecular ions $(M + H^+)$ are usually the dominant species in positive ionisation mode. These can be accompanied by salt adducts, a trace of the doubly charged molecular ion at about half the m/z value, and/or a trace of a dimeric species at about twice the m/z value. Positive ionisation is used in general for protein and peptide analyses. A positive ionisation MALDI spectrum of a peptide mixture using alpha-cyano–4–hydroxycinnamic acid as matrix is shown in Fig. 18.15.

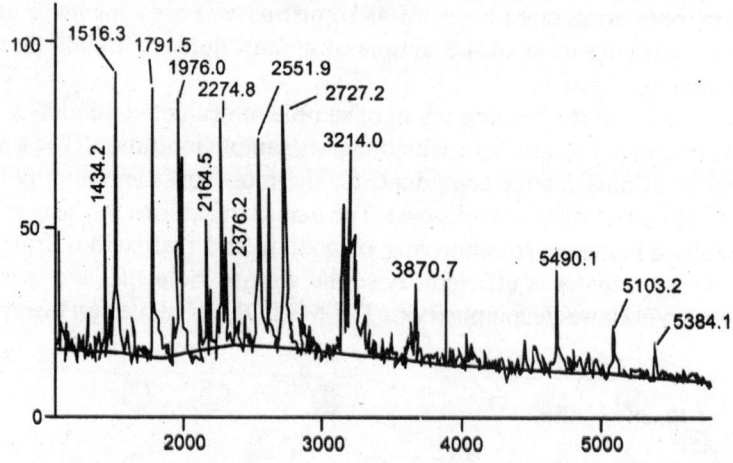

Fig. 18.15. MALDI positive ionisation mass spectrum of a peptide mixture.

The deprotonated molecular ions $(M – H)^-$ are usually the most abundant species in negative ionisation mode. These are accompanied by some salt adducts and possibly traces of dimeric or doubly charged materials. This is used for the analysis of oligonucleotides and oligosaccharides.

18.15 THERMOSPRAY IONISATION (TPSI)

What is done in this method is that the aqueous solution of the test sample is conducted through hot capillary into the ion source. A very fine spray i.e. a supersonic jet of vapour is produced. This spray actually contains small electrically charged droplets. The formed small droplets are next ionized by field-assisted ion evaporation of the solvent. These are now allowed to enter via s small orifice straight into the evacuated mass analyzer – the quadrupole or magnetic sector mass analyzer.

This technique may be used with high performance liquid chromatography (HPLC) because it is capable of dealing with high solvent flow rates. A thermospray ion source can be represented as shown in Fig. 18.16.

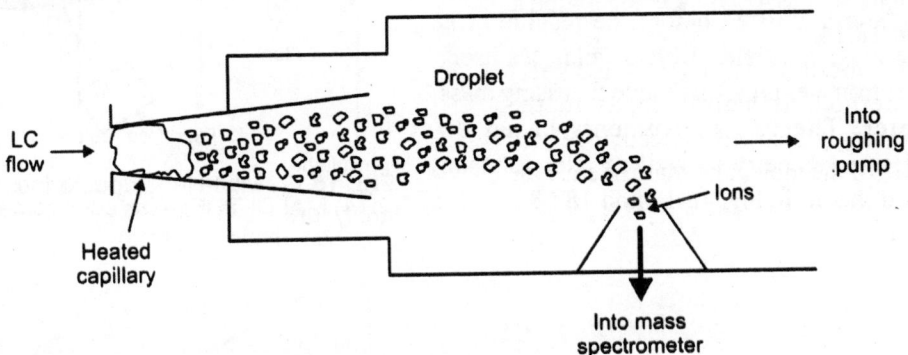

Fig. 18.16. A schematic thermospray.

18.16 TYPES OF MASS ANALYZERS

These are mainly of the following types :

1. Magnetic Sector (MS)
2. Time-of-Flight (TOF)
3. Quadrupole (Q)
4. Ion Cyclotron Resonance (ICR)
5. Fourier Transfer Ion Cyclotron (FTICR)

The highlights of these systems are collected in Table 18.4.

Table 18.4. Comparative account of various ionizational methods used in mass spectrometry

Method	Nature of analytes	Sample insertion	MW	Hard/Soft
Electron Impact (EI)	Small volatile	GC or liquid/ solid probe	Upto 1000 Daltons	Hard structure information
Chemical Ionization (CI)	Small volatile	GC or liquid/ solid probe	Upto 1000 Daltons	Soft molecular ion peak $[M + H]^+$
Electrospray (ESI) Naonspray (NSI)	Peptides Proteins nonvolatile	LC or syringe	Upto 200000 Daltons	Soft ions often multiply charged
Fast Atom Bombard-ment (FAB)	Carbohydrates Peptides nonvolatile	Sample in viscous matrix	Upto 6000 Daltons	Soft (harder than ESI and MALDI)
Matrix Assisted Laser Desorption (MALDI)	Peptides, Proteins, Nucleotides	Sample in solid matrix	Upto 500000 Daltons	Soft

18.17 MAGNETIC SECTOR MASS ANALYZER

We have already learnt about this in some details. In this analyzer, the molecular ions are separated according to their mass (m) to charge (z) ratio m/z in the presence of a magnetic field when they follow a curved flight path. In order to improve the resolution, an electric field is utilized before the resolution is done by the magnetic field. As two fields are used, the mass spectrometer is called double focussing mass spectrometer. The two instruments based on Mattauch-Hertz geometry as well as Nier-Johnson geometry are shown in Fig. 18.17 and 18.18.

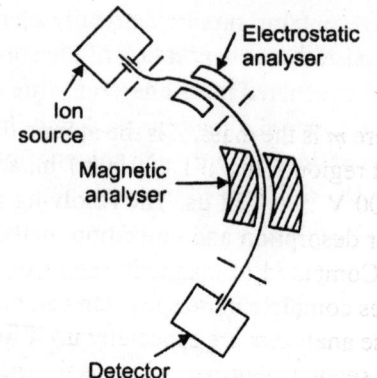

Fig. 18.17. Matt-Hertz double focussing mass analyser.

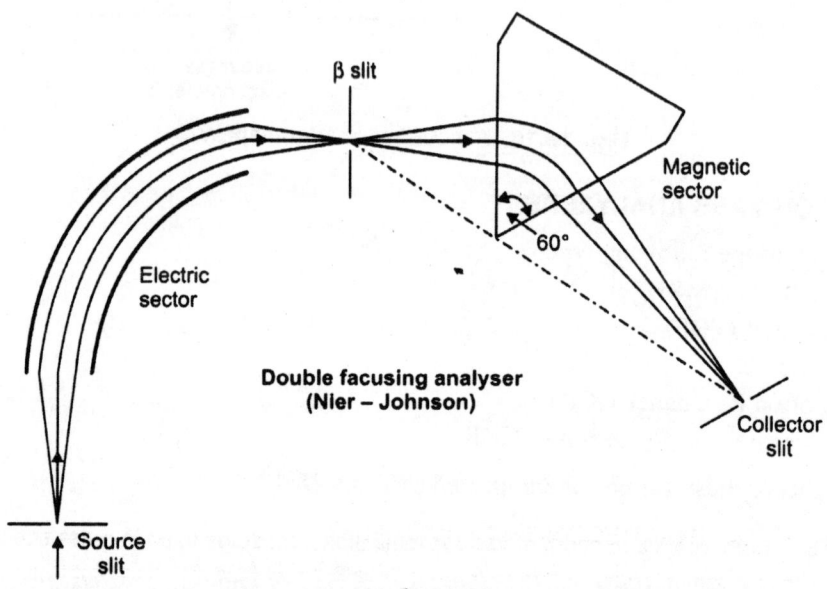

Fig. 18.18. The Nier-Johnson double focussing analyzer.

18.18 TIME-OF-FLIGHT (TOF)/MASS ANALYZER

This mass analyzer differs from the magnetic sector analyzer in that it does not use any magnetic sector (field) for resolving ions.

The TOF analyzers resolve ions having different masses on the basis of their velocities after accelerating them through a potential (V). As different ions have different velocities (V_1, V_2, V_3 etc.) due to different masses (the lighter ones move fast while the heavier ones move slowly) so they arrive at the detector at different time (t_1, t_2, t_3 etc.) intervals. Of course, the time intervals are very short, of the order of tens of μs. Hence, the m/z spectrum has to be displayed on a cathode ray tube.

The time of interval is given as :

$$t = \left(\frac{m}{2\,ZeV}\right)^{1/2} L_{TOF}$$

where m is the mass, Z is the atomic number, e is the electronic charge and L is equal to the length of the drift region. Thus if L_{TOF} is 0.1 m, $z = e = 1.602 \times 10^{-19}$ C, m = 10 kDa = 10 kg/6.0221 $\times$ 10^{23} and V = 100 V $\therefore$ $t = 72$ μs. The resolving power of modern TOF mass analyzer is of the order of 10^4 when laser desorption and ionization methods are used.

Compared to magnetic sector or quadrupole instruments, TOF analyzers have very fast response times complete mass spectrum can be repeated 2000 times in just a second! This has the advantage that these analyzers are especially used for investigations of fast reactions. Separations are of the order of a few seconds. Further, whereas the magnetic sector or quadrupole analyzers can detect only a fraction of the ions generated at any particular point in time, the TOF analyzers can detect all the generated ions simultaneously to give what is called "multi-channel" advantage. A TOF analyzer is shown in Fig. 18.19 and a TOF mass spectrometers are shown in Fig. 18.20 and 18.21.

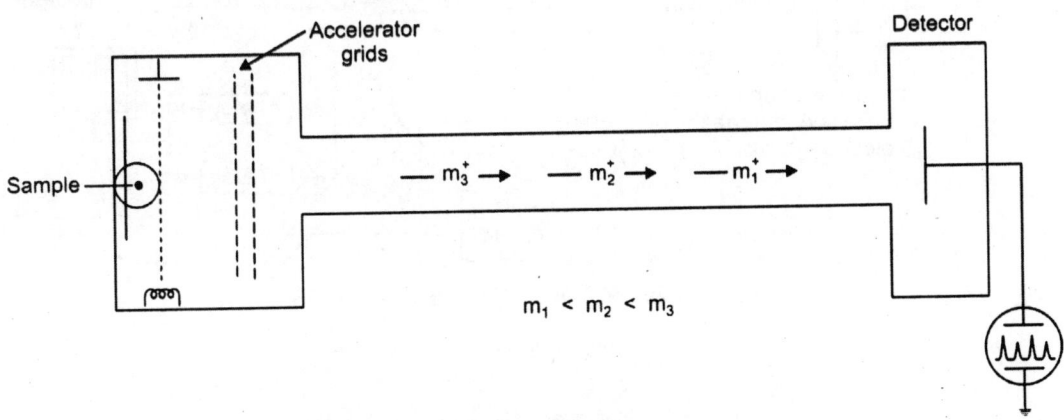

Fig. 18.19. A schematic time-of-flight analyzer.

18.19 ION-CYCLOTRON RESONANCE (ICR) ANALYZER

In this analyzer, the ions formed in an open ion source are subjected to the crossed electric and magnetic fields and are allowed to travel with the same drift velocity to the ion collector via a cycloidal path. The analyzer is only a few cm long, yet the time taken by an ion to traverse the analyzer is 5–10 milliseconds. Even though all ions have the same drift velocity, their individual cyclotron frequencies are proportional to their m/z values. In other words, the cyclotron frequency is a function of m/z value of the ion. So, when the frequency of the applied radio frequency becomes equal to the cyclotron frequency of the ion, resonance occurs, this frequency is measured. This reflects the m/z value of the ion. Or the total ion current generated can be measured to reflect m/e value.

The advantage of this method is that as the flight times in cyclotron spectroscopy are long, the probabilities of ion-molecule collisions are high. Consequently ion-molecule reactions can be investigated. Considerable information can thus be obtained about the ion-structures. Further via double resonance spectroscopy technique i.e. by irradiating one ion at its own cyclotron frequency, it is possible to observe the effect on the abundance of the another ion having different frequency.

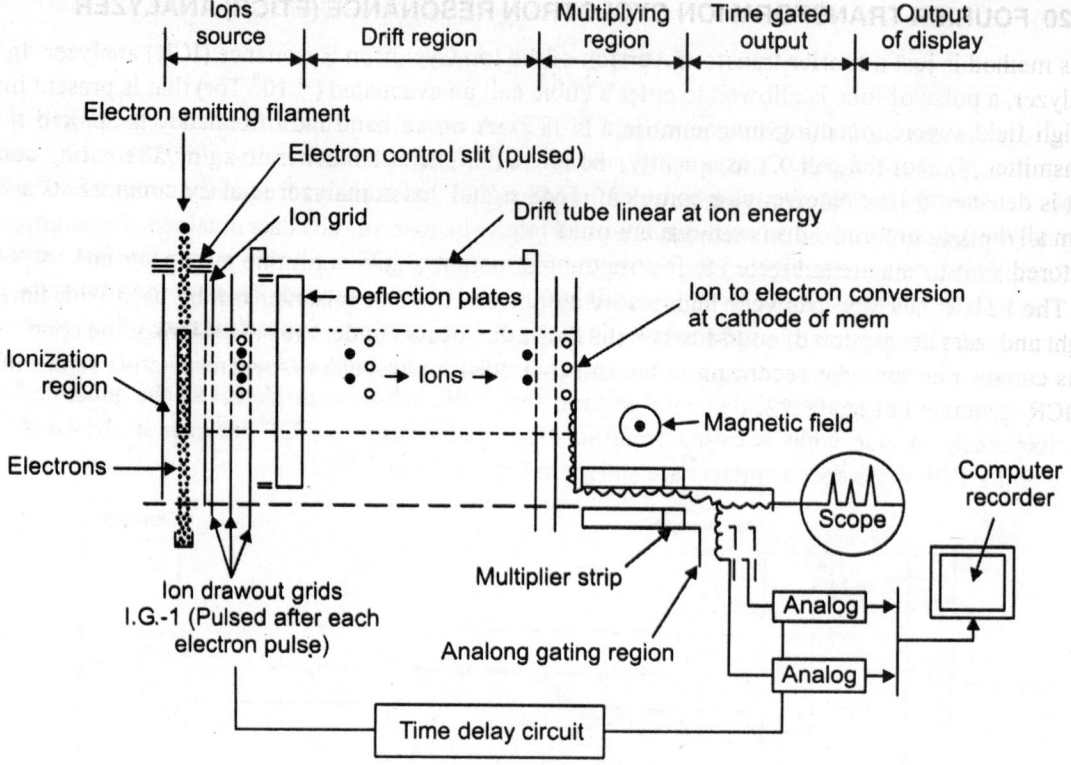

Fig. 18.20. A TOF mass spectrometer.

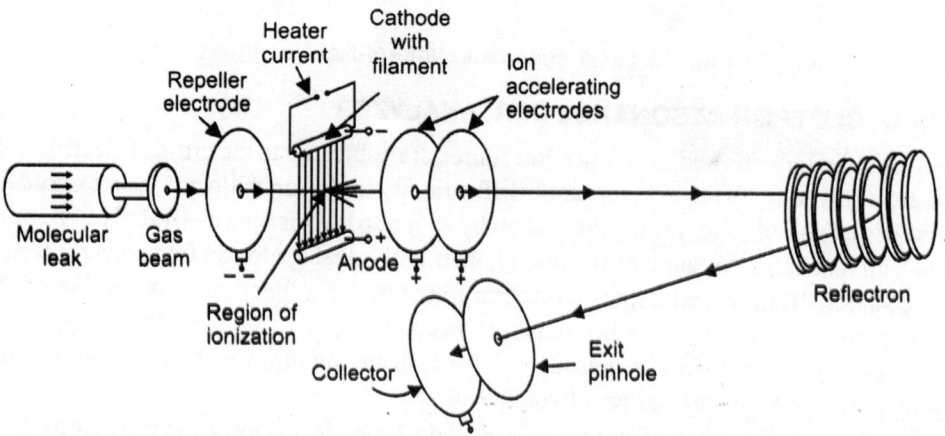

Fig. 18.21. Schematic reflection time-of-flight high-resolution mass spectrometer. The reflection is a series of rings or grids that act as an ion mirror. This mirror compensates for the spread in kinetic energies of the ions as they enter the drift region. The mirror thus improves the resolution of the instrument.

18.20 FOURIER TRANSFORM ION CYCLOTRON RESONANCE (FTICR) ANALYZER

This method is just a fourier transform version of the Ion Cyclotron Resonance (ICR) analyzer. In this analyzer, a pulse of ions is allowed to enter a cubic cell an evacuated ($< 10^8$ Tor) that is present inside a high field superconducting magnetic field (1–8T). A broad band radiofrequency is applied to the transmitter plate of the cell. Consequently, the ions after excitation generate a tiny alternating current that is detected by the receiver as a complex FTMS signal that contains frequency components arising from all the ions present. This is now transformed into voltage form. The data obtained after digitization is stored. Now, data are subjected to fourier transformation to give a routine m/z spectrum.

The FTICR (FTMS) has very high resolving power 10^6. This analyzer can be used with time-of-flight and laser desorption of course, when the ionization occurs under the pulsed ionization conditions. This can also be used for recording in tandem (MS/MS) mass spectra. A representative figure of the FTICR is shown in Fig. 18.22.

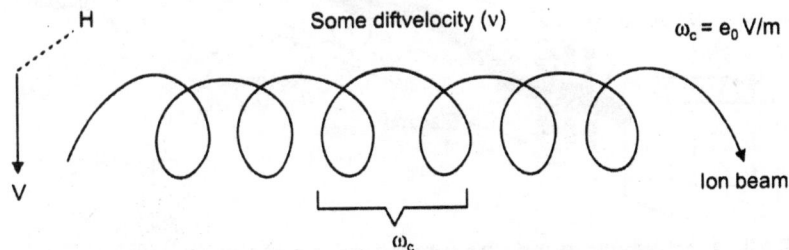

Fig. 18.22a. Ion beam path in ICR spectroscopy.

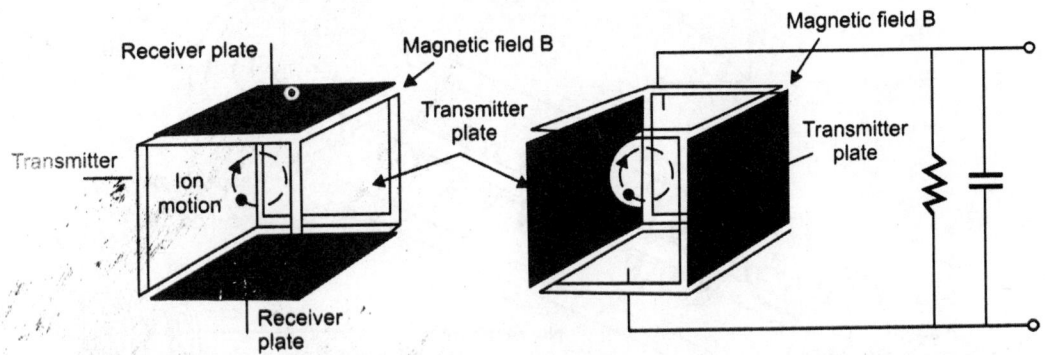

Fig. 18.22b. Block diagram of a FT ion cyclotron resonance mass spectrometer.

18.21A QUADRUPOLE ANALYZER ("MASS FILTER")

This analyzer does not use a magnetic sector. Instead, a radiofrequency quadrupole field is used, hence the name.

A quadrupole mass analyzer consists of four parallel electrodes (electric rods or poles) (separated by 6 cm) between which the ions are allowed to pass from the top parallel to the rods (2-direction). What is done in this method is that any mass is selected by arranging direct current (DC), voltage (V_{DC}) and radiofrequency fields between the electrodes such that all other ions having different masses are prevented from entering the passage i.e. they are filtered off, hence the name a mass filter. Radiofrequency used is of the order of a few hundred kilohertz. No focussing slits are required which means resolution is dependent only on the number of cycles an ion spends in the field so that the resolving power is around one part in 15000. Among other advantages the quadrupole analyzers are of small size, robust and compact and can be used with the bench-top GC/MS spectrometers. Further, they are inexpensive. A quadrupole mass analyzer is shown in Fig. 18.23 and 18.24 and a quadrupole mass spectrometer is shown in Fig. 18.25.

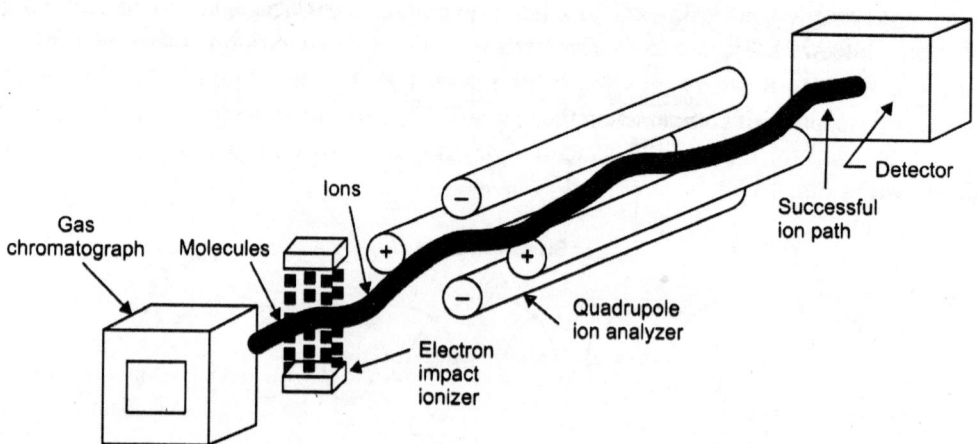

Fig. 18.23. A schematic quadrupole mass spectrometer in combination with GC.

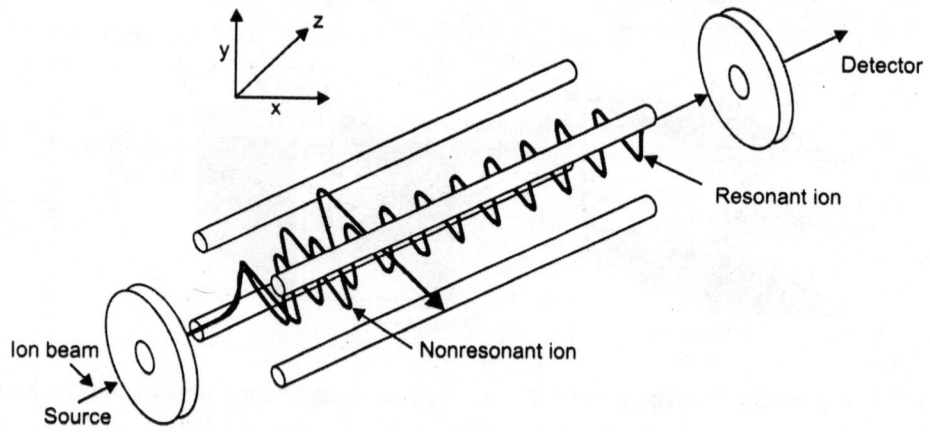

Fig. 18.24. A schematc quadrupole mass spectrometer.

18.21B ION-TRAP ANALYZER OR QUADRUPOLE ION STORAGE

An ion-trap mass analyzer is shown in Fig. 18.26. With the aid of different ratio frequency signals applied to the ring electrode and the endcaps, all ions are trapped in the cavity and sequentially ejected as per their m/z.

A high frequency octopole (Fig. 18.27) ion guide is used for injection of ions into an ion trap MS in preference to a quadrupole ion guide as it permits a higher precision of guidance.

used is of the order of a few hundred kilo... ...cusing slits are required which means resolution is dependent only on the number of turns at any ... ...es in the field and the resolving power is now ... as roughly ... of ... advantages ... small size, robust... ...expensive. ...... spectrometer is

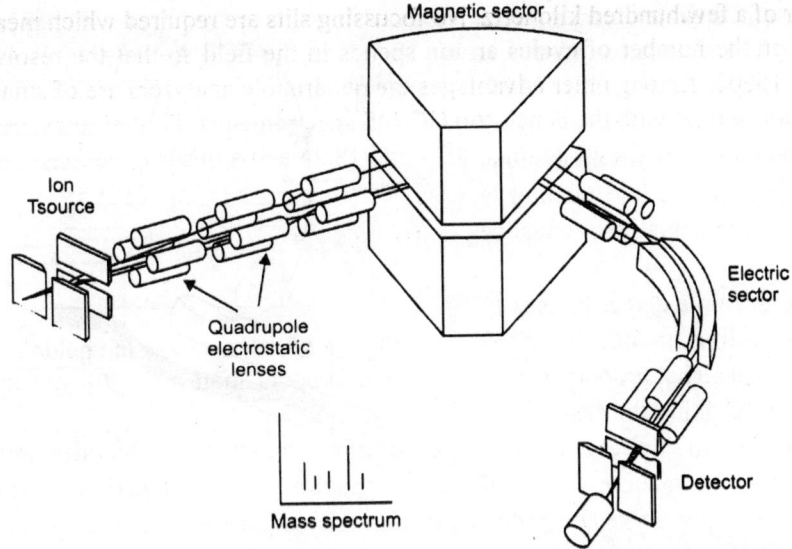

Fig. 18.25. A schematic quadrupole benchtop single-sector mass spectrometer.

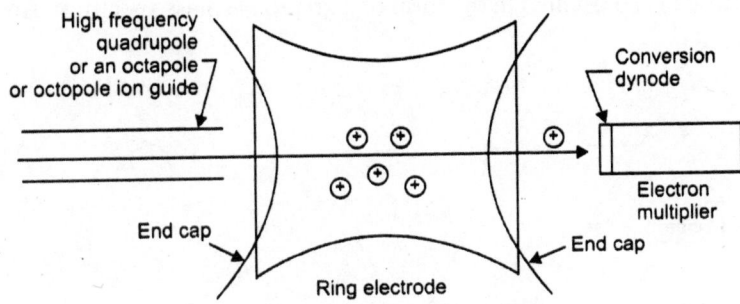

Fig. 18.26. An ion-trap analyzer.

The highlights of various types of analyzers are shown in Table 18.4.

Table 18.4. The highlights of various mass analyzers

Type	Characteristics
Quadrupole	Unit mass resolution, fast scan
Sector (magnetic and/or electrostatic)	High resolution, precise mass
Time-of-flight (TOF)	Theoretically, no limitation for m/z maximum, high throughput

18.22A ION DETECTION

Two methods can be used for the detection and recording of ions, one the photographic plates detection method (also called spectrographs) or by electric method (also called spectrometer).

In the first method, a photographic plate is kept perpendicular to the path of the ions consequently ions of successive m/z values form a linear series of images. The abundance of ions is observed by measuring the intensity of each image with a densitometer. The beauty of this detector is that it can detect all the ions almost simultaneously. But the method is less accurate in recording relative abundance ratios of ions.

The ions impinge on a detector, usually an electron multiplier in the electrical method. An electrical signal proportional to the number of ions striking the detector is

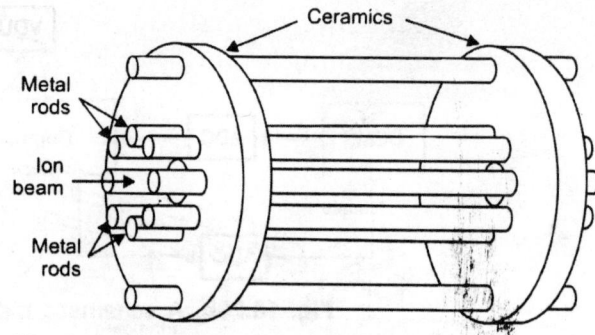

Fig. 18.27. An octopole ion guide for an ion trap MS. It is superior then a quadrupole ion guide.

generated. An electron multiplier consists of a series of electrodes called dynodes linked close to each other and enclosed in a vacuum jacket. The ions are allowed to hit the first dynode. A shower of electrons is released which strikes the second dynode which in turn releases a large shower of electrons that strike the third dynode. Such a cascading effect continues through the whole series of dynodes. As a result, the small electrical current generated when the ions hit the first dynode is generally amplified by factors of upto 10^6 and is presented in the form of a graph, the mass spectrum. An electron multiplier is shown in Fig. 18.28a.

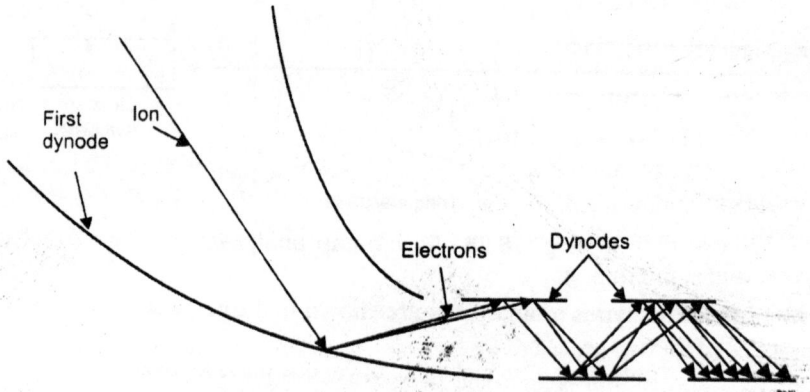

Fig. 18.28a. An electron multiplier.

18.22B DATA ACQUISITION AND PROCESSING

The electron multiplier relays the amplified signal to an on-line system, the whole system being called a Data System. It consists of a computer, an interface to the mass spectrometer, a VDU and a printer-plotter, shown in Fig. 18.28b.

Digital computers are used to acquire and process mass spectrometric data. The data system is shown in Fig. 18.28b.

The continually varying electric current or voltage output of the detection system is sampled by ADC. It produces discrete digital samples that are suitable for computer processing i.e. conversion to

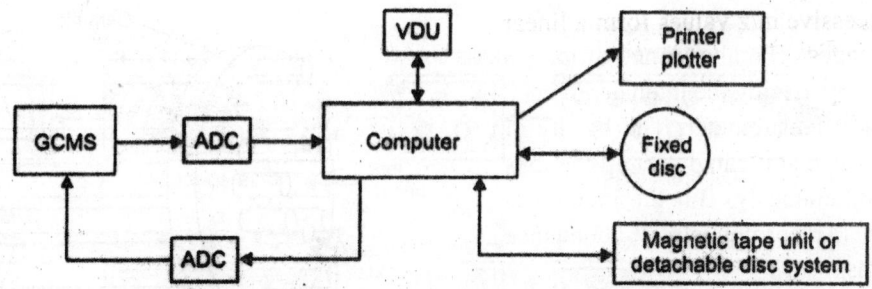

Fig. 18.28b. A schematic mass spectrometer data system.

mass and intensities. The high sampling rate is as shown in Fig. 18.29a produces well defined peak shapes. The edited output is designed on the visual display unit (VDU) during dat acquisition. Thus, the progress of a sample run can be mentioned. The output either plot of total ion current or mass chromatogram against scan number of abbreviated tabular or bar graph data.

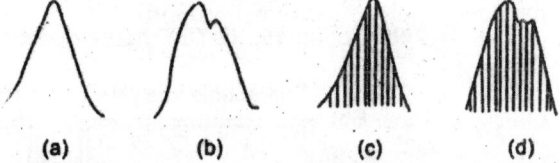

Fig. 18.29a. Peaks in analogue form a and b and in digital form c and d in a mass spectrum.

The computer is used to control the ionization methods, focussing, resolution, temperatures, the GC system and the scan speed etc.

18.23 TANDEM MASS SPECTROMETRY (MS/MS)

This technique is used for getting structural and sequence information by fragmenting specific sample ions within the mass spectrometer followed by the identification of the formed fragment ions. This technique is very effective for small organic molecules as well as for generating peptide sequence. MS/MS is of great value for monitoring of organic compounds present in a mixture that undergo fragmentation to generate common fragment ions. For example, aliphatic hydrocarbons in an oil sample, glycosylated peptides in tryptic digest mixture etc.

A tandem mass spectrometer is a mass spectrometer that has more than one analyser two, three or even four. In practice often two are used. The two analysers are separated by a collision cell into which an inert gas such as argon, xenon is admitted to collide with the selected sample ions and to assist in their fragmentation. This process is called Collision-Induced Decomposition (CID) or Collisionally-Activated Decomposition (CAD). Hence, the spectrum is also called CID or CAD mass spectrum. The analysers can be of the same or of different hybrid types. The most common combinations are:

(i) quadrupole - quadrupole

(ii) magnetic sector - quadrupole

(iii) magnetic sector - magnetic sector

(iv) quadrupole-time-of-flight (Q-TOF)

A Q-TOF mass spectrometer is shown in Fig. 18.29a and Fig. 18.29b, 18.29c, 18.29d and Fig. 18.4b.

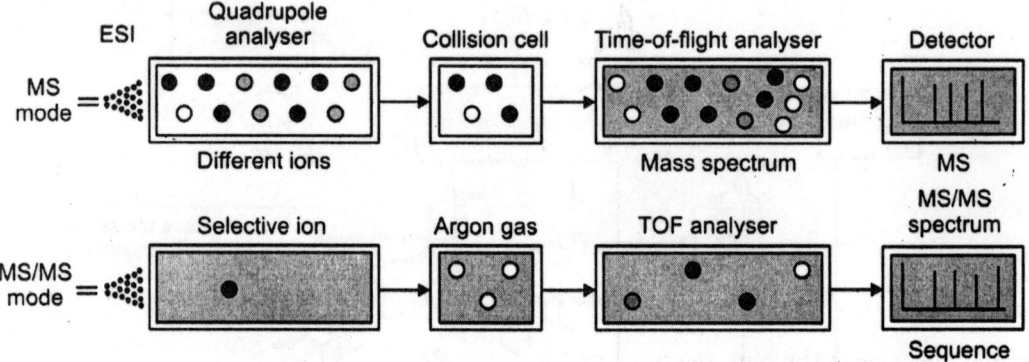

Fig. 18.29b. Schematic Q-TOF mass spectrometer in MS (upper) and MS/MS mode (lower).

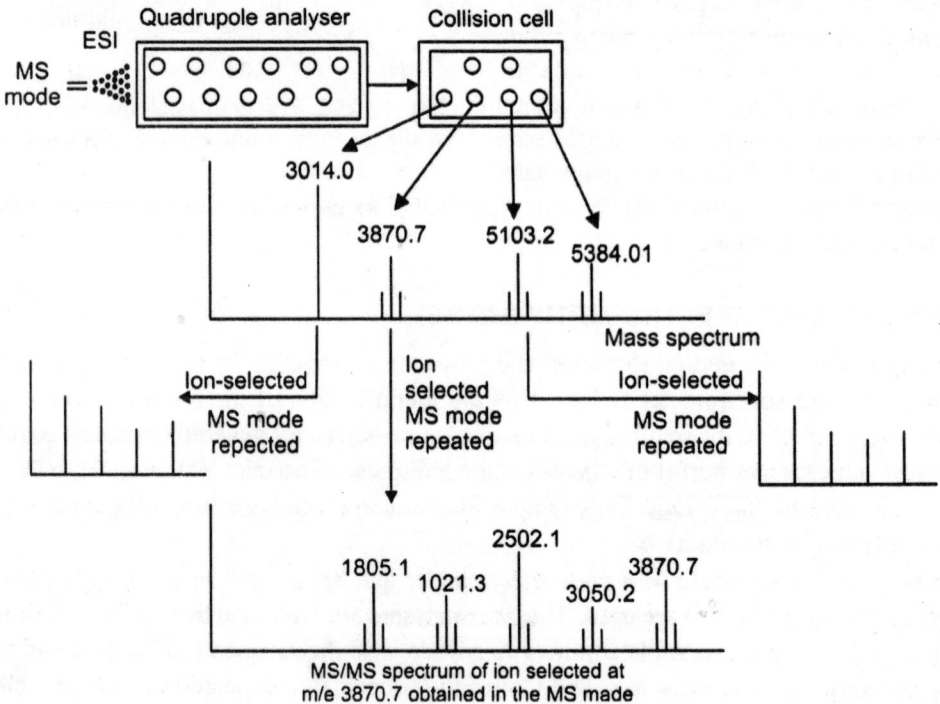

Fig. 18.29c. This fig. shows schematically how a selected ion contributing to peak at 3870.7 is again subjected to another MS operation to give the fragmentation pattern.

Role of First Analyser (Quadrupole)

It performs two functions:

(i) **Precursor or parent ion scanning:** The first analyser selects super-specified sample ions arising from a particular component. These are the molecular-related i.e. $(M + H)^+$ or $(M - H)^-$ ions. It scans the selected ions to pass into the collision cell wherein they are bombarded by the Xe or Ar gas molecules. Fragment ions are formed. These fragment ions daughter or product are separated according to their mass to charge ratios, by the second analyser.

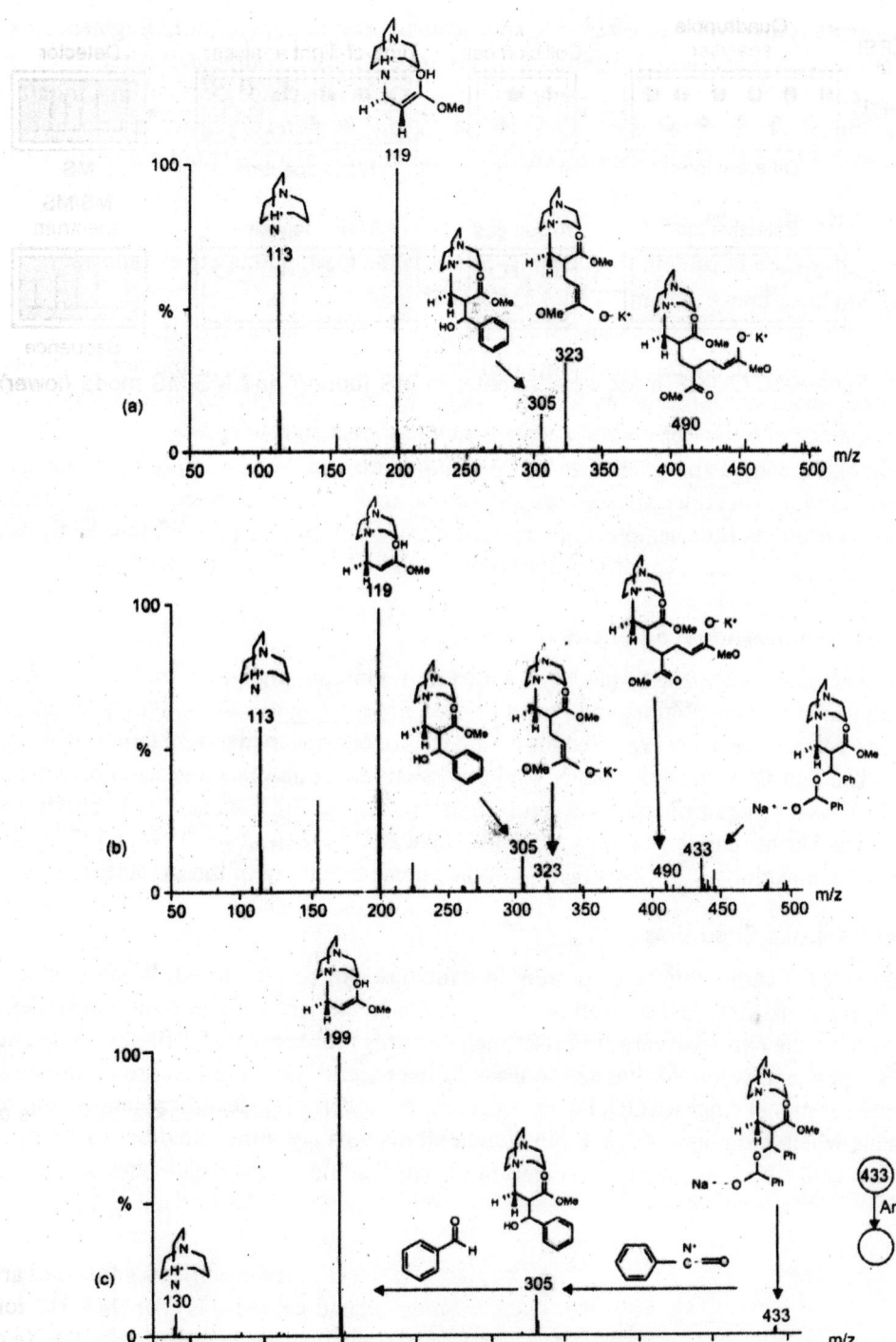

Fig. 18.29d. ESI(+)-MS of the Morita-Baylis-Hillman reaction of methyl methacrylate with benzaldehyde (a and b); ESI-MS (IMS) of the ion with m/z 433(c).

(ii) **Product or daughter ion scanning:** The second analyser monitors specific fragment ions. This type of experiment is particularly useful for monitoring groups of compounds present in a mixture which fragment to produce common fragment ions, e.g. glycosylated peptides in a tryptic digest mixture, aliphatic hydrocarbons in an oil sample, or glucuronide conjugates in urine. The information obtained is pieced together to generate structural information about the whole molecule.

Advantages of MS/MS Technique

MS/MS is commonly used in protein frequencing. Some of the main points are as follows:
- Peptides fragment along the amino acid backbone.
- Peptides with molecular mass about 2500 Da or less produce the most useful data.
- The amount of sequence information obtained varies from one peptide to another. Some peptides can generate sufficient information for a full sequence to be determined. Others may generate a partial sequence of only 4 or 5 amino acids which has great significance.
- A protein digest can be analysed as an entire reaction mixture. Separation of the products is not required. Individual peptides are selected and can be analysed. MS/MS sequencing is a sensitive technique consuming little sample. Only about 4 µL of solution is required for the analysis of the digest mixture, with a concentration based on the original protein of ca. 1–10 pmol/µL.

Special use in Pharmaceutical Sciences

Tandem mass spectroscopy (MS-MS) has been called an important, analytical tool for **'needle-in-a-haystack'** analytical problems. Plather and Powell, J. Nat. Prod. 1986, 49, 475 in Photochemistry. This type of mass spectrometry has been exploited for the analysis of cocaine in plants materials, Pyrralozidine in Senecio, afloxatoxin B$_1$ in peanut butter. Similarly, steroids, antibiotics and xanthones have also been analysed. Similarly, determination of taxol, cephalomannine and baceatin in T. brevifolia bark and needle extracts has been carried out by MS/MS (Hoke et al., J. Nat. Prod. 1994, 57, 277). Further this method has been exploited for investigation of the chemotaxonomy of the cactaceae.

Constant Neutral Loss Scanning

By this method, all the carboxylic acids present in a mixture can be monitored. What is done in this special experiment is that the first as well as the second analyzer are used to scan across the whole m/z range. However, the two analyzers are offset such that only those ions that differ by a fixed number of atomic mass units equivalent to the atomic mass of the neutral fragment lost are permitted by the second analyzer for monitoring. RCOOH acids fragment by undergoing decarboxylation (loss of CO_2 neutral molecule which has mass 44 Da. Even though all the ions are transmitted by the first analyzer into the collision cell, the second analyzer selects or detects just those ions which have undergone loss of 44 Da:

1st analyzer   2nd analyzer

18.24 FRAGMENTATION PATTERNS

Why does a molecule fragment in a mass spectrometer? High-energy electrons in the ionization chamber bombard a molecule. As a result the molecule after losing an electron form an ion, the molecular ion, $M^{\ddagger}$ which is often stable enough to be detected. Some energy is transferred to the molecule by the incident electrons which puts the $M^{\ddagger}$ in an excited vibrational state. As the mass spectra are recorded under very low pressure condition, there occur very few collisions. Consequently the $M^{\ddagger}$ ion dissipates energy by disintegration into smaller fragments. Depending upon the stability of the M^{+} radica ion may undergo fragmentation. If a molecular ion can live for a period greater than 10^{-6} sec, it contributes a peak in the mass spectrum. But the molecular ions which live for a period lesser than 10^{-6} sec, undergo fragmentation and give rise to their own signals as per their m/e in the mass spectrum. All peaks other than the molecular ion peak result from fragments.

Some **important fragmentation patterns** are as follows:

1. In saturated cyclic compounds, side chains are lost at the α-carbon. Further, the peaks that arise as a result of loss of the atoms are more intense than the peak arising from the loss of one atom.

2. Cleavage occurs at the bond β to the ring when the cyclic compound possesses a double bond next to the side chain.

3. Cleavage occurs β to the double bond in alkenes.

4. Cleavage in carbonyl compounds occurs at the carbonyl group such that positive charge remains on the fragment that contains the carbonyl group.

5. Positive charge remains on the branched fragment in hydrocarbons. Further, the ease of cleavage follows the order $3° > 2° > 1°$.

Carbocation

6. Small stable neutral molecules like H_2O, HCl, HCN, CO, NO, etc. can be lost from $M^{\ddagger}$.

7. α,β-cleavage is noted to occur in case of carbonyl compounds etc. wherein the bonds between the atoms which are α and β with respect to a heteroatom or a β bond show show heterocyclic cleavage. The driving force for such a cleavage is the resonance stabilisation of the resultant cation:

8. Rearrangements can also occur. One common rearrangement is called McLafferty arrangement. The occurrence of a rearrangement can be detected on the basis that a $M^{+\cdot}$ having an even mass cleaves to yield fragment ions which have odd masses (and of course, the reverse is true as well) when a rearrangement does not occur. Thus, in case if fragments have the same parity as the parent $M^{+\cdot}$, then this indicates the strong possibility of a rearrangement having taken place. By parity, we mean both the fragments and the molecular ion will have either the even or the odd mass values.

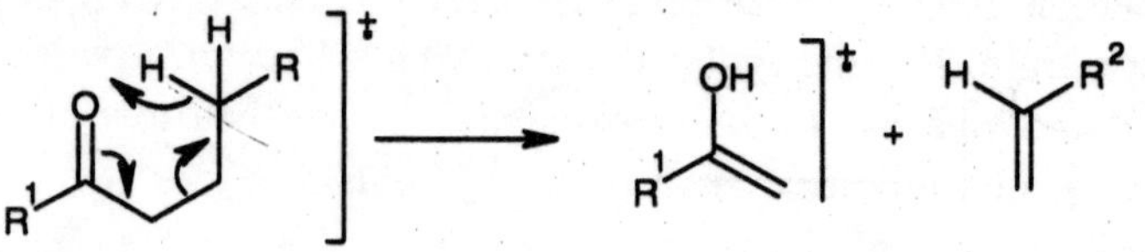

9. C—C bond cleavages: Cleavage occurs preferentially at allyl-substituted carbon.

(i) $\left[R-\overset{|}{\underset{|}{C}}-\right]^{+\cdot} \longrightarrow R^{+} + \cdot\overset{|}{\underset{|}{C}}-$

(ii) $R-\overset{|}{\underset{|}{C}}-\overset{|}{\underset{|}{C}}+ \longrightarrow R^{+} + \overset{|}{\underset{|}{C}}=\overset{|}{C}-$

Of course, the stabilities of carbocation, R^{+} rises in the following order:

$CH_3 < R_1CH_2 < R_2CH < R_3C < CH_3—CH=CH_2 <$ C_6H_5–CH_2

(iii) $\left[R-\overset{O}{\overset{\|}{C}}-R\right]^{+\cdot} \longrightarrow R^{\cdot} + R-\overset{+}{C}\equiv O$

(iv) $R-\overset{+}{C}\equiv \longrightarrow \overset{+}{R} + C=O$

10. Cleavages involving heteroatoms, X (OR^1, SR^1, N^1R_2, X). These types of such cleavages are encountered:

(i) $\left[-\overset{|}{\underset{|}{C}}-X\right]^{+\cdot} \longrightarrow -\overset{|}{\underset{|}{C}}^{\oplus} + \dot{X}$

(ii) $\left[R-\overset{|}{\underset{|}{C}}-X\right]^{+\cdot} \longrightarrow R^{\cdot} + \overset{|}{\underset{|}{C}}\overset{+}{=\!=}X$

During the cleavage, it is the heaviest substituent that is lost to general extent. For example, $CH_3\dot{C}H_2 > \dot{C}H_3$.

11. Concerted cleavages are proposed to explain away the formation of the products:

(i)

$$\xrightarrow[\text{Diels-Alder reaction}]{\text{Retro-}}$$

(ii)

(iii)

12. It also needs to be noted that whether it is the cleavage of bond(s) in an ion-radical or ion, the positive charge may go with either fragment:

$$n[AB]^+ \longrightarrow m(A^+ + B) + n - m(A + B^+)$$

Of course, the relative intensities being controlled by the relative stabilities of the ions.

Intext Exercise

1. Cyclic compounds give intense molecular ion peaks compared to their acyclic analogues. Why?

   Hint: This is because cleavage of a bond in a cyclic structure does not lead to splitting off of a fragment having lower mass.

18.25 PARAMETERS THAT AFFECT FRAGMENTATION AND GOVERNING REACTION PATHWAYS

The following parameters predominantly affect the course taken by fragmentation.

1. Thermal decomposition

Compounds that are thermolabile undergo thermal decomposition in the ion source before ionization. That causes hassles in interpretation of the m/z spectra. For example, the loss of water in alcohols may give rise to a peak at (M–18) irrespective of the loss occurring before or after ionization. Further, the thermal dehydration may entirely do away with the appearance of a molecular ion in the spectrum. Under these circumstance, the test sample should be ionized in a cooled ion source, so as to allow the electron bombardment of the entire molecule. Another solution is to convert the sample into a more volatile derivative. See the section on sample volatility (directed fragmentation).

2. Bombardment energies

At 70 eV, the molecular ions are formed. These possess a maximum of 6 eV in excess of their ionization potentials. It has been observed that if the energy is 20 eV down to the ionization potential of the molecule, then only the most favoured fragmentations occur. Thus, recording low energy spectra is a valuable tool in the study of bond energy to get progressively simple m/z spectra.

The important parameters that affect reaction pathways in mass spectrometry are as follows :

(a) Product stability

Stabilities of ions, radicals and neutral molecules, the fragmentation products is very significant. Thus, a particular ion may be abundant due to its greater stability effects on the rate of its formation as well as the rate of its subsequent decomposition pathways.

The stability of an ion is linked with its odd or even electron nature. The presence of unpaired electrons in an ionic or neutral species decreases their stability compared to species with paired electrons. This is a very important factor indeed.

Stability is dependent upon more parameters like :
- Electron sharing from a neighbouring group in alcohols etc.
- Inductive effect
- Resonance effects
- Chain branching
- Polarizability

Thus, the pathway that gives rise to the formation of the most stable product ion is generally preferred if many competing fragmentation mode are present. Further, the rate of an ion decomposition reaction is governed by its activation energy E_{act}. Furthermore, the structure of the transition state appears to resemble more the structure of the product ion relative to the structure of the decomposition ion.

(b) Active site

By an active site we mean either a localized positive charge or an unpaired electron radical. In fact, it represents the reaction centre in the molecule. In many cases both the charge and radical sites are located on the same atom in many molecules. However, these appear to be separated in decomposition of other molecules like the cyclic molecules as well as rearrangement reactions. It should be noted that the positive charge and unpaired electron display quite different reactivities. This happens due to the molecular orbital description of the ion and also on the relationship that exists between the site activity and the activation energy, E_{act}.

The skeletal rearrangements of even electron fragment ions appear to take place on electron deficient positive centres. On the other hand, hydrogen transfer rearrangement processes often take place on radical sites.

(c) Radical site induced reactions

These are most favourable for molecular and other odd-electron ions. Thus radical site induces the simply homolytic cleavage is caused by the radical site as shown for ethyl alcohol and phthalic anhydride molecules.

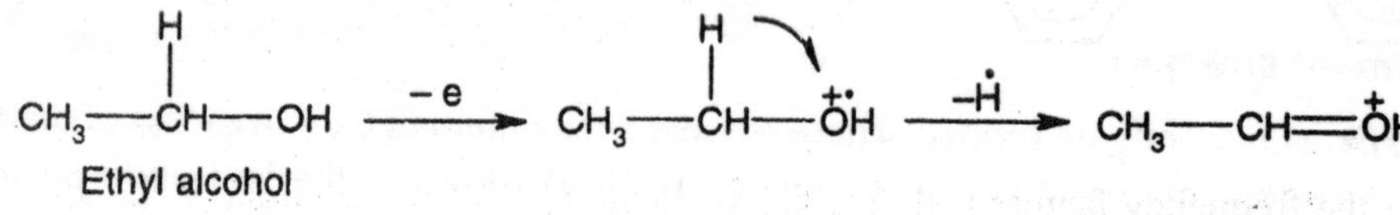

Ethyl alcohol

Phthalic anhydride

McLafferty rearrangement is also caused to occur as shown in an acidic molecular ion.

(d) Cationic sites induced reactions

Heterolytic bond cleavage as well as a rearrangement process are often caused by the cationic sites as shown in alkyl halides :

$$R - CH_2 - \overset{..}{C}l \xrightarrow{\ e\ } R - CH_2 - Cl^{+} \rightarrow R - \overset{+}{C}H_2 + \overset{.}{C}l$$

3. Structural factors

Any change in structure of a molecule naturally may bring about a change in the ionization potential of the molecule. This influences the molecular ion abundance. This also changes the pattern of the internal energy distribution in the molecule as well as the precursor ions. Electron releasing groups like $-NO_2$, $-OH$ etc. decrease the ionization potential of the parent aromatic. On the other hand, the electron withdrawing $-CN$, $-NO_2$ groups increase the ionization potential of the molecule. Furthermore, a substituent can modify the energy rate curve for a particular pathway. It can even generate a new pathway that was impossible in the original structures of the molecule.

4. Bond strengths

The bond strengths also form an important factor. Thus, the introduction of an amino group into a benzene ring, increases the electron density of the bond to be broken in substituted benzophenones that leads to the formation of $C_6H_5CO^{+}$.

5. Steric factors

These alternate the frequency factors and thus direct fragmentation modes in the molecule.

18.26 SAMPLE VOLATILITY (DIRECTED FRAGMENTATION)

Many organic compounds have to be heated in order to generate a sufficiently high vapour pressure even at 10^{-6} torr. However, there are dangers of these undergoing decomposition or rearrangement so that it is preferable to convert them into some suitable volatile derivatives to prevent these.

Examples :

1. Acids are converted into methyl esters :

$$\text{RCOOH} \xrightarrow{\text{CH}_2\text{N}_2} \text{RCOOCH}_3$$

2. Alcohols into trimethyl silyl ethers :

$$\text{ROH} \xrightarrow{\text{Me}_3\text{SiCl}} \text{R} - \text{O} - \text{SiMe}_3$$

Alcohols can get dehydrated easily, so that molecular ion is often weak.

This reaction is used for sugars and glycosides.

3. **Acetylation :** Phenols, amines are converted into volatile derivatives under mild conditions, often trifluoroacetylation is preferred.

4. **Reduction :** Amides and acids are reduced entirely to more volatile amines and alcohols respectively.

5. Ketone into ketals :

6. Location of double bonds :

This reaction fixes the double bond in alkenes as there occurs migration of the double bond after EI.

As in above examples derivatives are specifically made from the point of view of inducing a particular mode of ion decomposition, this fragmentation is called **directed fragmentation**.

18.27 MASS FRAGMENTATION PATTERNS OF CHEMICAL CLASSES

1. Alkanes

Normal alkanes exhibit peaks corresponding to their molecular ion, M^+. With branching, the intensity of the observed molecular ion peaks gets diminished. More the branching the lesser the intensity. What could be the possible reason for this? The normal alkanes undergo fragmentation due to cleavage carbon-carbon bonds so that a homologous series of fragmentation products is obtained. Thus, cleavage of the C_1 and C_2 bond in butane, leads to the loss of a methyl radical along with the formation of the propyl carbocation. Similarly, C_2 to C_3 bond cleavage, leads to the formation of the ethyl carbocation with the loss of an ethyl radical.

On the other hand, the carbon-carbon bond cleavage in branched-chain alkanes often forms the secondary or tertiary carbocations, more stable than primary ions. Spectrum (m/e) of n-octane is shown in Fig. 18.29e.

Further, it needs to be noted that straight chain alkanes do not lose methyl groups so that (M–15) peaks are not seen in their mass spectra. The mass spectra of 3–ethyl–2–methylpent–1–ene and n-butylbenzene are shown in Fig. 18.29f and 18.29g respectively.

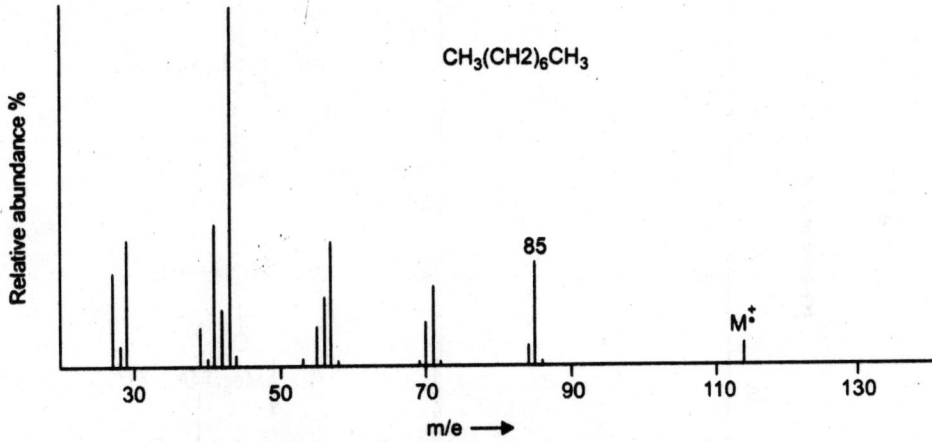

Fig. 18.29e. Mass spectrum of m/e of n-octane.

Cycloalkanes

- They generally form strong molecular ion peaks.
- As fragmentation involves fission of two bonds to form a fragment, fragmentation occurs to a smaller extent in cycloalkanes.
- The loss of a molecule of ethene is very common, either from the parent molecule or from the intermediate radical-ions. For example, the peak observed (M–28) at m/e = 42 in cyclopentane occurs due to loss of an ethene molecule from the parent molecule.
- The loss of the side chain if present is a favourable mode of fragmentation. For example, the peak seen at m/z 69 seen in the mean spectrum of methyl cyclopentane is due to loss of the methyl group, the side chain.

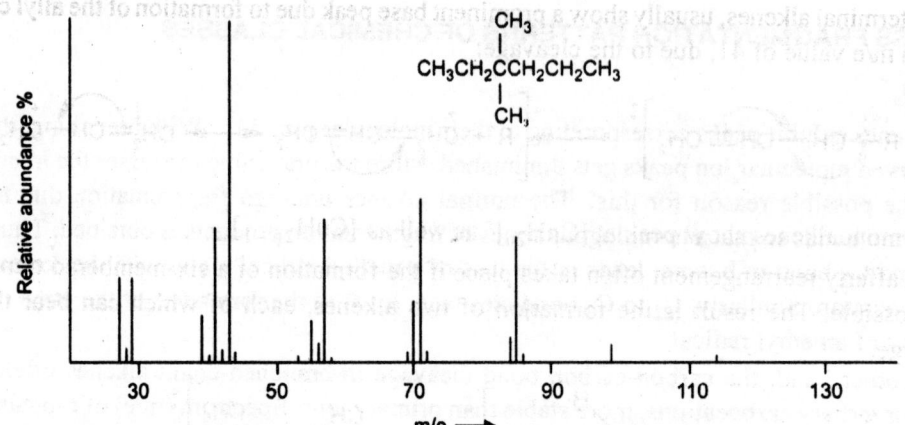

Fig. 18.29f. Mass spectrum of 3,3–dimethylhexane.

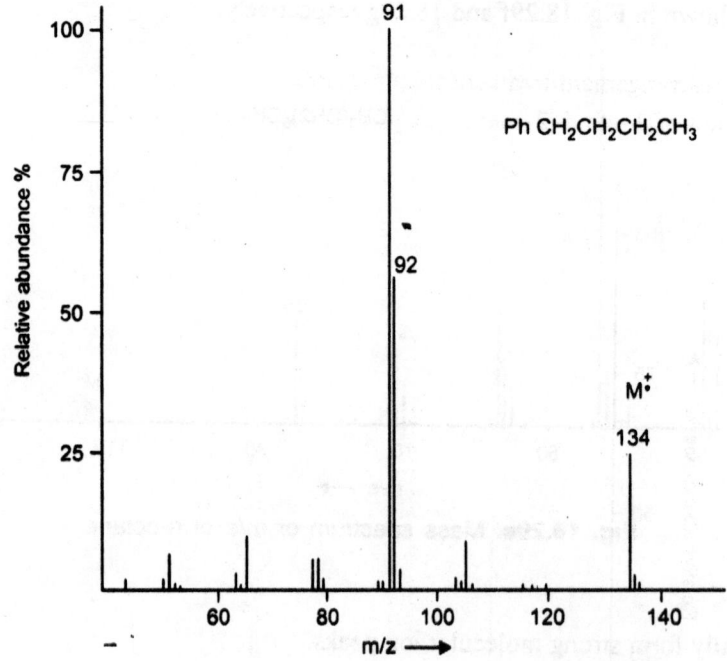

Fig. 18.29g. Mass spectrum of n-butylbenzene.

2. Alkenes

- It is the removal of the π-electrons apparently, that gives rise to the molecular ion peak in alkenes.
- The mass spectra of alkene isomers are similar. For example, the mass spectra of two isomers of the formula C_4H_8. The two mass spectra are very nearly identical. This is because after the electron impact, the double bond migrates readily.

- The terminal alkenes, usually show a prominent base peak due to formation of the allyl carbocation at an m/e value of 41, due to the cleavage:

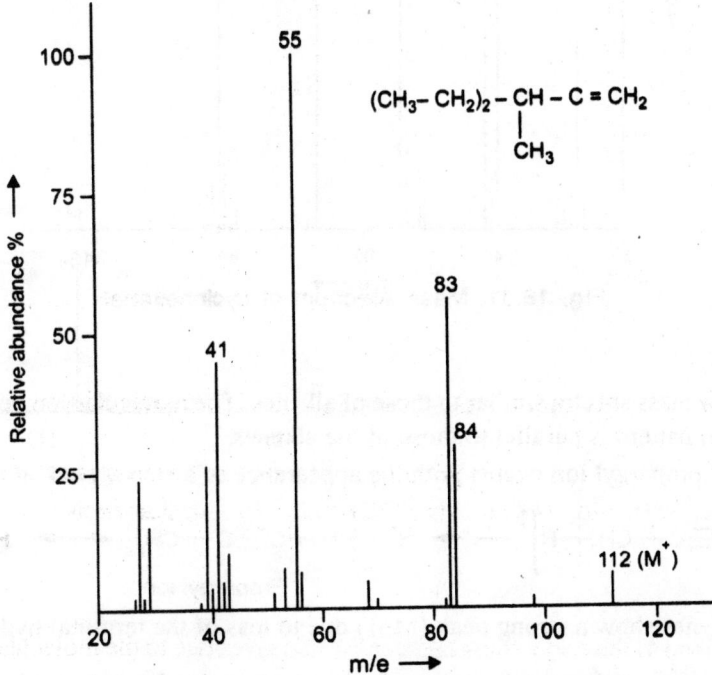

- The monoalkenes show peak at $[CnH_{2n}]^+$ as well as $[CnH_{2n-1}]^{+\cdot}$.

- McLafferty rearrangement often takes place if the formation of a six-membered transition state is possible. The result is the formation of two alkenes, each of which can bear the positive charge.

McLafferty rearrangement in alkenes: an example.

Mass spectrum of 3–ethyl–2–methyl pent–1–ene is shown in Fig. 18.30.

Fig. 18.30. Mass spectrum of 3–ethyl–2–methyl pent–1–ene.

3. Cycloalkynes

- Due to presence of a double bond, they undergo a fragmentation pattern that is equivalent to a reverse or retro-Diels-Alder reaction. m/e spectrum of cyclohexene is shown in Fig. 18.31.

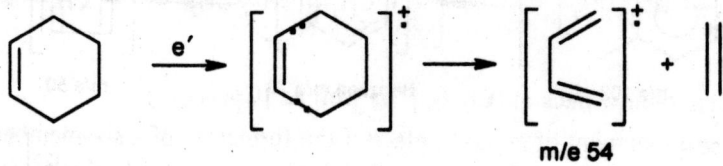

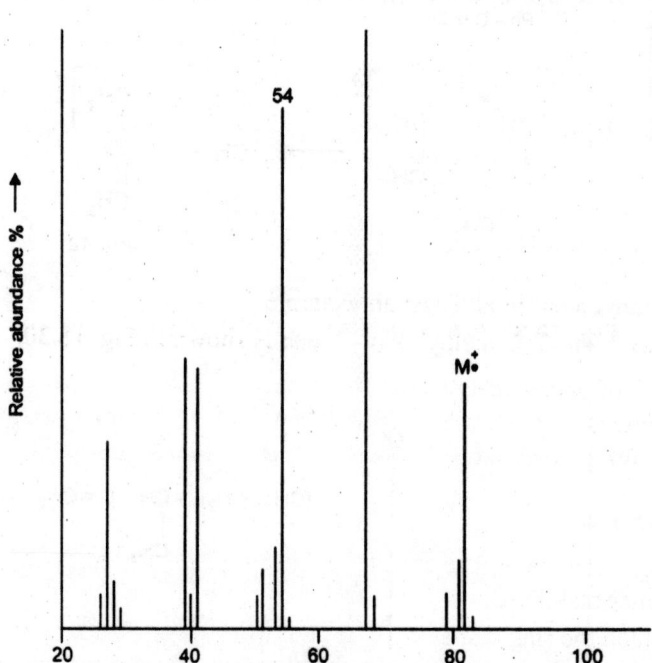

Fig. 18.31. Mass spectrum of cyclohexene.

4. Alkynes

- Alkynes show mass spectra similar to those of alkenes. The molecular ion peaks are intense. The fragmentation pattern is parallel to those of the alkenes.
- Formation of propargyl ion occurs with the appearance of a strong peak at m/e 39.

$$\left[H-\underset{2}{C}\equiv\underset{3}{C}-\underset{4}{CH_2}\!\!\mid\!\!R \right]^{\dot{+}} \longrightarrow R^{\bullet} + \left[H-\underset{9}{C}\equiv\underset{10}{\overset{+}{C}}-CH_2 \longleftrightarrow H-\underset{13}{\overset{+}{C}}=\underset{14}{C}=CH_2 \right]$$

Propargyl ion

- Terminal alkynes show a strong peak (M−1) due to loss of the terminal hydrogen.

$$\left[R-C\equiv C-H \right]^{\dot{+}} \longrightarrow R-C\equiv\overset{+}{C} + H^{\circ}$$

[M−1]

- m/e values of prominent peaks in the group of the homologous series of ions correspond to $CnH_{(2n-3)}$ as is shown for phenylacetylene (see mass spectrum in Fig. 18.32).

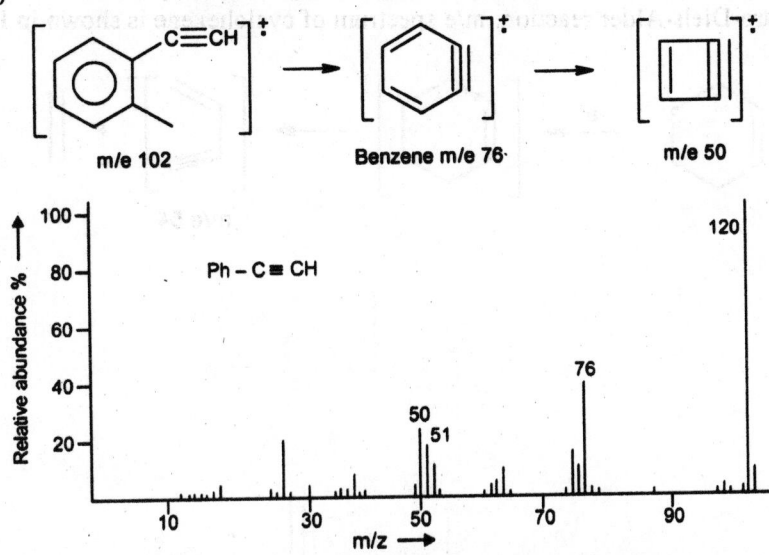

Fig. 18.32. Mass spectrum of Phenylacetylene.

The mass spectrum of phenylacetylene shows strong peak, the base peak (also the M^+ peak) at m/e 102. A low-intensity peak is also seen at m/e 103. The peak at m/e 76 corresponds to a benzyne radical-ion that loses a C_2H_2 molecule to give a peak at (76–26) m/e 50.

5. Aromatic Hydrocarbons

- These show strong molecular ion peaks. This is because the $M^{\ddagger}$ that is formed due to loss of a π-electron is resonance stabilised.
- Compounds in which the ring contains a side chain show a peak at m/e 91 due to fragmentation at the benzylic position. The formed benzyl cation rearranges spontaneously to a tropylium cation.

Toluene
(m/e 92)

Benzyl carbocation
(m/e 91)

Tropylium ion
(m/e 91)

- Mc-Lafferty rearrangement can also occur when an alkyl group attached to benzene ring has γ-H_x.

n-Butyl benzene

m/Z = 92

The mass spectrum of benzene and toluene is shown in Fig. 18.33 and 18.34 respectively, while that of ethyl benzene and naphthalene are shown in Fig. 18.35 and 18.36 respectively.

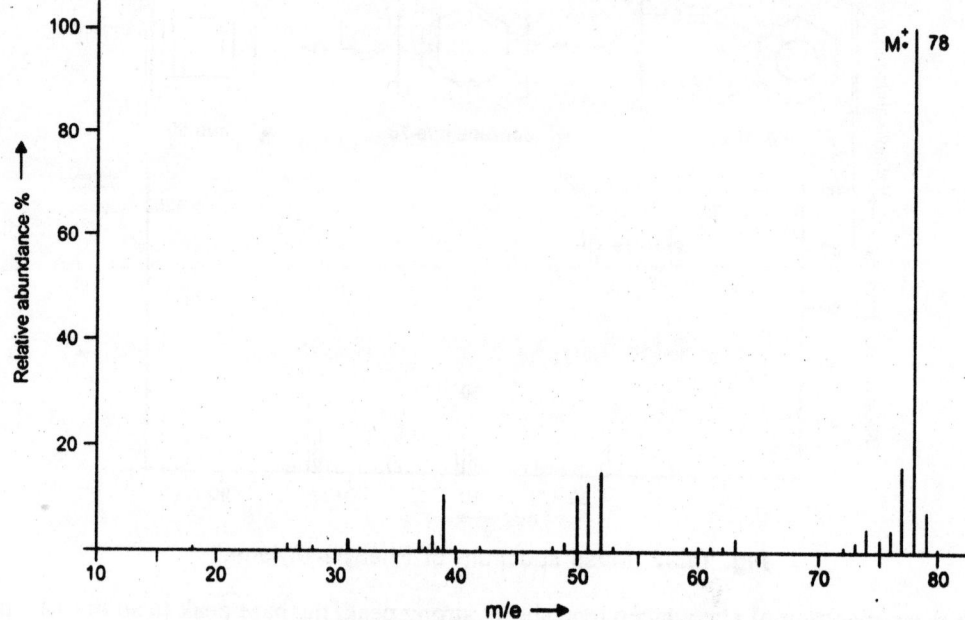

Fig. 18.33. Mass spectrum of benzene.

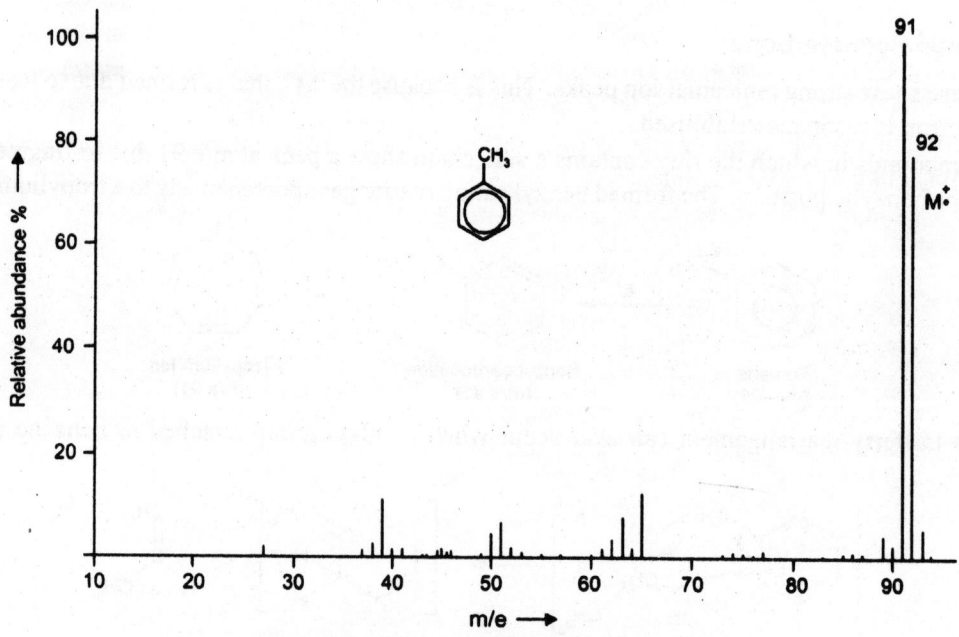

Fig. 18.34. Mass spectrum of toluene.

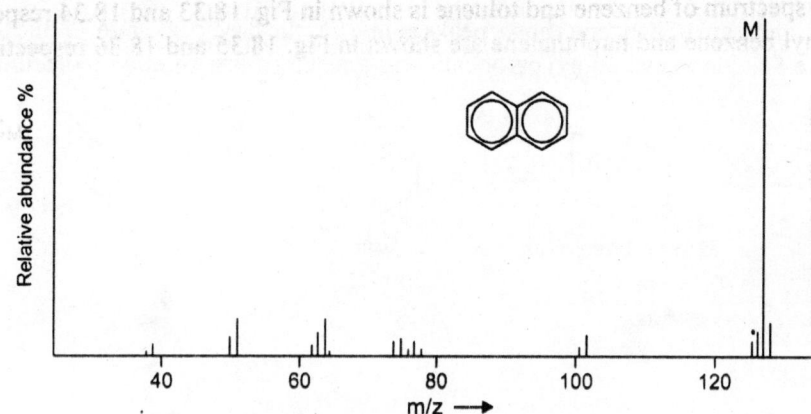

Fig. 18.35. Mass spectrum of naphthalene.

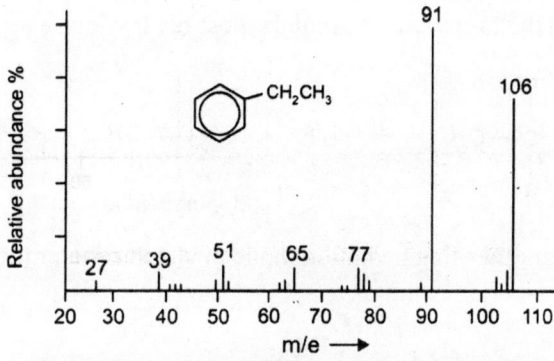

Fig. 18.36. Mass spectrum of ethylbenzene.

• The fragmentation in Ethylbenzene occurs as follows giving an intense peak due to tropylium cation at m/e 91 and a low-intensity peak at m/e 65 due to formation of cyclopentadienyl cation. The peak at m/e 105 arises due to loss of a H°.

CH₃
CH₂

−ĊH₃

⁺CH₂

Benzyl cation

Rearr

m/e 91 (tropylium ion)

−H°

CH₃
⊕CH

m/e 105

−C₂H₂

m/e 65
Cyclopentadienyl carbocation

- The mass spectrum of benzene shows peaks at m/e 78, the base peak, m/e 77 due to phenyl cation and at m/e 51, due to cyclobutyl carbocation as a result of loss of ethyl molecule:

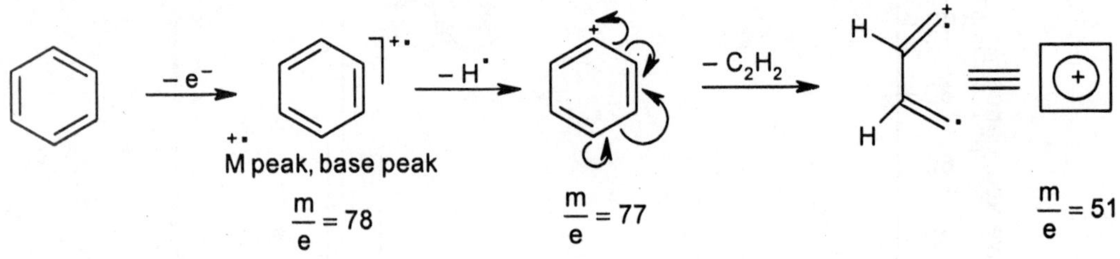

M peak, base peak

$$\frac{m}{e} = 78 \qquad\qquad \frac{m}{e} = 77 \qquad\qquad \frac{m}{e} = 51$$

6. Alcohols

(i) Aliphatic alcohols

- The molecule ion M^+ is either weak or absent. Loss of alkyl group cleavage occurs prominently in alcohols such that the largest alkyl group is most readily lost.

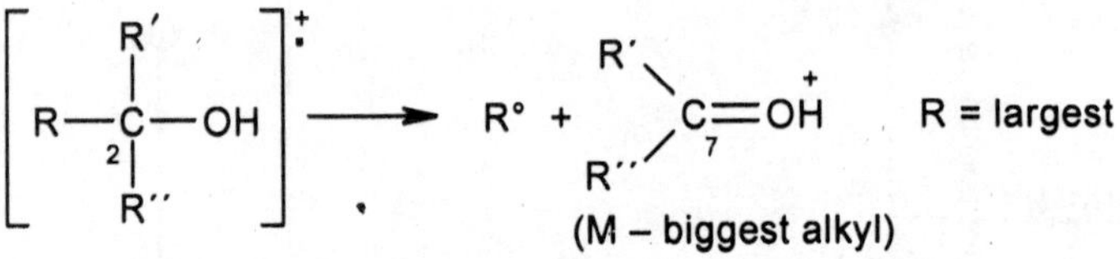

R = largest

(M – biggest alkyl)

- Alcohols also show another fragmentation mode in which a water molecule is eliminated. A δH is involved.

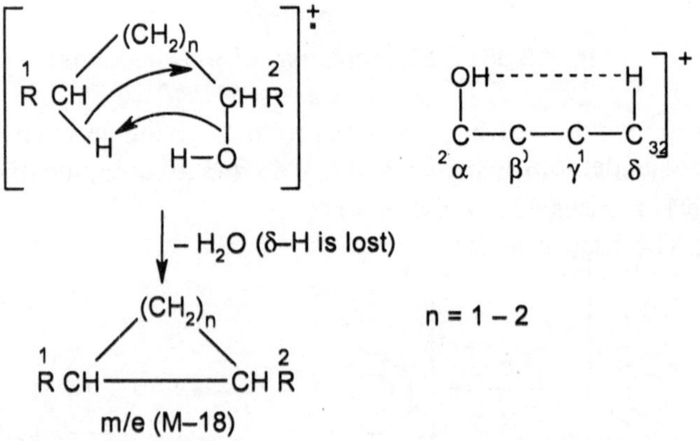

$- H_2O$ (δ–H is lost)

$n = 1 - 2$

m/e (M–18)

- Another mode involves simultaneous loss of a water molecule as well as an alkene to give an (M–46) ion. This happens in alcohols which contain more than four carbons.

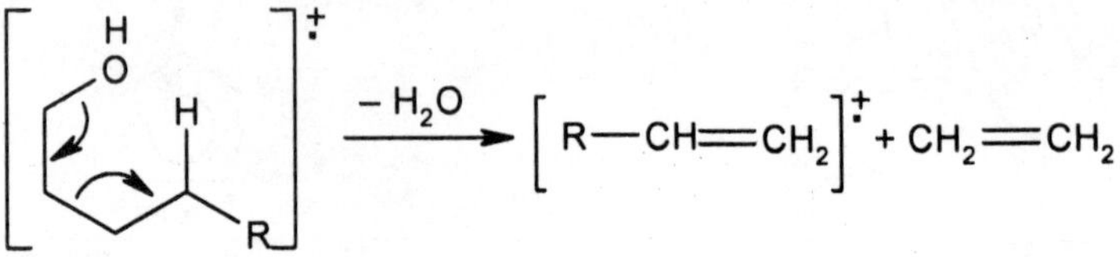

$- H_2O$

$$\left[R-CH\!=\!CH_2 \right]^{+\cdot} + CH_2\!=\!CH_2$$

Mass spectra of MeOH, n-pentanol and t-butanol are shown in Fig. 18.37, 18.38 and 18.39 respectively.

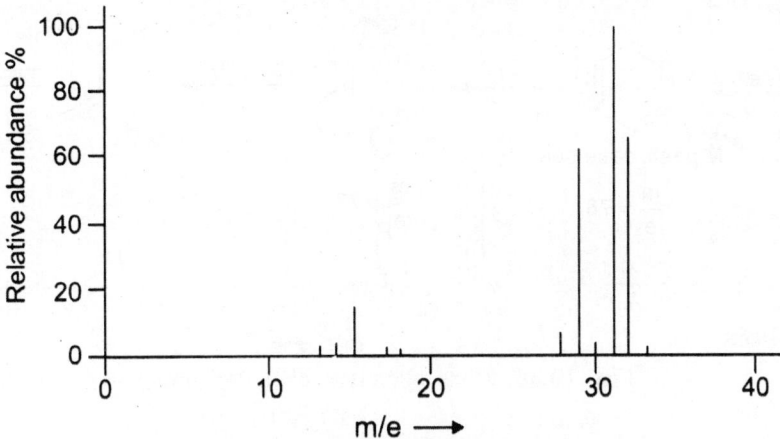

Fig. 18.37. Mass spectrum of MeOH.

Intext Exercise

2. Can you distinguish between these isomeric alcohols?

   1–Butanol, 2–Butanol and 2–Methyl–2–propanol

Ans. Yes, you can. Here I describe their main fragmentation patterns:

1. 1–Butanol

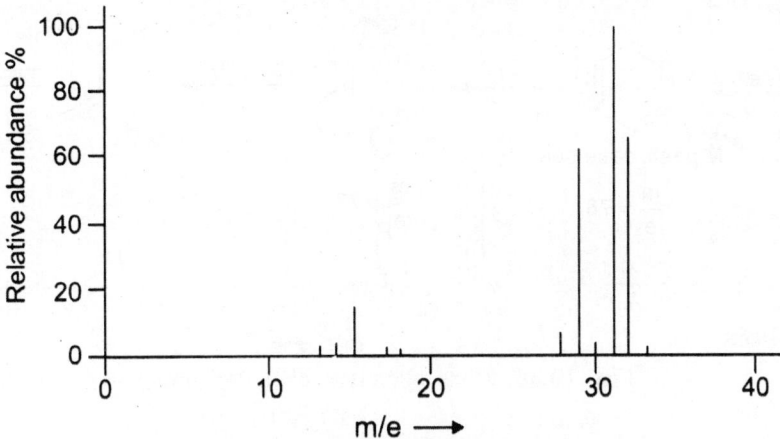

m/e 56

So, 1–Butanol undergoes loss of a water molecule to give a prominent peak, the base peak at m/e 56.

2. 2–Butanol : The base peak here occurs at m/e 45 that occurs due to loss of an ethyl radical:

$$CH_3—CH_2—\underset{\underset{\overset{+}{O}H}{|}}{C}H—CH_3 \longrightarrow CH_3—CH=\overset{+}{O}H + CH_3\dot{C}H_2$$

m/e 45

3. 2–Methyl–2–propanol : This alcohol gives base peak at m/e 59 due to loss of a methyl radical.

$$H_3C—\underset{\underset{CH_3}{|}}{\overset{\overset{CH_3}{|}}{C}}—\overset{+\bullet}{O}H \longrightarrow CH_3—\underset{\underset{CH_3}{|}}{C}=\overset{+}{O}H + \dot{C}H_3$$

m/e 59

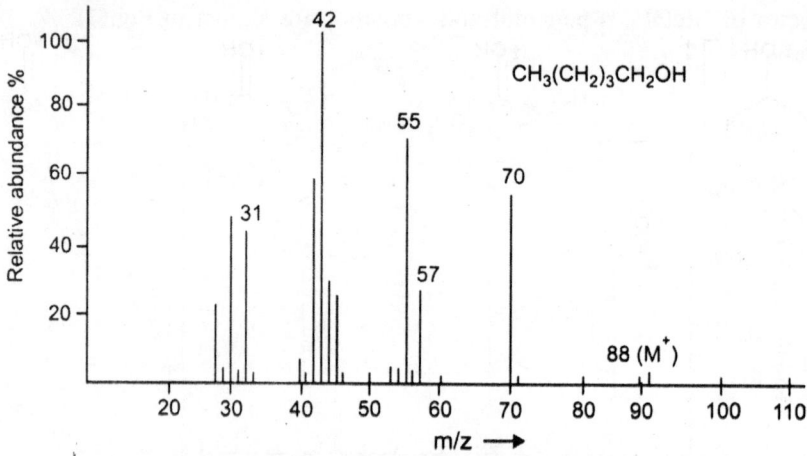

Fig. 18.38. Mass spectrum of n-Pentanol.

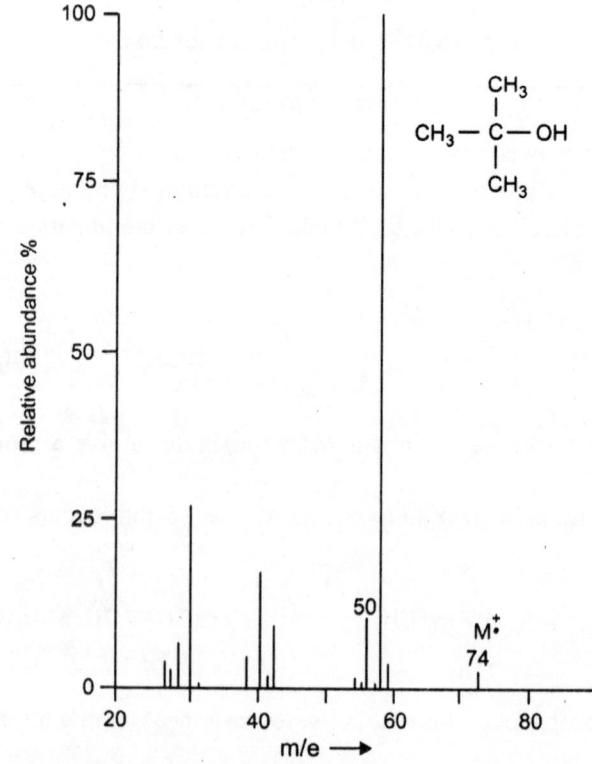

Fig. 18.39. Mass spectrum of tert-butyl alcohol.

(ii) Cyclic Alcohols

An illustration of the three different fragmentation pattern shown by cyclohexanol is as follows. The mass spectrum of this alcohol is shown in Fig. 18.40.

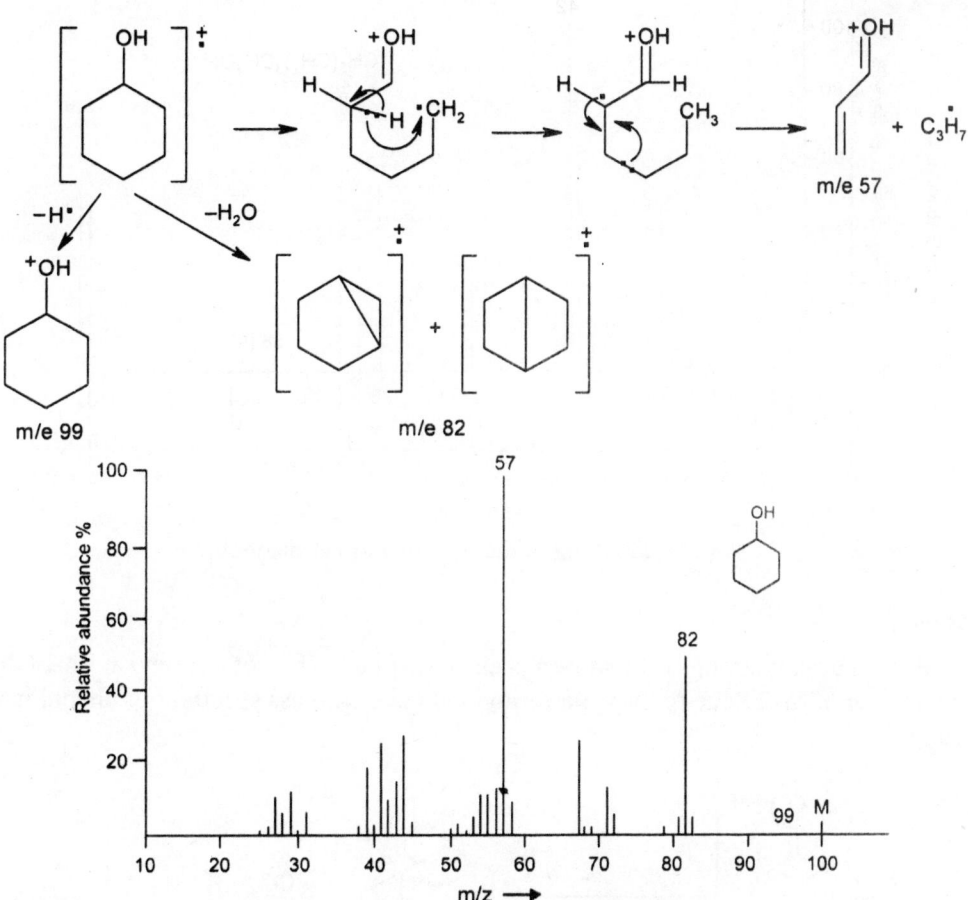

Fig. 18.40. Mass spectrum of Cyclohexanol.

(iii) Aralkyl alcohols

• Benzyl alcohol undergoes fragmentation as shown in Fig. 18.41.

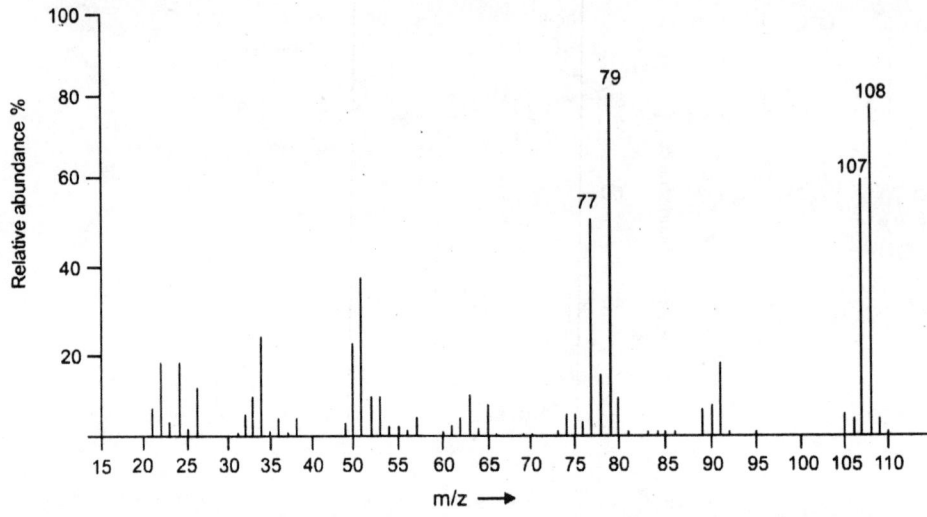

Fig. 18.41. Mass spectrum of Benzyl alcohol.

7. Phenols

The molecular ion peak is strong. They show a peak at M–1 due to loss of a H° and at M–28 due to loss of CO and another at M–29 due to loss of a formyl radical. The mass spectrum of phenol is shown in Fig. 18.42.

Fragmentation of phenol

M peak
m/e = 94

m/e = 66
(M–28)

m/e = 65
Base peak

8. Aliphatic Ethers

M/e spectrum of n-Butyl-ethyl ether is shown in Fig. 18.43.

- Ethers exhibit a fragmentation of ethers is somewhat similar pattern of to that of the alcohols.
- The C–C bond α to oxygen.
- α-cleavage may cleave to give ion positively charged fragment carbon instead of oxygen. For example the peak at m/e 45 in diethyl ether is due to α-cleavage.
- Cleavage of the C–O bond occurs giving a carbocation (29, 32, 57 .... R⁺). For example, the peak at m/e 43 in diisopropyl ether is due to generation of $C_3H_7^+$ fragment.
- Peaks at m/e 31, 45, 59, 73 are seen in the mass spectra of ethers (RO^+, $ROCH_2^+$). The fragmentation pattern of diethyl ether is like this:

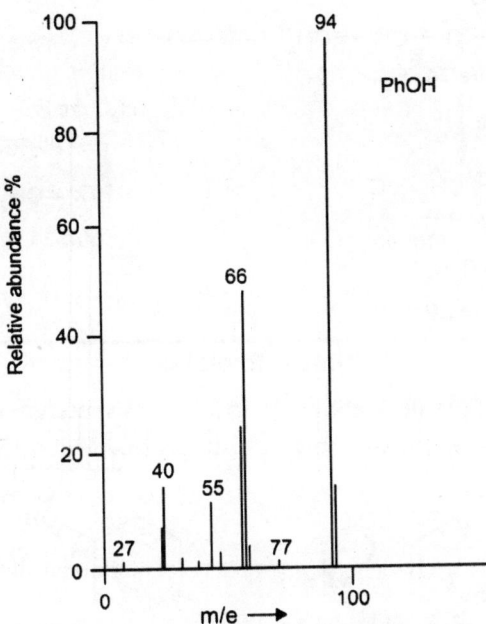

Fig. 18.42. Mass spectrum of Phenol.

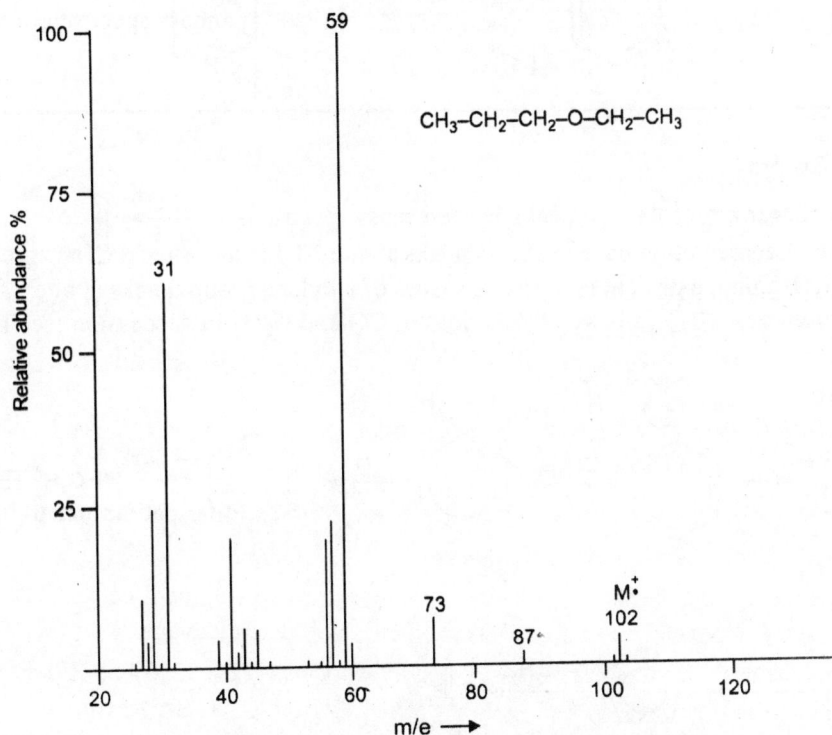

CH₃–CH₂–CH₂–O–CH₂–CH₃

Fig. 18.43. Mass spectrum of n-Butyl ethyl ether.

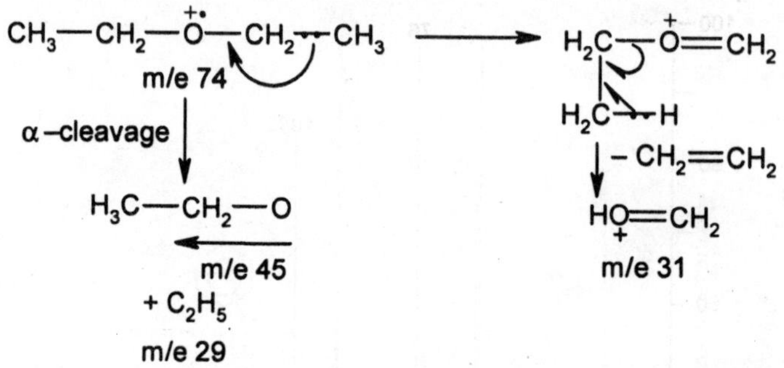

$$CH_3—CH_2—\overset{+\cdot}{O}—CH_2—CH_3 \longrightarrow H_2C—\overset{+}{O}=CH_2$$

m/e 74

α–cleavage

$$H_3C—CH_2—O$$

m/e 45

$$+ C_2H_5$$

m/e 29

$$H_2C—H$$

$$|-CH_2=CH_2$$

$$H\overset{+}{O}=CH_2$$

m/e 31

Intext Exercise

3. Explain the formation of the peak at m/e 94 in the mass spectrum of phenetole.

   Ans. This can be explained due to a four or a six-centred McLafferty rearrangement.

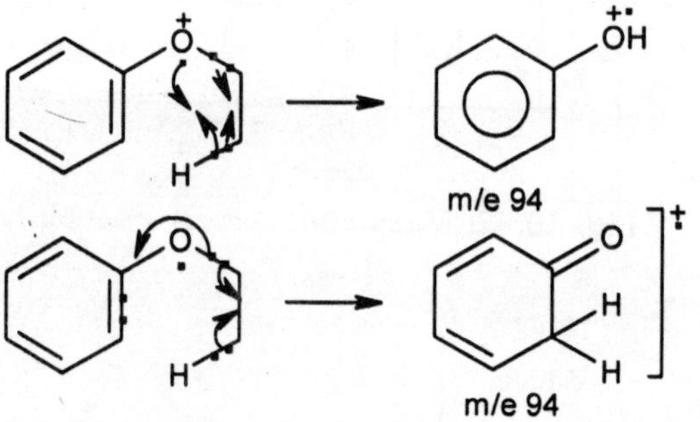

m/e 94

m/e 94

(ii) Aromatic Ethers

They exhibit stronger molecular ion peaks in their mass spectra.

   Anisole: The fragmentation pattern shows peaks at m/e 78 due to loss of a CH_2O group: m/e 77 due to loss of a $CH_3O^{\cdot}$ group, a peak at m/e 51 due to loss of ethylene group. Peaks at m/e 93, 65 and 39 are formed due to loss of a $CH_3^{\cdot}$ followed by the loss of CO and C_2H_2 in succession (see Fig. 18.44a).

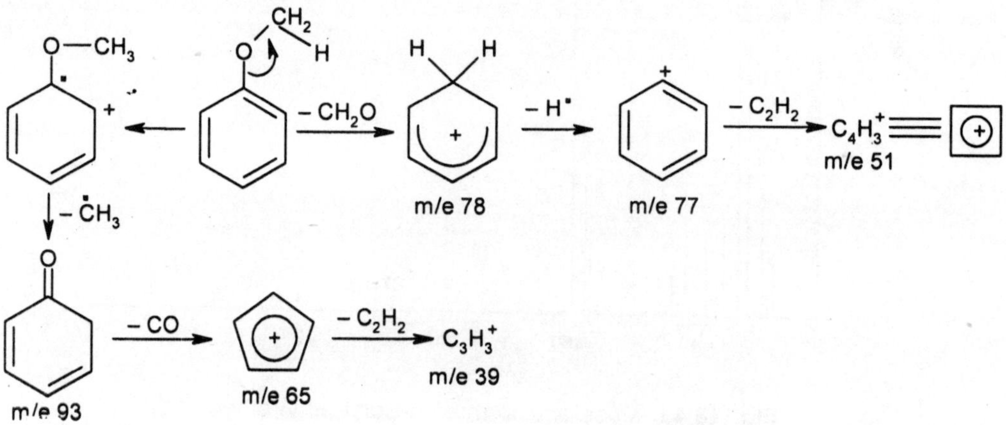

m/e 78

m/e 77

$$-C_2H_2 \longrightarrow C_4H_3^+ \equiv$$

m/e 51

$$-\overset{\cdot}{C}H_3$$

m/e 93

$$-CO \longrightarrow$$

m/e 65

$$-C_2H_2 \longrightarrow C_3H_3^+$$

m/e 39

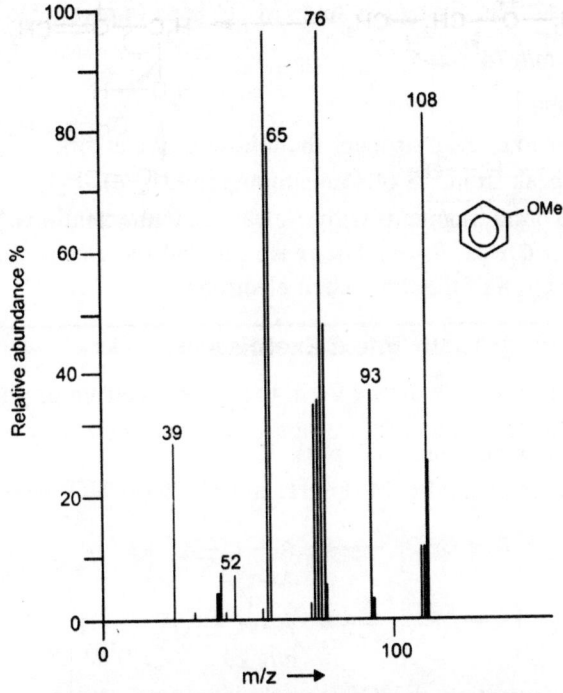

Fig. 18.44a. Mass spectrum of Anisole.

9. Thiols

Mass spectrum of 1–pentanethiol is shown in Fig. 18.45.

- Thiols show a more intense molecular ion peak compared to the corresponding alcohols.
- They show a significant M + Z peak, that arises due to the presence of the heavy isotope, ^{34}S (natural abundance of 44%).
- Thiols show fragmentation pattern similar to those of the alcohols.

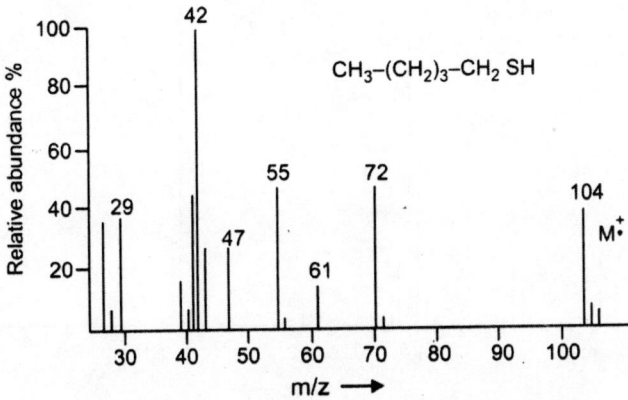

Fig. 18.45. Mass spectrum of 1–pentanethiol.

- They lose hydrogen sulfide, giving rise to an M–34 peak (a parallel to the elimination of H_2O in alcohols)

10. Thioethers

- They show molecular ion peaks stronger than those of the ethers.
- M + 2 is diagnostic peak from ^{34}S (4.4% natural abundance).
- α-cleavage: The C–S bond fragments with α-cleavage with retention of positive charge on sulfur, (RS^+) giving peaks at 47, 61, 75, ... The reason is that the electron deficiency is stabilised by sulfur due to participation of the inner shell electrons.
- β-cleavage: This occurs generally $R\overset{\oplus}{—CH=SH}$ ions. Peaks are seen at 46, 61, 75, 89, ...

11. Aldehydes

- Aliphatic aldehydes show a weak $M^{+\bullet}$ peak.
- α-cleavage is very common so that M–1 (–H) and M–29 (–CHO) peaks are characteristic peaks.

$$\left[R—CHO\right]^{+\bullet} \longrightarrow \underset{(M-1)}{R—C≡O^+} + H$$

$$\left[R—CHO\right]^{+\bullet} \longrightarrow \underset{m/e\ 29}{H—C≡O^+} + \underset{(M-29)}{R^\bullet}$$

The peak due to the formation of HCO^+ can be observed at m/e = 29. The mass spectrum of Benzaldehyde are shown in 18.46.

$$\left[R—CH_2—CHO\right]^{+\bullet} \longrightarrow \underset{m/e\ 43}{CH_2=CH—O} + \underset{M-43}{R^+}$$

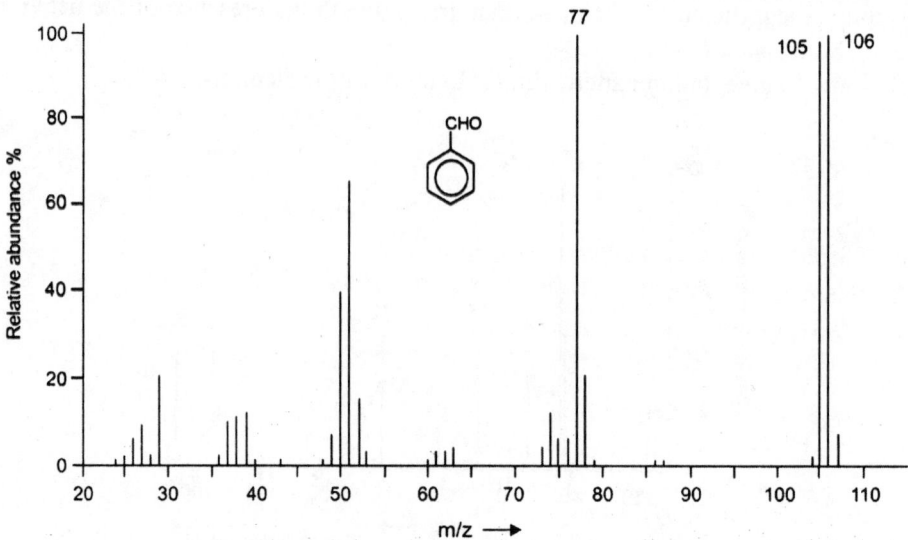

Fig. 18.46. Mass spectrum of benzaldehyde.

- McLafferty rearrangement also occurs when γ-hydrogen is present to give peaks at 44/58/72 due to –R–CH=CH$_2$. The peak at m/e 44 is also a characteristic peak of aldehydes.

12. Aromatic aldehydes

Aldehydes show the following features:
- These show intense M$^+$ peaks.
- α-cleavage with the loss of a hydrogen gives a M–1 peak.
- Peak at m/e 77 is due to the loss of the CHO group occurs yielding the phenyl cation.

Benzaldehyde: The mass spectrum of benzaldehyde is shown in Fig. 18.46. Benzaldehyde shows the following fragmentation pattern.

13. Ketones

(i) Aliphatic Ketones

- These show strong M$^+$ peaks.
- α-cleavage is a common fragmentation path such that the larger alkyl group is lost preferentially giving the base peak.

- McLafferty rearrangement can also occur:

2–Butanone (Ethylmethyl ketone): The spectrum is shown in Fig. 18.47. The fragmentation pattern occurs as follows:

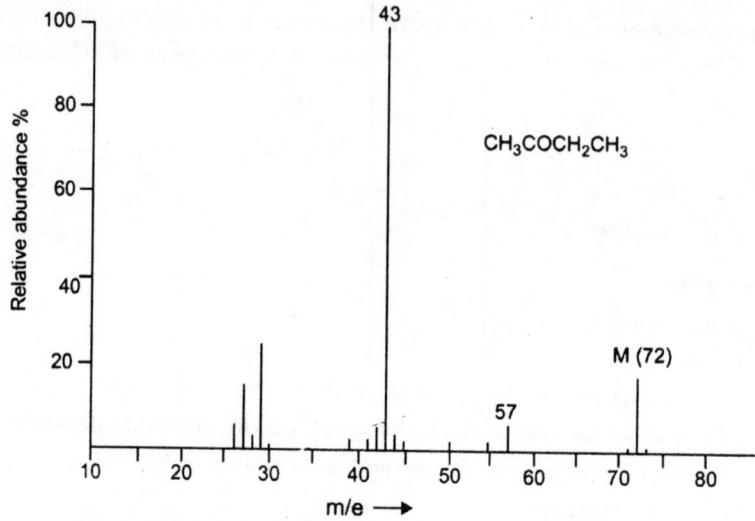

Fig. 18.47. Mass spectrum of 2–Butanone.

(ii) Cycloketones

These follow many fragmentation and rearrangement patterns.

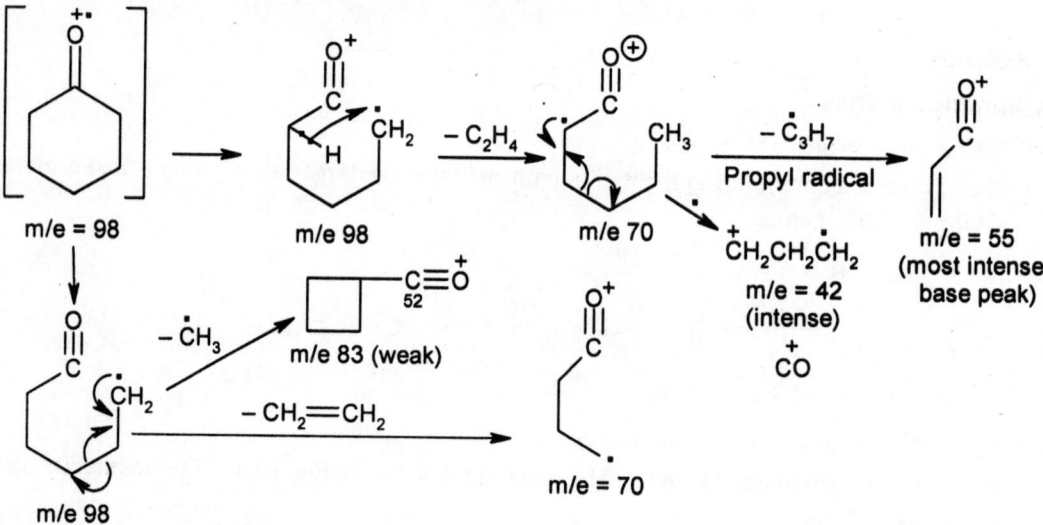

Mass spectrum of cyclohexanone is shown in Fig. 18.48.

(iii) Aromatic Ketones

- M^+ peaks are intense.
- These commonly show α-cleavage pattern to yield benzoyl cation (m/e 105) that is stabilised via resonance.
- When γ-hydrogen is available, McLafferty rearrangement occurs.

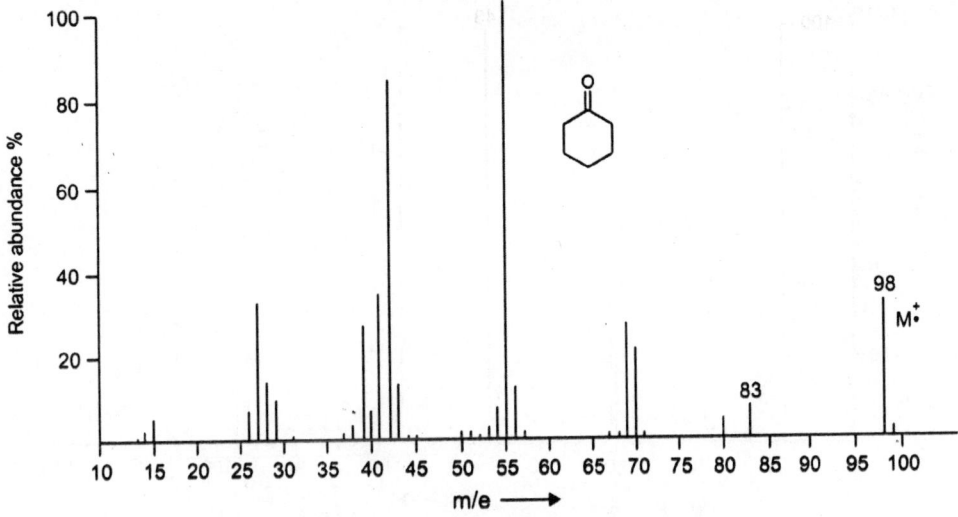

Fig. 18.48. Mass spectrum of Cyclohexanone.

Acetophenone: The mass spectrum of acetophenone is shown in Fig. 18.49. The ketone undergoes fragmentation as follows:

14. Carboxylic Acids

(i) Aliphatic carboxylic acids

- Aliphatic carboxylic acids show weak M^+ peak.
- a-cleavage involving loss of OH and CHOH occurs on either side of the carboxyl group.

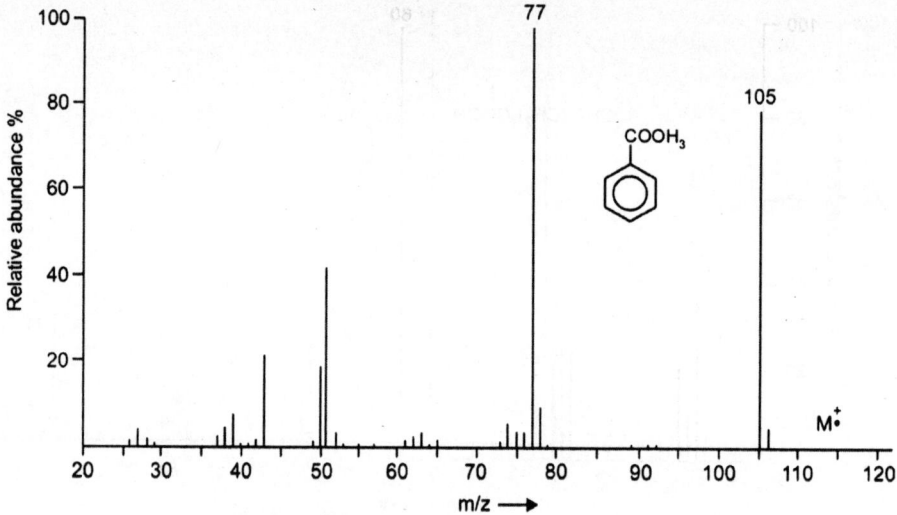

Fig. 18.49. Mass spectrum of acetophenone.

$$R-\underset{\underset{OH}{|}}{\overset{\overset{+\cdot}{O}}{\overset{||}{C}}} \xrightarrow{-\overset{\cdot}{O}H} R-C\equiv\overset{+}{O} \longrightarrow R^+ + CO$$

- McLafferty rearrangement occurs in acids containing γ–H giving the base peak.

1. **Butanoic Acid:** The mass spectrum of Butanoic acid is shown in Fig. 18.50. The fragmentation pattern is as follows. The peaks at m/e 45 arises due to α-cleavage and the base peak at m/e 60 is due to McLafferty rearrangement.

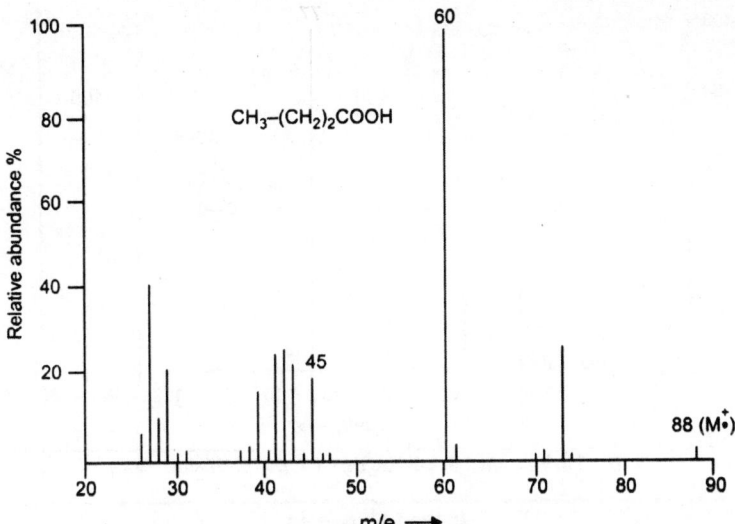

Fig. 18.50. Mass spectrum of Butanoic acid.

2. **Ethanoic Acid:** Ethanoic acid shows peak at m/e 45 due to α cleavage and at m/e 43 due to $\dot{O}H$ loss and at m/e 25 due to $\dot{C}H_3$ loss from the CH_3CO^+ (m/e 45).

$$
\begin{array}{c}
\overset{\bullet+}{O} \\
\parallel \\
CH_3-C-O-H \\
m/e = 60
\end{array}
\begin{array}{l}
\xrightarrow{-CH_3} \quad {}^+O\equiv C-OH \\
\qquad\qquad m/e = 45 \\
\\
\xrightarrow{-OH} \quad CH_3-C\equiv O^+ \xrightarrow{-CO} CH_3^+ \\
\qquad\qquad m/e = 43 \qquad\qquad m/e = 25
\end{array}
$$

Aromatic Acid

- These show intense M^+ peaks.
- Peaks at M–17, M–45 and M–18 are characteristics.
- Peak at M–17 is due to M–OH.
- Peak at M–45 is due to loss of ^+COOH (m/e 45).
- Peak at m/e 77 is due to phenyl cation [(M–OH)–CO].
- Peak at m/e 51 is due to loss of C_2H_2 from phenyl cation.

Example: p-Anisic acid.

The mass spectrum is shown in Fig. 18.51.

m/e = 122 $\xrightarrow{-OH}$ m/e = 105 (M–17) Base peak $\xrightarrow{-CO}$ m/e = 77 (M–45) $\xrightarrow{-C_2H_2}$ m/e 51 [(M–OH)–CO]

Fragmentation of benzoic acid

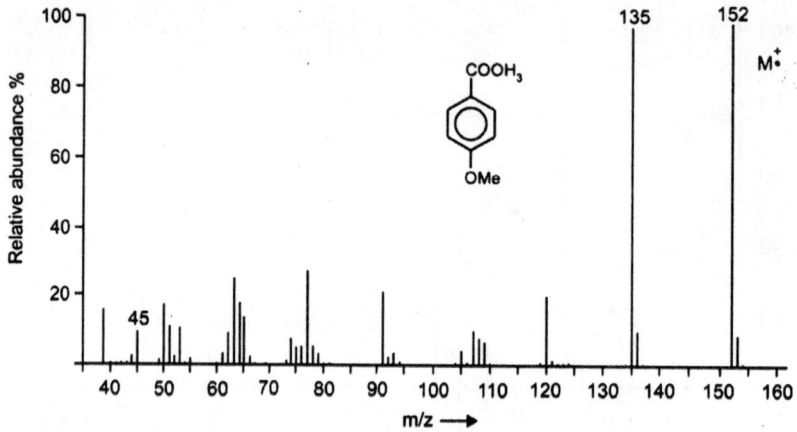

Fig. 18.51. Mass spectrum of para-anisic acid.

Intext Exercise

Q. What is the peak at m/e 149 due to in the mass spectra of phthalic acid esters?

Ans. The peak at m/e 149 arises from the following intermediate.

m/e 149

---

15. Esters

(i) Aliphatic esters

Esters show very weak M^{+} peak.

- The fragmentation of methyl esters is similar to those of carboxylic acids.
- Methyl esters show peaks at M–31, at m/e 59 and m/e 74.
- Acylium ion, RCO^{+} peak is a characteristic peak. Thus, the peak at m/e 71 in the mass spectrum of methyl butyrate is due to this cation.
- The peak at m/e 59 is due to $CH_3-O-C=\overset{+}{O}$ that is formed through loss of an alkyl group from the acyl part.

Mass spectrum of n-propyl acetate is shown in Fig. 18.52.

Examples

(i) **Methyl ethanoate:** It undergoes fragmentation as shown:

$$CH_3-\overset{\overset{\displaystyle O^{+}}{\|}}{C}-O-CH_3 \xrightarrow{-\dot{O}CH_3} CH_3-C\equiv O^{+} \xrightarrow{-CO} \overset{+}{C}H_3$$

$$\begin{array}{ccc} \text{M peak} & \text{m/e = 43} & \text{m/e = 15} \\ \text{m/e = 74} & & \end{array}$$

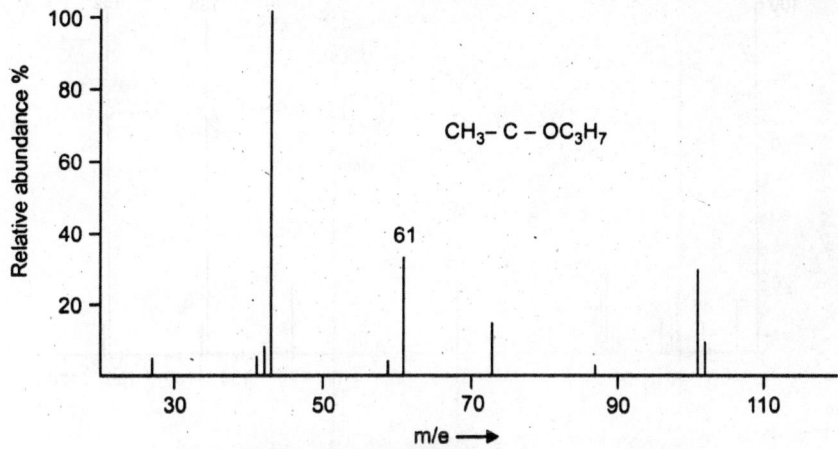

Fig. 18.52. Mass spectrum of n-propyl acetate.

(ii) Aromatic Esters

- They give intense $M^{\ddagger}$ peak, the intensity decreases with increasing size of the alcohol so that it is not observed when the alcohol has five carbons.
- A peak at m/e 105 is due to C_6H_5–CO^+ formed after loss of alkoxy moiety.
- A peak at m/e 77 is due to phenyl cation that is formed as a result of loss of CO from $C_6H_5CO^+$.
- McLafferty rearrangement in the presence of a γ–H occurs.
- When an alkyl group is present in the ortho position to the ester group, the alcohol molecule gets eliminated.

Example

The mass spectrum of methyl ester of toluic acid in Fig. 18.53a and that of Methyl benzoate in Fig. 18.53b.

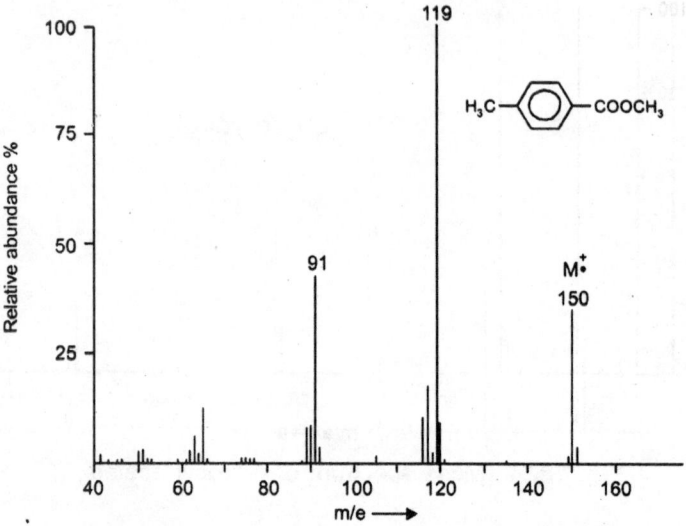

Fig. 18.53a. Methyl spectrum of Methyl ester of Toluic acid.

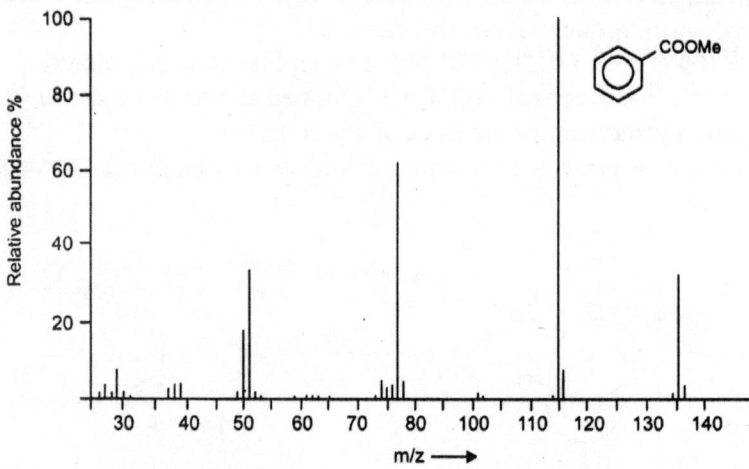

Fig. 18.53b. Mass spectrum of methyl benzoate.

16. Amines

(i) Aliphatic amines

$$\left[R-\overset{|}{\underset{|}{C}}-\ddot{N} \right]^{+} \longrightarrow \quad \nearrow C=\overset{+}{N} \diagdown \quad + R^{\bullet}$$

- M^{+} peak is weak and in aliphatic amines it is absent.

- The magnitude of molecular ion is very significant. If the molecular weight is odd, the amine must contain an odd number of nitrogen atoms.

  The base peak in aliphatic amines forms due to α-cleavage, with the largest R being lost preferentially.

  The mass spectrum of diethylamine is shown in Fig. 18.54.

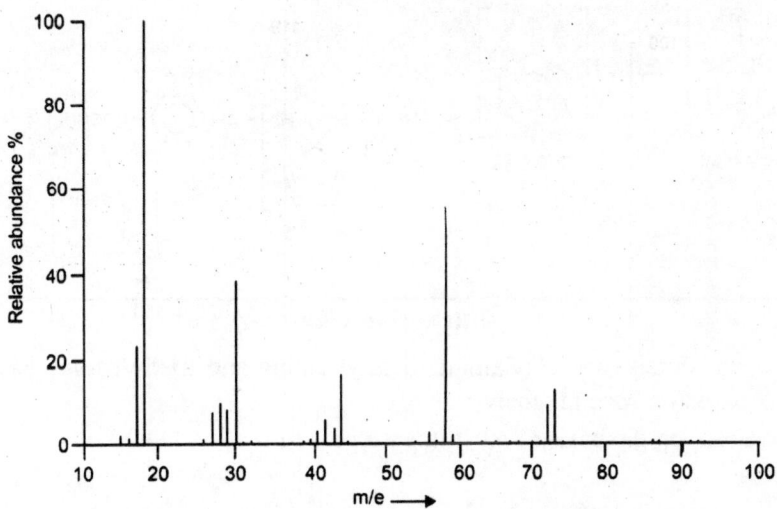

Fig. 18.54. Mass spectrum of diethylamine.

(ii) Aromatic Amines

- They give an intense $M^{\ddot{+}}$ peak.
- They show an M–1 peak due to loss of H atom.

Example: Aniline shows the following fragmentation pattern. The mass spectrum is of aniline is shown in Fig. 18.55.

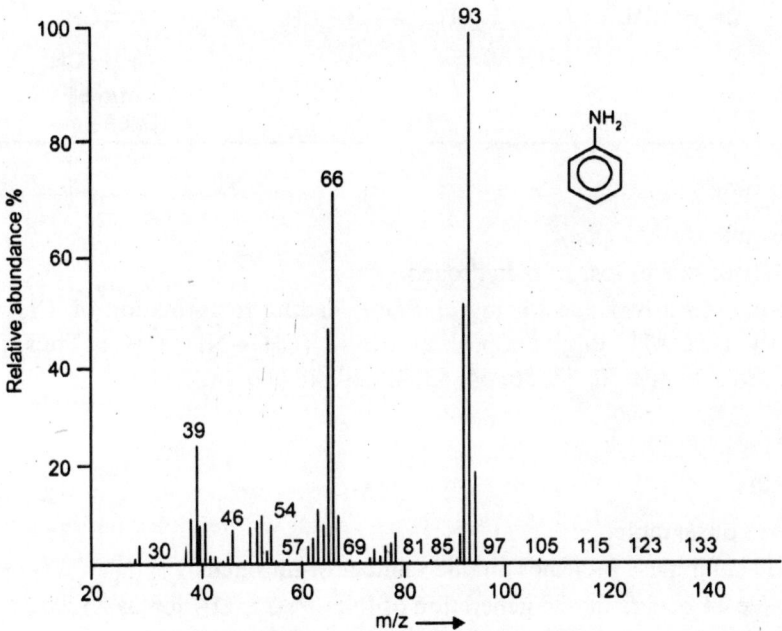

Fig. 18.55. Mass spectrum of aniline.

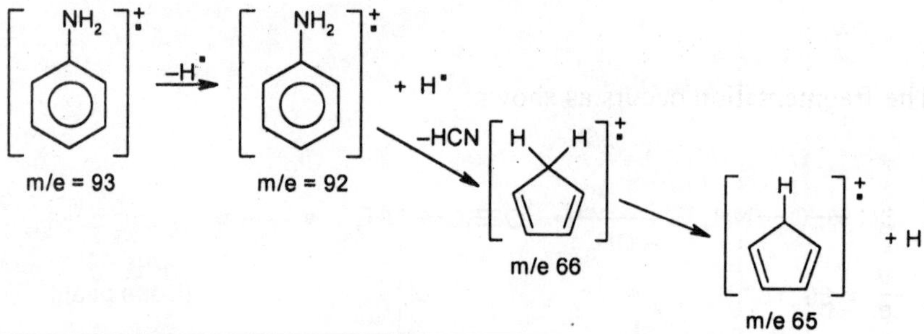

Scheme showing fragmentation: $m/e = 93 \xrightarrow{-H^\cdot} m/e = 92 \; (+H^\cdot) \xrightarrow{-HCN} m/e\; 66 \rightarrow m/e\; 65 \; (+H^\cdot)$

Intext Exercise

4. Can we distinguish between ethylamine, diethyl amine and triethylamine based upon most intense peak based on spectral analysis?

Ans. Yes, we can, on the basis of most intense peak

1. Ethylamine:

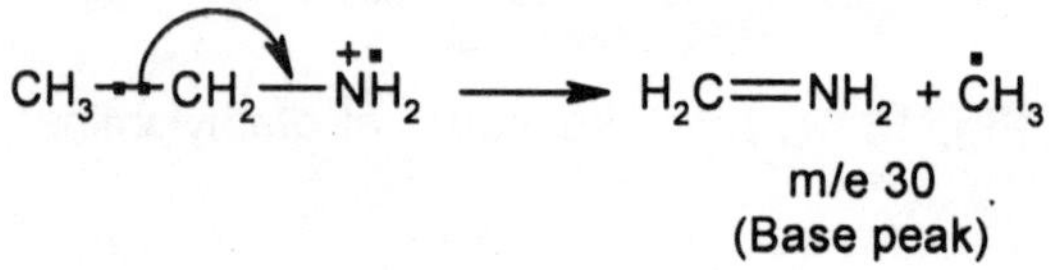

$$CH_3 \overset{+\cdot}{-}CH_2 - \overset{+\cdot}{NH_2} \longrightarrow H_2C = NH_2 + \dot{C}H_3$$

m/e 30
(Base peak)

2. Diethylamine:

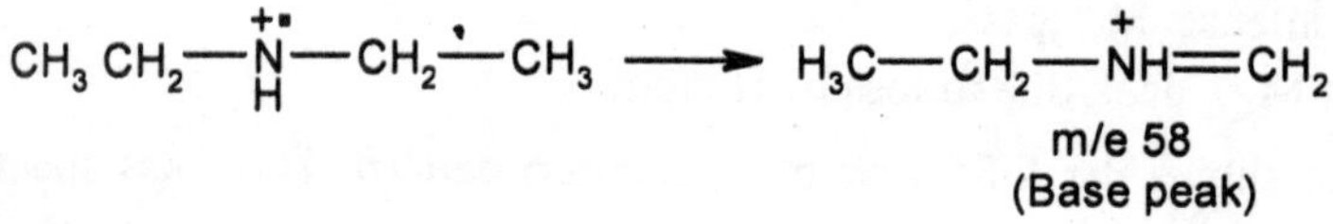

$$CH_3\,CH_2 - \overset{+\cdot}{\underset{H}{N}} - CH_2 \overset{\cdot}{-}CH_3 \longrightarrow H_3C - CH_2 - \overset{+}{N}H = CH_2$$

m/e 58
(Base peak)

3. Triethylamine:

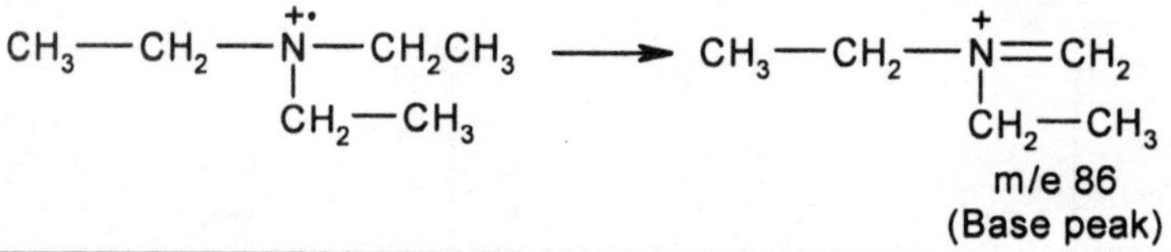

$$CH_3 - CH_2 - \overset{+\cdot}{\underset{\underset{CH_3}{|}}{N}} - CH_2CH_3 \longrightarrow CH_3 - CH_2 - \overset{+}{\underset{\underset{CH_3}{|}}{N}} = CH_2$$

m/e 86
(Base peak)

(iii) Cycloalkylamines

- These show intense $M^{+\cdot}$ peak.
- M–1 peak arises due to loss of α-hydrogen.
- A peak at m/e 43 arises due to ring cleavage leading to formation of $CH_2 = \overset{+}{N}H - \dot{C}H_2$ that subsequently loses a $H^\cdot$ to give a peak at m/e 42 ($CH_2 = NH - \dot{C}H_2$). Thus, piperidine shows diagnostic peaks at m/e 70, 57, 56, 44, 43, 42, 30, 29 and 28.

17. Amides

(i) Aliphtic amides

- $M^{+\cdot}$ peak are observable.
- An odd molecular mass indicates an odd number of nitrogens.
- A peak at m/e 44 occurs due to generation of $[NH_2 = C = O]^+$ ion as a result of α-cleavage.
- McLafferty rearrangement can also occur, giving a peak at m/e 59 in case of 1° amides.

Example

Ethanamide: The fragmentation occurs as shown:

$$CH_3 \overset{\overset{\displaystyle O^{+\bullet}}{\|}}{\underset{3}{C}} - NH_2 \xrightarrow{-CH_3} {}^+O \equiv C \text{-}\!\!\text{+}\!\!\text{o}\text{-} NH_2 \longleftrightarrow O = \underset{45}{C} = \overset{+}{N}H_2$$

$$\frac{M}{e} = 59 \qquad\qquad\qquad\qquad\qquad m/e\ 44$$
$$\text{(Base peak)}$$

(ii) Aromatic Amides

• These exhibit intense $M^{\ddagger}$ peak.

Example

Benzamide: The mass spectrum is shown in Fig. 18.56.

The fragmentation pattern:

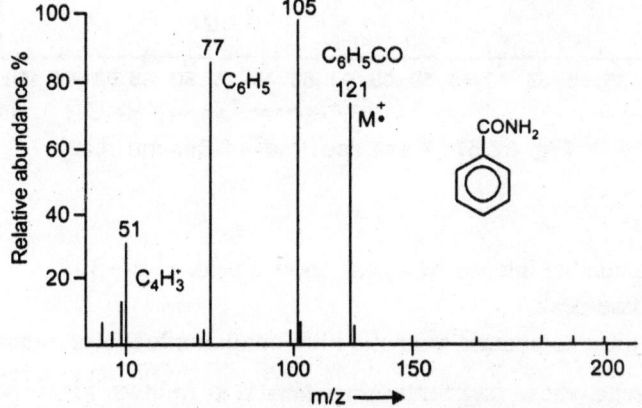

Fig. 18.56. Mass spectrum of Benzamide.

18. Nitriles

- In aliphatic nitriles, M^+ is very weak, practically not seen.
- M–1 peak is common due to loss of 1 H atom – a diagnostic peak.
- McLafferty rearrangement occurs in nitriles with γ–H.
- In aromatic nitrites M^{+} is intense. Spectrum of benzonitrile is shown in Fig. 18.57.

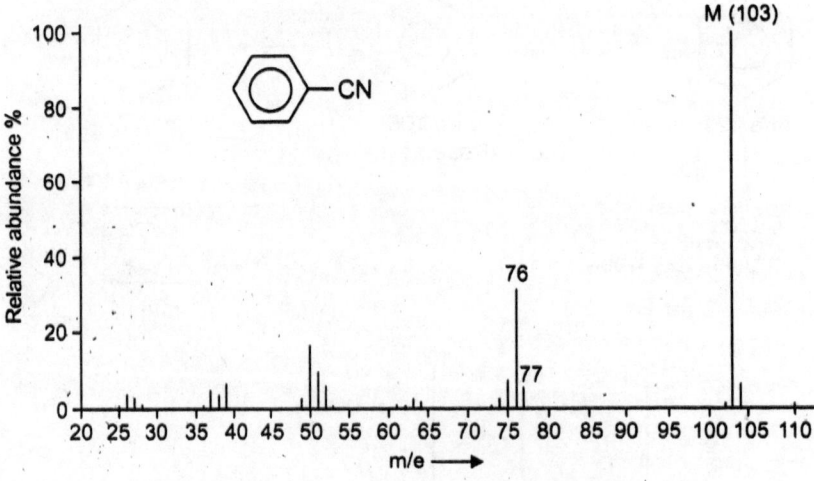

m/e 41 (Base peak)

$$\left[R—CH_2—C\equiv N \right]^{+\cdot} \longrightarrow R—CH=C\equiv N^+ + H^\bullet$$

m/e = 41 (Base peak)

Mass spectrum of benzonitrile.

Fig. 18.57. Mass spectrum of Benzonitrile.

19. Nitro compounds

- Aliphatic show moderate intense M^{+} peak show a peak at m/e 30.
- Show a weaker base peak.
- Unlike aliphatic nitro compound aromatic nitro compounds shows intense molecular ion peak.

Example: Nitrobenzene whose fragmentation pattern is as follows. Mass spectrum of nitrobenzene is shown in Fig. 18.58.

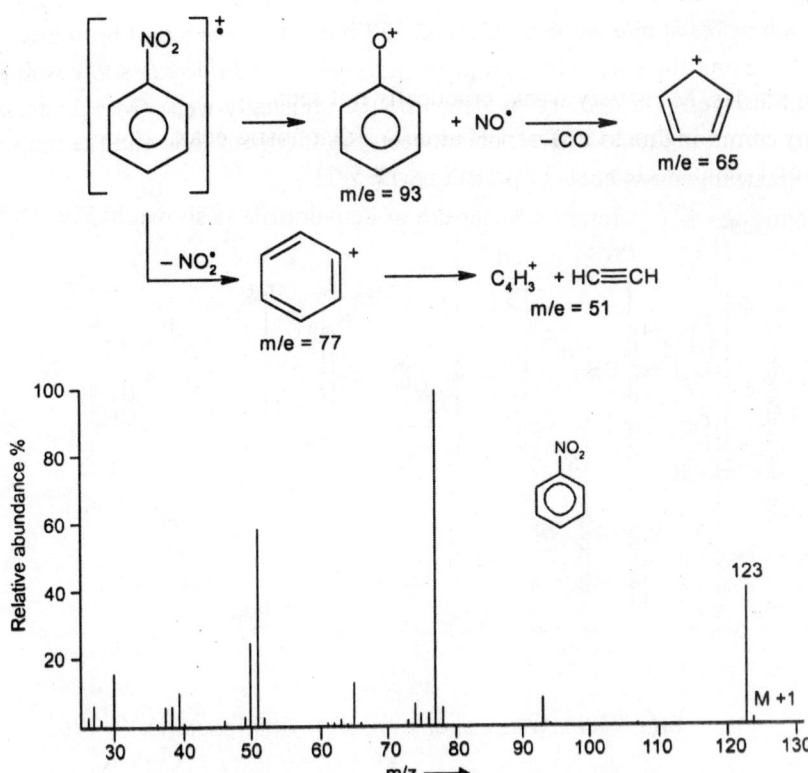

Fig. 18.58. Mass spectrum of Nitrobenzene.

20. Alkyl Halides

- Molecular ion M^{+} peak is strong.
- Most diagnostic peak is M + 2. M + 2 peak is also strong.
- The ratio M/M + 2 for Cl = 3:1.
- The ratio M/M + 2 for Br = 1:1.
- They fragment by losing a molecule of hydrogen halide.

$$\left[R-CH_2-CH_2-X \right]^{+\cdot} \longrightarrow \left[R-CH_2=CH_2 \right]^{+\cdot} + HX$$

- α-cleavage is also noted:

$$\left[R-CH_2-X \right]^{+\cdot} \longrightarrow R^{\cdot} + CH_2=X^{\oplus}$$

- An alkyl radical is also lost:

- Fragment ion peaks at m/e value of 135 and 137 indicate presence of bromine.
- As both iodine and fluorine exist isotope each in nature, they do not show isotopic peaks.
- Presence of halogen is elucidated by detecting the unusually weak (M + 1) peak. It can also be detected by observing mass difference between the fragment ions and the molecular ion. Mass spectrum of 1–chlorooctane is shown in Fig. 18.59.

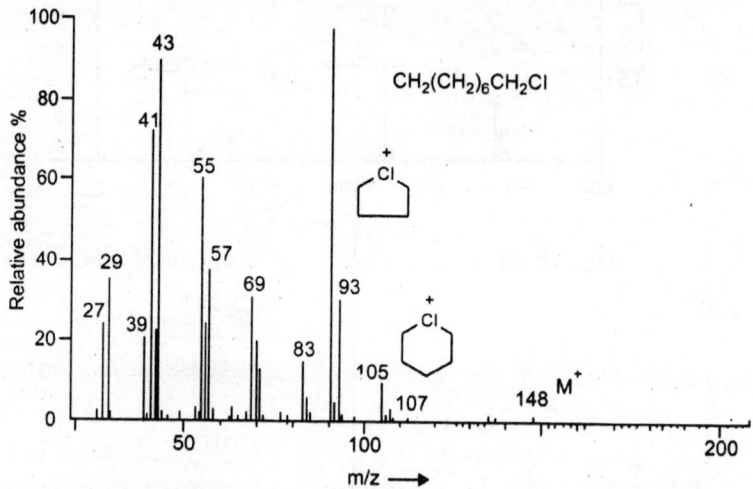

Fig. 18.59. Mass spectrum of 1–Chlorooctane.

21. Aryl Halides

- M^+ peak is sufficiently intense.
- Loss of halogen to Ar^+ is common.

$$C_4H_3^+ + C_2H_2$$
m/e 51

m/e 77

- Loss of halogen is common in benzyl halides to give $C_7H_7^+$ ion at m/e 91.

m/e 91   m/e 91

Mass spectrum of p-toluene iodide is shown in Fig. 18.60.

22. Peptide sequencing

By using MS peptide sequencing based upon Edman degradation can be achieved as shown in Fig. 18.61 and 18.62.

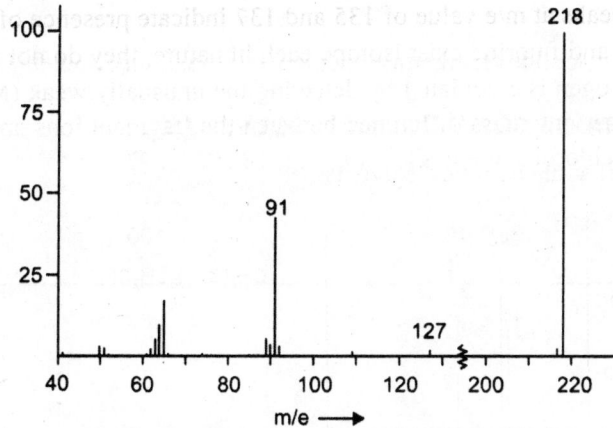

Fig. 18.60. Mass spectrum of p-toluene iodide.

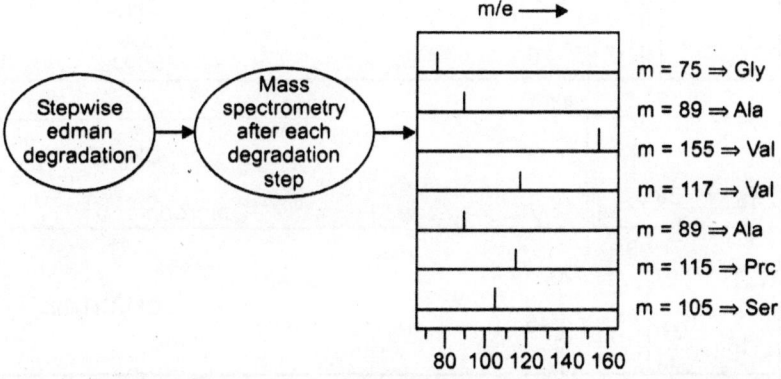

Fig. 18.61. Mass spectrometer in peptide sequencing by Edman degradation.

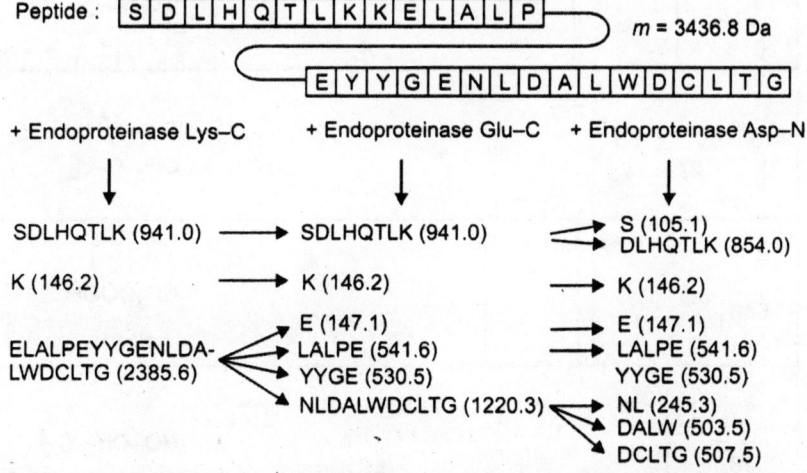

Fig. 18.62. Mass spectrometry and sequencing of the peptide SDLHQTLKKELALPEYYGENLDAL-WDCLTG. (proteolytic digestion).

23. DNA sequencing

Using Sanger dideoxynucleotide termination method and mass spectrometry.

18.28 MASS SPECTRA OF SOME COMMON SOLVENTS

Here are mass spectra of some common solvents:

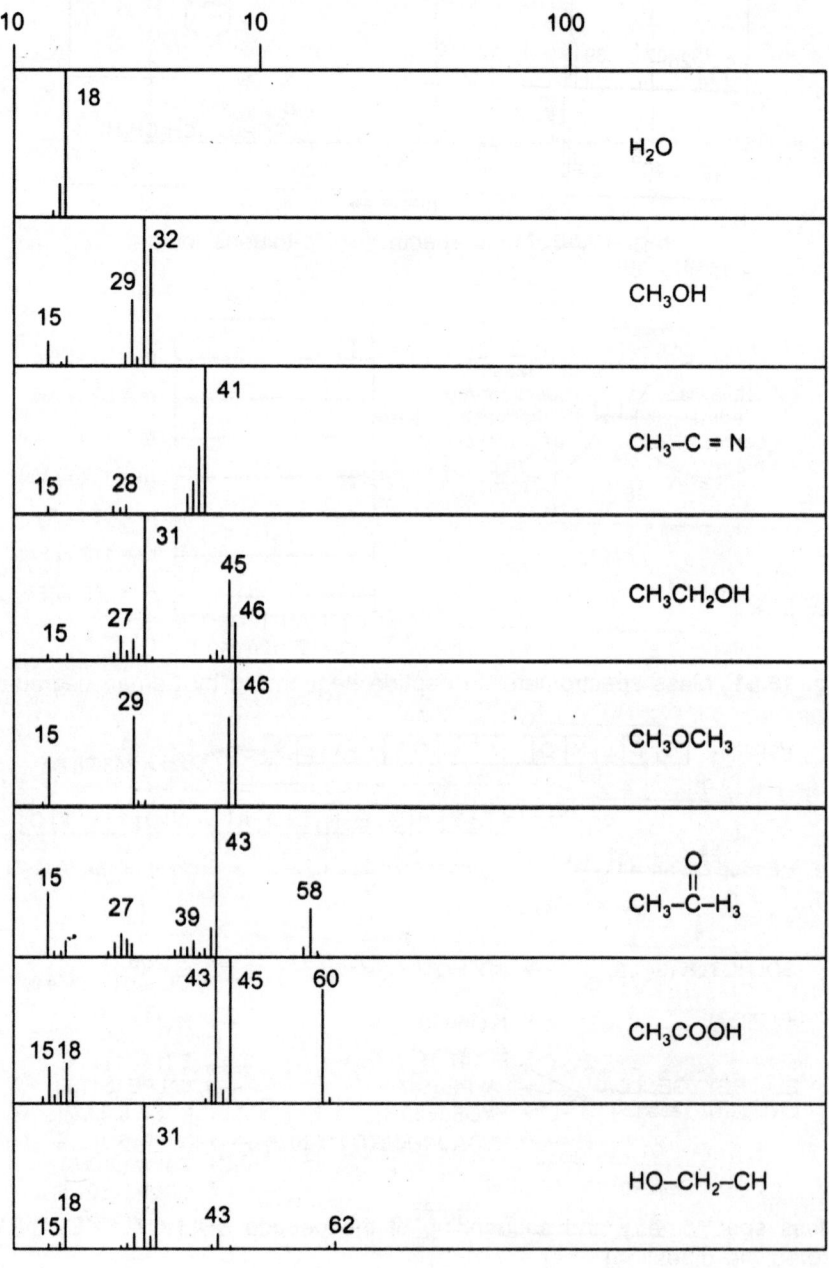

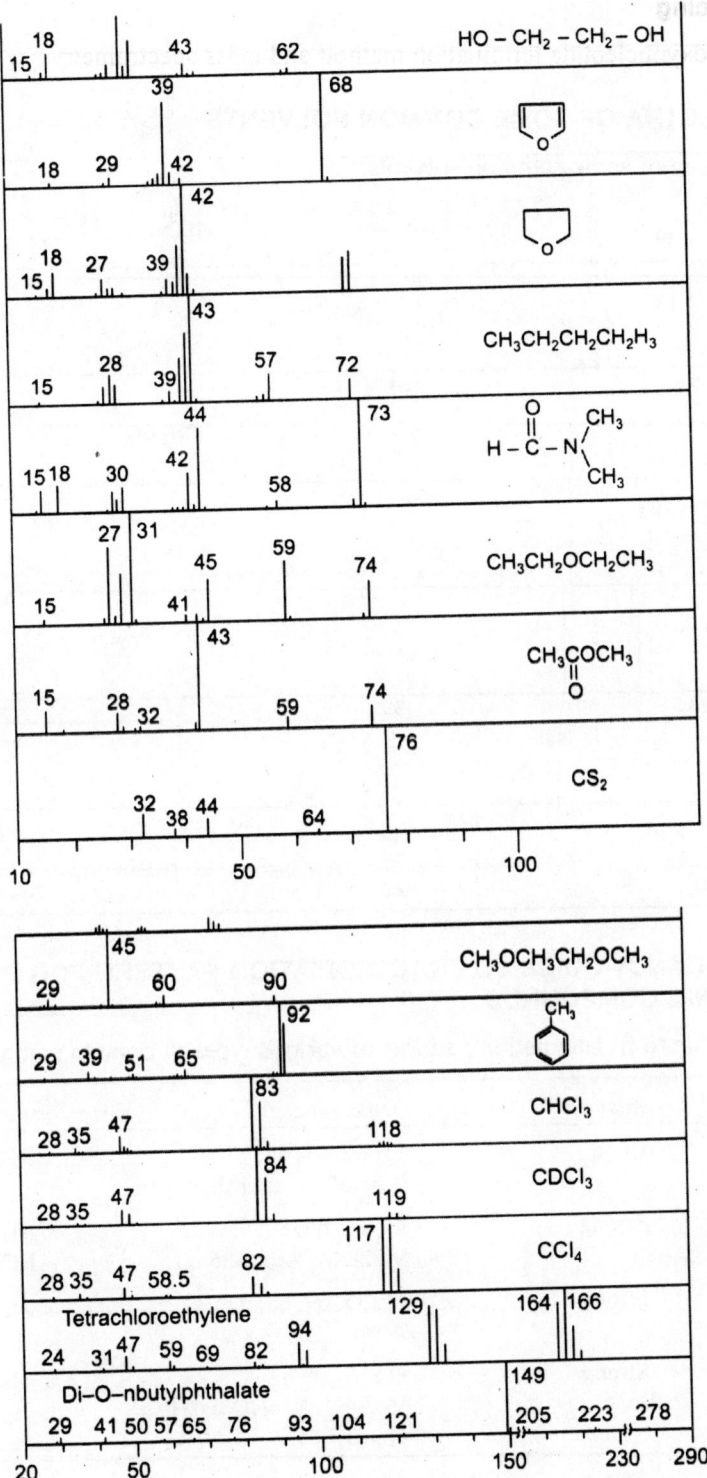

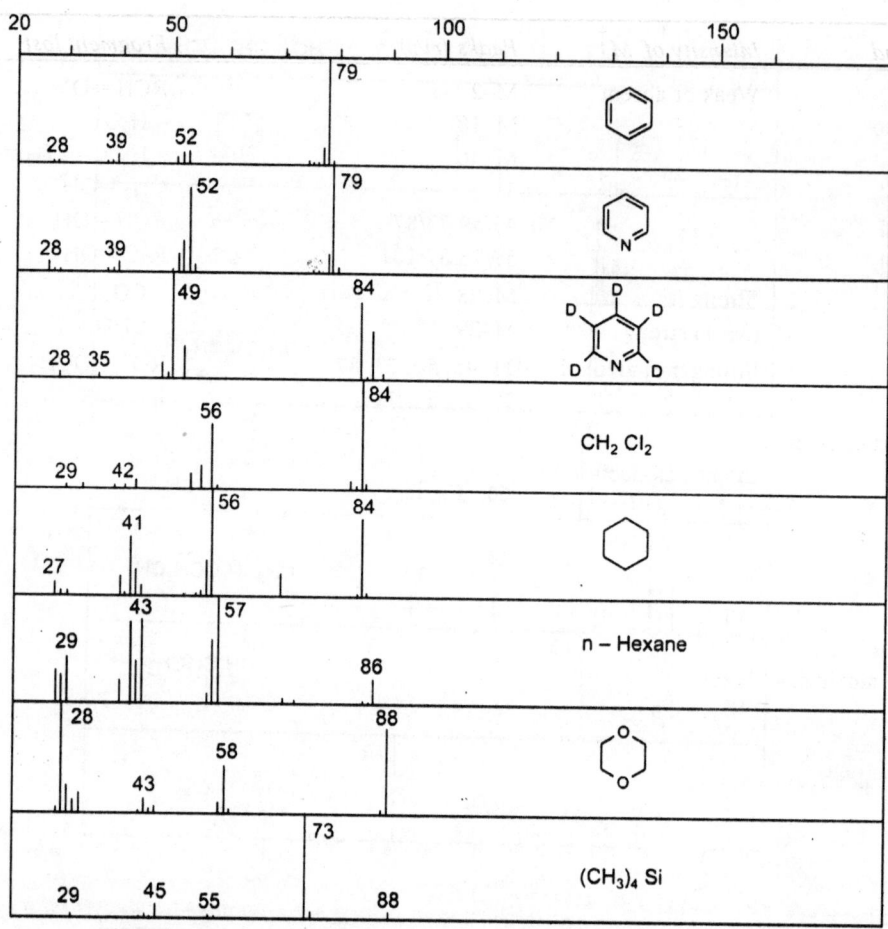

18.29 A HANDY-DANDY GUIDE TO FRAGMENTATION PATTERN FOR DIFFERENT TYPES OF ORGANIC COMPOUNDS

A handy-dandy guide to fragmentation patterns of various types in organic compounds is as follows:

Compound	Intensity of M^{+}	Peaks (m/z)	Fragment lost
1. Alkanes	Good	15, 29, 43, 57, 71 (loss of 14–amu fragments)	$C_nH_{2n+1}{}^+$
2. Cycloalkanes	Strong	41, 55, 69, 83, 97, ... M–28/M–42/M–56	$C_nH_{2n-1}{}^+$ $-RCN{=}CH_2$
3. Alkenes	Strong	41, 55, 69, 83, 97 77	$C_nH_{2n-1}{}^+$ $C_6H_5^+$
4. Aromatic (Benzenoids)	Strong	91 65 $\quad$ –HC ≡ CH 92	$C_7H_7^+$ $C_5H_5^+$ $C_7H_8^+$

(Contd.)

Compound	Intensity of M^{+}	Peaks (m/z)	Fragment lost
5. Alcohols	Weak or absent	M–2	$RCH{=}O^{+}$
		M–18	$-H_2O$
		M–46	$-H_2O, -CH_2{=}CH_2$
1° alcohol		31	$CH_2{=}OH^{+}$
2° alcohol		45/59/73/87	$RCH{=}OH^{+}$
3° alcohol		59/73/87/101	$R_2C{=}OH^{+}$
6. Phenols	Strong	M–28	$-CO$
	(M–1) strong	M–29	$-CHO$
7. Ethers	Stronger cf alcohols	31, 45, 59, 73, 87	$RO^{+}, ROCH_2{+}$
		29, 43, 57, 71	R^{+}
8. Thiols and sulfides			
Thiols	Intense cf alcohol	M–34	$-H_2S$
1°	M + 2 significant	47	$CH_2{=}SH^{+}$
2°		61/75/89/103	$RCH{=}SH^{+}$
3°		75/89/103/117	$R_2C{=}SH^{+}$
Sulfides		47/61/75/89	RS^{+}
9. Aldehydes			
Aliphatic aldehydes	Weak	M–1	$-H$
		M–29	$-CHO$
		44/58/72/86	$-RCH{=}CH_2$ (MCLafferty)
Aromatic aldehydes	Strong	M–1	$-H$
		M–29	$-H, -CO$
10. Ketones			
Aliphatic ketones	Intense	58/72/86/100	$-RCH{=}CH_2$ (MCLafferty)
Aromatic ketones		76 + mass of ring substituent(s)	$X{-}C_6H_{4+}$
		104 + mass of ring substituent(s)	$X{-}C_6H_4CO^{+}$
11. Carboxylic acids			
Acids	Weak	M–17	$-OH$
		M–45	$-COOH$
		M–28/M–42/M–56/M–70	$-RCH{=}CH_2$ (MCLafferty)
12. Methyl esters	Weak	M–31	$-OCH_3$
		M–59	$-CO_2CH_3$
		M–28/M–42/M–56/M–70	$-RCH{=}CH_2$ (MCLafferty)
13. Amines	Weak or absent		
Aliphatic amines		30, 44, 58, 72, 86	$RCHNH_{2+}$
Aromatic amines		M–1	$-H$
		M–2	$-$ⁿCN
		M–15/M–29/M–43	N-alkyl cleavage
14. Amides	Weak	M–15/M–29/M–43/M–57	N-alkyl cleavage
		M–28/M–42/M–56/M–70	$-RCH{=}CH_2$ (MCLafferty)

(Contd.)

Compound	Intensity of M^+	Peaks (m/z)		Fragment lost
15. Nitriles	Weak			
Aliphatic nitriles		M–1		– H
		M–28/M–42/M–56/M–70		– RCH=CH$_2$ (MCLafferty)
Aromatic nitriles		M–1		– H
		M–27		– HCN
16. Aromatic Nitro compounds	Seldom observed			
		M–30		– NO (with rearrangement)
		M–46		– NO$_2$
		M–58		– NO, – CO
		M–72		– NO$_2$, HC≡CH
17. Alkyl chlorides	Stronng doublet	M–36	M/M + 2 = 3:1	– HCl
		91		C$_4$H$_8$Cl$^+$
18. Alkyl bromides	(M$^+$, MH$_2$)	M–90	M/M + 2 = 1:1	–HBr
		135		C$_4$H$_8$Br$^+$

18.30 COMMON FRAGMENT IONS IN MASS SPECTROSCOPY

Here is the list of some common fragment ions observed in organic compounds.

m/e	Ions	Product ion
12	C$^+$	
13	CH$^+$	
14	CH$_2^+$, N$^+$, N$_2^{++}$, CO^{++}	
15	CH$_3^+$	M$^+$ – 15 (CH$_3$)
16	O$^+$, NH$_2^+$, O$_2^{++}$	M$^+$ – 16 (CH$_4$)
		(O)
		(NH$_2$)
17	OH$^+$, NH$_3^+$	M$^+$ – 17 (OH)
		(NH$_3$)
18	H$_2$O$^+$, NH$_4^+$	M$^+$ – 18 (H$_2$O)
19	H$_3$O$^+$, F$^+$	M$^+$ – 19 (F)
20	HF$^+$, Ar^{++}, CH$_2$CN^{++}	M$^+$ – 20 (HF)
21	C$_2$H$_2$O^{++}	
22	CO$_2^+$	
23	Na$^+$	
24	C$_2^+$	
25	C$_2$H$^+$	M$^+$ – 25 (C$_2$H)
26	C$_2$H$_2^+$, CN$^+$	M$^+$ – 26 (C$_2$H$_2$)
		(CN)
27	C$_2$H$_3^+$, HCN$^+$	M$^+$ – 27 (C$_2$H$_3$)
		(HCN)

(Contd.)

m/e	Ions	Product ion
28	$C_2H_4^+$, CO^+, N_2^+, $HCNH^+$	$M^+ - 28$ (C_2H_4)
		(CO)
		(N_2)
29	$C_2H_5^+$, CHO^+	$M^+ - 29$ (C_2H_5)
		(CHO)
30	CH_2O^+, $CH_2NH_2^+$, NO^+, $C_2H_6^+$, BF^+, $N_2H_2^+$	$M^+ - 30$ (C_2H_6)
		(CH_2O)
	N-indicator	NO
31	CH_3O^+, $CH_3NH_2^+$, CF^+, $N_2H_3^+$	$M^+ - 31$ (C_2H_6)
	O-indicator	(CH_3NH_2)
		(N_2H_3)
32	O_2^-, CH_3OH^+, S^+, $N_2H_4^+$	$M^+ - 32$ (CH_3OH)
	O-indicator	(S)
		(O_2)
33	$CH_3OH_2^+$, SH^+, CH_2F^+	$M^+ - 33$ ($CH_3 + H_2O$)
		(SH)
		(CH_2F)
34	SH_2^+ **S-indicator**	$M^+ - 34$ (SH_2)
		(OH + OH)
35	SH_3^+, Cl^+	$M^+ - 35$ (Cl)
		(OH + H_2O)
36	HCl^-, C_3^+	$M^+ - 36$ (HCl)
		($H_2O + H_2O$)
37	Cl^-, C_3H^+	
38	HCl^-, $C_3H_2^+$	
39	$C_3H_3^+$	$M^+ - 39$ (C_3H_5)
40	$C_3H_4^+$, CH_2CN^+, Ar^+	$M^+ - 40$ (CH_2CN)
41	$C_3H_5^+$, CH_3CN^+	$M^+ - 41$ (C_3H_5)
		(CH_3CN)
42	$C_3H_6^+$, $C_2H_2O^+$, CON^+, $C_2H_4N^+$	$M^+ - 42$ (C_3H_6)
		(C_2H_2O)
43	$C_3H_7^+$, $C_2H_3O^+$, $CONH^+$	$M^+ - 43$ (C_3H_7)
		(CH_3CO)
44	CO_2^+, $C_2H_6N^+$, $C_2H_4O^+$, $C_3H_8^+$, CH_4Si^+	$M^+ - 44$ (C_3H_8)
		(C_2H_6N)
		(C_2H_4O)
		(CO_2)
45	$C_2H_5O^+$, CHS^+, $C_2H_7N^+$	$M^+ - 45$ (C_2H_5O)
	O-indicator, S-indicator	(C_2H_7N)

(Contd.)

m/e	Ions	Product ion
46	$C_2H_5S^+$, NO_2^+	$M^{\ddagger} - 46$ (C_2H_6O)
		$(H_2O + C_2H_4)$
		$(H_2O + CO)$
		(NO_2)
47	CH_3S^+, CCl^+, $C_2H_5OH_2^+$, $CH(OH)_2^+$	$M^{\ddagger} - 47$ (CH_3S)
	S-indicator, 2 × O-indicator	
48	CH_3SH^+, $CHCl^+$, SO^+	$M^{\ddagger} - 48$ (CH_4S)
		(SO)
49	CH_2Cl^+, $CH_3SH_2^+$	$M^{\ddagger} - 49$ (CH_2Cl)
50	$C_4H_2^+$, CH_3Cl^+, CF_2^+	$M^{\ddagger} - 50$ (CF_2)
51	$C_4H_3^+$, CH_2Cl^+, CHF_2^+	
52	$C_4H_4^+$, CH_3Cl^+	
53	$C_4H_5^+$	
54	$C_4H_6^+$, $C_2H_4CN^+$	$M^{\ddagger} - 54$ (C_4H_6)
		(C_2H_4CN)
55	$C_4H_7^+$, $C_3H_3O^+$	$M^{\ddagger} - 55$ (C_4H_7)
56	$C_4H_8^+$, $C_3H_4O^+$	$M^{\ddagger} - 56$ (C_4H_8)
57	$C_4H_9^+$, $C_3H_5O^+$, $C_3H_2F^+$	$M^{\ddagger} - 57$ (C_3H_9)
		(C_3H_4O)
58	$C_3H_6O^+$, $C_3H_8N^+$	$M^{\ddagger} - 58$ (C_4H_{10})
	N-indicator, O-indicator	(C_3H_6O)
59	$C_3H_7O^+$, $C_3H_5ON^+$	$M^{\ddagger} - 59$ (C_3H_7O)
	O-indicator	
60	$C_2H_4O_2^+$, $CH_2NO_2^+$, $C_2H_7NO^+$	$M^{\ddagger} - 60$ (C_3H_8O)
	O-indicator	$(C_2H_4O_2)$
61	$C_2H_5O_2^+$, $C_2H_5S^+$	$M^{\ddagger} - 61$ $(C_2H_5O_2)$
	S-indicator, 2× O-indicator	(C_2H_5S)
62	$C_2H_6O_2^+$, $C_2H_3Cl^+$	$M^{\ddagger} - 62$ $(C_2H_6O_2)$
		(C_2H_6S)
63	$C_5H_3^+$, $C_2H_4Cl^+$, $COCl^+$	$M^{\ddagger} - 63$ (C_2H_4Cl)
		$(Cl + CO)$
64	$C_5H_4^+$, SO_2^+, S_2^+	$M^{\ddagger} - 64$ (SO_2)
		(S_2)
65	$C_5H_5^+$	$M^{\ddagger} - 65$ (S_2H)
66	$C_5H_6^+$	$M^{\ddagger} - 66$ (C_5H_6)
67	$C_5H_7^+$, $C_4H_3O^+$	$M^{\ddagger} - 67$ (C_4H_3O)
68	$C_5H_8^+$, $C_4H_3O^+$, $C_3H_6CN^+$	$M^{\ddagger} - 68$ (C_5H_8)
		(C_4H_4O)
69	$C_5H_9^+$, $C_4H_5O^+$, $C_3HO_2^+$, CF_3^+	$M^{\ddagger} - 69$ (C_5H_9)
		(CF_3)

(Contd.)

m/e	Ions	Product ion
70	C_5H_{10}	
	$C_4H_6O^+$	
	$C_4H_8N^+$	
71	$C_5H_{11}^+$	
	$C_4H_7O^+$	
72	$C_4H_8O^+$	
	$C_4H_{10}N^+$	
	C_6^+	
73	$C_4H_9O^+$	
	$C_3H_5O_2^+$	
	$C_3H_9Si^+$	
74	$C_4H_{10}O^+$	
	$C_3H_6O_2^+$	
75	$C_3H_7O_2$	
	$C_3H_7S^+$	
	$C_2H_7SiO^+$	
76	$C_6H_4^+$	
77	$C_6H_5^+$	
	$C_3H_6Cl^+$	
78	$C_6H_6^+$	
	$C_5H_4N^+$	
	$C_3H_7Cl^+$	
79	$C_6H_7^+$	
	$C_5H_5N^+$	
	Br^-	
80	$C_6H_8^+$	
	$C_5H_4O^+$	
	HBr^+	
81	$C_6H_9^+$	
	$C_5H_5O^+$	
82	$C_6H_{10}^+$	
	$C_5H_6O^+$	
	$C_5H_8N^+$	
	$C_4H_6N_2^+$	
83	$C_4H_{11}^+$	
	$C_5H_7O^+$	
84	$C_5H_{10}N^+$	
85	$C_6H_{13}^+$	
	$C_5H_9O^+$	

(Contd.)

m/e	Ions	Product ion
85	$C_5H_{10}O^+$	
87	$C_5H_{11}O^+$	
	$C_4H_7O_2$	
88	$C_5H_8O_2^+$	
89	$C_5H_9O_2^+$	
	$C_5H_9S^+$	
90	$C_7H_6^+$	
91	$C_7H_7^+$	
92	$C_7H_8^+$	
	$C_6H_6N^+$	
93	$C_6H_7O^+$	
	$C_6H_7N^+$	
	CH_2Br^+	
94	$C_6H_6O^+$	
	$C_5H_4NO^+$	
95	$C_5H_3O_2^+$	
96	$C_7H_{12}^+$	
97	$C_7H_{13}^+$	
	$C_6H_9O^+$	
	$C_5H_5S^+$	
98	$C_6H_{12}N^+$	
99	$C_7H_{15}^+$	
	$C_6O_{11}O^+$	
	$C_7H_7O_2^+$	
99	H_4PO^{+4}	
104	$C_8H_8^+$	
	$C_7H_4O^+$	
105	$C_8H_9^+$	
	$C_7H_5O^+$	
	$C_6H_5N_2^+$	
111	$C_5H_3OS^+$	
115	$C_9H_7^+$	
	$C_6H_{11}O_2^+$	
	$C_5H_7O_3^+$	
119	$C_9H_{11}^+$	
	$C_8H_7O^+$	
	$C_2F_5^+$	
	$C_7H_5NO^+$	

(Contd.)

m/e	Ions	Product ion
120	$C_2H_4O_2^+$	
	$C_8H_{10}N^+$	
121	$C_8H_9O^+$	
	$C_7H_5O_2^+$	
127	$C_{10}H_7^+ \cdot$	
	$C_7H_7O_3^+$	
	$C_6H_6NCl^+$	
	I^+	
128	$C_{10}H_8^+$	
	$C_6H_6OCl^+$	
	HI^+	
130	$C_9H_8N^+$	
	$C_9H_6O^+$	
131	$C_{10}H_{11}^+$	
	$C_5H_7S_2^+$	
	$C_3H_5^+$	
135	$C_4H_8Br^+$	
141	$C_{11}H_9^+$	
142	$C_{10}H_8N^+$	
149	$C_8H_5O_3^+$	

18.31 GAS CHROMATOGRAPHY–MASS SPECTROMETRY (GC–MS) AND 2D SPECTRA

This technique involves both gas chromatography and mass spectrometry wherein the latter essentially works as a detector. A GC/MS is shown in Fig. 18.63a, 18.63b, 18.63c and 18.63d. A mixture of the compounds to be separated is injected into the gas chromatograph. After the usual operation i.e. the mixture is vapourized in a heated chamber. The compound mixture now in the form of gas mixture is allowed to enter through a gas chromatograph column. The components get separated after interaction with the column. The fractions come out at different times. These fractions, as they exit from the GC are led into the ionization chamber of the mass analyzer that is usually a quadrupole mass analyzer which provides the mass spectra corresponding to the effluents. Mass spectro-meter based on this analyzer has high efficiency. This can fast scan the effluent before the next effluent is released from the GC. Thus, this is a very important analytical method. Fig. 18.63c shows the significance of GC/MS in biochemistry.

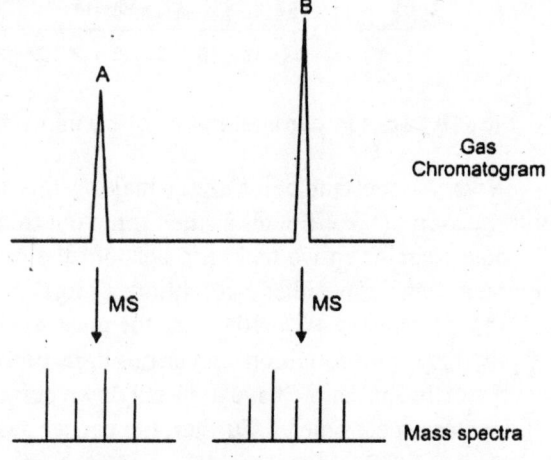

Fig. 18.63a. A GC/MS instrumental technique.

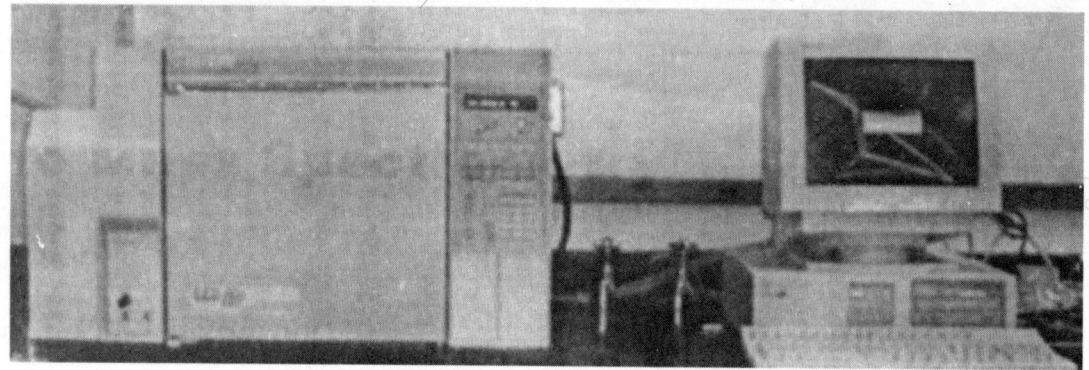

Fig. 18.63b. A GC-MS instrument.

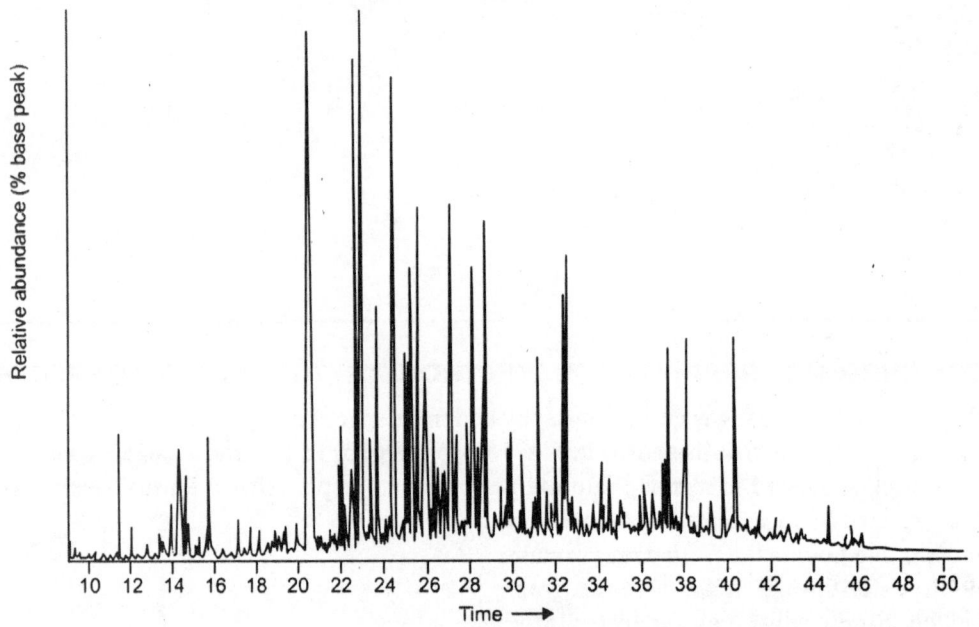

Fig. 18.63c. Ion chromatogram of human urine sample containing 1582 well identified peaks.

A very important point about making this combination of GC and MS work is related to the introduction of the effluents as they come out from GC into the MS such that the MS works. This would become clear when we take into account the conditions of pressure in both GC and MS. While GC operates under atmospheric conditions (1 torr), the MS operates at 10^{-5} torr as in EI or at 10^{-6} torr as in CI and typically at 10^{-6}–10^{-7} torr for mass analyzers. Therefore, it is very essential to maintain the required pressure conditions in various parts of the MS. In other words, the carrier gas flow rates which are typically 5 ml/min^{-1} have to be cut down before they are allowed to enter into the ionization chamber of the mass spectrometer. Further, the carrier gas has to be removed from the fractions.

Commercially available systems for coupling of GC with MS achieve this via an interface, the separator. They not only maintain the required pressure conditions but also enrich the concentration of

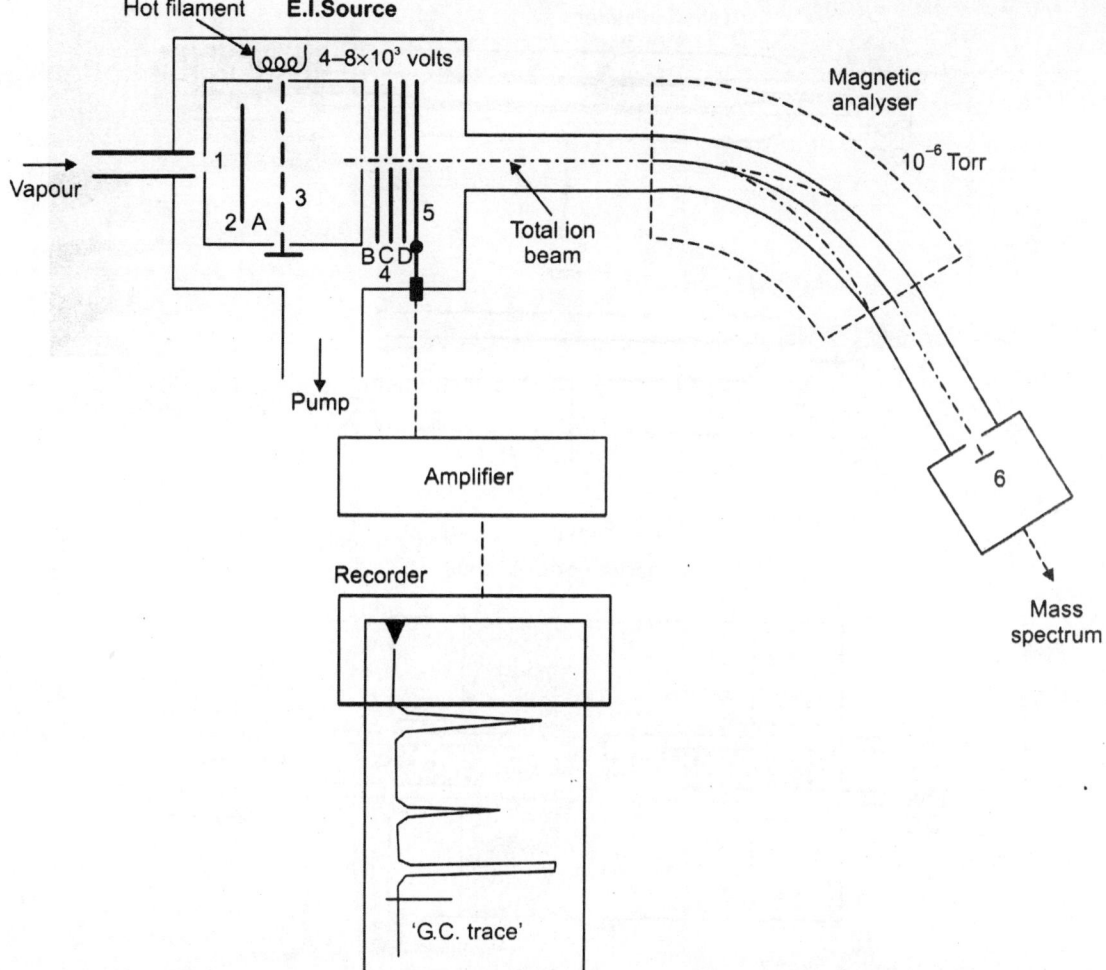

Fig. 18.63d. GC/MS functioning. Mass spectrometer : (1) sample inlet from GC/MS interface, (2) ion-repeller plate, (3) ionising electron beam, (4) plates for accelerating and focussing the ion beam, (5) total - ion monitor plate, (6) ion detector - usually an electron multiplier.

the fractions coming out of the GC before they enter the MS. The all glass single stage jet separator is a common interface among the various GC-MS interfaces available which are shown in Fig. 18.64.

Applications

- For separation of metabolites from natural compounds. This helps in investigating drug metabolism.
- Separation of barbiturates. A separation of all the twelve barbiturates has been demonstrated from a mixture.
- This is widely used for analysis of coffee containing food items.
- Pesticides and pollutants can be separated and identified.

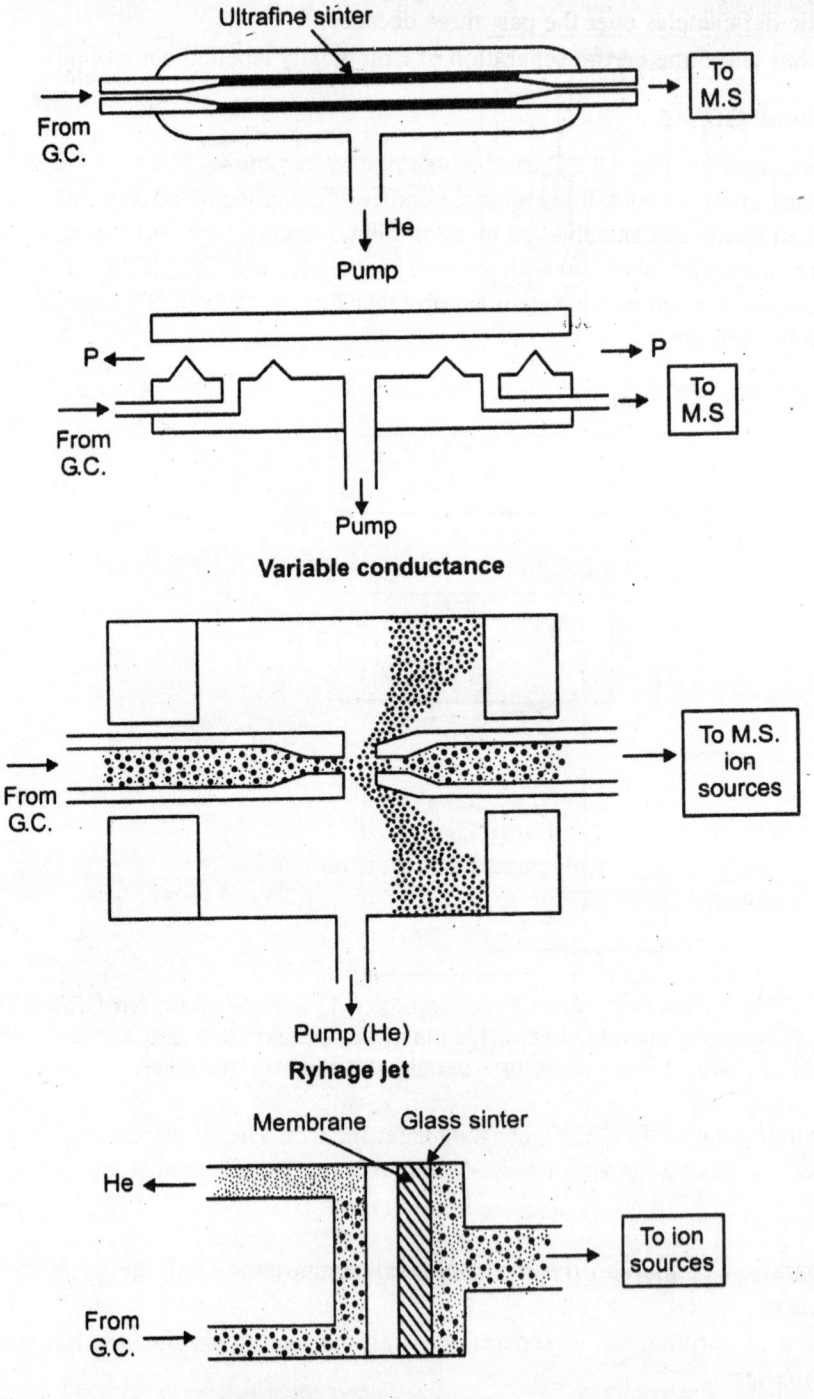

Variable conductance

Ryhage jet

Single stage membrane

Fig. 18.64. Various GC/MS interfaces.

- GC/MS technique for metabolic profiling has culminated in the discovery of many specific enzymatic deficiencies over the past three decades.
- GC/MS has led to the partial separation of isotopically labelled compounds.

Two-Dimensional GC/MS

Two-dimensional spectra (Fig. 18.65) can be obtained by combining MS with GC which enables us to study the complex mixtures containing a large number of components conveniently. A total resolution, R = 1000000 (ten lakh!) can be achieved by combining ion exchange chromatography on a crude cell extract with a resolution equal to 100 with a mass spectrometer with R = 10000. This has been achieved for small and medium-sized soluble cellular proteins for which both the methods are often largely independent from each other.

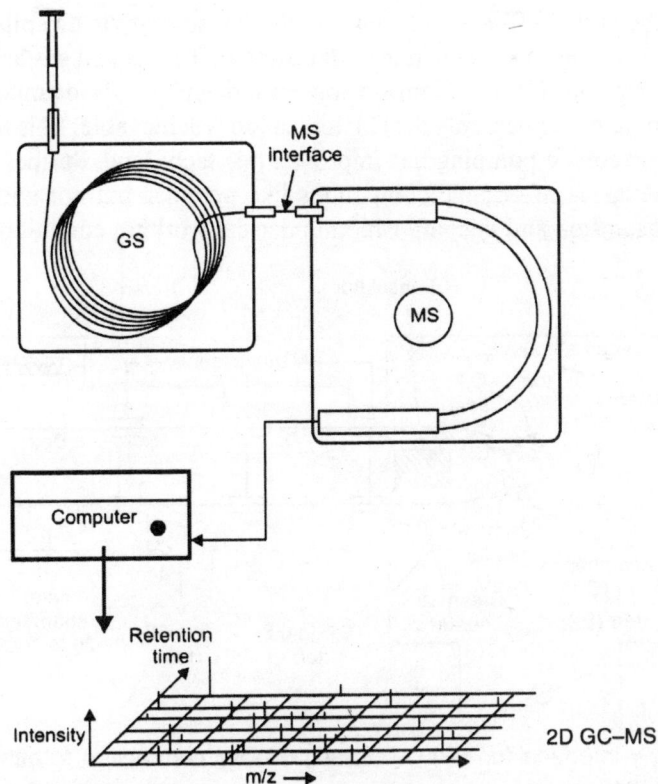

Fig. 18.65. GC/MS and two dimensional GC-MS spectrum.

18.32 HIGH PERFORMANCE LIQUID CHROMATOGRAPHY – MASS SPECTROMETRY (HPLC–MS)

In this technique, high performance liquid chromatography, one of the important separation method is combined with mass spectrometer. Consequently, this is used as a technique for separation as well as identification of constituents in mixtures. The mass spectrometer virtually serves as a detector. As in

GC-MS, the most important parameter for coupling HPLC with MS is to control the flow rates of the effluents from the HPLC column into the ionization chamber of the MS such that the MS is able to identify them. This is done through interface or separator. Many types of interfaces have been developed. The two main commercial interfaces are :

   1. Direct-insertion interface
   2. Moving belt (wire) interface

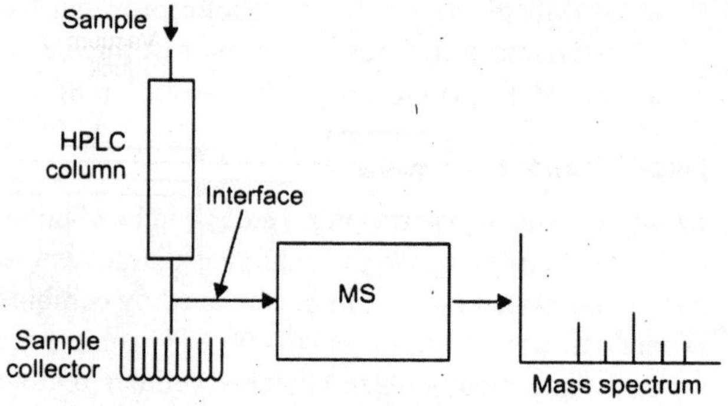

Fig. 18.66a. A schematic HPLC–MS instrument.

1. Direct-insertion interface

A proportion of the HPLC effluent is taken into the ion source via a capillary inlet (see Fig. 18.66b). The volatilized solvent becomes a chemical ionization (C.I.) reactant gas and the sample molecules are ionized by proton transfer from the ionized solvent molecules. Disadvantages are that only flow rates of 10–20 μL per minute. Further, only the C.I. ionization is achievable. EI is not workable here. Recently, however, cryogenic source pumping has improved this technique. Further, this technique works well only with certain classes of organic compounds like peptides but not with labile, in volatile solutes which undergo absorption and decomposition under the working conditions.

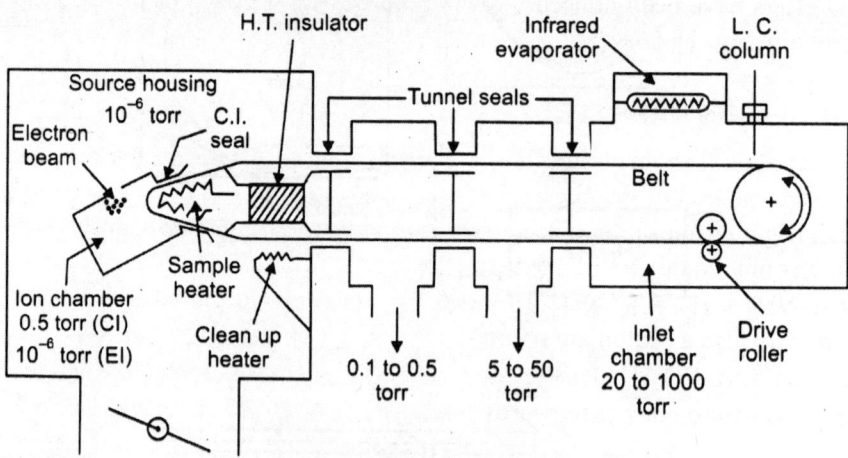

Fig. 18.66b. A new interface for HPLC-MS, suitable for connection to either quadrupole or magnetic sector spectrometers.

2. Moving belt (wire) interface

This is an endless moving belt as shown in Fig. 18.66c. What is done is that all the LC eluate is applied at one end of the belt. The solvent is evaporated off rapidly using an infrared heater. The analyte sample deposits are carried via a system of seals and vacuum chambers into the ion-source chamber. They are flash-evaporated from the belt surface in the ion source chamber.

   The advantage of this interface is that either CI or EI operations can be used with a choice of reactant gas in the CI mode. Either the quadrupole or the magnetic sector analyzer can be used.

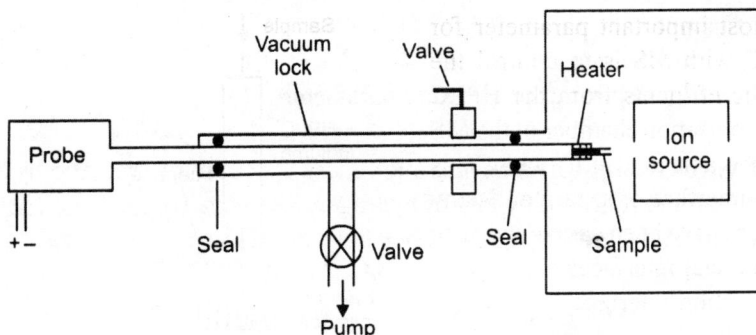

Fig. 18.66c. Direct insertion probe.

3. Thermospray interface

In this interface, partial or complete vaporization of a liquid occurs while it flows through the capillary tube, thereby generating a supersonic jet of vapour that contains a mist of fine particles plus the charges solvent droplets. The neutrals evaporate off from the droplets till the charge density of the droplets becomes very high making them unstable. The ions are evaporated from the surface. Evacuation of the ion chamber lowers down the pressure. As a result, this technique generates molecular and adduct ions of the involatile analyte. In fact, intact molecular ions for molecules like Vitamin B_{12}, dinucleotides, peptides and esters have been noticed in the m/z spectrum. A double sector MS in combination with HPLC is shown in Fig. 18.66a.

18.33 NEGATIVE ION MASS SPECTROMETRY AND APPLICATIONS

Although we have learnt about positive ion based mass spectrometry, the negative ions mass spectrometry based upon the formation of the negative ions is also known.

Positive or negative ionisation is decided by the nature of the functional groups present. For example, if the sample has functional groups that readily accept a proton (H^+) then positive ion ionization occurs.

Amines $R–NH_2 + H^+ = R–NH_3^+$ (proteins or peptides). On the other hand, when the functional groups that readily lose a proton are present, negative ion ionization occurs :

Carboxylic acids $R–CO_2H = R–CO_2^-$ and alcohols $R–OH = R–O–$ (saccharides or oligonucleotides).

When the negative ion m/z spectra are obtained, they often prove complementary to positive ion m/z spectra.

Modes of formation of negative ions

Three modes are known for the production of negative ions from a simple molecule when bombarded with electrons in the ionization chamber at 70 eV.

(i) Electron attachment also called resonance capture :

$$AB + e \longrightarrow AB^- \quad or \quad M + e \longrightarrow M^-$$

(ii) Dissociative resonance capture :

$$AB + e \longrightarrow A^{\bullet} + B^-$$

(iii) Ion-pair production:

$$AB + e \longrightarrow A^+ + B^- + e$$

All the three processes depend upon pressure parameter.

Example

1. **Aromatic Hydrocarbons :** The negative ion mass spectrum of aromatic hydrocarbons results from electron capture followed by loss of hydrogen. The negative ion mass spectra of anthracene and tetracene are shown in Fig. 18.64. Thus both of these show base peaks due to $(M)^-$. They also show peak at M + 15 which is due to $[(M - 1) O]^-$:

$$M + e \rightarrow [M - 1]^- \xrightarrow[+O]{H} [(M - 1) O]^- + H$$

2. Aldehydes, ketones, carboxylic acids, alcohols, esters, steroids show $[M - H]^-$ peaks.
3. Nitrocompounds show NO_2^- peaks.
4. Nitriles show CN^- peak.
5. Amino acids, peptides form very stable anions and so extensive fragmentation is prevented.

Note : Those molecules which do not form stable carbanions do not give interpretable mass spectra. Examples include thiophenes, ethers, lower mass hydrocarbons.

18.34 APPLICATIONS OF MASS SPECTROSCOPY TO PHARMACEUTICAL SCIENCES

1. Determination of Precise Molecular Mass

When the analyte molecular ion M^+ arrives at the detector intact i.e. without undergoing fragmentation, molecular ion peak whose m/e ratio corresponds to molecular mass of the original molecule is seen at the highest mass in the m/z spectrum. Further, as mass spectral patterns are reproducible, there is a library of published mass spectra for various types of functional groups. Thus, molecular mass of the investigated sample can be deduced on the basis of fragmentation. Instrument computers generally contain spectral libraries that can be searched for matches.

It should be noted that when atomic masses are determined even with sufficient precision, the molecular mass is not true. In fact, every isotopic mass is characterized by a small "mass defect". This is because the mass of each atom differs by some amount from a whole mass number. This is called nuclear packing fraction. High-resolution mass spectrometers take this into account and so give the precise molecular masses which help us in knowing the exact structure of the compound. The accuracy is 0.005% compared to $\pm$ (0.1–1%) by chemical method.

Further as mass spectral patterns are reproducible, there is a library of published mass spectra for various categories of functional groups. Thus, mass of the investigated sample can be deduced on the basis of fragmentation pattern. Instrument computers generally contain spectral libraries which can be searched for matches.

2. Determination of Molecular Formula

By Isotope Clusters

Molecular formula of an analyte sample can be determined by examining relative intensities of peaks due to M^+ molecular ion and the related ions containing more heavy isotopes. This is based on the fact that isotopes occur in compounds analyzed by mass spectrometry in the same abundances that they occur in nature.

Illustration

Example 1: Methylbromide: Methylbromide, CH_3Br which contains the common isotope of bromine with mass 79, shows a M^+ peak at m/z 94. Let us now imagine that the molecule contains a heavy isotope Br–81. Therefore, it should show another peak at m/z 96 ($M + 2$) and with a relative abundance of 98% compared to 100% per the peak at m/e 94. This is because the isotopes occur in the same abundance as they occur in nature. And indeed the mass spectrum shown in Fig. 4., shows two peaks at m/z 94 and m/z 96 in the relative ratio of 1.020 (100/98).

CH_3–Br	Observed	Natural abundance
79BrCH$_3$ m/z 94	100	100
81BrCH$_3$ m/z 96	98	98

Thus, it is evident that the m/z spectrum is due to methyl bromide, CH_3Br. This is how isotopic peak ratio helps us in identifying the M^+ ion and in deducing the molecular formula. An $M + 1$ peak appears at m/e 95 with a relative abundance of 6.1.

Example 2 : Ethane containing most common isotopes of C and H has molecular mass of 30, as per its molecular formula C_2H_6. Its m/z peak at m/z 30. Let us now imagine one carbon atom is a heavy isotope C–13. So the m/z spectrum should contain a peak at m/z 31 and its relative intensity would be 1.08% in mass spectra, the isotopes occur in the same abundances as they occur in nature. Now ethane molecule contains two carbons, therefore, we will see a peak at m/z 31 with a relative abundance of 2.16%. This is induced so.

Similarly, let us imagine a H atom of ethane being replaced by a deutrium atom ^2_1H (D), the molecule should show an additional peak at M + 1 value i.e. 30 + 1 = 31. What would be its intensity like? Because the natural abundance of deutrium is just 0.016% of that of a H atom, the intensity of the peak at m/e 31 should be 0.016 multiplied by six i.e. 0.096% of that of molecular ion (M^+) peak. Further as the molecule may contain one C–13, the total intensity of M + 1 peaks should be (0.096 + 2.16%) = 2.26% to that of molecular ion peak, M^+.

Molecular formula by comparison of intensities of M^+, M + 1 and M + 2 peaks (isotopic ratio) :

1. Number of carbon atoms in the analyte sample can be obtained from the relative heights say h of M^+ and h + 1 of (M + 1) ions respectively. This is given by the formula :

$$\text{No. of C atoms} = \frac{100(h + 1)}{1.1h}$$

This is because the natural abundance of C–13 relative to C–12 is 1.1%.

2. An odd molecular weigh points out at the presence of odd number of nitrogen atoms.
3. An intense M + 2 peak hints at the presence of chlorine and bromine. A less intense M + 2 peak points out the presence of sulfur.
4. When a compound has two chlorine or bromine atoms, M + 4 peak, a very clear cut peak is observed along with an intense M + 2 peak.
5. When two molecules have about the identical molecular mass, the relative intensities of the M + 1 and M + 2 peaks would clearly prove them different.
6. In order to deduce molecular formula of the sample analyte, it is necessary to know the accurate mass of M^+, the molecular ion. Tables or calculations can be used on Beynon and Withams

work. For an illustration consider the M^+ peak at m/e 100 in a m/z spectrum. This can correspond to the following elemental compositions.

M^+	Mass (accurate)
$C_3H_6N_3O$	100.0511
$C_4H_8N_2O$	100.0637
$C_5H_{10}NO$	100.0762
C_7H_{16}	100.1251

In the accurate mass was found to be 100.0760, the precise M.F. would be $C_5H_{10}NO$.

For all combinations of common elements having M.F. upto mass of 500, relative values of M + 1 and M + 2 ion peaks are available in the tables.

3. Warfare agents

The armies use mass spectrometers to detect the presence of chemical warfare agents in the war-zone. Thus, poisonous gases can be detected well on time.

4. Biotechnology

The analysis of proteins, peptides and oligonucleotides.

5. Pharmaceutical

Drug discovery, combinatorial chemistry and pharmacokinetics, drug metabolism.

6. Clinical

Neonatal screening, haemoglobin analysis and drug testing.

7. Environmental

Pollutants like PCBs, PAHs, water quality, PCDDs, PCDFs, food contamination etc.

8. Geological: Oil composition

This is based on the fact that there occurs small change in the isotopic composition of elements with time. For instance, as dead organisms cease to take up C–14, the date of death of the organisms can be found out by determining C–14 content in the fossil materials. Similarly pure tropical fruit juice is distinguished from the concentrations diluted locally by determining H/D ratio of water which is latitude dependent. Further S–34 isotope enables us to find out the origin of the fossil fuels.

9. Biochemistry

(i) **Precise molecular weight measurements:** These help us to determine the purity of a sample, amino acid and the number of disulphide bridges.

(ii) **Reaction monitoring:** This includes enzyme reactions, chemical modification, protein digestion.

(iii) **Amino acid sequencing:** This includes sequence confirmation, de novo characterisation of peptides and identification of proteins by database searching with a sequence "tag" from a proteolytic fragment.

(iv) **Oligonucleotide sequencing:** This means the characterisation or quality control of oligonucleotides.

(v) **Protein structure:** This implies protein folding monitored by H/D exchange, protein-ligand complex formation under physiological conditions and macromolecular structure determination.

10. Investigation of Metabolism

Mass spectrometry is a particularly sensitive technique for detection of metabolites at low concentrations. Fig. 18.67 illustrates the use of desorption electrospray ionization mass spectra (DESI-MS) for urine samples from individuals with inborn metabolism errors such as Phenylketonuria (PKU), homocystinuria (HCY), maple syrup urine disease (MSUD).

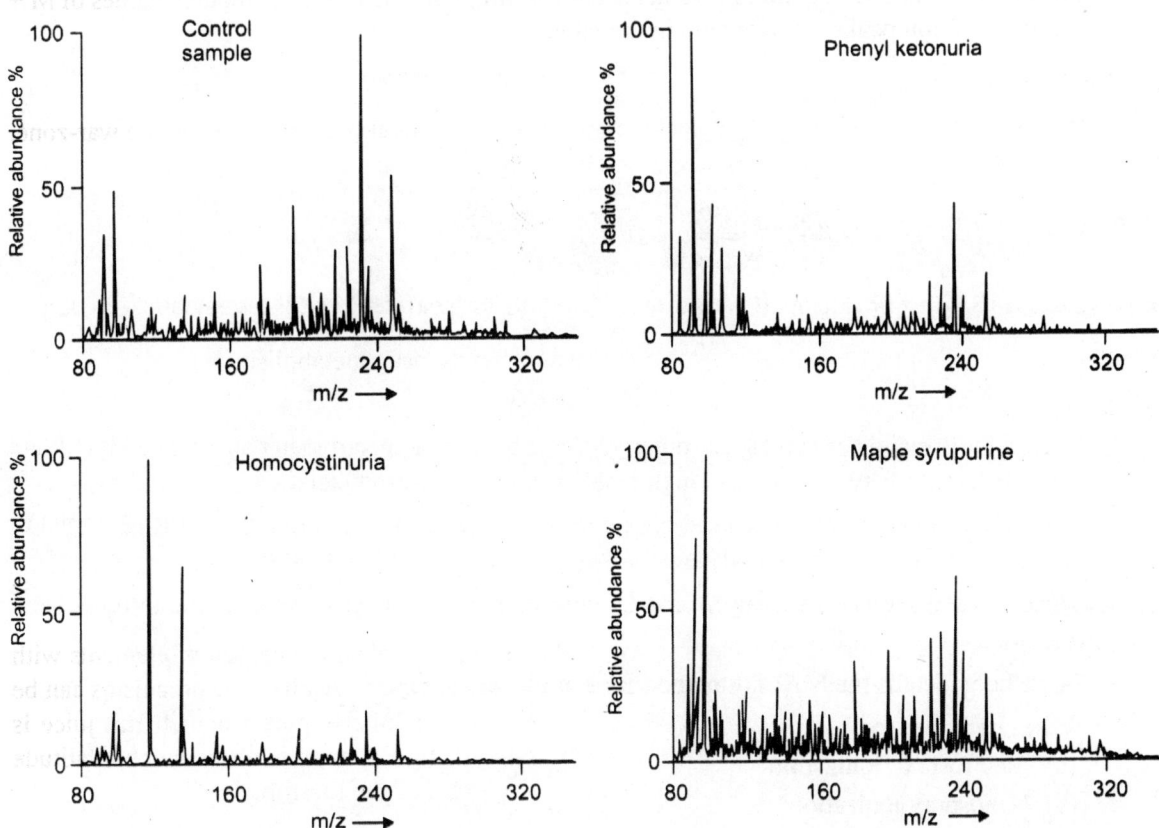

Fig. 18.67. Mass spectroscopy in abnormal metabolism.

Further, the combination of mass spectrometry with gas chromatography (GC-MS) enables us to resolve as well as identify hundreds of metabolites.

11. Investigation of Metabolism

Already mass spectrometry has been in use for searching extraterrestrial life in meteorites shows the use of Rovers fitted with mass spectrometers by NASA in this connection 18.68.

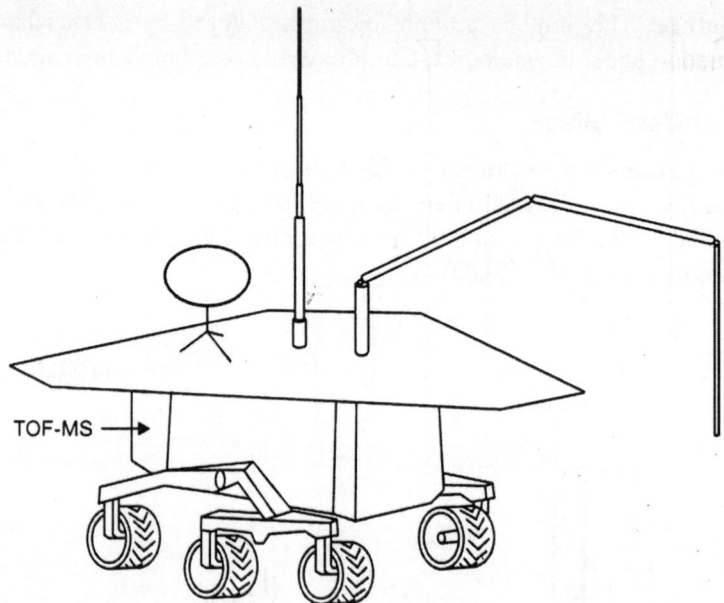

Fig. 18.68. NASA's rover equipped with a mini TOF–MS for searching extra-terrestrial life in space.

PROBLEMS

1. What is the principle of mass spectrometry? Describe a mass spectrometer and its working. What is the difference between low and high resolution mass spectrometers?

2. Name the eight commonly used sample ionization methods and describe CI and FAB methods. Which are hard and soft methods among these?

3. What is the difference between EI and CI ionization methods? Give an example to prove your reasoning.

4. Describe in details the MALDI method for sample ionization.

5. Write short notes on :
   (a) Electrospray ionization
   (b) Nanospray ionization
   (c) Thermospray ionization
   (d) Field desorption (field ionization)

6. Which is superior between EI and CI methods for ionization? Give an example to support your answer. Compounds that are either involatile or thermally unstable, these cannot be analyzed by the EI or CI methods. What technique would you prefer to use in order to get their m/z spectra.

7. What is Tandem mass spectrometry (MS/MS)? Explain in details.

8. What is an analyzer? Enlist all the analyzers available with their highlights.

9. The m/e spectrum of the hydrocarbon (A) is shown below. Explain its fragmentation pattern.

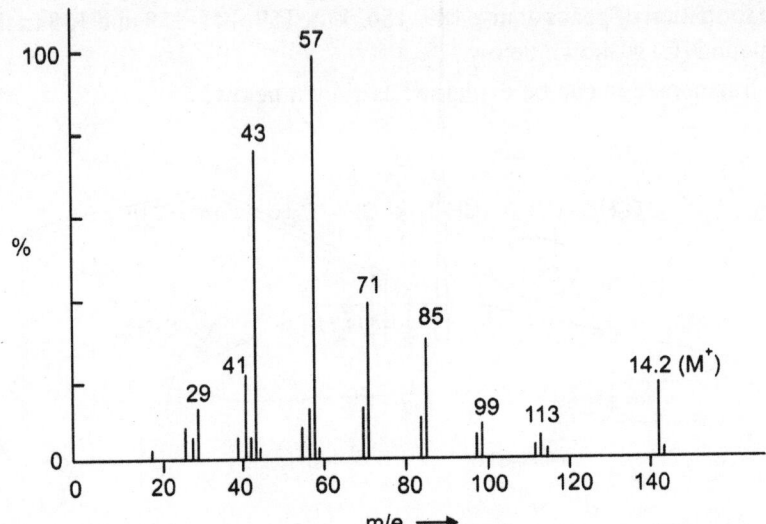

Hint :

$$CH_3 \;\; CH_2 \mid CH_2 \mid CH_2 \mid CH_2 \mid CH_2 \mid CH_2 \mid CH_2 \mid CH_2 \;\; CH_2$$

$$29 \quad 43 \quad 57 \quad 71 \quad 85 \quad 99 \quad 113$$

10. Explain fragmentation pattern of the m/e spectrum of the ketone (B) is shown below.

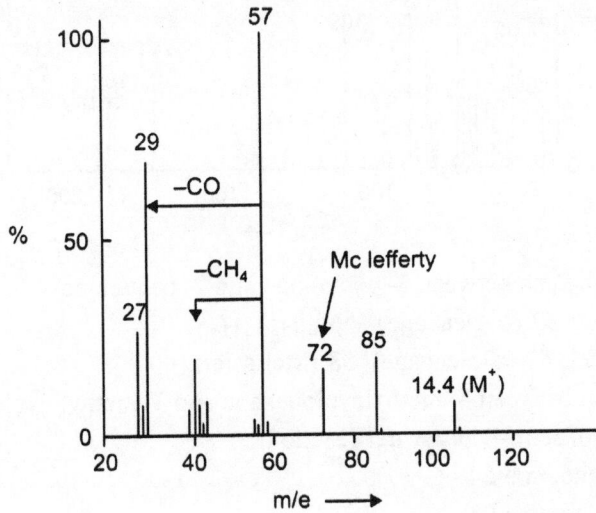

Hint :

$$\overset{57}{} \qquad \overset{85}{}$$

$$CH_3 \;\; CH_2 \mid \overset{}{\underset{\underset{O}{\parallel}}{C}} \mid CH_2 \;\; CH_2 \mid CH_2 \;\; CH_3$$

$$\underset{85}{} \qquad \qquad O \;\; 57$$

11. Explain the formation of peaks at m/e 189, 186, 171, 157, 141, 139 and 138 in the mass spectrum of the compound (C) is shown below.

    Ans. : The fragmentation can be explained as shown below.

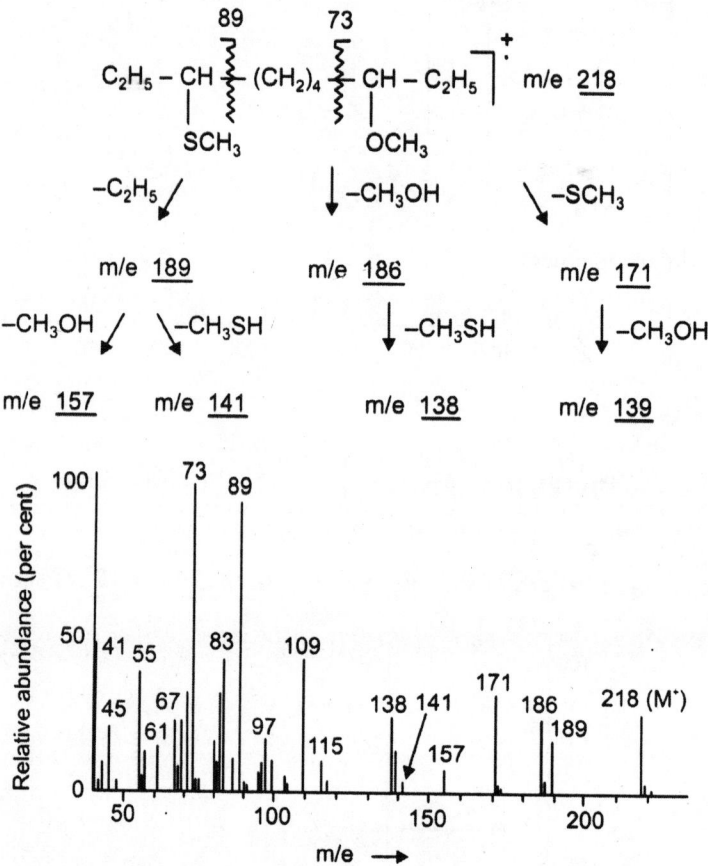

12. How will you distinguish between 3–pentanone and 2–pentanone?

    Hint: 3–Pentane: m/e 57 (α-cleavage), $29(CH_3 \overset{+}{C}H_2)$.

    2–Pentanone: m/e 71, 43 (α-cleavage), 58 (McLafferty).

13. Can you distinguish between 4–methylcyclohexane and 3–methyl cyclohexane.

    Hint: On the basis of retro-Diels-Alder reaction:

    4–methylcyclohexane: m/e 54

    3–methylcyclohexane: m/e 98

14. A bromo organic compound shows two equal intensity peaks at m/e 122 (M^+) and 124 in the highest mass region. Assign a suitable M.F. to this compound.

    Hint: As $M^+/M + 2$ ratio is 1:1, therefore, this indicates the presence of Bromine. If we deduct 79 from molecular mass 122, we are left with 43 mass units to be accounted for. Hence, the compound should be C_3H_7Br.

15. Explain the fragmentation pattern of 1–pentanol and Diethylamine.

16. Depict the fragmentation pattern of 2–pentene and pentanoic acid.

17. How will you distinguish among the following isomeric compounds on the basis of mass spectroscopy.

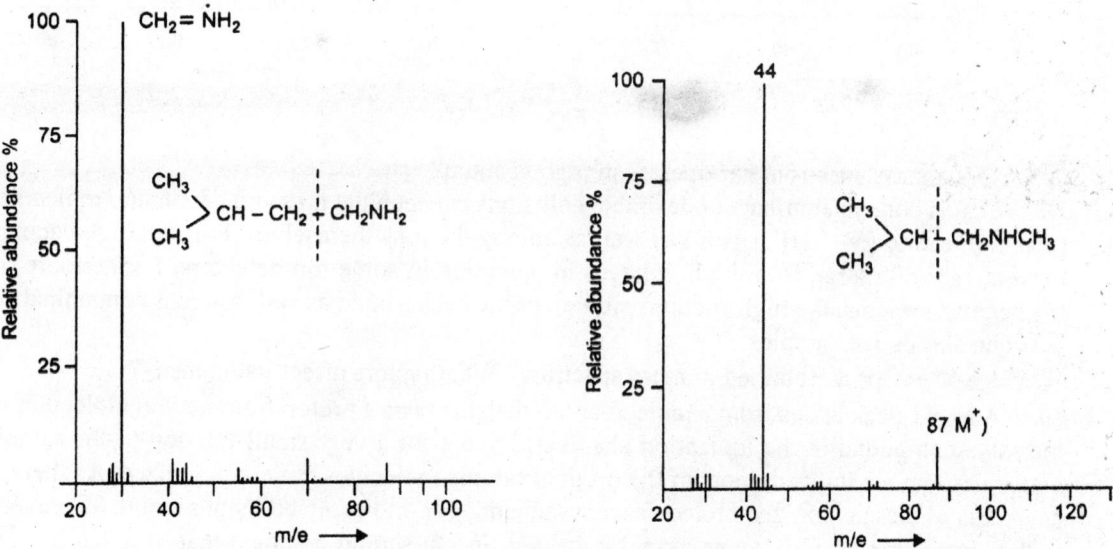

Hint: McLafferty rearrangement.

18. How will you distinguish between the following on the basis of mass spectroscopy:

$$\begin{array}{c} H_3C \\ \diagdown \\ H_3C \diagup \end{array} CHCH_2CH_2NH_2 \quad and \quad \begin{array}{c} H_3C \\ \diagdown \\ H_3C \diagup \end{array} CH-CH_2NHCH_3$$

Hint: See their mass spectra given below.

19. How can mass spectroscopy enable us to distinguish between the following isomeric alcohols.

$$CH_3CH_2CH_2CH_2OH \quad and \quad CH_3-CH_2-\underset{\underset{OH}{|}}{CH}-CH_3$$

Hint: Write their fragmentation patterns and compare the results on the basis of their spectra given below.

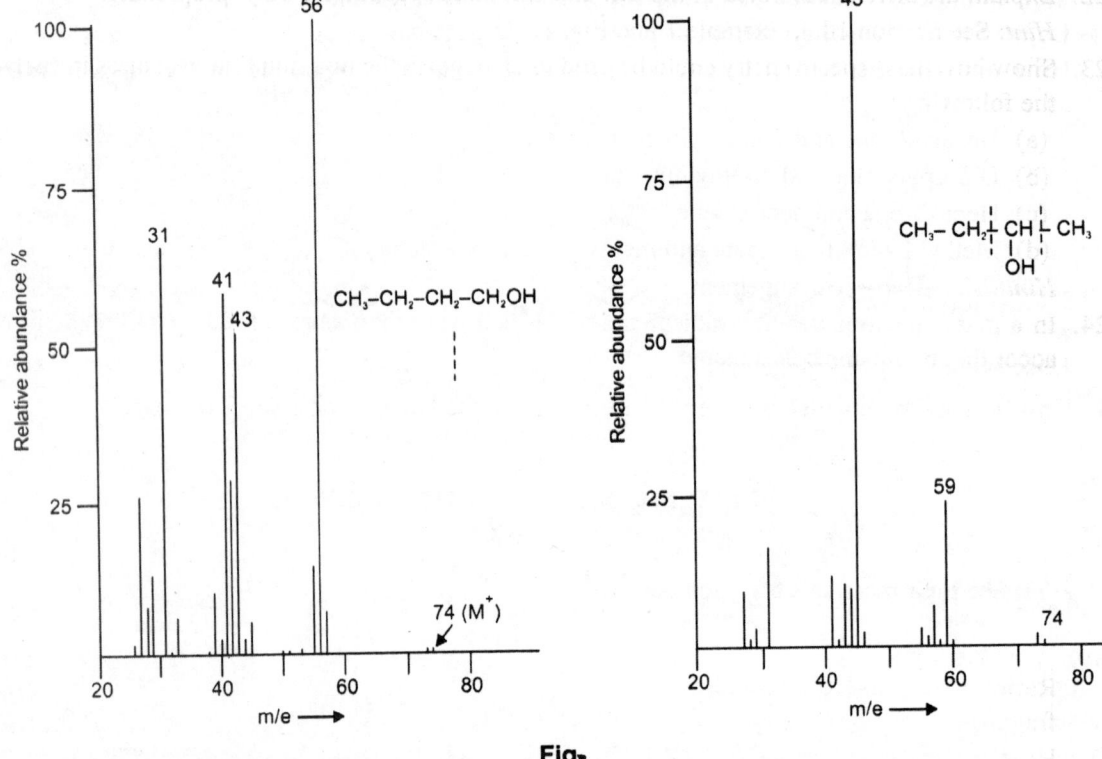

Fig.

20. Why does a mass spectrometer operate in high vacuum?

Hint: That is done to eliminate undesirable collisions between the ions and the neutral molecules (that can lead to $[M + H]^+$ signal) as well as among the ions themselves. Further, high vacuum prevents gas discharge from high voltages in operation in some ion detectors. Furthermore, in hyphenated systems, the high vacuum minimizes the background as well as cross contamination between successive samples.

21. Why is a M + 1 peak obtained in mass spectrum? What factors affect its intensity?

Hint: A M + 1 peak arises from a molecular ion that abstracts a proton from neutral molecules of the same compound in the ionization chamber. Except for a very small fraction of the sample molecules that are ionized, most of the original sample molecules remain unionized. As there is an excess of these unionized molecules, consequently ion-molecule collisions result. These lead to the abstraction of a hydrogen atom by the M^{+} ion. It should be noted that M + 1 peaks are very important in compounds like ethers, esters, nitriles, amines etc. whose M^{+} ions are unstable compared to protonated M + 1 ions. Among the factors which govern the intensity of the M^{+} ion, sample pressure in the ionization chamber is an important parameter. The intensity of the M + 1 $[M + H]^+$ peak is proportional to the square of the sample pressure as it is formed in a bimolecular process. With increase in the sample pressure, the intensity of the M + 1 peak relative to other peaks increases. Further, as the repeller plate potential increases, the intensity of the M + 1 peak decreases, as the probabilities of collisions between molecular ion and the neutral (un-ionized) sample molecules decreases.

22. Explain the differences noted in the E.I. and C.I. mass spectra of n-butyl propionate.

    Hint: See Section 18.9, Example 2 and Fig. 18.7.

23. Show how mass spectrometry could be used to distinguish the two isomeric structures in each of the following pairs:

    (a) Hexan–2–one and 3–methylpentan–2–one

    (b) Dipropylamine and N-ethylbutylamine

    (c) Hept–2–ene and hept–3–ene

    (d) Methyl 2–aminobenzoate and methyl 3–aminobenzoate

    Hint: McLafferty rearrangement.

24. In a mass spectrometer, the radical-cation derived from the natural product (A) breaks down according to the annexed scheme:

$$m/z \quad 314 \xrightarrow{-CH_3} 299$$

$$314 \xrightarrow{-C_4H_8} 258$$

$$314 \xrightarrow{-C_5H_8} 246 \xrightarrow{-CH_3} 231$$
$$\text{(Base peak)}$$

(A); M = 314

Rationalise these observations in terms of commonly encountered mass spectrometric fragmentation processes.

How could it be shown that the m/z 231 ion is formed by the route shown above rather than by an alternative route involving loss of CH_3 followed by loss of C_5H_8?

25. The EI mass spectrum of an alkaloid believed to possess structure A, show prominent ion peaks at m/z 273 ($C_{17}H_{23}NO_2$; M^+), 258, 216 ($C_{14}H_{13}NO$), 152 ($C_9H_{14}NO$), 110 and 94 (base peak). Show how these ions could be formed from structure A according to well-known types of mass spectrometric cleavage processes.

26. How would you know whether or not halogens are present in the given sample by Mass Spectrometry?

    Hints:

    (i) **Monohalogenated compounds**: The mass spectrum readily shows whether or not halogens are present in the given test compound. As chlorine is present as either of two isotopes ^{35}Cl and ^{37}Cl, the mass spectrum of monochlorinated compound contains two parent peaks, $[M + 1]^+$ and $[M + 2]^+$, separated by two atomic mass units and of heights in the ratio 3:1 (note this is also the ratio of their natural abundances). Similarly, bromine shown two parent peaks $[M + 1]^+$ and $[M + 2]^+$, corresponding to two isotopes ^{79}Br and ^{81}Br separated by two atomic mass units but in the ratio of 1:1 in their heights (Note: This is also the ratio of their natural abundances).

(ii) **Polyhalogenated compounds:** (n + 1) Peaks are observed for polyhalogenated compounds containing (n) halogens, their ratio being dependent upon the halogens being present. For two bromine atoms, a 1:2:1 triplet of peaks is observed; for two chlorine atoms the ratio is 9:6:1; for one chlorine and one bromine atom, the ratio observed is 3:4:1.

MULTIPLE CHOICE QUESTIONS FOR NET, SLAT, GAIT, GPAT, CSE, HCS, GRE ETC. COMPETITIVE EXAMS

1. The electromagnetic rays used in mass spectroscopy are:
   (a) IR
   (b) Microwaves
   (c) Radiowaves
   (d) None
   Hint: (d).

2. Which does not apply to mass spectrometry?
   (a) Ionization of molecules and vacuum
   (b) Magnetic field
   (c) Acceleration of charged particles
   (d) Microwaves
   Hint: (d).

3. The fundamental equation that makes detection of charged particles possible in mass spectrometry is:

   (a) $\dfrac{m}{e} = \dfrac{rH^2}{V}$

   (b) $\dfrac{m}{e} = \dfrac{r^2H}{2V}$

   (c) $\dfrac{m}{e} = \dfrac{r^2H^2}{2V^2}$

   (d) $\dfrac{m}{e} = \dfrac{r^2H^2}{2V}$

   Hint: (d).

4. Mass spectrometry requires a minimum sample size of:
   (a) Micrograms
   (b) Nanograms
   (c) Picograms
   (d) None of these
   Hint: (c).

5. Which technique in mass spectrometry is based on an acid-base reaction for generation of ions in the ion source?
   (a) Electron ionization
   (b) Chemical ionization
   (c) Fast atom bombardment
   (d) Electron spray ionization
   Hint: (b).

6. Which is incorrect about Electron Impact (E.I.).
   (a) It is a "hard" technique
   (b) It always leads to appearance of the parent peak in the mass spectrum
   (c) It involves more fragmentation of the parent peak compared to the chemical ionization (CI) technique
   (d) It involves a potential of 50–70 eV for ionization
   Hint: (b).

7. C.I. technique is preferred to E.I. technique in mass spectrometry because:
   (a) It involves more fragmentation of the ions but does not lead to the appearance of parent peak
   (b) It involves less fragmentation of the ions and does not lead to the appearance of the parent peak
   (c) It involves more fragmentation and appearance of the parent peak
   (d) It involves less fragmentation and appearance of the parent peak
   Hint: (d).

8. Which of the following ionization techniques involves the use of a matrix in mass spectrometry.
   (a) EI   (b) CI
   (c) FAB   (d) ESI
   Hint: (c).

9. A molecule ion in mass spectrometry is observed if it lives for:
   (a) 10^{-8} s   (b) 10^{-7} s
   (c) 10^{-6} s   (d) 10^{-5} s
   Hint: (c).

10. A metastable peak in m/e spectrum, m* is related to m_1^+ and m_2^+ in the following conversion:

$$m^+ \longrightarrow m_2^+ + \text{fragment}$$

(a) $m* = \dfrac{(m_1)^2}{m_2}$ (b) $m* = \dfrac{m_1}{m_2}$

(c) $m* = \dfrac{m_2}{(m_1)^2}$ (d) $m* = \dfrac{(m_2)^2}{m_1}$

Hint: (d).

11. As per the nitrogen rule in mass spectrometry which is correct.
   (a) When a compound has an odd number of nitrogens, its molecular ion will appear at an even value
   (b) When a compound has an even number of nitrogen, its molecular ion will appear at an odd value
   (c) When a compound has an even number of nitrogens, its molecular ion will appear at an even value and when a compound has an odd number of nitrogens, its molecular ion will appear at an odd value
   (d) When a compound has an even number of nitrogen, its molecular ion will appear at an odd value and when a compound has an odd number of nitrogens, its molecular ion will appear at an even value
   Hint: (c).

12. The presence of a chlorine is indicated in a compound if its mass spectrum show M + 1 and M + 2 peaks in the intensity ratio.
   (a) 2:1   (b) 3:1
   (c) 1:1   (d) 1:2
   Hint: (b).

13. The presence of a bromine is indicated in a compound if its mass spectrum shows M + 1 and M + 2 peaks in the intensity ratio.

    (a) 2:1   (b) 3:1

    (c) 1:1   (d) 1:2

    Hint: (a).

14. For a polyhalogenated compound, the number of peaks observed in the highest mass region is:

    (a) n + 2   (b) n + 3

    (c) n + 1   (d) 2n + 2

    Hint: (c).

15. The mass spectrum of 2–bromobutane shows two major peaks at 136 and 138 because:

    (a) Bromine forms both Br^+ and Br^- ions

    (b) 2–Bromobutane exists in eclipsed and staggered conformations

    (c) Bromine exists in two isotopic forms

    (d) 2–Bromobutane exists as R– and S–enantiomers

    (e) The molecular ion may carry one or two positive charges

    Hint: (b).

19

Ultraviolet Spectroscopy

19.1 PRINCIPLE

That part of electromagnetic spectrum which gives a spectrum using ultraviolet radiation is called the ultra-violet region. This extends from 190 nm to 380 nm (Fig. 19.1). Although organic compounds, in general, do not absorb in this

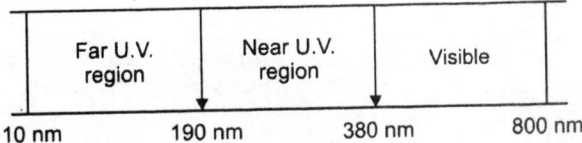

Far U.V. region	Near U.V. region	Visible
10 nm	190 nm	380 nm	800 nm

Fig. 19.1. UV and visible regions of electromagnetic spectrum.

region, this branch of spectroscopy does have some limited utility and we will discuss this in some details although some modern textbooks have done away with this Chapter.

19.1.1 Electronic Transitions

Absorptions of radiation in UV or UV-visible (190–800 nm) region occurs due to transitions between the electronic energy levels. When radiation is absorbed by a molecule, there occurs transition from the

Highest Occupied Molecular Orbital (HOMO) to the Lowest Occupied Molecular Orbital (LUMO). In general, lowest occupied molecular orbitals are the σ-orbitals which have lower energy than π-orbitals. The π-orbitals have lower energy than the orbitals having non-bonded electron pairs (n) called non-bonding orbitals.

Of all the orbitals, the antibonding orbitals (unoccupied) are orbitals with the highest energy. Important transitions are shown in Figs. 19.1–19.6.

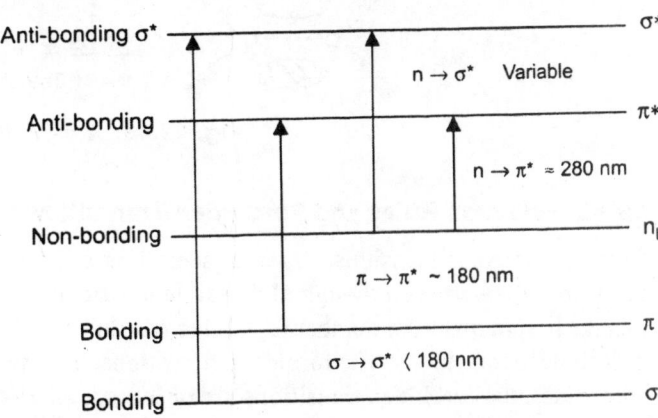

Fig. 19.2. Electronic transitions between electronic levels.

581

It is obvious from the Figs. 19.1–19.6, the energy required for transition from HOMO in ground state to LUMO is lower compared to the energy required for a transition from lower occupied energy level.

Thus an n→π* transition requires lower energy than a π–π* transition.

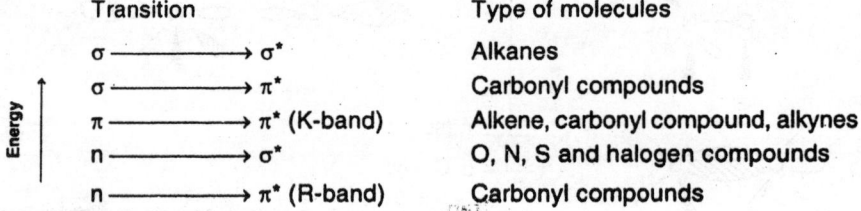

Transition	Type of molecules
σ ⟶ σ*	Alkanes
σ ⟶ π*	Carbonyl compounds
π ⟶ π* (K-band)	Alkene, carbonyl compound, alkynes
n ⟶ σ*	O, N, S and halogen compounds
n ⟶ π* (R-band)	Carbonyl compounds

Fig. 19.3. Order of increasing energies for the electronic transitions.

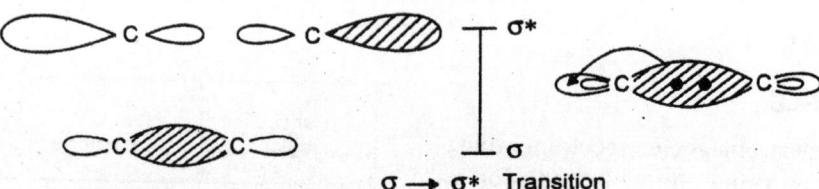

σ ⟶ σ* Transition

Fig. 19.4a. A σ–σ* transition.

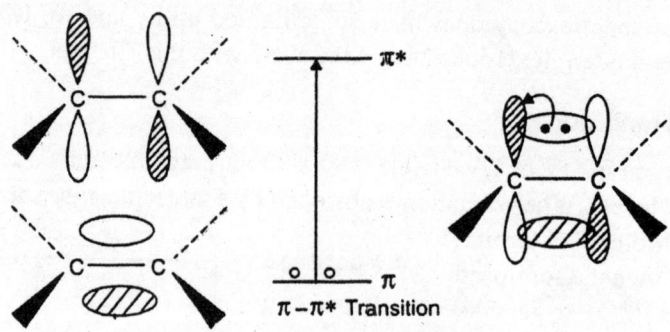

π–π* Transition

Fig. 19.4b. A π–π* transition.

19.1.2 Selection Rules and Forbidden Transitions

From the above discussions, it would seem that all transitions can occur. However, certain selection rules are followed even though all possible transitions may seem to occur. Transition which involve a change in spin quantum number (s) of electron during the transition, are forbidden and therefore known as forbidden transitions. The forbidden transitions, in general are not observed in the spectrum. However, sometimes, the forbidden transitions are observed; when observed, the intensity of these absorptions is much lower compared to that of the allowed ones. A most common example of forbidden transition is n–π* transition as in carbonyl compounds.

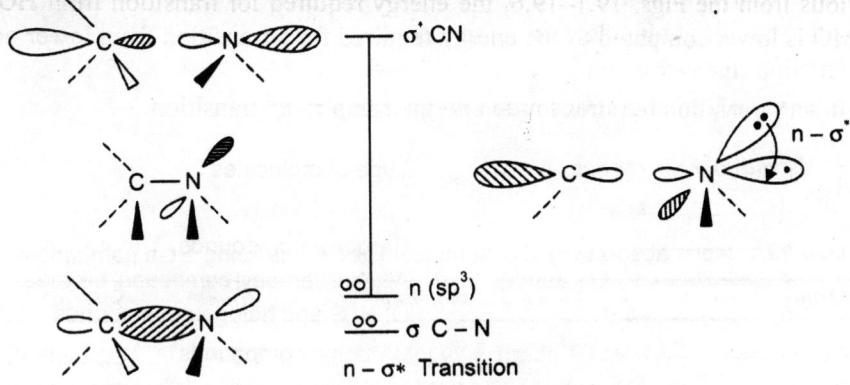

Fig. 19.5. A n–σ* transition.

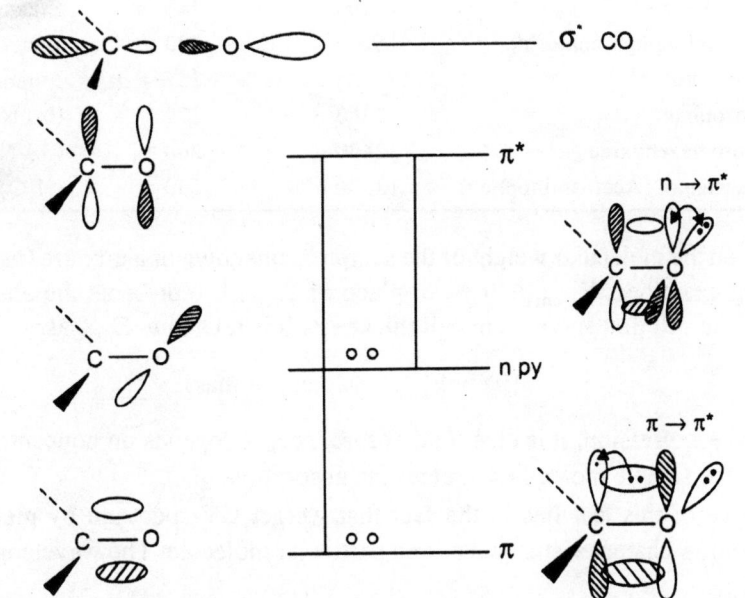

Fig. 19.6. Carbonyl group: the electronic transitions.

19.1.3 Lambert-Beer Law and Factors affecting Molar Absorptivity

A UV spectrum we talk about is nothing but a plot of log Σ versus wavelength (nm) called molar absorption or log Σ. It is the term that forms the basis of Lambert-Beer or the Beer-Lambert law:

$$\text{Log} \frac{I}{I_0} = \Sigma \, c.l$$

where $\Sigma = \dfrac{K}{2.303}$ = molar absorptivity (earlier called optical density or extinction. Molar absorptivity data of some selected drugs (using 1 cm path-length) are collected in Table 19.1

c = molar concentration

I = intensity of light incident on sample cell

l = length of the cell in cm

I = Intensity of radiation transmitted by the sample

$\text{Log} \dfrac{I}{I_0}$ is called Absorbance, A

Table 19.1. Molar absorptivity Σ of some selected drugs using 1 cm path-length cell

Drugs	$\Sigma L\ mol^{-1}\ cm^{-1}$	λ_{max} (nm)	Solvent
Colchicine	29200	243	Ethanol
Reserpine	14500	267	Chloroform
Riboflavin	35500	222	Water
Prednisolone	17500	263	Ethanol
Tetracycline-hydrochloride	16200	380	Water
Tolazoline	24	257	Ethanol
Dextrophan	2360	279	$(0.1\ N\ H_2SO_4)$
Chlorodiazepoxide	32400	260	$(0.1\ N\ NaOH)$
Paracetamol (Acetoaminophen)	13500	250	(H_2O)

However, when the molecular weight of the sample is unknown or a mixture (usually impure natural product) is being examined, $E_{1\ cm}$ is used in place of Σ_{max}. It represents the absorbance of 1% w/v concentration of the solution and a 1 cm cell thickness. It is related to Σ_{max} as:

$$10\Sigma = E_{1\ cm}^{1\%} \times \text{Molecular mass}$$

From the above expression, it is clear that absorbance, A depends on concentration i.e. greater the concentration of the sample molecules, greater the absorption.

The importance of this law lies in the fact that we get UV spectrum by plotting Absorbance A versus λ which shows characteristic peaks for a particular molecule. The wavelength corresponding to Σ_{max} is called λ_{max}.

Further, molar absorptivity, earlier called molar extinction coefficient Σ is a characteristic of the molecule that yields the UV-spectrum. It is a measure of the chromophore group that stands responsible for absorption of UV light present in the molecule. **It does not depend upon the variable parameters which can have their effect in preparing a sample solution.** Value of Σ can tell us whether the transitions are allowed or forbidden. Absorptivity can have values $0-10^6$. Absorptions with Σ more than 10^4 are termed high-intensity absorptions, those with Σ less than 10^3 are known as low-intensity absorptions. Transitions with Σ in between 0 to 10^3 are the forbidden transitions. In case forbidden transitions occur, they give sharp peaks.

Limitations: (i)The law is not followed if the absorbing molecules occur in different forms that exist in equilibrium, (ii) when the solute and the solvent undergo association, (iii) it does not take into account the effects of pH, (iv) temperature, (v) water length. So, it only applies to dilute solutions.

19.1.4 Transition Probability (Factors affecting Σ_{max})

The molar absorptivity Σ_{max} depends upon transition probability (P) and the target area (α) of the absorbing system called chromophore.

$$\Sigma_{max} = 0.87 \times 10^{20}.P.\alpha$$

where P = 0–1

Thus Σ_{max} for a chromophore with a length of the order of 10^{-7} cm (10Å) having unit probability (P = 1) will be ~ 10^5. As transition probability also depends on some other effects like geometries of the lower and higher energy molecular orbitals as well as symmetry of the molecule as a whole, therefore Σ_{max} also depends on these factors. Thus, symmetrical molecules display more restrictions on their transitions compared to less symmetrical molecules. That is why you will find that symmetrical molecules such as benzene show simple electronic absorption spectra whereas highly unsymmetrical molecules show complex electronic absorption spectra.

Intext Exercise

1. One tablet of colchicine taken from a chemist shop has to be analysed. It is dissolved in 100 mL ethylalcohol when it shows λ_{max} at 243 nm with absorbance equal to 0.438 in a 1 cm path length cell. If colchicine has molar absorptivity $\Sigma = 29200$ at λ_{max} 243 nm, what is the quantity in mg of colchicine in that tablet? MW of colchicine is equal to 399.4 g mol^{-1}.

    Solution:

    We know $\qquad \Sigma = \dfrac{A}{b \times c}$

    or $\qquad c = \dfrac{A}{\Sigma\, b}$

    Now $\qquad A = 0.438$ per 100 mL $= \dfrac{0.438 \times 1000}{100} = 4.38\ \text{L}^{-1}$

    $\Sigma = 29200 \qquad b = 1$

    $\therefore \qquad c = \dfrac{4.38}{29200 \times 1}\ \text{mol L}^{-1}$

    or $\qquad = \dfrac{4.38}{2920 \times 1} \times 399.4 = 0.60\ \text{g L}^{-1}$

    $\qquad\qquad = 0.060 \times 1000 = 60\ \text{mg L}^{-1}$

    $\qquad\qquad = 60\ \text{mg per tablet}$

2. Chlordiazepoxide, a tranquilizer has a concentration of 2×10^{-5} moles L^{-1} in 0.1 N NaOH. The solution shows absorbance of 0.648 in a 1 cm path-length cell. What is its molar absorptivity?

    Solution:

    $$\Sigma = \frac{A}{b \times c} = \frac{0.648}{2 \times 10^{-5} \times 1} = 3.24 \times 10^4\ \text{L mol}^{-1}\ \text{cm}^{-1}$$

19.1.5 Typical UV Spectrum

Typical UV spectra are shown in Fig. 19.7. As can be seen, the peaks are broad rather than sharp in nature. Why? This is because a molecule contains electronic, vibrational and rotational energy levels with less energy separations. Further, each vibrational level is actually associated with a set of rotational levels which have even lesser energy separation. Furthermore, each vibrational level is actually associated with a set of rotational levels which have even lesser energy separation. Consequently, there occur a large number of possible transitions which are responsible for change from one electronic level in one vibrational level to another electronic level in another vibrational level. This is shown in Fig. 19.8.

19.2 UV DOUBLE BEAM SPECTROPHOTOMETER

Fig. 19.9 shows a schematic diagram of a spectrophotometer which is double-beam type. It has the following six features:

1. Radiation source

It is in general, a deuterium lamp. This lamp emits electromagnetic radiation in the u.v. region (180–200 nm). Another light source which is a tungsten lamp is used for visible region of the spectrum.

2. Monochromator and chopper

It is a diffraction grating whose function is to divide the beam of light coming from the source into two component beams, one for reference, another for sample. This is done with the help of the chopper (also called Beam Divider) which is actually a rotating mirror.

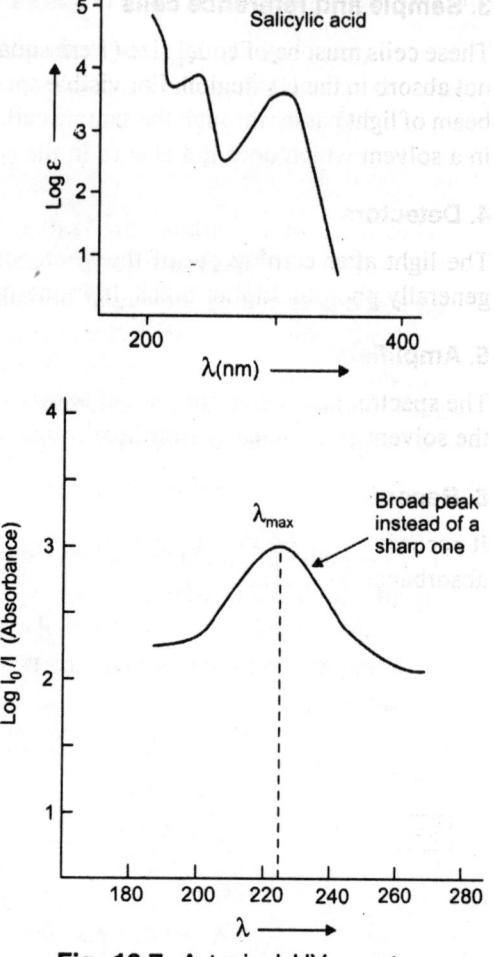

Fig. 19.7. A typical UV spectra.

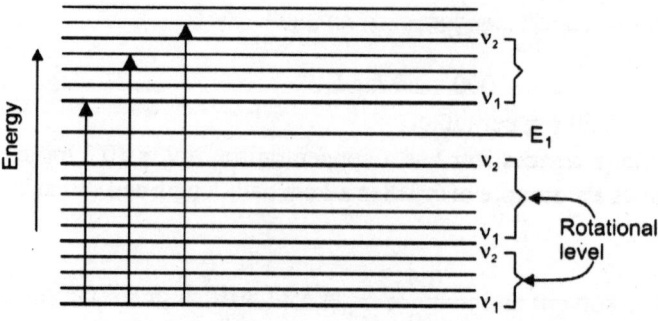

Fig. 19.8. Molecular energy levels-electronic, rotational and vibrational and the transitions.

3. Sample and reference cells

These cells must be of equal size (1 cm square) and made up of the same material i.e. quartz which does not absorb in the UV region. For visible spectrum region, cells are usually made of glass or plastic. One beam of light passes through the sample cell, the other through the reference cell. The sample is dissolved in a solvent which does not absorb in the spectrum (water, ethanol etc.).

4. Detectors

The light after coming out of the reference and sample cells is detected by the detectors. These are generally photomultiplier tubes. In modern instruments, photodiodes are used.

5. Amplifiers

The spectrophotometer consists of balancing amplifier whose function is to subtract the absorption of the solvent electronically from that of the solution.

6. Recorder

It records the spectrum by plotting wavelength of light absorbed against molar absorptivity, ε or absorbance, A.

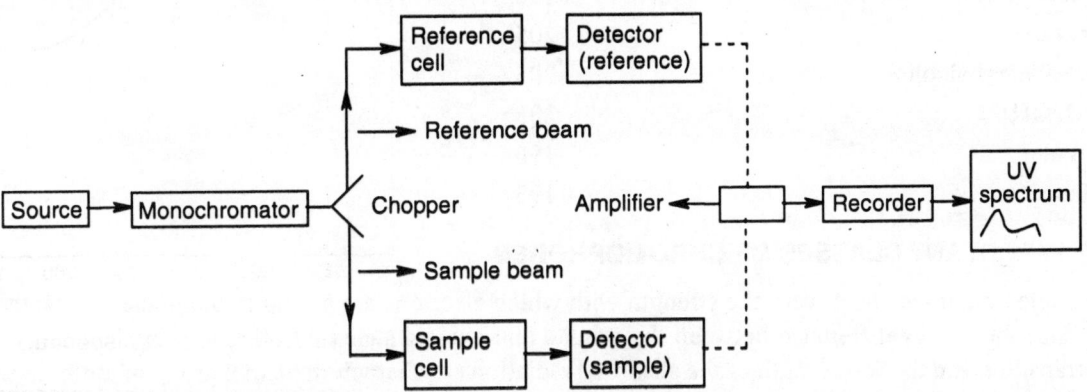

Fig. 19.9. Block diagram of a double-beam UV-visible spectrophotometer.

19.3 SAMPLE HANDLING AND SOLVENTS

(a) Sample handling

In general, the concentration of the solutions should be 10^{-5} to 10^{-2} molar. The per cent transmittance should be 20-25% for many organic compounds, a solution containing 10 mg in 100 mL is satisfactory although 0.1 to 100 mg of the sample may be required.

(b) Solvents

The choice of a suitable solvent as in any spectroscopy is always very significant. One of the main criterion is that the solvent selected should be transparent in the same UV region in which the substance under consideration absorbs. Evidently, the solvents that do not possess conjugated system would be most suitable as they will not absorb in the UV radiation. This is indeed the case in practice.

Compared to the situation in infrared spectroscopy, the choice of solvents for UV spectroscopy is much wider. Few simple solvents absorb strongly in the UV above 200 mμ.

Water, the most transparent solvent for the UV and visible regions is often used. Organic solvents for use down to 200 mμ are limited in practice to saturated hydrocarbons such as *n* hexane, cyclohexane, alcohols (methanol and ethanol) and ethers such as dioxan, tetrahydrofuran. The most common as well as most useful solvent, which in 1 cm cells, transmits sufficient light to give reliable spectra above 215 mμ is 95% (benzene free) ethanol. Commercial alcohol is avoided as it contains traces of a benzene as an impurity.

Hydrocarbon solvents are useful for non-polar substances. Being opaque to UV radiation below 245 mμ, chloroform is unsatisfactory. Chloroform and pyridine are avoided as these absorb at 200–260 nm. In fact, these can be used as better solvents for coloured compounds that absorb in the visible region e.g. carotenoids.

The solvent cutoffs are as described below:

Solvent	λ_{max}
Cyclohexane	195
Acetonitrile	190
n–hexane	205
95% ethyl alcohol	205
MeOH	205
Water	190
Isooctane	195

19.4 IMPORTANT CLASSES OF CHROMOPHORES

The nuclei in a molecule govern the strength with which electrons are bound to the nuclei. Thus, they influence the energy difference between the ground and excited states. In other words, the energy of any transition and the wavelength of the absorbed radiation are characteristic of a group of atoms in the molecule. These groups of atoms are known as chromophores. Because different classes of molecules possess different chromophore structures, so the energy and intensity of absorption change for all associated transitions. The UV spectral data of some non-conjugated chromophores are recorded in Table 19.2.

Alkanes

Here the only transition possible is $\sigma \rightarrow \sigma^*$ type as they contain only the single bonds and no unpaired electrons. These transitions require high energy so they absorb at very short wavelengths.

Saturated alcohols, ethers and amines

They possess nonbonding pair of electrons (n). Obviously transition of $n \rightarrow \sigma^*$ type are involved. These are also high energy transitions which occur in the region 175 to 200 nm in sulphur compounds like thiols and sulfides absorb in the slightly higher region of 200 and 220 mμ.

Table 19.2. The ultraviolet spectra of some non-conjugated chromophores

Compound	Chromophore	Transition	λ_{max}	ε_{max}	Solvent
Olefins	$-\overset{\displaystyle |}{C}=\overset{\displaystyle |}{C}-$	$\pi \rightarrow \pi^*$	180-200	5-10,000	–
Oct-3-ene	$H_3CHC=CHC_2H_5$	$\pi \rightarrow \pi^*$	185	8,000	n-Hexane
Acetylenes	$-C\equiv C-$	$\pi \rightarrow \pi^*$	173	–	Vapour
Ketones	$\overset{\diagdown}{\underset{\diagup}{}}C=O$	$\pi \rightarrow \pi^*$	Far UV		
		$\pi \rightarrow \pi^*$	270-285	15-30	–
Acetone	$\overset{H_3C}{\underset{H_3C}{\diagdown\diagup}}C=O$	$\pi \rightarrow \pi^*$	188	900	Ethanol
		$\pi \rightarrow \pi^*$	279	15	
Aldehydes	$H-\overset{\displaystyle |}{C}=O$	$\pi \rightarrow \pi^*$	Far UV		–
		$\pi \rightarrow \pi^*$	280-300	15-30	–
Acetaldehyde	$H-\overset{CH_3}{\overset{|}{C}}=O$	$\pi \rightarrow \pi^*$	Far UV		
		$\pi \rightarrow \pi^*$	293	11.6	Ethanol
Acetic acid	$HO-\overset{CH_3}{\overset{|}{C}}=O$	$\pi \rightarrow \pi^*$	Far UV	60	Water
		$\pi \rightarrow \pi^*$	204		

Alkenes and alkynes

These exhibit $\pi \rightarrow \pi^*$ transition which require rather high energy. Alkenes absorb at a slightly higher wavelength (175 nm) than alkynes (170 nm) (Fig. 19.3b).

Aldehydes, ketones, carboxylic acids

These compounds undergo $n \rightarrow \pi^*$ transitions around 280 to 290 nm. Of course, these transitions as expected are sensitive to substitution on the basic chromophoric structure. As per the selection rules, these transitions, in general are forbidden but those which occur have low intensity. The second category of transitions in such molecules are $\pi-\pi^*$ transitions that are noticed around 190 nm (Σ 900) as shown in Fig. 19.6.

19.5 AUXOCHROMES AND SHIFTS

A substituent alters the absorption of the main chromophore. Those substituents such as CH_3, OH, X, NH_2, NHR, NR_2 etc. that enhance the intensity of absorption and the wavelength are called auxochromes. Substituents other than auxochromes can cause any of the following observed effects regarding intensity or wavelength of the absorption (see Fig. 19.10).

1. Bathochromic shift (or red shift): This means a shift of the absorption to lower energy or longer wavelength.
2. Hypsochromic shift (or blue shift): This means a shift of the absorption to higher energy or shorter wavelength.

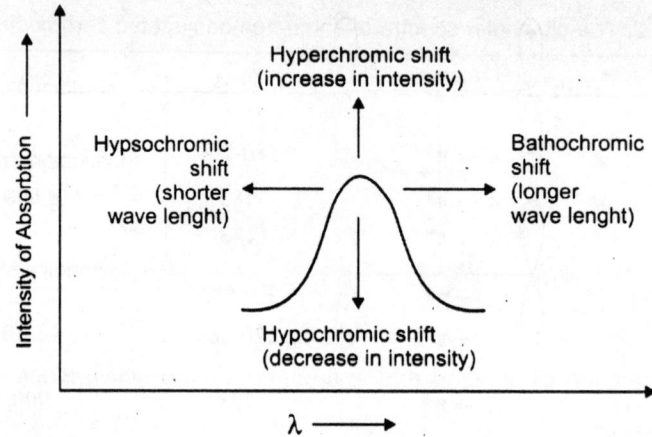

Fig. 19.10. The four types of shifts observed in UV spectroscopy.

3. Hyperchromic effect: This means an increase in intensity.
4. Hypochromic effect: This implies a decrease in intensity.

19.6 THE PARAMETERS THAT AFFECT SHIFTS : CONJUGATION AND SOLVENT SHIFTS

The effect of conjugation

The conjugation parameter that affects shifts leads to lowering of energy or increase in λ (bathochromic shift) w.r. to $\pi-\pi^*$ transition. Greater the extent of conjugation in a double bonded system, greater the bathochromic shift. Due to conjugation, what happens is that electronic energy levels of a chromophore move close together with the result that energy required for transition is lowered down. Further, conjugation of two chromophores leads to red shift besides enhancing the intensity of the absorption. We will now discuss the **effect of conjugation in alkenes** in details.

As per this theory, the atomic p orbitals on each carbon atom in the molecule combine to π molecular orbitals – the bonding and anti-bonding MOs form (Fig. 19.11a). Thus in ethene, the two atomic p orbitals, ϕ_1 and ϕ_2 give rise to two π MO, ψ_1, the bonding MO and ψ_2^* the antibonding MO are formed (Fig. 19.11a). As per the LCAO approach, the bonding orbital ψ_1 is a consequence of additive overlap and thus has lower energy. The antibonding orbital, π_2^* being a consequence of the subtractive overlap has higher energy. Because each of atomic p orbital possesses one electron, therefore, ψ_1 will have 2 electrons and it will form a new π bond. Electronic transition in this system is a $\pi-\pi^*$ transition from π_1 to π_2^* :

$$\psi_1 \xrightarrow[\text{transition}]{\pi-\pi^*} \psi_2^*$$

In case of 1,3 butadiene, there are four energy levels which give rise to four MOs (Fig. 19.11b). In this case $\pi-\pi^*$ transition occurs from $\psi_2 \rightarrow \psi_3^*$. This transition requires lower energy compared to $\pi-\pi^*$ transition in ethene. With the increase in the number of P orbitals making up the conjugated system, the transition from HOMO to LUMO require less energy. Consequently, the increased conjugation leads to an increase in the wavelength as shown in Fig. 19.12 for dimethyl polyenes. When there are 8 or more conjugated double bonds, the compound absorbs in the visible region so that it is

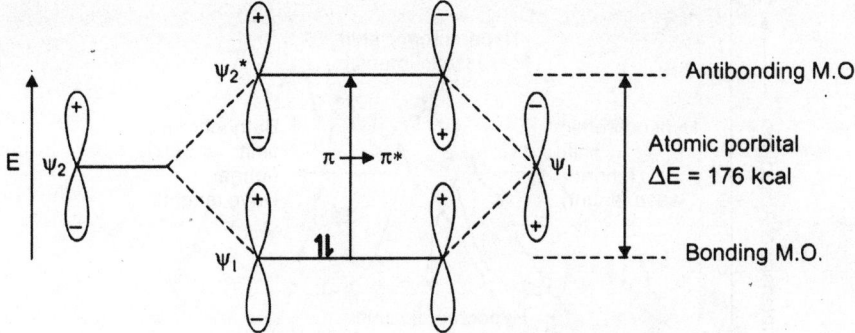

Fig. 19.11a. Formation of bonding and anti-bonding molecular orbitals in ethene.

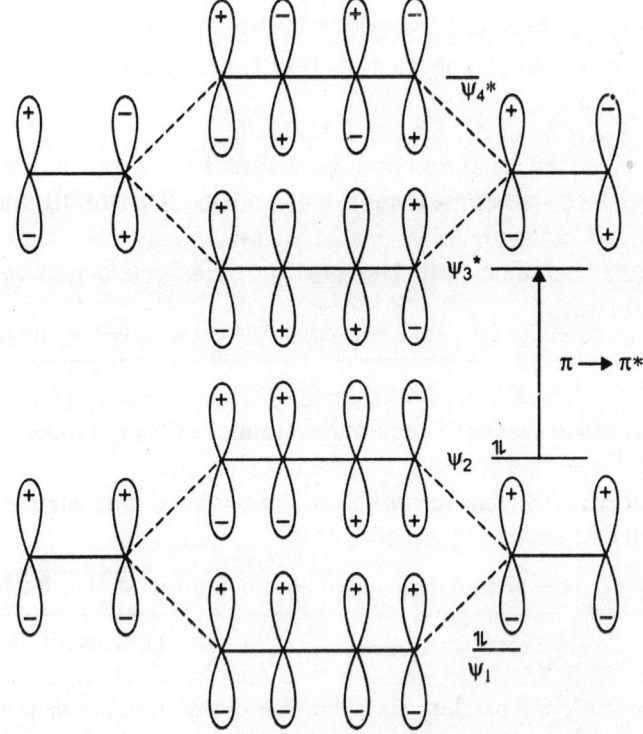

Fig. 19.11b. M orbitals and $\pi-\pi^*$ transition in butadiene.

coloured. For example, β-carotene (orange coloured) contains 11 double bonds. The auxochromes which possess a pair of non-bonded electrons on the atom directly bonded to the double bond system, cause a resonance interaction that increases the length of the conjugated system as shown:

A = Auxochrome
= OCH_3, OH
= $N(CH_3)_2$, NH_2
= X

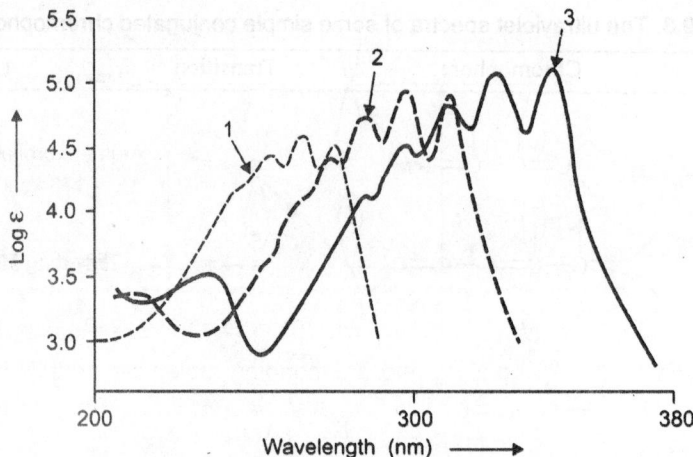

Fig. 19.12. UV spectra of dimethyl polyenes, $CH_3-(CH=CH)_n-CH_3$, with (1) n = 3, (2) n = 4, (3) n = 5.

In other words, the nonbonded electrons become a part of the π-system of the MO. This leads to an increase in the length by one orbital. Consequently, the transition from the highest occupied orbital, ψ_2 to the antibonding orbital ψ_3^* always requires relatively lower energy now than before. Thus $\pi-\pi^*$ and $n-\pi^*$ transitions show a bathochromic shift. The $n-\pi^*$ transition gets buried under the $\pi-\pi^*$ intense bond as conjugated chain length.

Intext Exercise

1. Why does a methyl group produce a red (bathochromic) shift even though it does not possess unshared electrons?

   Solution: This is because it interacts with the double bond by hyperconjugation given the overall effect of an extension of π-system.

The UV spectral data of some simple conjugated chromophores is recorded in Table 19.3.

Solvent shifts

Solvents can shift the absorption depending upon the type of electronic transition involved.

1. n-π^* and n-σ^* transition

In case a group is more polar in ground state than in its excited state, H-bonding or dipole-dipole interactions stabilise the n-electrons in the ground state relative to excited state. Consequently, the energy difference between the excited state and ground state increases. This shifts the band towards shorter wavelength (Fig. 19.13a).

For example, this happens in case of carbonyl group. A carbonyl group is more polar in the ground state than in its excited state. The absorption maxima of acetone at 279 nm in hexane, a non-polar solvent shifts to shorter wavelength with increasing polarity of the solvent:

Table 19.3. The ultraviolet spectra of some simple conjugated chromophores

Compound	Chromophore	Transition	λ_{max}	ε_{max}	Solvent
1,3–Butadiene	$\underset{/}{\overset{\backslash}{C}}=\overset{|}{C}-\overset{|}{C}=C$	$\pi \to \pi^*$	217	20,900	–
1,3,5–Hexatriene	$\underset{/}{\overset{\backslash}{C}}=\overset{|}{C}-\overset{|}{C}=C-\overset{|}{C}=\overset{/}{\underset{\backslash}{C}}$	$\pi \to \pi^*$	258	35,000	–
Cyclopentadiene		$\pi \to \pi^*$	239	3,400	–
Methyl Vinyl ketone	$-\overset{\overset{O}{\|}}{C}-\overset{|}{C}=\overset{/}{\underset{\backslash}{C}}$	$\pi \to \pi^*$	212	6,500	Ethanol
$(CH_2 = CH.CO.Me)$		$n \to \pi^*$	320	24	–
Mesityl oxide	$-\overset{\overset{O}{\|}}{C}-\overset{|}{C}=\overset{/}{\underset{\backslash}{C}}$	$\pi \to \pi^*$	224	9,750	–
$\left(\underset{H_3C}{\overset{H_3C}{>}}C=CH.CO.Me\right)$		$n \to \pi^*$	315	38	–
Methyl isopropenyl ketone	$-\overset{\overset{O}{\|}}{C}-\overset{|}{C}=\overset{/}{\underset{\backslash}{C}}$	$\pi \to \pi^*$	235	14,000	–
$\left(\underset{H_3C}{\overset{H_3C}{>}}C.CO.Me\right)$		$n \to \pi^*$	314	60	–
Acrolein	$-\overset{\overset{O}{\|}}{C}-\overset{|}{C}=\overset{/}{\underset{\backslash}{C}}$	$\pi \to \pi^*$	208	10,000	–
$(CH_2 = CH.CHO)$		$n \to \pi^*$	328	13	–
Crotonaldehyde	$-\overset{\overset{O}{\|}}{C}-\overset{|}{C}=\overset{/}{\underset{\backslash}{C}}$	$\pi \to \pi^*$	220	15,000	Ethanol
$(Me.CH=O.CHO$		$n \to \pi^*$	322	28	
Crotonic acid	$HO-\overset{\overset{O}{\|}}{C}-\overset{|}{C}=\overset{/}{\underset{\backslash}{C}}$	$\pi \to \pi^*$	205	15,000	–
Diethyl maleate	$RO-\overset{\overset{O}{\|}}{C}-\overset{|}{C}=\overset{|}{C}-\overset{\overset{O}{\|}}{C}-OR$	$\pi \to \pi^*$	205	8,000	–
Diethyl fumarate	$RO-\overset{\overset{O}{\|}}{C}-\overset{|}{C}=\overset{|}{\underset{|}{C}}-\overset{\overset{O}{\|}}{C}-OR$	$\pi \to \pi^*$	211	16,000	–

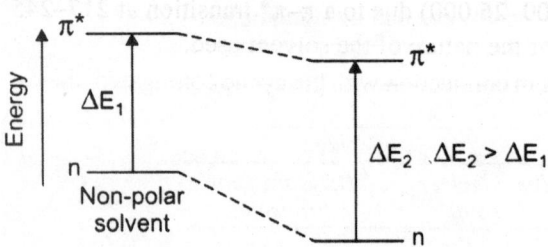

Fig. 19.13a. Solvent shifts towards shorter λ.

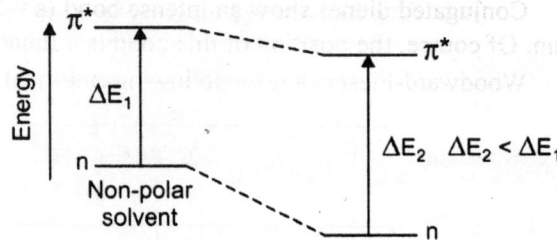

Fig. 19.13b. Solvent shift towards higher λ.

$$\overset{\delta+ \quad \delta-}{\underset{}{C}=O}$$

$$\overset{\delta- \quad \delta+}{\underset{}{C}=O}$$

Ground state, more polar   Excited state, less polar

Increasing polarity →

Solvent	C_6H_{14}	$CHCl_3$	C_2H_5OH	CH_3OH	H_2O
λ_{max}	279	277	272	270	264.5

Greater magnitude of the shift, indicates that the H-bonding becomes stronger increasingly. In other words, the extent of H-bonding decreases in the order:

water > methanol > ethanol > chloroform

In a similar manner, the polarity of solvent shifts n → σ* transition towards shorter wavelength.

2. π → π* transition

In case a group is more polar in the excited state compared to in the ground state, the H-bonding and dipole dipole interactions with the solvent stabilize the excited state more than they stabilize the ground state. This has the effect of decreasing the energy gap between the ground state and the excited state. Consequently absorption shifts towards longer wavelength:

An example is ethylene molecule. In the ground state, the molecule is non-polar as π electrons are equally distributed between the two carbon atoms. In the excited state with one carbon atom becoming electron-rich and the other electron deficient, the molecules becomes polar. This makes, ethylene more polar in the excited state.

Ground state, non-polar   E. state, more polar

As discussed above in a polar solvent, π* orbitals are more stabilized relative to π-orbitals, thereby shifting the absorption to longer wavelength.

19.7 WOODWARD-FIESER RULES FOR DIENES

Woodward and Fieser correlated the observed maxima with some empirical rules in order to make quantitative predictions for absorptions of unsaturated hydrocarbons such as dienes.

Conjugated dienes show an intense bond (ε = 20,000–26,000) due to a π–π* transition at 217–245 nm. Of course, the position of this bond is a function of the nature of the solvent used.

Woodward-Fieser gave the following empirical rules in connection with the cyclic conjugated dienes.

Value	Type of diene	
	Homonuclear (cisoid)	Heteronuclear (transoid)
Base value increments	253	214
Double bond extended conjugation	30	30
Exocyclic double bond	5	5
Alkyl group or residue	5	5
Other groups		
OR	6	6
Halogen (Cl, Br)	5	5
NR$_2$	60	60
SR	30	30

Note: An exocyclic double bond is one which lies outside with respect to a given ring, even if it is present inside another ring. Usually it lies at the junction points on rings as is shown in the examples herein.

Examples

1.

This is not an exocyclic double bond

This is an exocyclic double bond

Transoid	214 nm
Three ring residues	15 (5 × 3)
One exocyclic double bond	5
Predicted value	= 235 nm (obs 234 nm)

2.

$H_3CH_2CH_2CO$

This is an exocyclic double bond

Transoid	214 nm
Three ring residues	15 (5 × 3)
One exocyclic double bond	5
–OCH$_2$CH$_2$CH$_3$	6
Predicted value	= 240 nm (obs 239)

3.

Cisoid   253 nm
Three ring residues   25 (5 × 5)
Double bond extending conjugation   60 (2 × 30)
Three exocyclic double bond   15 (3 × 5)
Predicted value   = 353 nm (obs 354 nm)

4.

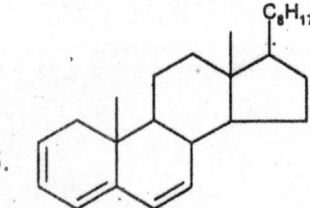

Ring residues

Cisoid   253 nm
3 ring residues   15 (5 × 3)
One alkyl substituent   5
One exocyclic double bond   15
Predicted value   = 278 nm (obs. 276)
Observed value   = 275 nm

5.

Homoannular diene   = 253 nm
Double bond extended conjugation   = 30
Three ring residues   = 15 (5 × 3)
One exocyclic double bond   = 5
Predicted value   = 303 nm
Observed value   = 305 nm

19.8 WOODWARD'S RULE FOR ENONES

Similar rules for prediction of absorption were workout in case of enones as well. Thus, double bond conjugated with a carbonyl group gives intense absorption (ε = 8000 to 20000). This absorption corresponds to a $\pi \to \pi^*$ transition of the carbonyl group. Simple enones show this absorption at 220 to 250 nm. On the other hand, the n $\to \pi^*$ shows at 310 to 330 nm and is much less intense (ε = 50 to 100).

Of these two transitions only the $\pi \rightarrow \pi^*$ transitions show predictable dependance on structural modifications of the chromophore base. The base value for acyclic enone and six-membered enone was set at 215 nm while that for the five-membered was assigned 202 nm.

Rules for α,β-unsaturated Enones

Rules for a,b-unsaturated ketones (enones):

$$\overset{\delta}{\underset{|}{C}}=\overset{\gamma}{\underset{|}{C}}-\overset{\beta}{\underset{|}{C}}=\overset{\alpha}{\underset{|}{C}}-\underset{|}{C}=O$$

$$\delta-C=C-C=C-C=O$$

Parent acyclic	= 215
5–membered cyclic	= 207
6–membered cyclic	= 202
Increments	
Double bond extended conjugation	= 30
α-alkyl group	= 10
β-alkyl group	= 12
γ and higher alkyl group	= 18
α OH	= 35
β OH	= 30
δ OH	= 50
α,β, δ OAC (OCOCH$_3$)	= 06
α OCH$_3$	= 35
β OCH$_3$	= 30
γ OCH$_3$	= 17
δ OCH$_3$	= 31
α Cl	= 15
β Cl	= 12
α Br	= 25
β Br	= 30
β SR	= 85
β NR$_2$	= 95
Exo double bond	= 05
Homoannular diene compound	= 39

1.

Six-membered	215 nm
One α-substituent	10 nm
One β-substituent	12 nm
Calculated	= 237 nm
Observed value	= 236 nm

2.

Six-membered	215 nm
Double bond extended conjugation	30 nm
One β substituent	12 nm
One d substituent	18 nm
One Exo double bond	5
Total	= 280 nm
Observed value	= 278 nm

3.

Six membered enone	215 nm
Double bond extended conjugation	30
Homocyclic diene	39
δ ring residue	18
	= 302 nm
Observed value	= 298 nm

4.

Six membered enone	215 nm
Double bond extended conjugation	30
δ ring residue	18
One exocyclic double bond	5
	= 280 nm
Observed value	= 278 nm

19.9 EMPIRICAL RULES FOR CARBONYL COMPOUNDS: α, β-UNSATURATED ALDEHYDES, ACIDS AND ESTERS

These compounds also follow the similar rules to those followed by enones.

Rules for α,β-unsaturated aldehydes, acids and esters

Aldehydes	Acid + Esters
Parent value = 208 nm	208 nm
With α or β alkyl = 220	208
With α, β or β, β dialkyl groups = 230	217
1 Exocyclio α, β-double bond	5
1 Endocyclic α, α double bond in 5 or 7 membered ring	5

Examples

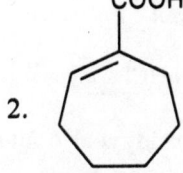

1.

α, β dialkyl base value	217 nm
Double bond in a six membered ring adds nothing	0
Observed value	= 217 nm

2.

α, β dialkyl base value	217 nm
Double bond in a seven membered ring	5 nm
Predicted value	= 222 nm
Observed value	= 222 nm

19.10 UV SPECTRA OF AROMATIC COMPOUNDS

The UV spectra data of some benzene derivatives are recorded in Table 19.4. Benzene shows (Fig. 19.14a) three absorption bands containing fine structure. The electronic transitions are π–π* type. Although one absorption peak is predictable due to four possible transitions of same energy based on the MO diagram of benzene, however, owing to electron-electron repulsions and symmetry

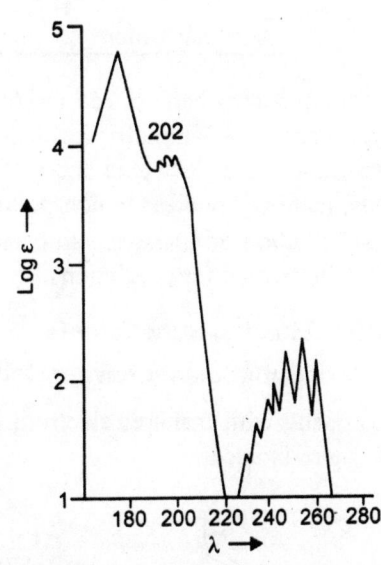

Fig. 19.14a. The ultraviolet spectrum of benzene.

considerations, only three electronic transitions occur. The primary bands at 184 and 202 nm and the secondary band at 255 nm. The allowed band (ε = 47000) is not seen in the spectrum because it lies in vacuum region of UV. The band at 202 nm is much weaker (ε = 7400). Obviously it is forbidden.

Table 19.4. The ultraviolet spectra of simple benzene derivatives

Compound	Transition	λ_{max}	ε_{max}	Solvent
Benzene	$\pi \longrightarrow \pi^*$	19	7493	Hexane
		25	251	
Toluene	$\pi \longrightarrow \pi^*$	207	6910	Methanol
		261	224	
Ethylbenzene	$\pi \longrightarrow \pi^*$	208	7762	Ethanol
		260	219	
o-xylene	$\pi \longrightarrow \pi^*$	210	8318	Methanol
		263	302	
m-xylene	$\pi \longrightarrow \pi^*$	212	7244	Methanol
		205	302	
p-xylene	$\pi \longrightarrow \pi^*$	216	7586	Ethanol
		268	501	
Chlorobenzene	$\pi \longrightarrow \pi^*$	210	7413	Methanol
		264	191	
Phenol	$\pi \longrightarrow \pi^*$	219–225	1000–4786	Ethanol
		272–275	724–2692	
Phenolate anion	$\pi \longrightarrow \pi^*$	290	3162	0.1 N NaOH
Anisole	$\pi \longrightarrow \pi^*$	217	6457	Methanol
		269	1459	
Aniline	$\pi \longrightarrow \pi^*$	234	6310	Ethanol
		284	1585	
Anilinium cation	$\pi \longrightarrow \pi^*$	254	159	0.1 N HCl

The secondary band at 255 nm (ε = 250–300) also called benzenoid band (B-band) is also intense corresponds to a symmetry forbidden electronic transition. This secondary band, the result of the interaction of the electronic energy level with vibrational modes, has a fine structure (six vibrational bands) that is quite clear in non-polar solvents.

Substitution on benzene can cause hyperchromic and bathochromic shifts so that empirical rules cannot be framed for predictions.

19.10.1 Effect of Substituents

Effect of Substituents having Non-bonded Electrons

Substituents with unshared electrons lead to shift in 1° and 2° absorption bands. They cause an increase in λ via resonance:

Evidently, greater the availablity of these n electrons, greater the shift. Examples include –OH, –OCH$_3$, –NH$_2$ groups etc. Consequently the 1° and 2° absorption bands of benzene are shifted to longer wavelength. Further these n electrons also lead to $n \rightarrow \pi^*$ transitions. How? The n electron gets excited and goes into the extended N* chromophore. This leads to charge separation in the excited state. The UV spectrum of phenol is recorded in Fig. 19.14b.

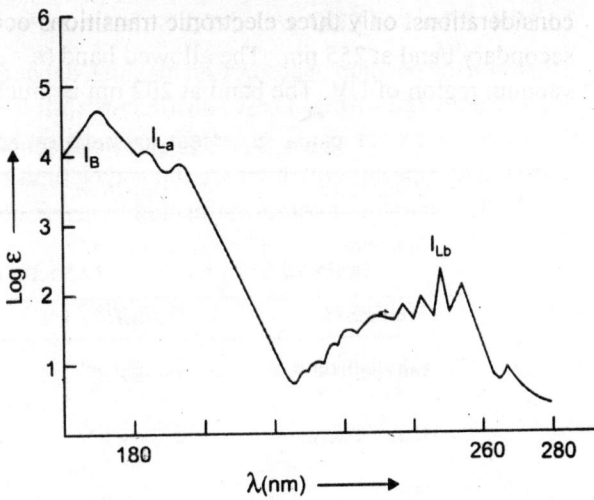

Fig. 19.14b. UV spectrum of phenol in ethyl alcohol.

19.10.2 Effect of pH

pH exerts considerable effects on the position of both 1° as well as 2° bands. For example, there is a shift from 203.5 in benzene to 210.5 nm – 1.7 nm shift – in the primary band in phenol. The secondary band also shifts from 254 to 270 nm showing a 16 nm shift. In aniline, 1° band shifts from 203.5 to 230 nm and the 2° band shifts from 254 to 280 nm. Can we see such shifts in anilinium ion? No, because the lone pair on nitrogen is used up as N gets protonated.

Isobestic or Isoabsorptive Point

This is a characteristic of a system containing two chromophores that are interconvertible e.g. aniline-anilinium and phenol-phenolate systems. When absorbance (%) is plotted against λ(nm), then a common point appears in the curves produced at various pH values. This point is called isobestic point.

19.10.3 Effect of Substituents having π Electrons

The π electrons of these substituents interact with the benzene electrons. This leads to a new electron transfer band. The resultant band is intense and obscures the secondary band of benzene system.

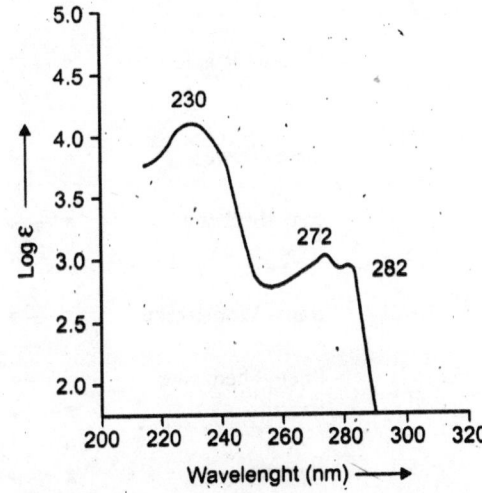

Fig. 19.15. Ultraviolet spectrum of benzoic acid in cyclohexane.

Thus, the 1° and 2° bands in benzoic acid are shifted when compared to those for benzene (Fig. 19.15).

19.10.4 Effect of EDG and EWG Substituents

Effects on the position of absorption maxima, depend upon whether the substituents are electron releasing or electron withdrawing. These substituents shift the 1° absorption band to longer wavelength. Electron withdrawing groups cause no effect on position of 2° absorption band. On the other hand, electron releasing groups not only increase the wavelength but also the intensity of secondary absorption band.

The UV spectra of some conjugated benzene derivatives are recorded in Table 19.5.

Table 19.5. The ultraviolet spectra of conjugated benzene derivatives

Compound	Transition	λ_{max}	ε_{max}	Solvent
Benzonitrile	$\pi \longrightarrow \pi^*$	224	12880	Ethanol
		271	1000	
Benzoic acid	$\pi \longrightarrow \pi^*$	226	9300	
		272	832	Ethanol
	$n \longrightarrow \pi^*$	280	646	
Benzaldehyde	$\pi \longrightarrow \pi^*$	244	19950	
		290	1000	Ethanol
	$n \longrightarrow \pi^*$	321	32	
Acetophenone	$\pi \longrightarrow \pi^*$	244	12590	
		280	1585	Ethanol
	$n \longrightarrow \pi^*$	317	63	
Benzophenone	$\pi \longrightarrow \pi^*$	252	19950	Ethanol
		330	182	
Nitrobenzene	$\pi \longrightarrow \pi^*$	260	7943	Ethanol
		333 (sh)	200	
Styrene	$\pi \longrightarrow \pi^*$	245	15850	Ethanol
		275	1000	
		285	1000	
		297	631	
Cannamic acid	$\pi \longrightarrow \pi^*$	204	39610	Ethanol
		222	14450	
		273	19950	
cis-Stilbene	$\pi \longrightarrow \pi^*$	222	22910	Ethanol
		280	13490	
trans-Stilbene	$\pi \longrightarrow \pi^*$	226	15140	Ethanol
		295	26920	
		310	25120	
trans-Azobenzene	$\pi \longrightarrow \pi^*$	315	50120	Ethanol
		445	7493	
Phenyl benzoate	$\pi \longrightarrow \pi^*$	265	1995	Ethanol
Benzil	$\pi \longrightarrow \pi^*$	259	20420	Ethanol
	$n \longrightarrow \pi^*$	370	78	
Benzoin	$\pi \longrightarrow \pi^*$	248	13800	Ethanol
	$n \longrightarrow \pi^*$	318	275	
Biphenyl	$\pi \longrightarrow \pi^*$	250	17380	Ethanol

19.10.5 Disubstituted benzenes

(i) In para-disubstituted benzenes, if both substituents are electron withdrawing either, they cause effects which we see in monosubstituted benzenes, shift being determined by the group with stronger effect.

(ii) On the other hand, if there are two electronically complementary substituents i.e. one is electron releasing while the other is e⁻ withdrawing then the magnitude of the observed shift in the position of 1° band is greater than the sum of shifts that occur due to individual groups. This is due to resonance interaction which leads to an extension of the chromophore via the intermediacy of the benzene ring. This effect is not seen when these groups are ortho or meta w.r. to each other. In fact, the observed magnitude of the shift is almost equal to the sum of the observed shifts effected by these individual groups. Furthermore, there is steric hinderance in case of ortho groups that does not allow resonance to occur.

19.10.6 Polynuclear Aromatic Hydrocarbons (PAH)

UV spectral data for some PAH are recorded in Table 19.6. The UV spectra of anthracene and phenanthrene are shown in Fig. 19.16. The 1° and 2° band shift to longer wavelength in these compounds. This band is noticed at 220 nm in case of Naphthalene. With the extent of conjugation increasing, the magnitude of bathochromic shift increases. This happens due to decrease in the energy gap between

Table 19.6. The ultraviolet spectra of polynuclear aromatic compounds

Compound	Transition	λ_{max}	ε_{max}	Solvent
Naphthalene	$\pi \longrightarrow \pi^*$	222	10000	Ethanol
		257	3981	
		265	5012	
		275	5012	
		286	3981	
Phenanthrene	$\pi \longrightarrow \pi^*$	245	39810	Ethanol
		250	50120	
		274	12590	
		282	6310	
		293	10000	
Anthracene	$\pi \longrightarrow \pi^*$	245	100000	Ethanol
		252	199500	
		324	2884	
		338	1585	
		355	7943	
		374	7943	

HOMO and LUMO, with increase in the number of p-orbitals as the number of linearly fused benzene ring increases. The UV spectra of PAH have characteristic intensity, shapes as well as fine structure. The spectrum of PAH is identified by comparison with the spectrum of unsubstituted hydrocarbon. The nature of chromophore in PAH is often identified on the basis of observed similarity of peak shapes and fine structure with those of the unsubstituted polynuclear hydrocarbon (PAH).

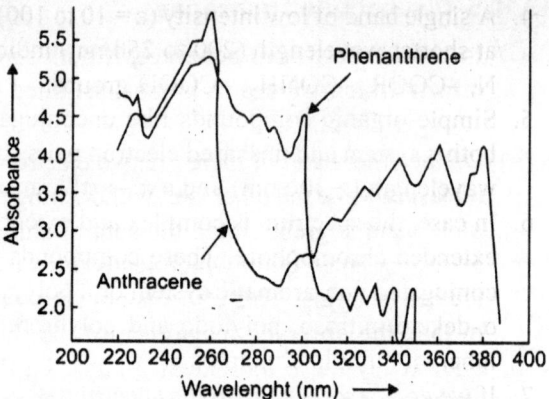

Fig. 19.16. UV spectra of anthracene and phenanthrene in cyclohexane solvent.

19.10.7 Heterocyclic molecules

These compounds show complex electronic transitions which also include combination of $\pi \to \pi^*$ and $n \to \pi^*$ transitions. UV spectrum of pyridine is shown in Fig. 19.17.

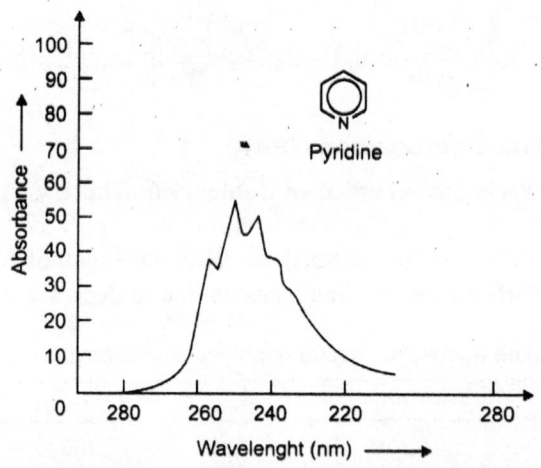

Fig. 19.17. Ultraviolet spectrum of pyridine in 95% ethanol.

19.11 A HANDY-DANDY GUIDE TO INTERPRETATION OF UV SPECTRA IN LAB

The following generalizations are helpful, should be taken only as guidelines:

1. Two bands having $\lambda_{max} > 200$ nm of medium intensity ($\varepsilon = 1000$ to 10000), generally indicate the presence of an aromatic system. Further, a good deal of fine structure is observed in longer wavelength band.

2. If the spectrum is simple and shows high intensity bands ($\varepsilon = 10000$ to 20000) above 210 nm, this indicates either an α, β unsaturated ketone, a diene or a polyene.

3. A single band of low to medium intensity ($\varepsilon = 100$ to 10000) at $\lambda_{max} < 220$ nm, indicates $n \to \sigma^*$ transition. This means the presence of amines, alcohols, ether (of course, an exception is the $n \to \pi^*$ transition in cyano group that also appears in this region).

4. A single band of low intensity (ε = 10 to 100) in the range 250 to 360 nm but no major absorptions at shorter wavelength (200 to 250 nm) indicates n $\rightarrow$ π^* transition of C = O, C = N, $-NO_2$, N = N, $-COOR$, $-CONH_2$, $-COOH$ groups.

5. Simple organic compounds like unconjugated ketones, acids, esters, amides etc. that contain both π system and unshared electron pairs show two absorptions at an n $\rightarrow$ π^* transition at longer wavelength (> 300 nm) and a π $\rightarrow$ π^* transition at (< 250 nm) shorter wavelength.

6. In case, the spectrum is complex and extends to visible region, the sample molecule contains an extended chromophore. These compounds that are highly coloured often contain a long chain conjugated non-aromatic system or a polycyclic aromatic chromophore. Some simple azo, nitro, α-deketo, nitroso, polyiodo and polybromo compounds may also exhibit colour, due to their inherent quinoid structures.

7. If we do not see a peak in the spectrum, this is giving us a useful message regarding the structure of the compound. This indicates the presence of saturated lipids, alkanes, aliphatic amino acids and sugars etc.

19.12 SOME SPECIAL APPLICATIONS OF UV SPECTROSCOPY

1. **Geometrical isomerism, coplanarity and steric factor:** This is exemplified by stilbenes. UV spectroscopy shows that the cis isomer absorbs at λ_{max} 274 nm while the trans λ_{max} 294 nm. This reflects the steric strain. In the cis-form the complete coplanarity is prevented, so it absorbs at smaller λ_{max} whereas complete complanarity in the trans isomer allows conjugation to occur readily.

trans-stilbene
λ_{max} 294 nm
co-planarity leads to conjugation

cis-stilbene
λ_{max} 274 nm
steric factor prevents coplanarity

A similar behaviour is noted in cis- and trans-azobenzenes as well.

Intext Exercise

2. Explain the reason for the differences in the UV spectra of cis and trans azobenzenes.

cis-azobenzene
π–π^* 281 (5260)
n–π^* 433 (1520)

trans-azobenzene
320 (21300)
443 (510)

Ans.: Steric factor force the rings out of coplanarity and hence conjugation.

2. **Steric hindrance:** This is exemplified by biphenyl derivatives. While biphenyl exhibits intense absorption at 252 nm (ε max 19000) but 2,2′–dimethyl biphenyl shows absorption almost similar to O-xylene (λ_{max} 262, ε 270). The reason is steric inhibition of resonance in 2,2′–dimethyl biphenyl. The presence of the two methyl groups forces the rings out of coplanarity that is seen in biphenyl (although biphenyl is not exactly planar as the two rings are at an angle of 45° w.r. to each other).

Biphenyl	2,2′–dimethyl biphenyl
Co-planar resonance	The two methyls force the rings out of copoalarity : no resonance

---

Intext Exercise

3. What is the reason for the differences noted in the UV spectra of ortho and para-methyl-acetophenone?

λ_{max} 243 nm	λ_{max} 252 nm
(ε_{max} = 9500)	(ε_{max} = 15800)

Ans.: The methyl ortho to the $COCH_3$ forces the CO group out of conjugation with the benzene.

---

3. **Investigation of charge-transfer complexes:** When electron-rich (donor) and electron-deficient (acceptor) molecules are mixed, they permit the transfer of electron charge between them through space. Two new molecular orbitals are generated when filled π- or non-bonded orbitals of the donor molecule overlap with the depleted orbitals of the acceptor. It is the transitions between these newly generated orbitals that gives rise to new absorption hands noticed in the charge transfer complexes.

Example

Benzene-Iodine charge-transfer complexes: It is common observation that hexane is violet in *n*-hexane but brown in benzene. The reason is that the brown colour is due to the formation of benzene-iodine charge-transfer complex as a result of interaction between the π-cloud of benzene and the outer electrons of iodine. A new band is noticed at λ_{max} 290 nm (15000) that is different from λ_{max} of benzene at 255 nm and that of iodine is 500 nm (visible).

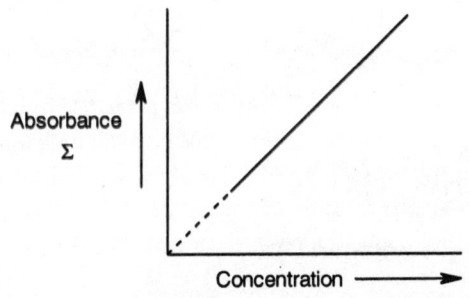

Charge-transfer complex
λ_{max} 290 (ε 15000)

19.13 APPLICATIONS OF UV SPECTROSCOPY IN PHARMACEUTICAL SCIENCES

1. Quality Control

1. The British Pharmacopoeia (BP) uses characteristics as quality control standards for benzyl penicillin, lanatoside C and alkaloids like emetine, morphine, reserpine, cocaine, colchicine, tubocuraine chloride and lobeline.
2. The United State Pharmacopoeia (USP) includes UV absorbance test for absence of foreign oils in oils of lemon and orange.
3. The BP includes UV absorbance test for the extinction limit test (between 268 and 270 nm) for castor oil.

2. Quantitative Applications of UV Spectroscopy

This is done on the basis of Beer-Lambert law (molar extinction coefficient):

$$\text{Log } I_o/I = \Sigma Cl$$

whereby Σ is the molar absorptivity, C is the concentration, l is the thickness in cm of the medium. Thus absorbance versus concentration standard plot can be drawn for a known pharmaceutical sample as shown in Fig. 19.18. Then, by knowing the absorbance of the known sample. Concentration of the sample can be known. Of course, the above law is not followed if there are solute-solute or solute-solvent interactions or chemical reactions.

Absorbance
Σ

Concentration ⟶

Fig. 19.18.

3. Quantitative Assay

First of all, a standard curve is obtained by determining the absorbances ($\text{Log}_{10} I_o/I$, earlier called optical density) of a series of the standard solutions of the pure compound by using a UV radiation of a suitable wavelength, which is usually the value at which the compound gives an absorption maximum (i.e. λ_{max}). It is essential that dilute solutions are used otherwise the Beer-Lambert law is not obeyed.

Next, the absorbance of the test sample solution is measured and its composition is ascertained from the standard curve already in hand. Further, it is possible to determine the individual components by UV absorption if different absorption maxima are shown by the different components. For example strychnine and brucine show different λ_{max} at the same UV wavelength:

λ	Brucine	Strychnine
262 nm	322 ($E_{1\,cm}^{1\%}$)	312 ($E_{1\,cm}^{1\%}$)

Similar is the situation at UV wavelength of 300 nm:

300 nm	5.16 ($E_{1\,cm}^{1\%}$)	216 ($E_{1\,cm}^{1\%}$)

Here it should be noted that $E_{1\,cm}^{1\%}$ represents absorbance for a 1% w/v solution with a layer thickness of 1 cm. This is how, the mixed solution of the above two alkaloids can be assayed for both the individual components. In fact, the European pharmacopoeia (EP) uses a similar type of assay for quinine-type and cinchona-type alkaloids in cinchona bark wherein the determinations are carried out at 316 and 348 nm wavelengths, giving in our hand a two-point spectrophotometric assay.

4. Determination of protein concentration

No amino acids absorbs in the visible region. However, several amino acids absorb UV light. Only the aromatic amino acids like tryptophan, tyrosine and phenylalanine show significant absorption above 250 nm. Thus, these absorptions are used for the determination of protein concentration.

5. Determination of Concentration of Vitamin A₁ and Vitamin A₂ in Natural Oils and Fats

Vitamin A_1 that has five conjugated double bonds absorbs at λ_{max} 325 nm, while vitamin A_2 having six conjugated double bonds absorbs at λ_{max} 351 nm. Thus the intensities of these two peaks are measured and then compared with those observed in the standard solutions of these vitamins to have their quantitative estimations.

Vitamin A₁
λ_{max} 325 nm

Vitamin A₂
λ_{max} 351 nm

6. Estimation of Ergosterol (Provitamin D)

Ergosterol present in fats is estimated in a manner similarly.

7. Estimation of Chlorophyll

The estimation of chlorophyll present in plant material is also done similarly as described in point 4.

8. Detection of Impurities

In case, the UV spectrum of a known pharmaceutical compound or a blend contains extra absorption, it is clear that there is present an impurity in it.

PROBLEMS

1. Explain the principle of UV-spectroscopy based upon electronic transitions, the selection rules and Beer-Lambert law. Why are the peaks broad in a UV spectrum?

2. Discuss the working of a double-beam UV spectrophotometer with the help of a block diagram. Discuss sample handling and solvents in UV spectroscopy.

3. What factors affect shifts peak position in UV spectroscopy? Explain with suitable examples.

4. Explain the effect of following in UV spectra of aromatic compounds:
   (a) Effect of substituents having non-bonded electrons.
   (b) Effect of substituents with p-electrons.
   (c) Effect of EDG and EWG substituents.

5. How does UV spectroscopy help us to study?
   (a) the geometric isomerism
   (b) extent of conjugation
   (c) steric hindrance

6. (a) Write notes on chromophore.
   (b) What is an auxochrome?

7. (a) Explain how does an auxochrome exert Bathochromic shift on a chromophore?
   (b) What is meant by the terms bathochromic shift and hypsochromic shift?

8. Write a note on solvent shifts in UV spectroscopy.
   Hint: See Section 5.6.

9. 2,2′–Dimethylbiphenyl exhibits a UV spectrum similar to o-xylene, λ_{max} 262 (ε 270) whereas biphenyl shows a very intense band at 252 nm (ε 19000). Why?
   Hint: See answer to Intext Exercise 2.

10. p-Methyl acetophenone shows λ_{max} at 252 nm (ε 15800) while ortho-methyl acetophenone shows λ_{max} at 243 nm (ε 9500).
    Hint: See answer to Intext Exercise 3.

11. Iodine in benzene is brown while it is violet in n-hexane. Why?
    Hint: See answer in Section 12.

12. While trans-stilbene absorbs at λ_{max} 294 nm, the cis isomer does at λ_{max} 274 nm. Explain why?
    Hint: See answer in Section 12.

13. Aniline has l_{max} 230 nm in neutral medium while 203 nm in acidic medium. Why?
    Hint: The N electron pair that is involved in resonance with the ring, is used up in making nitrogen protonated upon addition of acid, thereby removing resonance. Consequently the shift to smaller wavelength.

λ_{max} 230 λ_{max} 203

14. Acrylaldehyde (acrolein) shows λ_{max} at 217 nm (ε 16000). What weight concentration in g/ml will be required to obtain an absorbance of 0.8 when the cell length is 1 cm.

    Hint: $A = \varepsilon Cl$

    or $\quad C = \dfrac{A}{\Sigma l} = \dfrac{0.8}{16000 \times 1} = 5 \times 10^5$ mol L^{-1}

    $\qquad = 56.06 \times 5 \times 10^{-5}$

    $\qquad = 2.8 \times 10^{-6}$ g/ml

15. Why does polar solvent usually shifts the $\pi \rightarrow \pi^*$ transition to longer wavelength and n–π^* transition to shorter wavelength?

    Hint: See Section 19.6.

16. Explain as to why p-Nitroaniline shows in the K-band a pronounced red shift which is not observed in its ortho or meta isomers.

    Hint: See Section 5.10.4.

17. What is the reason for differences in the following:

	CH$_3$Cl	CH$_3$Br	CH$_3$I
l$_{max}$	173 nm	204 nm	258 nm

    Hint: As we move down the group (Cl $\rightarrow$ Br $\rightarrow$ I), the n electrons get removed from the nuclear attractive force. Hence, they are easily excited into so that λ_{max} goes on increasing.

18. Predict the λ_{max} values of these dienes.

    Hint:

Transoid	= 214 nm
Alkyl group	= 15 (3 × 5)
Predicted value	= 229 nm
Observed value	= 227 nm

    Hint:

Transoid	= 214 nm
Observed	= 217 nm

19. Predict the λ_{max} value of the following enone.

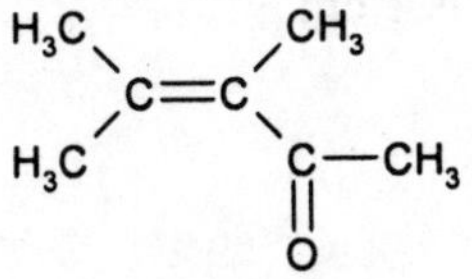

Acyclic enone

Hint:

Base Acyclic enone	215 nm
α CH$_3$	10
Two β CH$_3$	24 (12 × 2)
	= 249 nm
Observed value	= 249 nm

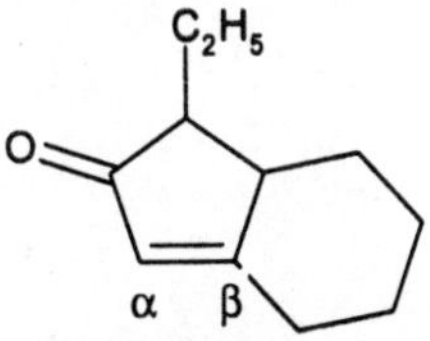

5 membered enone

Hint:

Five membered enone	202 nm
Two b ring residue	24 (12 × 2)
One exocyclic double bond	5
	= 231 nm
Observed value	231 nm

20. Using the empirical rules, predict the λ_{max} in these molecules.

(a)

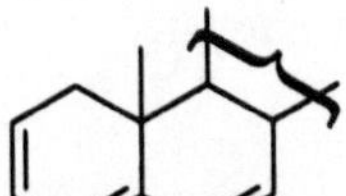

(b)

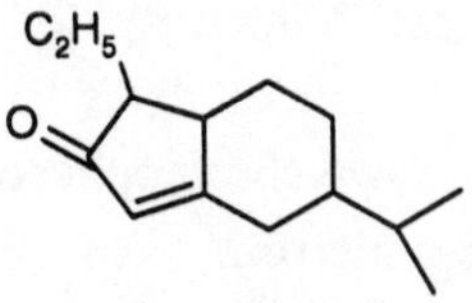

(c)

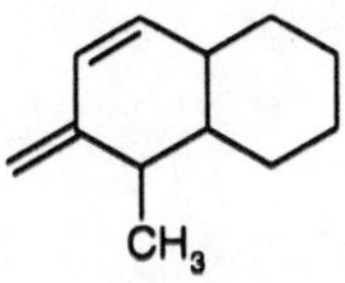

(d)

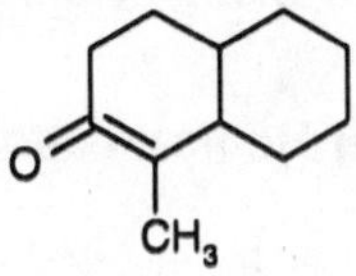

(e)

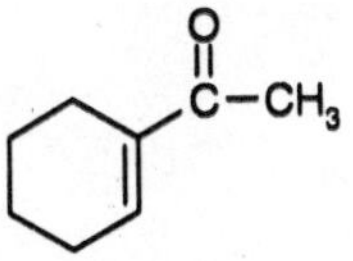

(f)

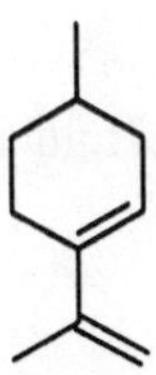

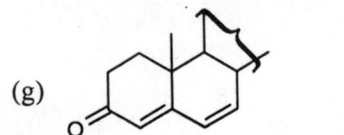

(g)

(h)

Multiple Choice Question for Competitive Exams—CSIR (UGC), NET, SLAT, GAIT, GPAT, CSE, HCS, GRE etc.

1. Alkanes show which transition?
   (a) $\sigma - \pi^*$
   (b) $\sigma - \sigma^*$
   (c) $\pi - \pi^*$
   (d) $n - \pi^*$
   Hint: (b)

2. Carbonyl compounds exhibit the transition:
   (a) $\sigma - \sigma^*, \pi - \pi^*$
   (b) $\sigma - \pi^*, \pi - \pi^*, n - \pi^*$
   (c) $\sigma - \sigma^*, n - \sigma^*, \pi - \pi^*$
   (d) None of these
   Hint: (b)

3. Molar absorptivity Σ is given by:
   (a) A.C.l.
   (b) A/Cl
   (c) C/Al
   (d) l/AC
   Hint: (b)

4. Bathochromic shift implies:
   (a) A shift to longer wavelength
   (b) A shift to smaller wavelength
   (c) An increase in intensity
   (d) A decrease in intensity
   Hint: (a)

5. Hyperchromic shift means:
   (a) A shift to longer wavelength
   (b) A shift to smaller wavelength
   (c) An increase in intensity
   (d) A decrease in intensity
   Hint: (c)

6. Conjugation of two chromophores leads to:
   (a) Bathochromic shift
   (b) Hyperchromic or hypochromic shift
   (c) Bathochromic and hyperchromic shift
   (d) Bathochromic and hypochromic shift
   Hint: (c)

7. The base value per Homoannular (cisoid) dienes (in nm) is:
   (a) 253
   (b) 214
   (c) 215
   (d) 202
   Hint: (a)

8. The base value for Heteroannular (transoid) diene (in nm) is:
   (a) 253
   (b) 214
   (c) 215
   (d) 202
   Hint: (b)

9. Diode-array is used in which spectrometer?

    (a) IR

    (b) UV

    (c) NMR

    (d) Mass

    Hint: (b)

10. The energy of the transitions in UV spectroscopy follows the order:

    (a) $\sigma - \sigma^* > \sigma - \pi^* > n - \pi^* > n - \sigma^* > \pi - \pi^*$

    (b) $\sigma - \sigma^* > \pi - \pi^* > n - \sigma^* > n - \pi^* > \sigma - \pi^*$

    (c) $\sigma - \sigma^* > \sigma - \pi^* > \pi - \pi^* > n - \sigma^* > n - \pi^*$

    (d) None of these

    Hint: (c)

11. Auxochromes are the substituents that:

    (a) Increase the intensity and wavelength

    (b) Decrease the intensity and wavelength

    (c) Increase the intensity and decrease wavelength

    (d) Decrease the intensity and increase wavelength

    Hint: (a)

12. Which aromatic band shows fine structure?

    (a) Primary

    (b) Secondary

    (c) Tertiary

    (d) None

    Hint: (b)

13. Σ and $A_{1\,cm}^{1\%}$ can be interconverted using which of the following formula?

    (a) Σ and $A_{1\,cm}^{1\%} \times$ mol. wt./100

    (b) Σ and $A_{1\,cm}^{1\%} \times$ mol. wt./10

    (c) Σ and $A_{1\,cm}^{1\%} \times$ eq. wt./1000

    (d) Σ and $A_{1\,cm}^{1\%} \times$ eq. wt./100

    Hint: (b)

14. An organic compound has a M.W. of 297 and an equivalent weight of 148.5 and an $A_{1\,cm}^{1\%}$ of 742 at 309 nm. Its molar absorptivity is:

    (a) 220.37

    (b) 1101.87

    (c) 110.18

    (d) 22037.5

    Hint: (d)

Combined Structural Problems

20.1 SOLVED PROBLEMS

No one spectrum of a compound alone can yield its exact structure. However, in the view of this author, NMR spectroscopy is the major technique that can take the lion's share of structural analysis. Other spectra, of course, are complementary in nature. ^1H and ^{13}C NMR spectra, combined together aid us tremendously in arriving at a right structure of compound. Mass spectrum gives us the exact molecular formula of the compound. Although i.r. spectra are complementary in nature, I also have a feeling that people in the field of chemistry, will not emphasise in near future upon the hitherto asked for i.r. data of a compound for publication, so that i.r. spectroscopy will become a technique of historical importance in organic chemistry. UV spectra have already almost met such a fate.

A wide variety of techniques such as NOE help us unambiguously in stereochemistry determination. Further tests like APT, DEPT, INEPT help us in distinguishing between the various types of carbons—CH_3, CH_2, CH. Techniques such as the 2D NMR, 3D NMR enable us to sort out the complete structure of complicated molecules. So, we will lay emphasis upon NMR analysis, ^1H and ^{13}C followed by mass spectral and infrared analysis and of course, double bond equivalents when required urgently.

Double Bond Equivalent, DBE

If we know the molecular formula of the unknown compound, it is always helpful to know the double bond equivalents, DBE in the compound. **DBE means number of double bonds and rings.** For a compound containing only C, H and O, DBE is given as:

$$DBE = \frac{(2a + 2) - b}{2}$$

whereby $(2a + 2)$ represents the number of hydrogens in a saturated hydrocarbon compound, a is the number of carbon atoms in the molecule. As for the formation of a π or double bond or a ring, two hydrogens are reduced, so the total number of double bonds and rings in the molecule can be obtained by subtracting the real number of hydrogens present, b from $(2a + 2)$ and dividing the figure obtained by two. So, in case of benzene, C_6H_6, DBE would be equal to:

$$C_6H_6 \ DBE = \frac{(2a+2)-b}{2}$$

$$= \frac{(2 \times 6 + 2) - 6}{2}$$

$$= \frac{14-6}{2} = 4$$

Obviously as benzene contains one ring, so it must contain 3 double bonds. So, we can say benzene hs 4 double bond equivalents.

Still better formula is:

$$N = \frac{\sum n_i(v_i - 2) + 2}{2}$$

where n_i is the number of atoms of any kind

v_i is the valence of atoms of any kind

Thus, for phenol, $C_6H_5OH \equiv C_6H_6O$

$$N = \frac{\sum 6(4-2) + 6(1-2) + 1(2-2) + 2}{2} = \frac{8}{2} = 4$$

Thus, phenol has four double bond equivalents i.e. one ring and so three double bonds.

We will now discuss some combined structural problems.

Problem 20.1.1. An organic compound has MF C_7H_9N. It exhibits the following spectra (^{1}H, IR, mass). C–13 NMR spectrum shows the following data:

$$56(q), \ 114(d), \ 122.9(s), \ 131.1(d), \ 167.2(s) \ \text{and} \ 172(s).$$

Assign a suitable structure to this compound.

1. ^{1}H NMR spectral analysis

There are two singlets in the relative ratio of 3:2 positioned at δ 2.2 and 3.45 ppm respectively. Clearly these are due to a CH_3 and CH_2 or NH_2 groupings respectively. As we see a pair of doublets in the aromatic region (at 6.81 ppm) that is a characteristic of p-disubstituted benzene ring, it is clear that the two substituents, one CH_3 and another 2H containing substituent must be present in p-position w.r. to each other. Further, it is clear that CH_2 alone cannot be present as a substituent directly attached to the ring as its valency cannot be satisfied. It cannot be a $O–CH_2$ group as the MF does not contain an oxygen group. Clearly, as the compound contains one nitrogen, it must be an amino group, $–NH_2$ group.

2. CMR analysis

The peak at 22.0 ppm which appears as a quartet upon H-coupling, must be an aliphatic methyl group. Out of the remaining 4 peaks seen in the aromatic region due to the benzene ring, two appear as doublets at 115.0 and 130 ppm. Obviously, these represent carbon (3, 4) and (2, 6) respectively. The latter will be more deshielded due to their closer proximity to the NH_2 group. The remaining peaks at 127.7 and 143.7 ppm which remain singlets upon H-coupling must be quaternary carbons to which substituents are attached. The most deshielded at 143.7 ppm will be the one to which electronegative nitrogen is attached. The carbon at 127.7 ppm must be attached to the CH_3 group.

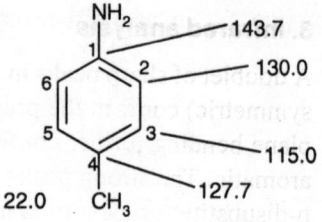

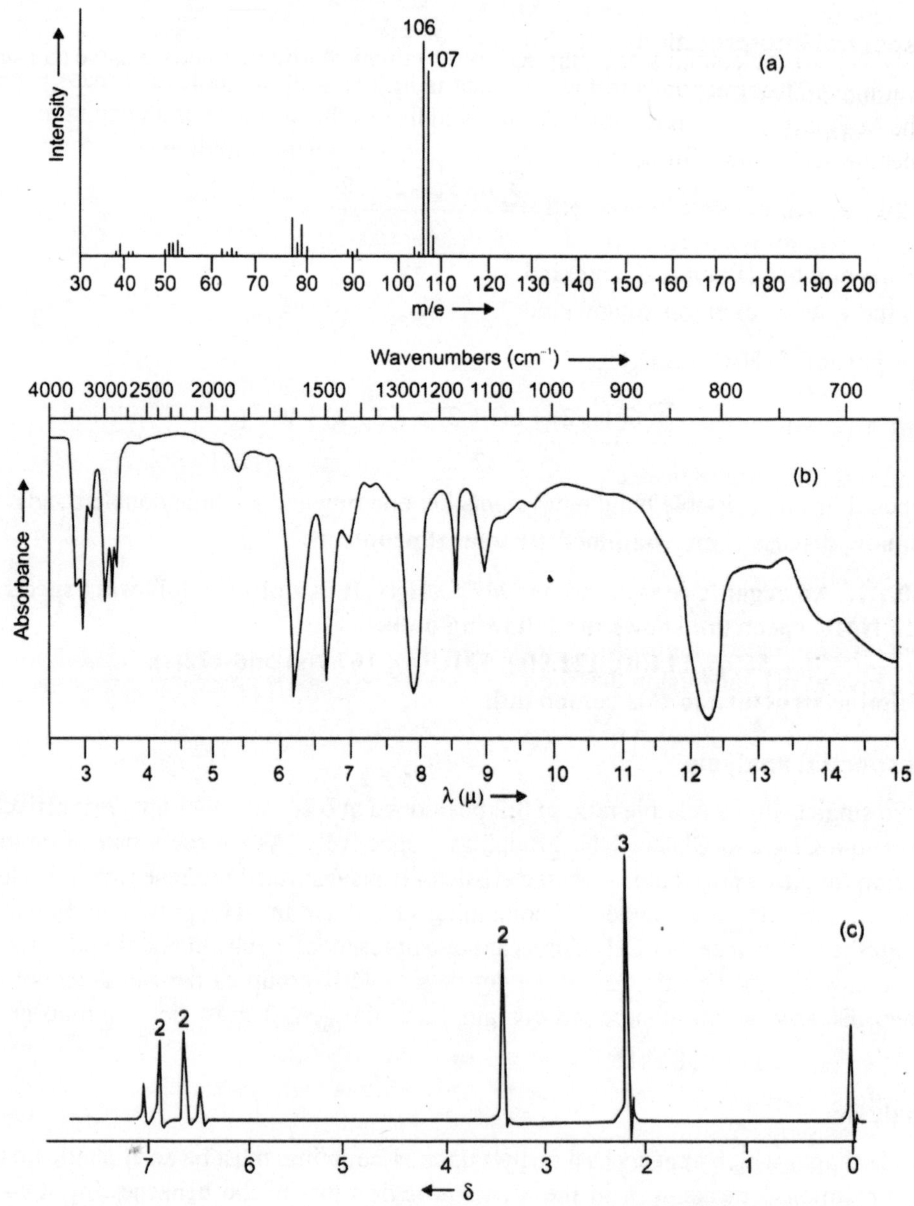

Fig. 20.1. (A) Mass spectrum, (B) i.r. spectrum and (c) ^1H NMR spectrum of Problem 20.1.1.

3. Infrared analysis

A doublet of sharp peaks in the expected region (3500–3300 cm^{-1}) for N–H stretching (asymmetric and symmetric) confirm the proposal of the presence of NH$_2$ group. A strong peak at 1575 due to NH – in plane bending further confirms the presence of the NH$_2$ group. The peak at 1260 cm^{-1} is due to C–N aromatic. The strong peaks at 1600 cm^{-1} and 1450 cm^{-1} confirm the presence of benzene nucleus. The p-disubstitution pattern is indicated by the presence of strong peak at 830 ppm.

4. Mass spectral interpretation

The peak at m/e 107 corresponds to the M$^{\dot+}$ that is in line with the molecular mass expected on the basis of the M.F. C$_7$H$_9$N. An odd molecular mass indicates the presence of an odd number of nitrogen in the molecule, as per the Nitrogen Rule. So, the compound is p-Toluidine.

Problem 20.1.2. An organic compound with M.F. C$_8$H$_8$O$_3$ gave the following ^{1}H NMR I.R. and mass spectra. Assign a suitable structure to the compound.

^{13}C NMR shows the following data:

$$172(s), 167.2(s), 131.1(d), 122.9(s), 114(d), 56.0(q).$$

Solution

1. ^{1}H NMR Analysis

The spectrum shows a sharp peak at 11.52 ppm equivalent to 1H. Obviously, the compound contains a –COOH group. As these are present peaks in the aromatic region (6–8.5), the presence of an aromatic ring is indicated. In fact, a symmetrical four-line pattern is present in this region that points out the presence of a p-disubstitution pattern on the aromatic ring. This is also indicated by the integral ratio of these peaks that is equivalent to 4H protons. One substituent is the –COOH group. What is the other substituent? A deshielded singlet at 3.85 ppm equivalent to 3H indicates the presence of a CH$_3$ group. Thus, we arrive at the conclusion that the above compound is p-Anisic acid.

COOH

OCH$_3$

2. IR Analysis

A broad band centred at 2980 cm^{-1} due to O–H stretching confirms the presence of carboxylic acid group. A strong band at 1675 cm^{-1} is due to the CO stretching. A medium band at 1320 cm^{-1} arises from C–O stretching. A strong band at 1250 cn^{-1} and a medium band at 1040 cm^{-1} are due to C–O stretching that are characteristics of phenyl alkyl ethers. The broad band due to O–H OOP is present at 940 cm^{-1}. The band at 835 cm^{-1} confirms the presence of p-substituted aromatic ring. The bands at 1600 cm^{-1} and 1450 cm^{-1} are due to ring skeletal C=C bands.

C–13 Analysis

The peak at 172.0 ppm is due to carbonyl carbon which appears as a singlet in the proton coupled spectrum. The carbon to which COOH group is attached contributes to the signal at 122.9 ppm and it also remains a singlet in the proton coupled spectrum as expected. The aromatic carbon to which –OCH_3 group is attached is clearly more deshielded at 167.2 and again appears as a singlet in the proton-coupled spectrum. The remaining signals at 131 ppm and 114.0 ppm respectively represent the carbon–2,6 and carbon–3,5.

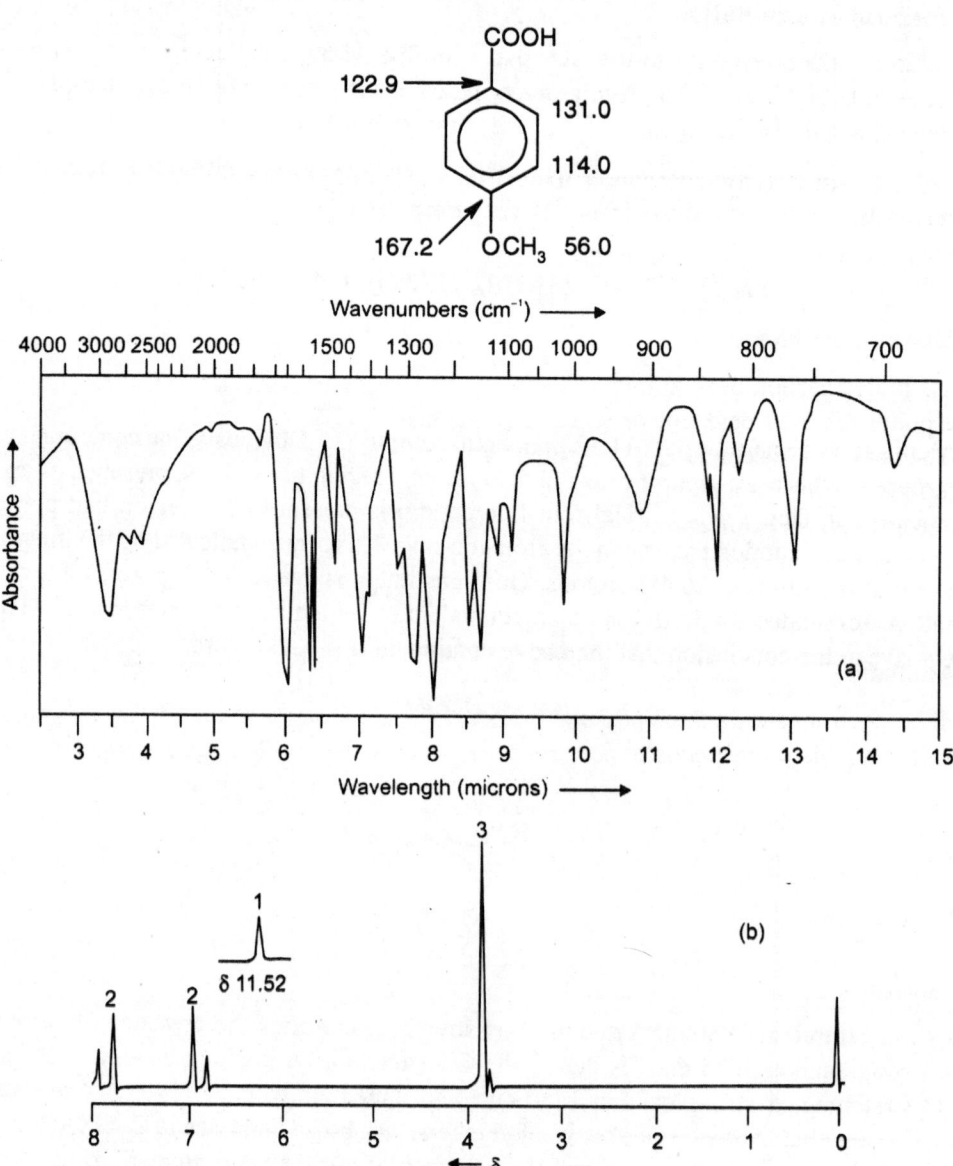

Fig. 20.2. IR (A), ^{1}H NMR (B) and mass (C) spectra for Problem 20.1.2.

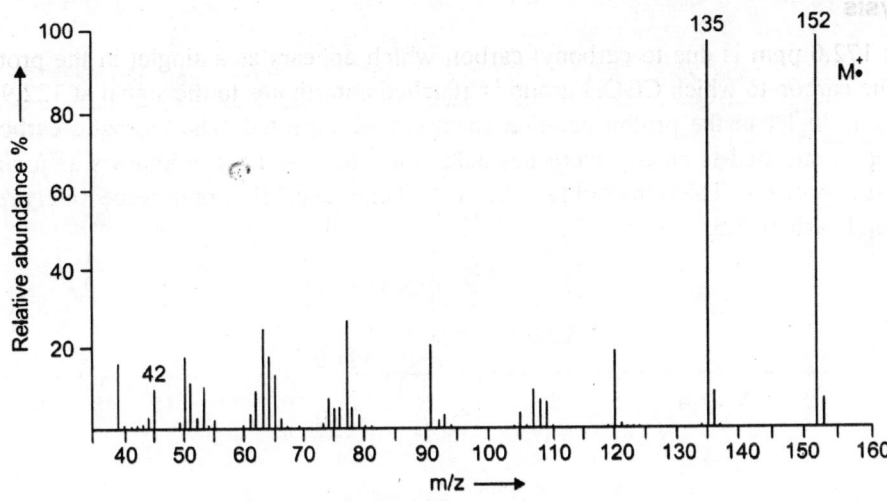

Fig. 20.2c. Mass spectrum of para-anisic acid.

4. Mass Spectral Analysis

The intense molecular ion peak at m/z 152 corresponds to the M.F. $C_8H_8O_3$. The strong peak at m/z 135 corresponds to M–17 peak due to loss of OH. Further loss of CO occurs to give a peak at m/z 107 (M–45). The peak at 77 is due to $C_6H_5^+$ ion. The loss of OCH_3 is indicated by the peak at m/z 121. See the detailed general mechanism in the chapter on mass spectrometry.

Problem 20.1.3. An organic compound with M.F. $C_9H_{10}O_2$ shows the following spectral analysis for NMR, infrared and mass spectra. Suggest possible structure of this compound.

Solution

1. PMR Analysis

The 60 MHz spectrum shows three peaks at δ 1.96, 5.01 and 7.22 ppm in the relative integral ratio of 3:2:5. Obviously, this corresponds to a total of ten protons. The peak at 7.22 in the aromatic region

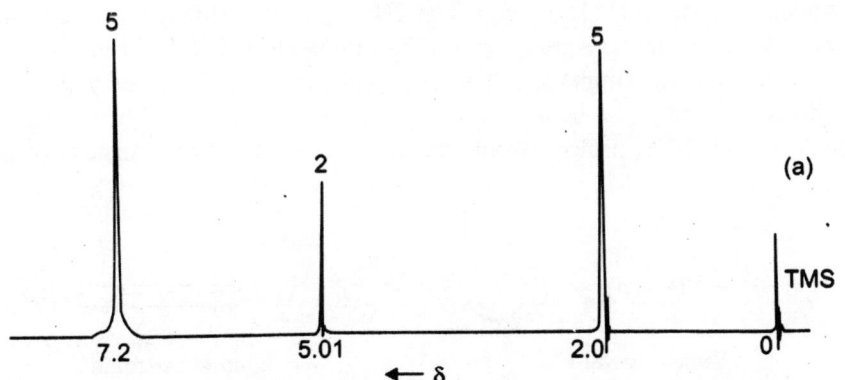

Fig. 20.3a. ^1H NMR spectrum (60 MHz) Problem 20.1.3.

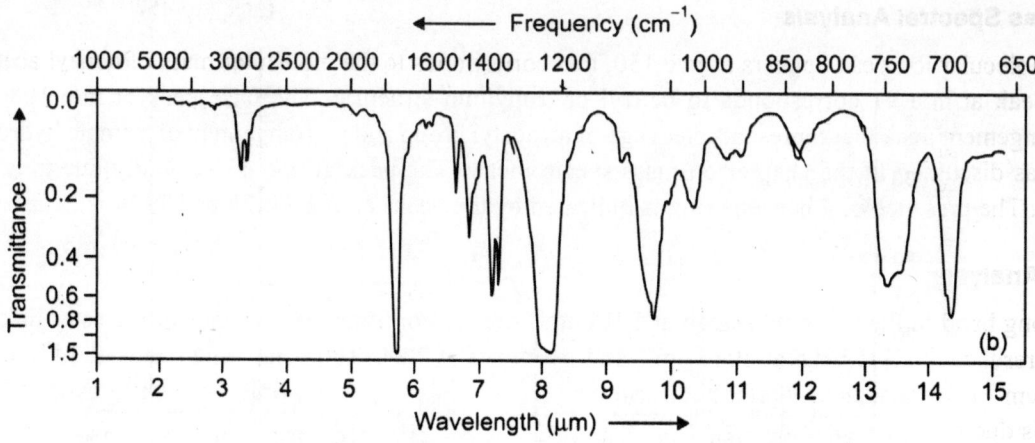

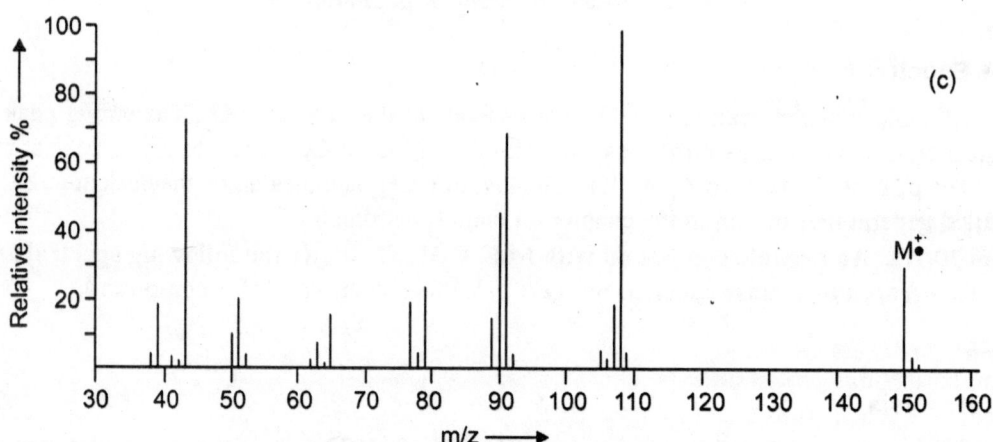

Fig. 20.3b. I.R. and mass spectra (Problem 20.1.3).

clearly corresponds to a phenyl (C_6H_5) group. The 2H singlet is deshielded as it appears at 5.00 ppm and is most likely to be a methylene grouping ($-CH_2-$) joined to the phenyl ring. It is not joined to an atom that has protons on it. The singlet at 1.96 ppm should correspond to a methyl group (CH_3-). These data indicate the compound to be benzyl acetate. The data do not fit with the structure of methyl benzoate as in that case OCH_3 protons would absorb at around 3.8 ppm instead of at 1.96 ppm as observed.

Benzyl acetate   Methyl benzoate

The 100 MHz spectra can shows the complicated splittings of the phenyl ring protons.

2. Mass Spectral Analysis

The molecular ion peak appears at m/e 150, that corresponds to the molecular mass of benzyl acetate. The peak at m/e 91 corresponds to benzyl or tropylium structure. The base peak at m/e 108 is a rearrangement peak that represents cleavage of an acetyl group and rearrangement of a single hydrogen atom as discussed in the chapter on mass spectrometry. The peak at m/e 43 is clearly due to acetyl group. The presence of a benzene ring is indicated by the peaks at m/e 77, 78 and 79.

3. IR Analysis

A strong band in the carbonyl region at 1715 cm^{-1} clearly confirms the presence of the ester linkage. The presence of C–H band at 3040 cm^{-1} and overtones at 2000–1667 cm^{-1} and bands at 1470 cm^{-1}, 1430 cm^{-1} (C=C skeletal stretch) confirm the presence of an aromatic ring. The strong band at 1055 cm^{-1} is due to C–O stretching.

Thus, it is clear from the above analysis that the compound is benzyl acetate.

Problem 20.1.4. A compound, C_9H_8O shows the following i.r., ^1H spectra. The C–13 spectral data are as follows:

190.0(d), 150.3(d), 134.9(s), 129.6(d), 128.4(d), 127.7(d) and 126.2(d).

Its mass spectrum shows M^+ at 148.

1. The ^1H NMR Spectrum

PMR spectrum does not contain peaks in the aliphatic region. The doublet at 9.7 ppm, equivalent to 1H indicates the presence of a formyl group (–CHO). As it is a doublet, it must be the result of splitting by nearby proton. As we do not find a signal in the aliphatic region, rather we find peaks in the region 6–7 ppm, clearly this proton must be olefinic in nature, =CH. In this region, there are two doublets equivalent to 1H each. Thus, there must be present a CH=CH–CHO unit. A multiplet equivalent to 5H in the aromatic region (7–8 ppm) indicates the presence of an aromatic nucleus. Thus, the proposed structure would be:

Two isomers are possible for this structure, cis and trans isomers. Which one is the right structure can be decided only by knowing the values of the coupling constants. As the ^3J is about 16 Hz, we have the trans rather than cis-cinnamaldehyde (as ^3J cis is about 8 Hz).

2. ^{13}C NMR Interpretation

The most deshielded carbon appears at 190 ppm which is the CHO as it becomes a doublet in a ^1H-coupled spectrum. A look at the δ values of the remaining carbons quite clearly indicates that these are all aromatic/olefinic carbons. Further, as there is only quaternary carbon, it will remain as singlet in proton-coupled spectrum. Therefore, it must be the carbon at 150.3 ppm. All remaining carbons appear

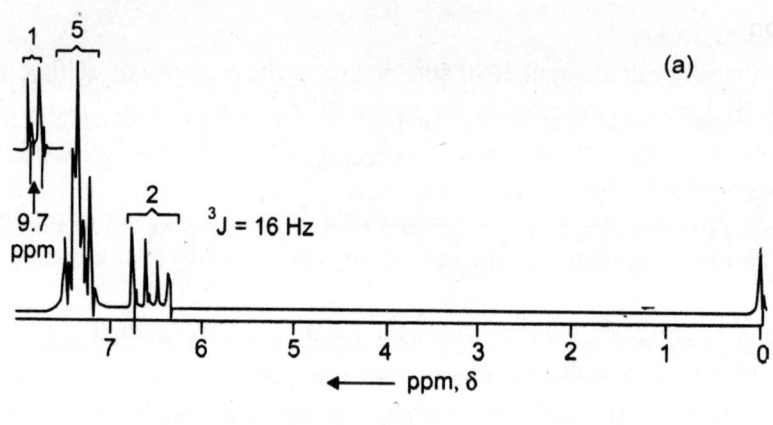

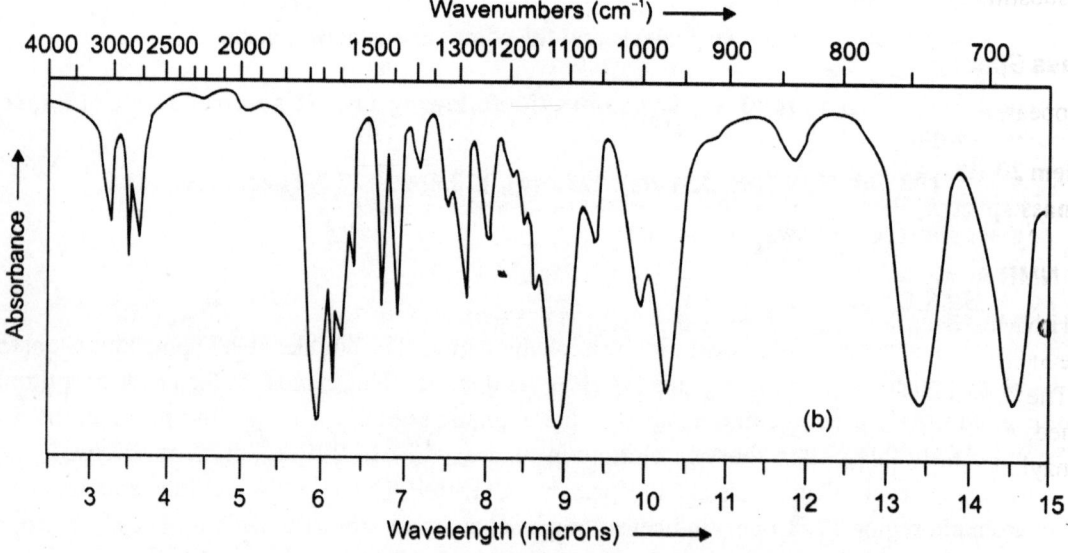

Fig. 20.4. IR(A), ^{1}H NMR (B) and mass (C) spectra for Problem 20.5.

as doublets in ^{1}H-coupled CMR spectrum and so are either aromatic or olefinic. The carbon to which CHO group is joined should be most deshielded of these. It will be the one at 150.3 ppm. The next deshielded will be the olefinic attached directly to the phenyl ring i.e. at 129.6 ppm. The carbon para to the substituent would be the most shielded at 126.2 ppm. The remaining signals at 128.4 and 127.7 must correspond to the two sets of carbons being ortho and meta respectively w.r. to the substituent.

3. IR Interpretation

The appearance of a weak peak at about 3090 cm^{-1} indicates the presence of olefinic system.

The presence of CHO group is indicated by the doublet at 2820 and 2750 cm^{-1} due to Fermi resonance.

A strong peak at 1685 cm^{-1} in the carbonyl region confirms the aldehydic carbonyl present in conjugation with the aromatic ring.

The band at 1630 cm^{-1} (m) due to C=C stretching confirms the presence of olefinic system.

The presence of aromatic system is confirmed due to presence of skeletal vibrations at 1610, 1580, 1500 and 1450 cm^{-1}.

The C–H in-plane bending at 1400 cm^{-1} further confirms the CHO group.

C–O stretch of the α,β-unsaturated system occurs at 1120 cm^{-1}.

A strong band due to C–H OOP, aromatic at 750 cm^{-1} indicates that the benzene ring is monosubstituted.

4. Mass Spectral Analysis

The appearance of M‡ peak at m/e 148 confirms the structure as trans-cinnamaldehyde.

Problem 20.1.5. An organic compound with M.F. C$_7$H$_8$O shows the following ^{1}H NMR, ^{13}C NMR and mass spectra. Propose a suitable structure of the compound.

1. ^{1}H NMR Analysis

The ^{1}H NMR spectrum contains three peaks at 7.35, 4.62 and 2.40 ppm, in the integral ratio of 5:2:1. As the 5H singlet appears in the aromatic region, it is clear that the compound C$_7$H$_8$O contains a phenyl ring. The 2H singlet at 4.62 means a methylene group. So, we are left only with an OH group to be assigned. As the OH can appear anywhere between 0.5 to 5.0 ppm, the compound, therefore, seems to be benzyl alcohol. Clearly the O–H group is not involved in spin-spin splitting with the CH$_2$ group.

CH$_2$OH

2. CMR Interpretation

The C–13 NMR shows the presence of five peaks at 64.5, 126.8, 127.2, 128.2 and 140.8. The presence of the last four peaks clearly confirms the presence of the aromatic ring. The methylene carbon attached to phenyl ring on one hand and to oxygen on the other gets deshielded and appears at 64.5 ppm.

3. IR Interpretation

The broad peak at 3300 cm^{-1} indicates O–H stretching (intermolecular hydrogen bonded). The peak at 2985 cm^{-1} indicates the presence of aromatic ring due to C–H stretching. The band at 2857 cm^{-1} implies the presence of methylene group. Bands in the region 2000–1667 cm^{-1} are the overtones

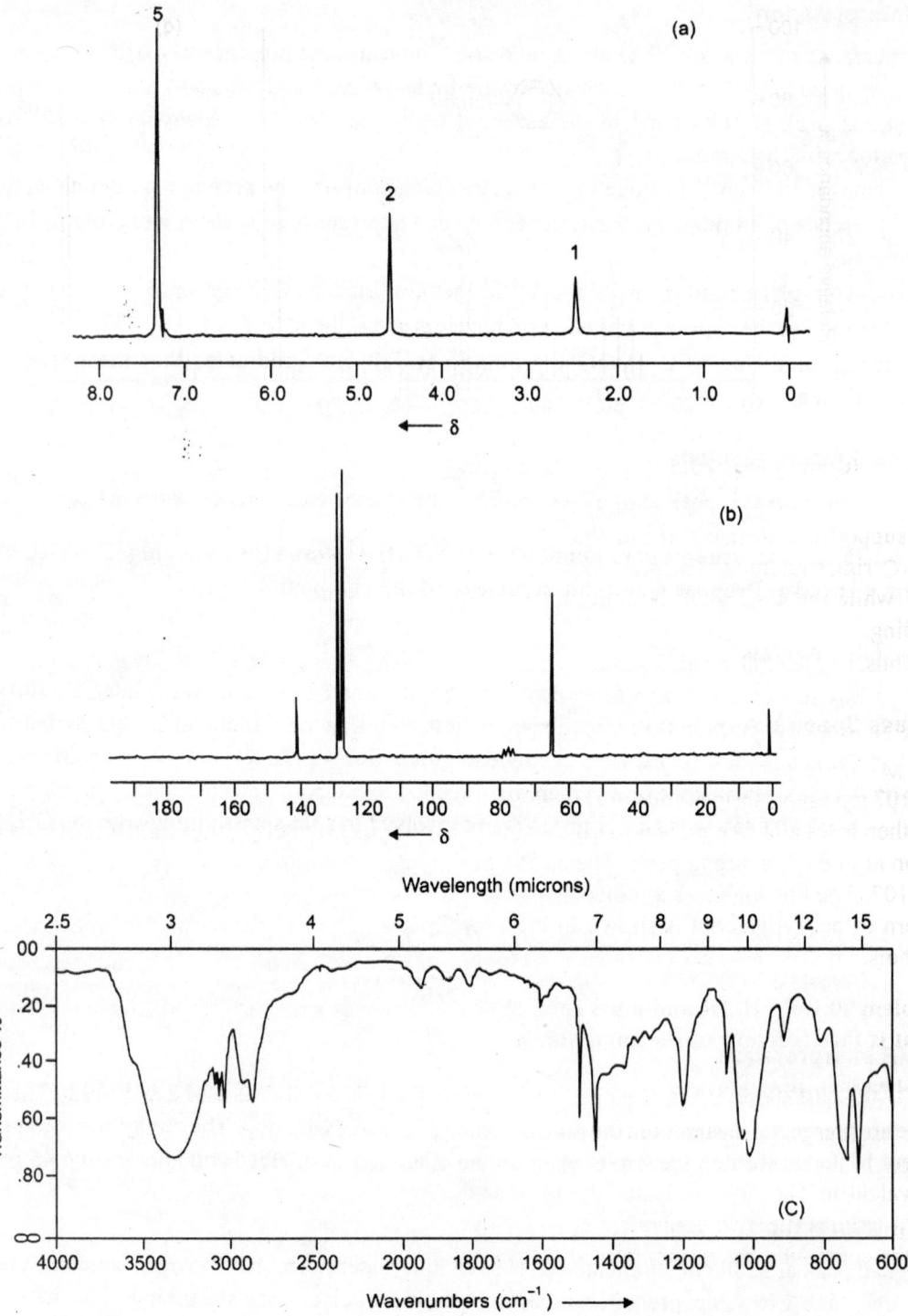

Fig. 20.5. (A) ^{1}H, (B) C–13, (C) IR, (D) Mass spectra for problem 20.1.5. (Contd.)

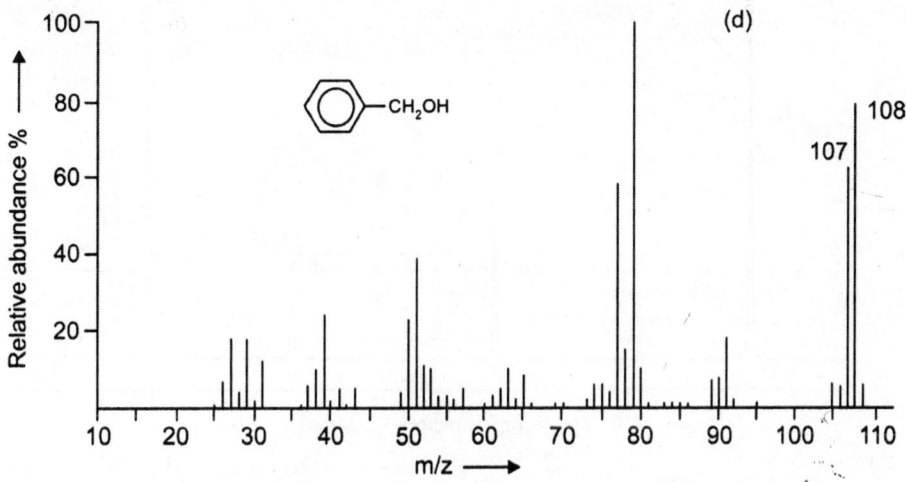

(Contd.) **Fig. 20.5.** (A) ^{1}H, (B) C–13, (C) IR, (D) Mass spectra for problem 20.1.5.

that support the presence of the phenyl ring. Bands at 1497 cm^{-1} and 1453 cm^{-1} are due to skeletal C$=$C ring stretching. The band at 1471 cm^{-1} is due to CH$_2$ scissoring. O–H bending occurs at 1208 cm^{-1} while the C–O OOP is noticeable at 735 cm^{-1}. The band at 697 cm^{-1} is due to ring C$=$C bending.

Thus, i.r. spectral analysis supports the structural elucidation done on the bases of ^{1}H NMR analysis.

4. Mass Spectral Analysis

The M^{+} corresponds to strong peak at m/e 108 which corresponds to M.F. C_7H_8O. The strong peak at m/e 107 represents the peak due to H radical loss (M – 1). The weak peak at m/e 106 is due to [Ph CHO]$^{+}$ that then loses a H free radical to give a small peak at m/e 105 which after loss of a CO yields phenyl cation at m/e 77, a strong peak. The strong peak at m/e 79 arises due to loss of CO from the peak at m/e 107. The Ph$^+$ ion loses a molecule of acetylene to give $C_4H_3^{+}$ ion, at m/e/ 51. The fragmentation pattern of benzyl alcohol is shown in the chapter on mass spectroscopy under the subtitle arylalkyl alcohols.

Problem 20.1.6. ^{1}H, IR and mass spectra of a compound with M.F. $C_4H_{11}N$ are recorded below. **What is the structure of the compound?**

1. ^{1}H NMR interpretation

There are present three signals in the ratio of 1:6:4 which counts for the total, eleven number of hydrogens present in the molecule. The triplet at 1.15 ppm is equivalent to 6H, while the quartet at 2.56 ppm is equivalent to 4H. This indicates the presence of two equivalent methyl groups and two equivalent –CH$_2$– groups (i.e. two equivalent ethyl groups). As the singlet at 0.65 ppm is equal to 1H, it is clear that the compound has a symmetrical structure, most probably, it is diethylamine, a secondary amine:

$$CH_3\ CH_2\ \underset{H}{N}\ CH_2\ CH_3$$

Further, we know that the NH proton lies in the range 0.5–5.0 ppm for this type of proton.

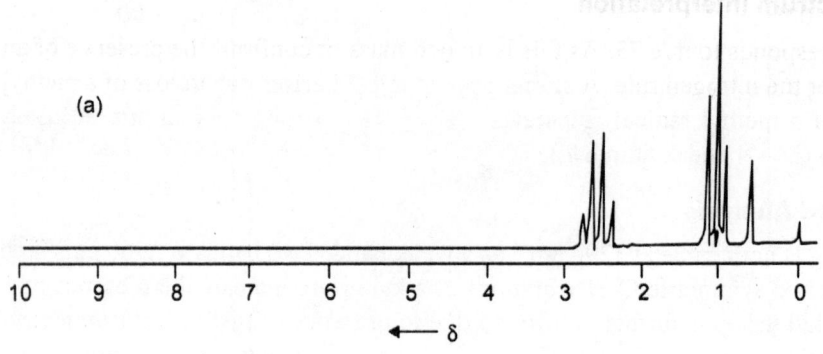

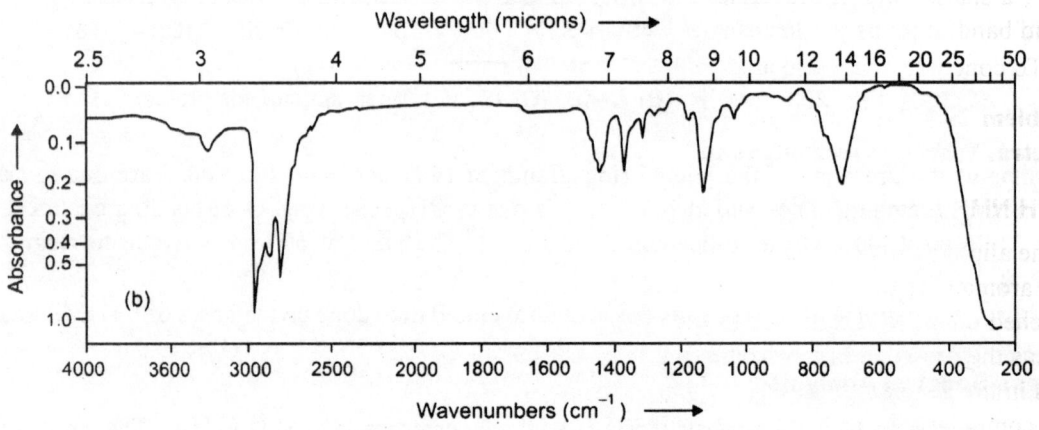

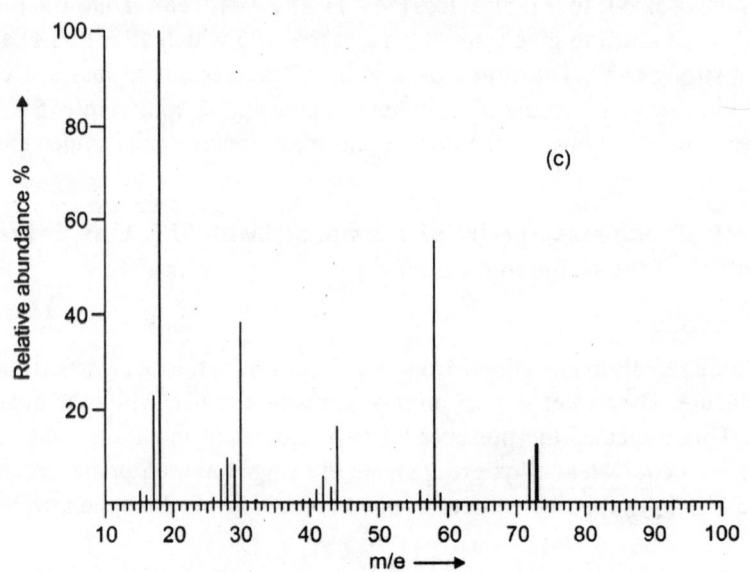

Fig. 20.6. PMR (a), IR (b), and mass spectra (c) (Problem 20.1.6).

2. Mass Spectrum Interpretation

$M^{\ddagger}$ peak corresponds to m/e 73. As this is an odd mass, it confirms the presence of an odd number of nitrogen, as per the nitrogen rule. A strong peak at m/e 58 arises due to loss of a methyl group (M–15). Further loss of a methyl radical, generates $CH_2=NH_2$ strong peak at m/e 30. Loss of a hydrogen radical gives a (M – 1) peak at m/e 72.

3. The Infrared Analysis

N–H stretching is noticeable at 3290 cm^{-1} as a weak band. Two bands at 2960 cm^{-1} and 2815 cm^{-1} due to asymmetric and symmetric C–H vibrations of alkyl group indicate the presence of alkyl group. The presence of alkyl group is further confirmed due to presence of respective asymmetric and symmetric N–H bands at 1450 and 1375 cm^{-1}. C–N stretching is indicated by the presence of a peak at 1140 cm^{-1}, a sharp band of moderate intensity. The N–H OOP bending is indicated by the presence of a broad band of moderate intensity at 725 cm^{-1}.

To conclude, the compound, in hand, is diethylamine.

Problem 20.1.7. Compound with M.F. C$_8$H$_9$NO exhibits the following ^{1}H NMR, IR and mass spectra. What is this compound?

1. ^{1}H NMR Interpretation

In the aliphatic region, we find two peaks as singlets at 3.15 and 2.15 ppm in the integral ratio of 1:3. The aromatic region shows a 5H multiplet. Obviously, the singlet at 2.15 ppm must be a methyl group attached either to the ring or to the nitrogen as it is a relatively deshielded methyl. The 5H protons means the presence of a benzene ring. The singlet at 3.15 ppm could be either OH or NH proton as it falls in the general range 0.5–5.0 ppm for such kinds of protons. Thus the most probable structure for this compound seems to be as shown below, particularly in view of the fact that two pairs of doublets, that characterize the presence of p-disubstituted benzene ring not present.

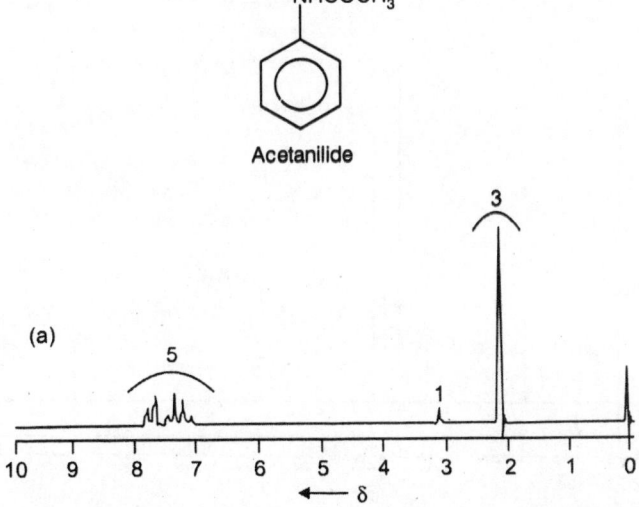

Acetanilide

Fig. 20.7. (A) ^{1}H NMR, (B) IR, (c) Mass, (d) CMR spectra for Problem 20.1.7. *(Contd.)*

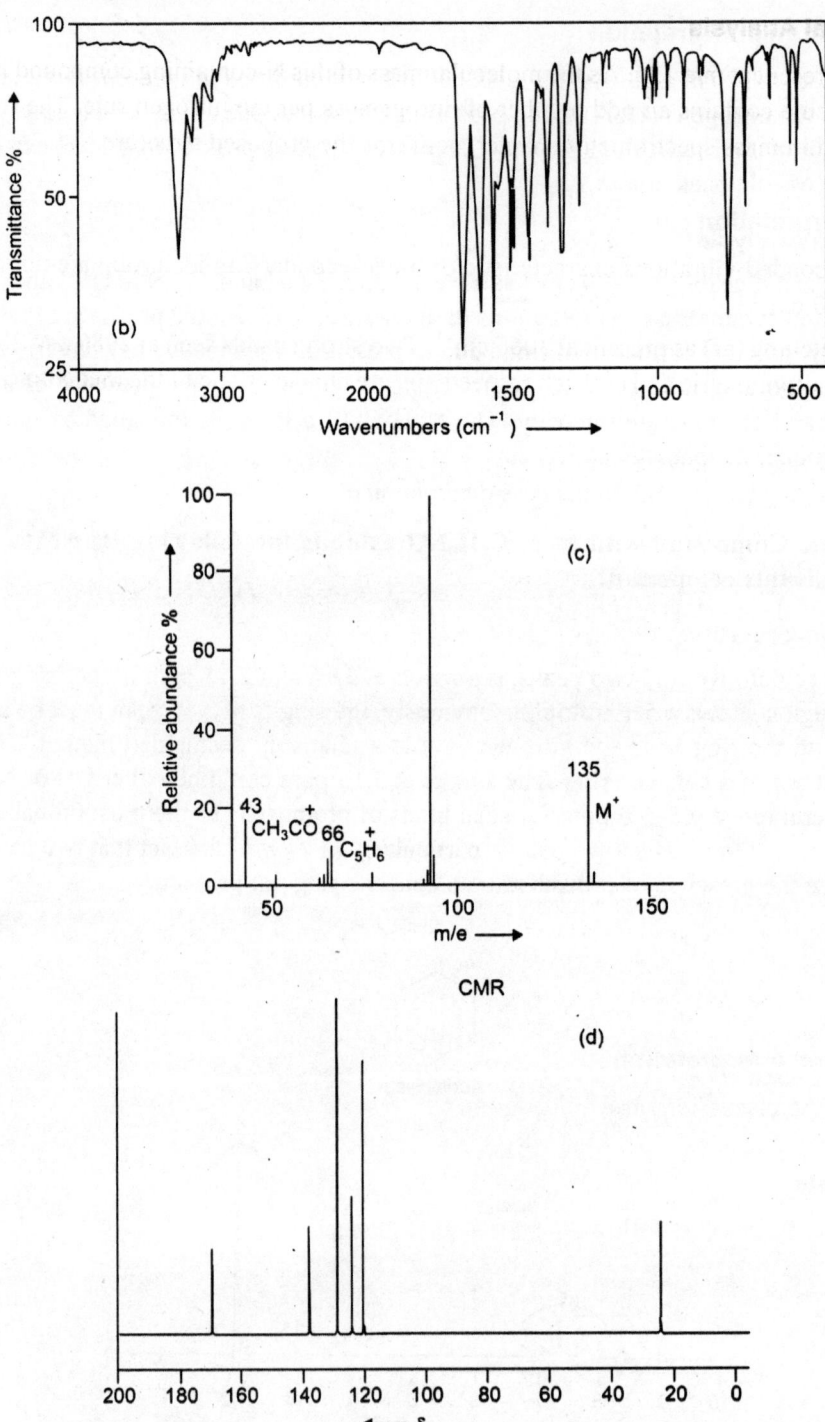

Fig. 20.7. (A) ^{1}H NMR, (B) IR, (c) Mass, (d) CMR spectra for problem 20.1.7.

2. Mass Spectral Analysis

The M^+ ion is present at m/e 135. As the molecular mass of this N-containing compound is odd, it tells us that the molecule contains an odd number of nitrogens as per the nitrogen rule. The fragmentation pattern discussed in mass spectrometry chapter, confirms the proposed structure.

3. Infrared Interpretation

N–H stretching bonded vibrations characteristic of trans secondary amide group are noticeable in the range 3300–3120 cm^{-1}.

The C–H stretching (ar) as present at 3065 cm^{-1}. Two strong bands seen at 2980 and 2800 cm^{-1} due to asymmetric and symmetric C–H stretch respectively are characteristic of the methyl group present in the molecule.

The carbonyl region shows a very strong band due to carbonyl group at 1670 cm^{-1}. This is also known as Amide I band.

The presence of aromatic ring is further indicated by the presence of overtones in the region 2000–1667 cm^{-1} as well as strong bands at 1600 and 1500 cm^{-1} (skeletal vibrations). Further, the presence of a band at 750 cm^{-1} due to C–H OOP indicates that the benzene ring is only monosubstituted. Amide II-band at 1550 cm^{-1} indicates the presence of N–H (ip) bending vibration.

From the above, we conclude the presence of an anilide unit in the molecule.

The ^{1}H NMR and IR analysis lead us to the following structure of the sample compound.

NHCOCH$_3$

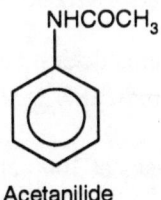

Acetanilide

4. Mass Spectral Interpretation

This is given in the discussion on Anilide in the chapter on mass spectrometry.

5. C–13 analysis

The peaks can be assigned as follows:

169.49	1
138.17	2
128.77	3
124.23	4
120.39	5
24.18	6

20.2 UNSOLVED PROBLEMS FROM VARIOUS INTERNATIONAL UNIVERSITIES

1. Elucidate the structure of the compound.
   (a) A compound C_4H_6O is not an alcohol
   (b) Does not show significant UV obsorption
   (c) Show absorption at 3300, 2950 cm^{-1} and 2200 cm^{-1}. No absorption at 1700 cm^{-1} is noticeable
   (d) ^1H NMR spectrum shows three singlets: d 3.0 (1H), 3.5 (3H) and 4.9 (2H)

   (University of Edinburgh)

2. $C_9H_{13}N$ is the molecular formula of an organic compound with the following spectral characteristics. What is its structure?
   (a) UV absorption occurs at λ_{max} 230 nm (Σ_{max} = 8000)
   (b) IR spectrum shows strong absorptions at 3000 cm^{-1} and 700 cm^{-1} but no absorption at 1700 cm^{-1} and in the region 3200–3600 cm^{-1}
   (c) ^1H NMR. δ 1.1 (t, 3H), 2.8 (s, 3H), 3.1 (q, 2H), 6.8–7.2 (m, 5H)

   (University of Edinburgh)

3. An organic compound C_5H_8O displays the following spectral characteristics. What is its structure?
   (a) UV absorption occurs at λ_{max} 228 nm (Σ 19000)
   (b) IR spectrum shows bands at 3000 cm^{-1} and at 1700 cm^{-1} but no absorptions in the region 3600–3200 cm^{-1}
   (c) NMR spectrum shows: δ 2.0 (s, 3H), 2.2 (s, 3H), 6.1 (d, 1H), 9.5 (d, 1H)

   (University of Wales)

4. An unknown molecule (A) has the formula $C_8H_{10}O$ and exhibits the following spectral data. Answer the following:
   (a) How many double band equivalents does it have?
   (b) The UV spectrum shows absorption at λ_{max} 223 nm (Σ = 5800). What information does it carry?
   (c) The infrared spectrum shows peaks at 3000 cm^{-1} and in the region 700–800 cm^{-1} but none near 1700 cm^{-1} or in the region 3600–3200 cm^{-1}. What information does it provide?
   (d) ^1H NMR spectrum shows absorptions at δ H 3.7, 4.9 and in the region 6.8–7.3 with corresponding integral steps of 4.8, 3.2 and 8.0 cm. Using these data and the M.F., calculate how many protons correspond to each absorption.
   (e) Draw two possible structures for (A) and indicate which proton in (A) correspond to the n.m.r. absorptions.
   (f) How might a closer examination of the n.m.r. spectrum reveal which structure was correct?

   (University of Bristol)

5. A compound yielded the following spectroscopic data. Deduce the structure of this compound and explain your reasoning.
   (a) IR spectrum shows absorption at 700, 1700 and 3000 cm^{-1}
   (b) The UV spectrum shows λ_{max} = 240 nm (Σ = 12000)
   (c) The mass spectrum shows a parent ion peak at m/z 120 and fragment ions at m/z 105 and 77

   (University of Edinburgh)

Note: This is an example which illustrates as to how sometimes even without the ^{1}H NMR data you can arrive at the structure of a compound. Anyway, ^{1}H NMR data of this compound is δ 2.5 (s, 3H), 6.5–8.0 (m, 5H).

6. A natural product A was shown by mass spectrometry to have the molecular formula $C_9H_{10}O_5$ and it gave deep red coloration with ferric chloride. The proton n.m.r. spectrum showed the following absorptions:

   δ = 7.0 (singlet, 2H); δ = 5–6 (broad resonance, 3H); δ = 4.2 (quartet, J = 7 Hz, 2H); δ = 1.2 (triplet, J = 7 Hz, 3H).

   The carbon–13 n.m.r. spectrum showed the following absorptions:

   δ = 14(q); δ = 63(t); δ = 110(d)*; δ = 122(s); δ = 139(s); δ = 145(s)*' δ = 170(s). The multiplicity of the peaks in the off resonance proton decoupled spectrum is given in brackets (s = singlet, d = doublet, t = triplet, q = quartet) and the resonances marked * each correspond to two carbon atoms. Deduce, giving your reasoning, two structures for A consistent with this data. Explain briefly how a knowledge of the carbon–13 chemical shifts of appropriate monosubstituted benzene derivatives would enable a choice to be made between your structures.

   (University of Washington)

7. An organic compound contains C = 36.9%, H = 5.67%, Br = 41%. It shows two strong peaks in its i.r. spectrum at 1735 and 1250 cm^{-1}. Its ^{1}H NMR shows the following multiplicities.

   d 4.1 (2H, q, J = 7.5 Hz)

   3.8 (2H, t, J = 7 Hz)

   2.4 (2H, t, J = 7.2 Hz)

   1.8 (2H, m)

   1.25 (3H, t, J = 7.5 Hz)

   Its mass spectrum shows two peaks at 194 and 196. Predict its structure.

   Hint: The compound is:

$$\underset{q}{\underset{1.25}{CH_3}}\ \underset{t}{\underset{4.1}{CH_2}}-O-\underset{\underset{O}{\|}}{C}-\underset{t}{\underset{2.4}{CH_2}}-\underset{m}{\underset{1.8}{CH_2}}-\underset{t}{\underset{3.8}{CH_2}}-Br$$

   The peak at 1735 cm^{-1} is due to CO stretching and that at 1250 cm^{-1} is due to $-\underset{\underset{O}{\|}}{C}-$ bending.

   The peak at m/e 194 represents the molecular ion while that at 196 is the M + 2 peak due to Br–81 isotope.

8. An organic compound with MF $C_4H_9NO_2$ shows two prominent peaks in i.r. at 1690 cm^{-1} and 1620 cm^{-1}. It shows M^{+} peak at 103. The ^{1}H NMR shows the following multiplicities. δ 1H s at 5.2 ppm, a 3H t at 1.2 ppm, a 2H q at 4.2 ppm, a 3H d at 1.3 ppm.

   Hint: The structure is:

$$\underset{1.3}{H_3C}-\underset{\underset{5.2}{\underset{H}{|}}}{N}-\underset{\underset{O}{\|}}{C}-O-\underset{4.2}{CH_2}-\underset{1.2}{CH_3}$$

9. Assign a suitable structure to the organic compound having M^{+} peak at 116 on the basis of following spectral data:

UV : λ_{max} 283 nm ($\Sigma = 22$)

IR: 3000–2500 (broad), 1715 (strong), 1342 cm^{-1} (weak)

NMR: δ 2.12 (3H, s), 2.60 (2H, t), 2.25 (2H, t), 11.9 (1H, s)

10. Assign a suitable structure to the organic compound whose i.r., ^{1}H NMR and mass spectra are recorded in the Fig. below.

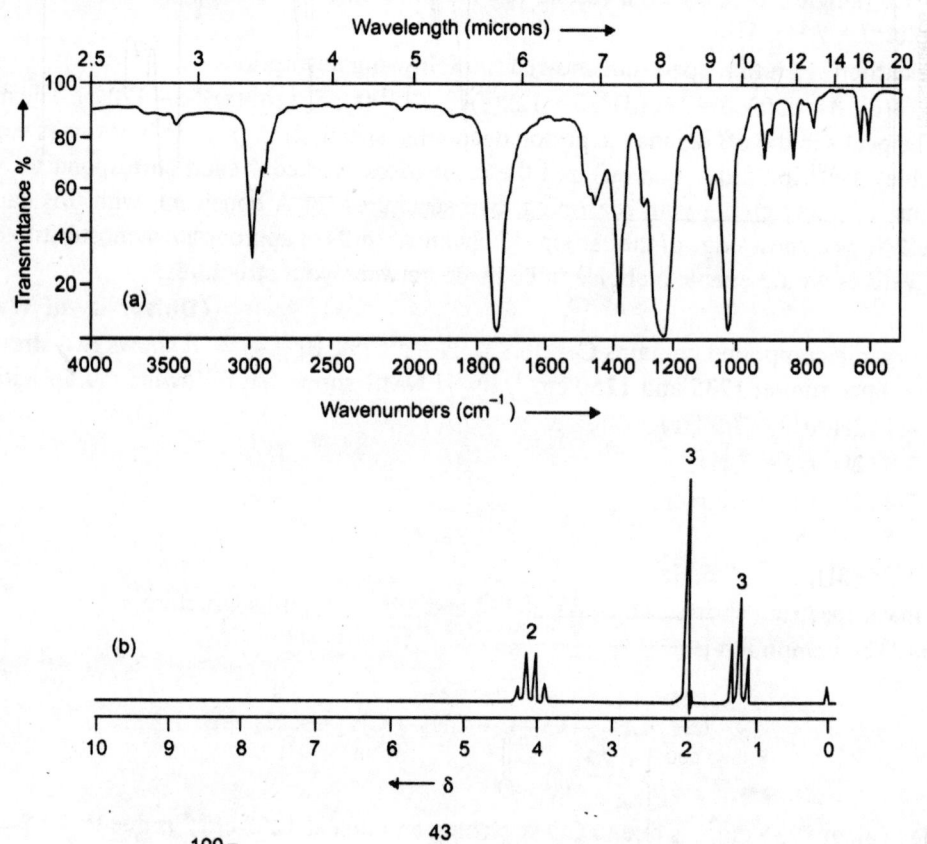

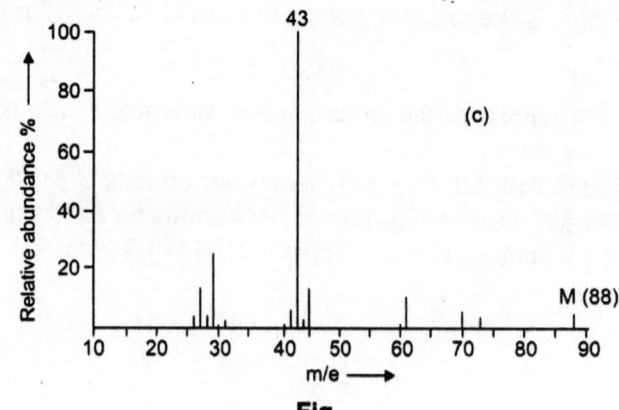

Fig.

11. Identify the compound whose, i.r. ^{1}H and mass spectra are given below.

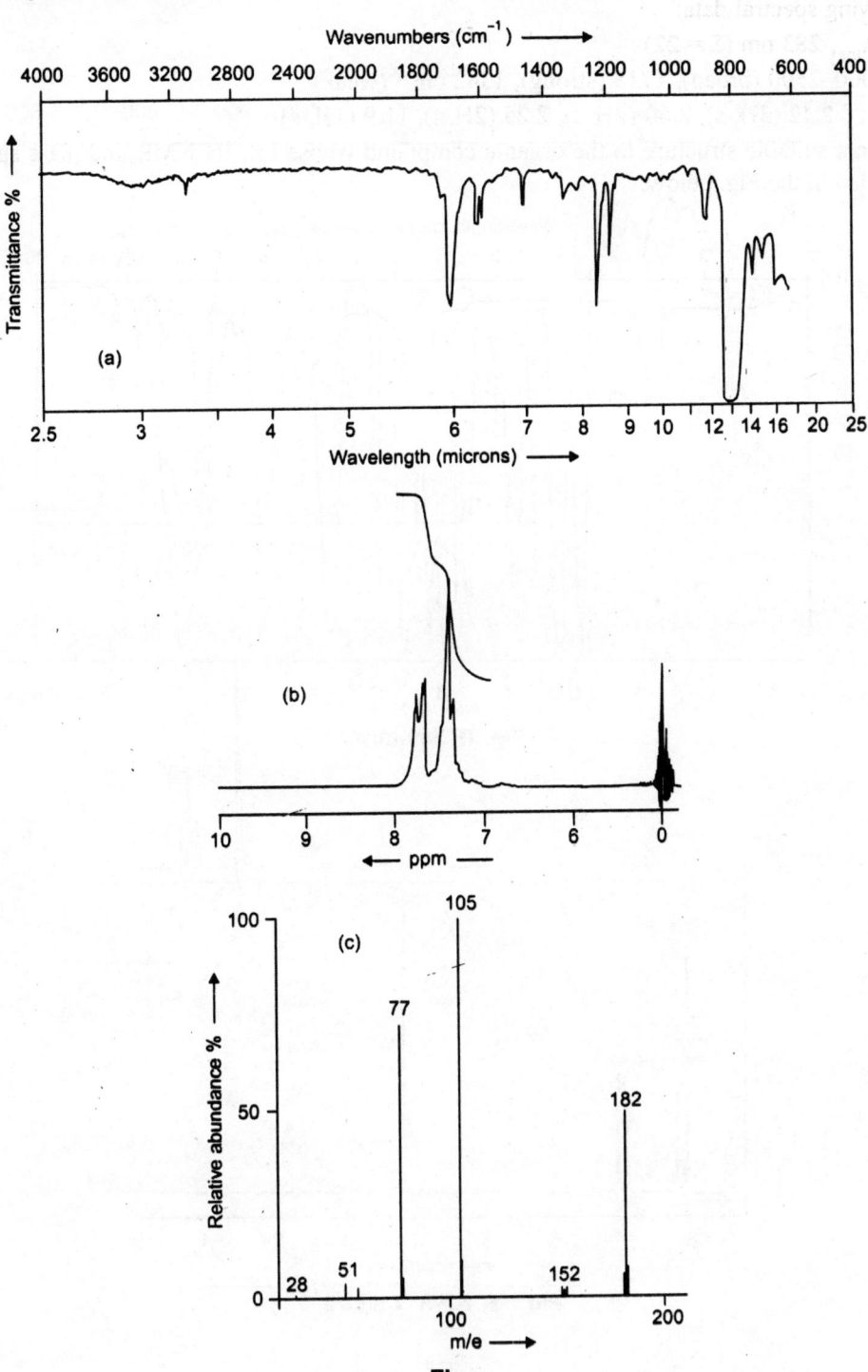

Fig.

12. Identify the compound with m/e = 136 $M^{\ddot{+}}$, whose i.r. and ^1H spectra are given below.

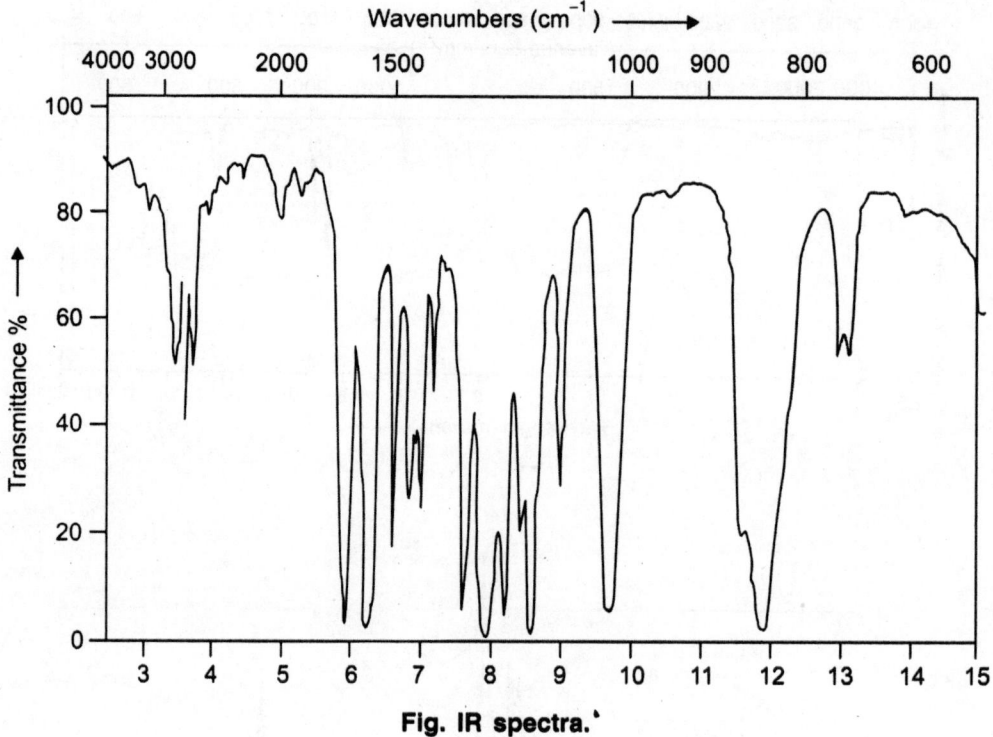

Fig. IR spectra.

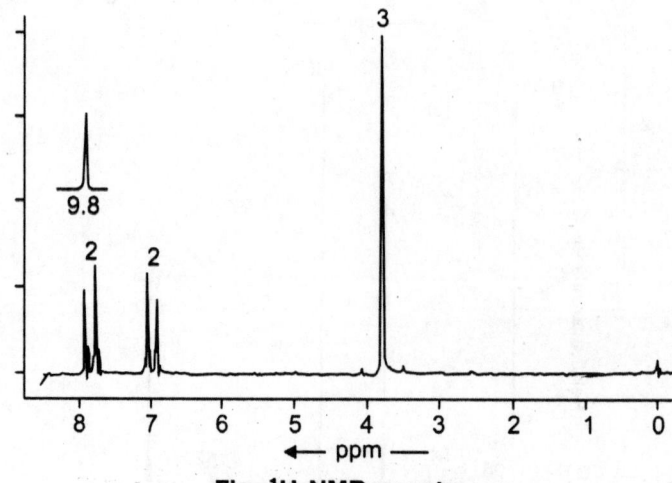

Fig. ^1H NMR spectra.

13. What is the structure of the organic compound having, MF $C_2H_5NO_2$, m/e = 75 (M^{+}) whose i.r. and ^1H NMR spectra (D_2O) are given below.

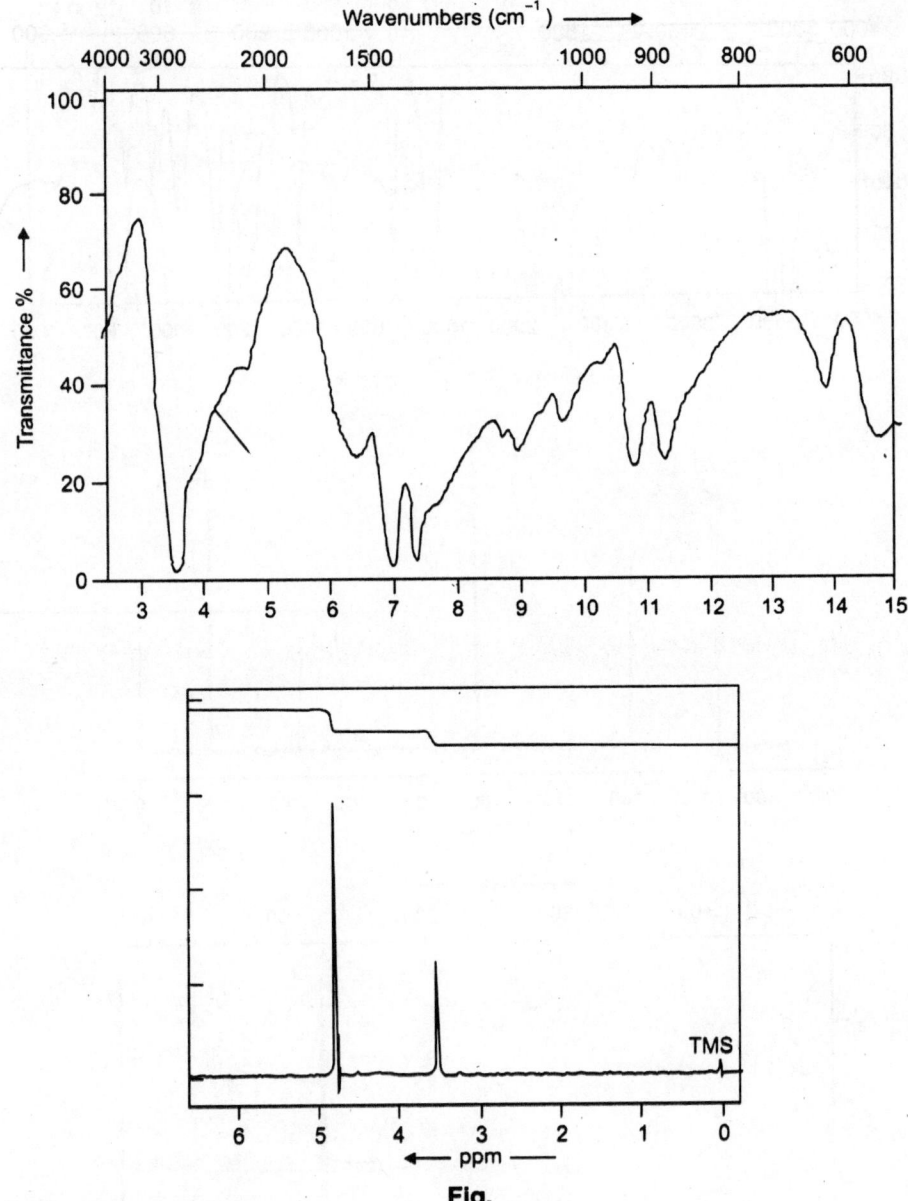

Fig.

Hint: NH_2-CH_2-COOH

$\downarrow D_2O$

$NH_2 - CH_2 - COOH$

14. What is the structure of organic compound with MF $C_4H_6O_2$ whose i.r. C–13 and ^1H spectra are recorded below.

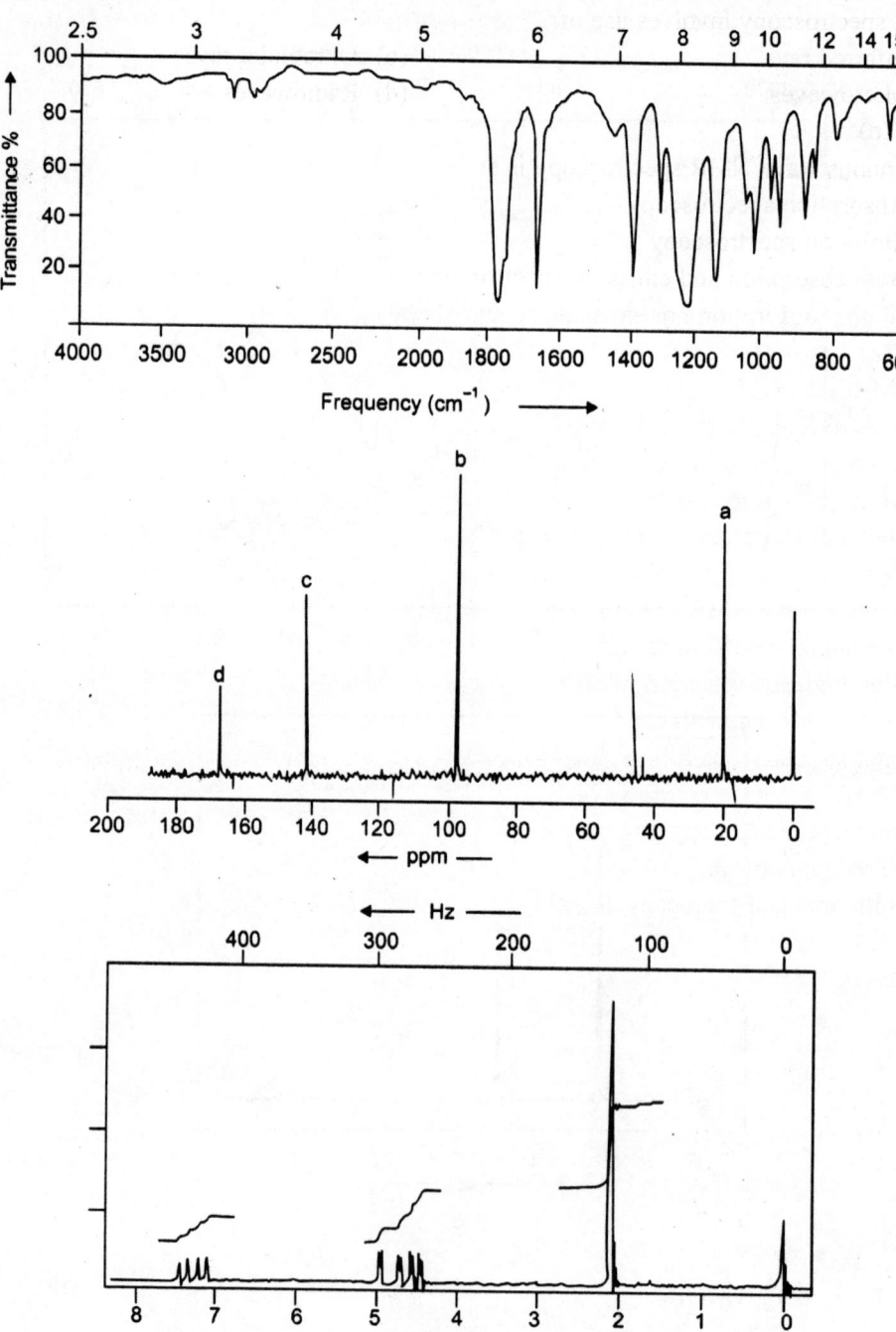

Fig. Infrared, CMR and proton NMR spectra (Problem 14).

20.3 MULTIPLE CHOICE QUESTIONS FOR NET, SLAT, GAIT, GPAT, GRE, CSE, HCS ETC. COMPETITIVE EXAMS

1. NMR spectroscopy involves use of:
   (a) Infrared rays
   (b) Ultraviolet rays
   (c) Microwaves
   (d) Radiowaves
   Hint: (d)

2. Continuous wave NMR spectroscopy is a:
   (a) Absorption spectroscopy
   (b) Emission spectroscopy
   (c) Both absorption and emission spectroscopy
   (d) Neither absorption nor emission spectroscopy
   Hint: (a)

3. FT NMR is a
   (a) Absorption spectroscopy
   (b) Emission spectroscopy
   (c) Both absorption and emission spectroscopy
   (d) Neither absorption nor emission spectroscopy
   Hint: (b)

4. Continuous wave NMR spectroscopy involves:
   (a) Sequential detection of resonances of nuclei
   (b) Simultaneous detection of all resonances of nuclei
   (c) Sometimes sequential and sometimes simultaneous detection of all resonances of nuclei
   (d) First simultaneous followed by sequential detection of resonances of nuclei
   Hint: (a)

5. Continuous spectroscopy gives a spectrum that is:
   (a) Time-domain
   (b) Frequency-domain
   (c) Both time and frequency domain
   (d) Neither of these
   Hint: (b)

6. I for B–11 is:
   (a) 1
   (b) 2
   (c) 1/2
   (d) 3/2
   Hint: (d)

7. I for P–31 is:
   (a) 1
   (b) 1/2
   (c) 2
   (d) 5/2
   Hint: (b)

8. I for N–15 is:
   (a) 1
   (b) 1/2
   (c) 2
   (d) 3/2
   Hint: (b)

9. I for N–14 is:
   (a) 1
   (b) 1/2
   (c) 2
   (d) 3/2
   Hint: (a)

10. I for C–12 is:
    (a) 1
    (b) 1/2
    (c) 2
    (d) 0
    Hint: (d)

11. I for C–13 is:
    (a) 1
    (b) 1/2
    (c) 3/2
    (d) 2
    Hint: (b)

12. I for H–1 is:
    (a) 1
    (b) 1/2
    (c) 3/2
    (d) 2
    Hint: (b)

13. I for D (H–2) is:
    (a) 1
    (b) 1/2
    (c) 3/2
    (d) 2
    Hint: (a)

14. I for F–19 is:
    (a) 1
    (b) 1/2
    (c) 3/2
    (d) 2
    Hint: (b)

15. Number of orientations w.r. to applied magnetic field for B–11 is:
    (a) 2
    (b) 3
    (c) 4
    (d) 5
    Hint: (c)

16. Number of orientations w.r. to applied magnetic field for D is:
    (a) 2
    (b) 3
    (c) 4
    (d) 1
    Hint: (b)

17. Number of orientation w.r. to applied magnetic field for P–31 is:
    (a) 1
    (b) 2
    (c) 3
    (d) 4
    Hint: (b)

18. General chemical shift range for protons is:
    (a) 0–12
    (b) 2–8
    (c) 3–30
    (d) 2–40
    Hint: (a)

19. General chemical shift range for C–13 is:
    (a) 0–12
    (b) 0–300
    (c) 0–200
    (d) 20–800
    Hint: (c)

20. General chemical shift range for P–31 is:
    (a) 0–700
    (b) 0–600
    (c) 0–500
    (d) 0–1000
    Hint: (a)

21. General chemical shift range for N–15 is:
    (a) 0–400
    (b) 0–500
    (c) 0–600
    (d) 0–700
    Hint: (c)

22. Internal reference for proton is:
    (a) $(CH_3)Si$
    (b) $(CH_3)_3Si$
    (c) $(CH_3)_5Si$
    (d) $(CH_3)_2Si$
    Hint: (a)

23. Internal reference for phosphorous is:
    (a) H_3PO_3 (85%)
    (b) H_3PO_5 (85%)
    (c) H_3PO_2 (85%)
    (d) None
    Hint: (b)

24. Internal reference for C–13 is:
    (a) $(CH_3)_4Si$
    (b) $CDCl_3$
    (c) $(CH_3)_2CO$
    (d) C_6D_6
    Hint: (a)

25. Internal reference for F–19 is:
    (a) $CFCl_3$
    (b) CF_2
    (c) NH_4F
    (d) NaF
    Hint: (a)

26. Internal reference for N–15 is:
    (a) Liq NH_3
    (b) NH_4OH
    (c) NH_4Cl
    (d) NH_4F
    Hint: (a)

12. G.C. Levy, *Topics in C-13 Spectroscopy*, John Wiley and Sons, N.Y., 1954.
13. G.C. Levy, R.L. Lichter, G.L. Nelson, *C-13 NMR Spectroscopy*, 2nd Ed., John Wiley and Sons, N.Y.

21

References for NMR, IR, Mass and UV

21.1 NUCLEAR MAGNETIC RESONANCE

Spin-Spin Coupling

1. J.O. Pople, W.G. Schneider and H.J. Bernstein, *High Resolution Nuclear Magnetic Resonance*, McGraw-Hill, NY, 1959.
2. M. Barfield and D.M. Grant, Ch. 4, *Theory of Nuclear Spin-Spin Coupling*, and A.A. Bothner, Ch. 5, *Geminal and Vicinal Proton-Proton Couplings in Organic Compounds, in Advances in Magnetic Resonance* (J.S. Wagh, Ed.), Academic Press, NY, 1965.
3. H. Booth, *Application of NMR Spectroscopy to Conformational Analysis of Cyclic Compounds in Progress in NMR Spectroscopy*, Vol. 5 (J.W. Emsley, J. Feeney and L.H. Suitcliffe, Ed.), Pergamon Press, Oxford, 1969.
4. J. Kowalewski, *Calculations of Nuclear Spin-Spin Coupling Constants in Progress in NMR Spectroscopy*, Vol. II (J.W. Emsky, J. Feeney, and L.H. Suitcliffe, Eds.), Pergamon Press, Oxford, 1977, pp. 1–78.
5. J.D. Roberts, *An Introduction to the Analysis of Spin-Spin Splitting in High Resolution NMR Spectra*, W.A. Benamin, NY, 1962.
6. K.B. Wiberg and B.J. Nist, *The Interpretation of NMR Spectra*, W.A. Benzamin, NY, 1962.
7. T.R. Hoye, P.R. Hanson, J.R. Vyvyan, *A Practical Guide to First-Order Multiplet Analysis in ^1H NMR Spectroscopy*, J. Org. Chem., 59, 4096, 1994.
8. L.F. Johnson and W.C. Jankowski, *Carbon–13 NMR Spectra, a Collection of Assigned, Coded and Indexed Spectra*, Wiley, NY, 1972.
9. A. Ditchfield and P.D. Ellis, Ch. 1, *Theory on ^{13}C Chemical Shifts in Topics in C–13 NMR Spectroscopy*, Vol. I (G.G. Levy, Ed.), Wiley, NY, 1974.
10. E. Breitmaier ad W. Voelter, *Carbon–13 NMR Spectroscopy, Method and Applications*, Verlag-Chemie, Bergstr, 1974.
11. N.K. Wilson and J.D. Stothers, *Stereochemical Aspects of ^{13}C NMR Spectroscopy in Topics in Stereochemistry*, Vol. 8, p. 1, Wiley, N.Y., 1974.

12. G.C. Levy, *Topics in C–13 Spectroscopy*, John Wiley and Sons, N.Y., 1984.
13. G.C. Levy, R.L. Lichter and G.L. Nelson, *C–13 NMR Spectroscopy*, 2nd Ed., John Wiley and Sons, N.Y., 1980.

Computer Programs for Learning C–13 NMR Shifts

14. F.W. Clough, *Introduction to Spectroscopy, Version 2.0 for MS-DOS and Mckintosh*, Trinity Software, 607, Tenney-Min. Highway, Suite 215, Plymouth, N.H., 03264, Web: www.trinitysoftware.com.
15. P.F. Schatz, *Spectrabook I and II, MS-DOS Version and Spectradeck I and II, Macintosh Version*, Falcon Software, One Hollis Street, Wellesley, MA 02481. Web: www.falconsoftware.com.

Pulse FT NMR Spectroscopy

16. T.C. Farrar and E.D. Becker, *Pulse and Fourier Transform NMR*, Academic Press, N.Y., 1961.
17. D. Shaw, *Fourier Transform NMR Spectroscopy*, Elsevier, Amsterdam, 1976.
18. K. Mullen and P.S. Pregosin, *Fourier Transform NMR Techniques, a Practical Approach*, Academic Press, N.Y., 1976.
19. E. Breitmaier, G. Jung and W. Voelter, *Pulse Fourier Transform ^{13}C NMR Spectroscopy, Principles and Applications*, Angur. Chem. Int., Ed., 10, 673, 1971.
20. E.D. Becker, *High Resolution NMR: Theory and Chemical Applications*, 3rd Ed., Academic Press, San Diego, CA, 2000.
21. F. Bloch, Phy. Rev., 70, 460, 1946.
22. F. Bloch, W.W. Hansen and M. Packard, Phy. Rev., 70, 474, 1946.
23. L.M. Jackman and S. Sternhell, *Applications of NMR Spectroscopy in Organic Chemistry*, Pergamon Press, 1969.
24. A. Autt, G.O. Dudek, *NMR—An Introduction to Nuclear Magnetic Resonance Spectroscopy*, Holden-Day, San Franscisco, 1976.
25. H. Fricbolin, *Basic One- and Two-Dimensional NMR Spectroscopy*, 2nd ed., VCH Publishers, N.Y., 1993.
26. R.S. Macomber, *A Complete Introduction to Modern NMR Spectrometry*, John Wiley and Sons, N.Y., 1997.
27. A. Autt and M.R. Autt, *A Handy and Systematic Catalog of NMR Spectra*, 60 MHz with some 270 MHz, University Science Books, Mill Valley, CA, 1980.
28. C.J. Pouchert, *The Aldrich Library of NMR Spectra*, 60 MHz, 2nd ed., Aldrich Chemical Company, Milwaukee, WI, 1983.
29. C.J. Pouchert and J. Blenke, *The Aldrich Library of ^{13}C and ^1H FT NMR Spectra*, 300 MHz, Aldrich Chemical Company, Milwaukee, WI, 1993.
30. E. Pretsch, T. Clerc, J. Seibl, W. Simon, *Tables of Spectral Data for Structure Determination of Organic Compounds*, 2nd ed., Springer-Verlag, Berlin and N.Y., 1989.

2D and 3D (Protein) NMR

31. N.E. Jacobsen, *NMR Spectroscopy Explained, Simplified Theory, Application and Examples for Organic Chemistry and Structural Biology*, Wiley-Interscience, John Wiley and Sons, Hoboken, 2007.

32. J. Cavanagh, W.J. Fairbrother, A.G. Palmer, N.J. Sketton, *Protein NMR Spectroscopy*, Academic Press, 1996.

33. J. Cavanagh, W.J. Fairbrother, A.G. Palmer III, R. Rance and N.J. Skelton, *Protein NMR Spectroscopy*, Elsevier Boston, MA, USA, 2007.

34. N.E. Jacobson, A.J. Abadi, M.X. Sliwkowski, D.Reilly, N.J. Skelton, W.J. Fairbrother, *High Resolution Structure of the EGF-like Domain of Heregulin-α, Biochemistry*, 1996, 35, 3402–3417.

35. K.E. Kay, D.R. Muhandiram, *Gradient-enhanced Triple-Resonance 3–D NMR Experiments with Improved Sensitivity*, J. Mag. Reson., B 1994, 103, 203–216.

36. E. Brunner, *Residual Dipolar Couplings in Protein NMR*, Concepts Magn. Reson., 2001, 13, 238–59.

37. G.S. Rule and T.K. Hitchens, *Fundamentals of Protein NMR Spectroscopy*, Springer, Dordrecht, The Netherlands, 2006.

38. Wuthrich, K., *NMR of Proteins and Nucleic Acids*, John Wiley and Sons, New York, USA, 1986.

39. K.A. Gardner and L.E. Kay, *The Use of ^{2}H, ^{13}C, ^{15}N Multidimensional NMR to Study the Structure and Dynamics of Proteins*, Annual Review of Biophysics and Biomolecular Structure, 27, 1998, 357–406.

HSQC

40. G. Bodenhausen and D.J. Ruben, *Natural Abundance Nitrogen–15 NMR by Enhanced Heteronuclear Spectroscopy*, Chemical Physics Letters, 69, 1980, 185–189.

41. N.E. Jacobsen, *NMR Spectroscopy Explained*, John Wiley and Sons, Hoboken, New Jersey, 2007.

HMQC

42. A. Bax, R.H. Griffey and B.L. Hawkins, *Correlation of Proton and N–15 Chemical Shifts by Multiple Quantum NMR*, J. Mag. Res., 55(2), 1983, 301–315.

43. N.E. Jacobson, *NMR Spectroscopy Explained*, John Wiley and Sons, Hoboken, New Jersey, 2007.

HMBC

44. N.E. Jacobsen, *NMR Spectroscopy Explained*, John Wiley and Sons, Hoboken, New Jersey, 2007.

HN (CO) CA, HNCA, HNCO

45. S. Grzesiek and A. Bax, *Improved 3D-Triple/Resonance NMR Techniques Applied to a 31kD Protein*, J. Mag. Res., 96, 1992, 432–440.

46. S.M. Pascal, *NMR Primer: An HSQC-Based Approach*, I.M. Publications, Chichester, 2008.

47. N.E. Jacobson, *NMR Spectroscopy Explained*, John Wiley and Sons, Hoboken, New Jersey, 2007.

48. L.E. Kay, M. Ikura, R. Tschudin and A. Bax, *3–D Triple Resonance NMR Spectroscopy of Isotropically Enriched Proteins*, J. Mag. Res., 89, 1990, 496–514.

Tocsy, Tocsy-HSQC-Tocsy

49. L. Braunschweiler and R.R. Ernst, *Coherence Transfer by Isotopic Mixing, Application to Protein Correlation Spectroscopy*, J. Mag. Res., 53, 1983, 521–528.
50. A.D. Bax and D.G. Davis, MLEV–17 *Based Two-Dimensional Homonuclear Magnetization Transfer Spectroscopy*, J. Mag. Res., 65, 1985, 355–360.
51. N.E. Jacobson, *NMR Spectroscopy Explained*, John Wiley and Sons, Hoboken, 2007.
52. S.M. Pascal, *NMR Primer, An HSQC-Based Approach*, I.M. Publications, Chichester, 2008.

Trosy, Trosy-HSQC

53. K. Pervushin, R. Rick, G. Wider and K. Wuthrich, *Attenuated T_2 Relaxation Macromolecules in Solution*, Proceedings of the National Academy of Sciences, USA, 94(23), 1997, 12366–12371.
54. N.E. Jacobsen, *NMR Spectroscopy Explained*, John Wiley and Sons, Hoboken, 2007.
55. S.M. Pascal, *NMR Primer, An HSQC-Based Approach*, I.M. Publications, Chichester, 2008

NMR Spectroscopy

56. H. Gunther, *NMR spectroscopy*, 3rd edn., Georg Thieme, Stuttgart, New York, 1992.
57. M.H. Levi H, *Spin Dynamics – Basic Principles of NMR Spectroscopy*, J. Wiley & Sons, Chichester, 2001.
58. M. Hesse, H. Meier, B. Zech, *Spectroscopic Methods in Organic Chemistry*, Georg Thieme, Stuttgart, New York, 1997.
59. G.C. Levy, R.L. Lichter, G.L. Nelson, *Carbon–13 Nuclear Magnetic Resonance Spectroscopy*, 2nd edn., Wiley-Interscience, New York, 1980.
60. E. Breitmaier, W. Voelter: *Carbon–13 NMR Spectroscopy – High Resolution Methods and Applications in Organic Chemistry and Biochemistry*, 3rd edn., VCH, Weinheim, 1990.
61. J.L. Marshall, *Carbon-Carbon and Carbon-Hydrogen NMR Couplings: Applications to Organic Stereochemistry and Conformational Analysis*, Verlag Chemie International, Deerfield Beach, FL, 1983.
62. H. Friebolin, *One and Two-dimensional NMR spectroscopy, An Introduction*, 3rd edn., VCH, Weinheim, 1997.
63. J.K.M. Sanders, B.K. Hunter, *Modern NMR Spectroscopy. A Guide for Chemists*, 2nd edn., Oxford University Press, Oxford, 1993.
64. S. Braun, H.O. Kalinowski, S. Berger, 150 *and More Basic NMR Experiments*. A Practical Course, 2nd edn., Wiley-VCH, Weinheim, 1998.
65. *Structure Elucidation by NMR in Organic Chemistry*, a Practical Guide, E. Breitmaier, 3rd edn., John Wiley & Sons Ltd., Chichester.

Dynamic NMR Spectroscopy

66. M. Oki (Ed.), *Applications of Dynamic NMR Spectroscopy to Organic Chemistry*, VCH, Deerfield Beach, FL, 1985.
67. J. Sandstrom, *Dynamic NMR Spectroscopy*, Academic Press, New York, 1982.
68. G.C. Ley, R.L. Lichter, *Nitrogen–15 Nuclear Magnetic Resonance Spectroscopy*, Wiley-Interscience, New York, 1979.

APT, J-Modulated Spin Echo

69. D.W. Brown, T.T. Nakashima, D.I. Rabenstein, J. Magn. Reson., 45 (1981), 302.

70. C. LeCocq. J.T. Lattemand, J. Chem. Soc. Chem. Commun. 1981, 150.

J-Resolved 2D CMR

71. A. Bax, *Two-Dimensional Nuclear Magnetic Resonance in Liquids*, Reidel, Dordrecht, 1984.

72. R.R. Ernst, G. Bodenhausen, A. Wokaun, *Principles of Nuclear Magnetic Resonance in One and Two Dimensions*, Oxford University Press, Oxford, 1990.

H-H Cosy, Inadequate

73. W. Ane, E. Bartholdi, R.R. Ernst, J. Chem. Phy. 64 (1976), 2229.

74. A. Bax and R. Freeman, J. Mag. Reson., 42 (1981), 164.
Ibid, 44 (1981), 542.

75. A. Bax, R. Freeman, S.P. Kempsell, J. Am. Chem. Soc., 102 (1980), 4581.

HN NOESY, ROESY

76. G. Bodenhausen, R.R. Ernst, J. Am. Chem. Soc. 104 (1982), 1304.

DEPT

77. D.M. Dodrell, D.T. Pegg, M.R. Bendall, J. Magn. Reson. 48 (1982), 323.
Ibid, J. Chem. Phys. 77 (1982), 2745.
M.R. Bendall, D.M. Dodrell, D.T. Pegg, W.E. Hull, DEPT., Information brochure with experimental details, Bruker Analytische Messtechnik, Karlsruhe, 1982.

NOE

78. D. Nenhas, M.P. Williamson, The Nuclear Overhauser Effect in Structural and Conformational Analysis, 2nd edn., Wiley-VCH, Weinheim, 2000.

79. M. Kinns, J.K.M. Sanders, J. Mag. Reson. 56 (1984), 518.

21.2 MASS SPECTROMETRY

1. J.H. Beynon, *Mass Spectrometry and its Applications to Organic Chemistry*, Elsevier, Amsterdam, 1960.

2. K. Biemann, *Mass Spectrometry: Organic Chemical Applications*, McGraw-Hill, N.Y., 1962.

3. J.R. Chapman, *Practical Organic Chemistry*, John Wiley, N.Y., 1985.

4. E.A. Constatin, A. Schnett and M. Thompson, *Mass Spectrometry*, Prentice-Hall, Englewood Cliffs, N.J., 1990.

5. E.T. Pretsch, J. Cleve, J. Siebl, and W. Simon, *Tables of Spectral Data for Structure Determination of Organic Compounds*, 2nd ed., Springer-Verlag, Berlin and N.Y., 1989, Translated from the German by K. Biemann.

6. F.W. Lafferty and F. Turecek, *Interpretation of Mass Spectra*, 4th ed., University Science Books, Mill Valley, Calif., 1993.

7. R.M. Silverstein, F.W. Webster, *Spectrometric Identification of Organic Compounds*, 6th ed., John Wiley, N.Y., 1998.

8. National Institute of Standards and Technology, NIST Chemistry Web Book: http:/webook.nist.gov/chemistry.

9. National Institute of Materials and Chemical Research, Tsukuba, Ibaraki, Japan, Integrated Spectra.

10. Data Base System for Organic Compounds (SDBS). http://www.aist.go.jp/KIODG/SDBS/menu-e.html.

11. D.L. Pavia, G.M. Lampman, G.S. Kriz, *Introduction to Spectroscopy*, Ch. 8, 3rd ed., Brooks/ Cole, Cengage Learning, 2001.

12. S. Shrader, *Introductory Mass Spectrometry*, Allyn and Bacon, Boston, 1971.

13. R.A.W. Johnstone, *Mass Spectrometry of Organic Chemists*, Cambridge University Press, 1982.

LC-ToF MS, TOF-MS-MS

14. *Liquid Chromatography Time-of-flight Mass Spectrometry*, Ed. I. Ferrer and E.M. Thurman, John Wiley and Sons, N.J.

LC-MS

15. *Liquid Chromatography – Mass Spectrometry*, Niessen, W.M.A., Marcel, Dekker Inc: NY, 1999.

16. *A Global View of LC/MS*, Second Edition, Global View Publishing, Pittsberg, PA, 2002.

ESI, MS/MS

17. C.M. Whitehouse, R.N. Dryer, M. Yamashita, J.B. Fenn, Anal. Chem., 1985, 57, 675–679.

18. Amarante et al., JOC, 74(8), 2009, 3034.

19. J.B. Fenn et al., Science, 1989, 246, 64–71.

20. R.B. Cole in Electrospray Ionization Mass Spectroscopy, John Wiley and Sons, Inc., N.Y., 1997.

21.3 UV SPECTROSCOPY

1. Stern, E.S. and T.C.J. Timmons, *Electronic Absorption Spectroscopy in Organic Chemistry*, St. Martin's Press, N.Y., 1971.

2. L. Lang, *Absorption Spectra in the Ultraviolet and Visible Region*, McGraw-Hill Book Co. (U.K.) Ltd., 1987.

3. C. Sandorfy, *Electronic Spectra and Quantum Chemistry*, Englewood Cliffs, N.J., Prentice-Hall, 1964.

4. R.B. Woodward, J. Am. Chem. Soc., 1952, 64, 72.

5. S.F. Mason, *Molecular Electronic Absorption Spectroscopy*, Quart. Revs., 1961, 15, 287.

6. H.H. Jaffe and M. Orchin, *Theory and Applications of Ultraviolet Spectroscopy*, John Wiley, N.Y., 1962.

7. K. Hiryama, *Handbook of Ultraviolet and Visible Absorption Spectra of Organic Compounds*, N.Y., Plenum Data Division, 1967.

8. R.P. Bauman, *Absorption Spectroscopy*, N.Y., John Wiley and Sons, 1962.

21.4 ONE DIMENSIONAL I.R.

1. J.R. Dyer, Organic Special Problems, Prentice-Hall, Englewood Cliffs, N.J., 1972.
2. J.R. Dyer, Application of Absorption Spectroscopy of Organic Compounds, Prentice-Hall, Englewood Cliffs, N.J., 1965.
3. L.J. Bellamy, the Infrared Spectra of Complex Molecules, 2nd ed., Methuen, London, 1958.
4. J.R. Durig, Chemical, Biological and Industrial Applications of Infrared Spectra, Wiley, N.Y., 1965.
5. N.P.G. Roeges, Guide to Interpretation of Infrared Spectra of Organic Structures, Wiley, N.Y., 1984.
6. H.A. Szymanski, Interpreted Infrared Spectra, Vol. I–III, Plenum Press, N.Y., 1964–1967.
7. Aldrich Library of FTIR Spectra, 3 Vols., Milwankee, WI, 1984.
8. R.F. Silverstein and F.X. Webster, Spectrometric Identification of Organic Compounds, in Chapter on Infrared Spectroscopy, John Wiley and Sons, 2002.
9. F.F. Bentley, L.D. Smithson and A.L. Rozek, Infrared Spectra and Characteristic Frequencies – 700 to 300 cm^{-1}, A Collection of Spectra, Interpretation and Bibliography, Wiley-Interscience, N.Y., 1988.
10. B.C. Smith, Fundamentals of Fourier Transform Infrared Spectroscopy, CRC Press, Boca Raton, F.L., 1999.
11. J.R. Ferraro and L.J. Basile, Eds., Fourier Transform Infrared Spectroscopy, 4 Vols., Academic Press, N.Y., 1985.
12. D. Pavia, G. Lampman and Kriz, Introduction to Spectroscopy in Chapter on Infrared Spectroscopy, Harcourt, Inc., 2001.
13. http//webbook.nist.gov/chemistry.

2D FTIR Spectroscopy

14. P. Hamm, M.H. Lim, R.M. Hochstrasser, Structure of amide I band of peptides measured by Fentosecond nonlinear infrared. Spectroscopy, J. Phy. Chem. B., 102, 6123, 1998.
15. S. Mukamel, "Multidimensional Femtosecond Correlation Spectroscopies of Electronic and Vibrational Excitations", Annual Review of Physics and Chemistry, 51, 691, 2000.
16. N. Demirdoven, C.M. Cheatum, H.S. Chung, M. Khalil, J. Knoester, A. Tokmakoff, Two-dimensional infrared spectroscopy of antiparallel beta-sheet secondary structure", J. Am. Chemo. Soc., 126, 7981, 2004.
    – For Use in Semi-conductor Microelectronics Industry – W.S. lau, Infrared Characterization for Microelectronics. World Scientific (1999).

646 Organic Spectroscopy

21.4 ONE DIMENSIONAL I.R.

1. J.R. Dyer, Organic Spectroscopy, Prentice-Hall, Englewood Cliffs, N.J., 1972.

Index